ADVANCED SURGICAL RECALL

ADVANCED SURGICAL RECALL

RECALL SERIES EDITOR AND SENIOR EDITOR

LORNE H. BLACKBOURNE, M.D.
General Surgeon
Fayetteville, North Carolina

SENIOR EDITOR

KIRK J. FLEISCHER, M.D.
Chief Resident
Department of Surgery
The Johns Hopkins Hospital
Baltimore, Maryland

EDITORS

OLIVER A.R. BINNS, M.D.
Resident in General Surgery
University of Virginia
Charlottesville, Virginia

TANANCHAI A LUCKTONG, M.D.
Resident in General Surgery
Mercy Hospital of Pittsburgh
Pittsburgh, Pennsylvania

JOSEPH WELLS, M.D.
Resident in General Surgery
University of Texas, Parkland
Dallas, Texas

LIPPINCOTT WILLIAMS & WILKINS
A **Wolters Kluwer** Company
Philadelphia · Baltimore · New York · London
Buenos Aires · Hong Kong · Sydney · Tokyo

Editor: Elizabeth A. Nieginski
Manager, Development Editing: Julie Scardiglia
Managing Editor: Amy G. Dinkel
Marketing Manager: Rebecca Himmelheber
Development Editor: Carol Loyd
Production Coordinator: Danielle Hagan
Text/Cover Designer: Karen Klinedinst
Typesetter: Port City Press, Inc.
Printer/Binder: Port City Press, Inc.

Figures 46–1 and 46–2 were redrawn with permission from Moore KL: *Essential Clinical Anatomy.* Baltimore, Williams & Wilkins, 1995.

Accurate indications, adverse reactions and dosage schedules for drugs are provided in this book, but it is possible that they may change. The reader is urged to review the package information data of the manufacturers of the medications mentioned.

Printed in the United States of America

First Edition

Library of Congress Cataloging-in-Publication Data
Advanced surgical recall / senior editors, Lorne H. Blackbourne, Kirk Fleischer. — 1st ed.
   p.   cm.
  Includes index.
  To be used in conjunction with: Surgical recall. c1994.
  ISBN 0-683-00834-X
  1. Surgery—Examinations, questions, etc. I. Blackbourne, Lorne H. II. Fleischer, Kirk. III. Surgical recall.
  [DNLM: 1. Surgery, Operative—examination questions. WO 18.2 A244 1997]
RD37.2.A39 1997
617'.0076—dc20
DNLM/DLC
for Library of Congress   96-35097
                                                          CIP

The publishers have made every effort to trace the copyright holders for borrowed material. If they have inadvertently overlooked any, they will be pleased to make the necessary arrangements at the first opportunity.

To purchase additional copies of this book, call our customer services department at **(800) 638-3030** or fax orders to **(301) 824-7390**. For other book services, including chapter reprints and large quantity sales, ask for the Special Sales Department. International customers should call **(301) 714-2324**.

Visit Lippincott Williams & Wilkins on the Internet: http://www.lww.com. Lippincott Williams & Wilkins customer service representatives are available from 8:30 am to 6:00 pm, EST.

02 03
4 5 6 7 8 9 10

David Holt, M.D.
Attending
Division of Transplant Surgery
Fairfax Hospital
Falls Church, Virginia

Brian Jones, M.D.
Attending
Summa Health Care Center
Akron, Ohio

Scott Langenburg, M.D.
Fellow in Pediatric Surgery
Children's Hospital of Michigan
Detroit, Michigan

John Minasi, M.D.
Assistant Professor
University of Virginia
Charlottesville, Virginia

Stanley L. Minken, M.D.
Attending
Division of Vascular Surgery
The Johns Hopkins Hospital
Baltimore, Maryland

Michael A. Mont, M.D.
Attending
Department of Orthopedic Surgery
The Johns Hopkins Hospital
Baltimore, Maryland

Marcia Moore, M.D.
Attending
Department of General Surgery
University of Virginia
Charlottesville, Virginia

Paul J. Mosca, M.D., Ph.D.
Resident in General Surgery
Duke University
Durham, North Carolina

Kate Willcutts
Nutritionist
University of Virginia
Charlottesville, Virginia

Leslie Wong, M.D.
Attending
Division of Plastic Surgery
Johns Hopkins Bayview Medical Center
Baltimore, Maryland

Jeffrey Young, M.D.
Attending
Department of Surgery
University of Virginia
Charlottesville, Virginia

Contributors

Gina Adrales, M.D.
Resident in General Surgery
University of Florida
Jacksonville, Florida

Stephen Bayne, M.D.
Resident in General Surgery
Akron City Hospital
Akron, Ohio

Gauri Bedi, M.D.
Senior Resident in General Surgery
The Johns Hopkins Hospital
Baltimore, Maryland

Oliver A.R. Binns, M.D.
Resident in General Surgery
University of Virginia
Charlottesville, Virginia

Lorne H. Blackbourne, M.D.
General Surgeon
Fayetteville, North Carolina

Carol Bognar
Nutritionist
Charlottesville, Virginia

Lee Butterfield, M.D.
Resident in Internal Medicine
Yale University
New Haven, Connecticut

Sung W. Choi, M.D.
Resident in Internal Medicine
New England Medical Center
Boston, Massachusetts

Jeffery Cope, M.D.
Resident in General Surgery
University of Virginia
Charlottesville, Virginia

Jennifer Deblasi, B.S.
Medical Student
University of Virginia
Charlottesville, Virginia

Matthew Edwards, M.D.
Resident in General Surgery
Bowman-Gray University
Winston-Salem, North Carolina

Brian Ferris, M.D.
Resident in General Surgery
Oregon Health Sciences University
Portland, Oregon

Anne C. Fischer, M.D.
Chief Resident in General Surgery
The Johns Hopkins Hospital
Baltimore, Maryland

Kirk J. Fleischer, M.D.
Chief Resident in General Surgery
The Johns Hopkins Hospital
Baltimore, Maryland

Cynthia Gingalewski, M.D.
Chief Resident in General Surgery
Yale–New Haven Hospital
New Haven, Connecticut

Thomas Gleason, M.D.
Resident in General Surgery
University of Virginia
Charlottesville, Virginia

David D. Graham, M.D.
Resident in General Surgery
University of Virginia
Charlottesville, Virginia

Sean P. Hedican, M.D.
Chief Resident in Urology
The Johns Hopkins Hospital
Baltimore, Maryland

Stanley "Duke" Herrel, M.D.
Resident in Urology
University of Virginia
Charlottesville, Virginia

Jason Lamb, M.D.
Resident in General Surgery
Allegheny General Hospital
Pittsburgh, Pennsylvania

Scott London, M.D.
Resident in Otolaryngology—Head
    and Neck Surgery
University of Virginia
Charlottesville, Virginia

Tananchai A Lucktong, M.D.
Resident in General Surgery
Mercy Hospital of Pittsburgh
Pittsburgh, Pennsylvania

Peter Mattei, M.D.
Chief Resident in General Surgery
The Johns Hopkins Hospital
Baltimore, Maryland

Addison May, M.D.
Fellow in Trauma, Critical Care
University of Pennsylvania
Philadelphia, Pennsylvania

Joseph R. McShannic, M.D.
Resident in General Surgery
Summa Health System
Akron, Ohio

Paul Mosca, M.D.
Resident in General Surgery
Duke University
Durham, North Carolina

David Musante, M.D.
Resident in Neurosurgery
University of Washington
Seattle, Washington

Mark J. Pidala, M.D.
Fellow in Colon and Rectal Surgery
UMDNJ/Robert Wood Johnson
    Medical School
Department of Surgery
New Brunswick, New Jersey

John Pilcher, M.D.
Attending Surgeon
United States Air Force
San Antonio, Texas

Philip Pollice, M.D.
Chief Resident in Otolaryngology,
    Head and Neck Surgery
The Johns Hopkins Hospital
Baltimore, Maryland

Naveen Reddy, M.D.
Resident in General Surgery
Ohio State University
Columbus, Ohio

Brian Romaneschi, M.D.
Chief Resident in Otolaryngology,
    Head and Neck Surgery
The Johns Hopkins Hospital
Baltimore, Maryland

Janice Ryu, M.D.
Associate Professor of Radiation
    Oncology
University of California at Davis
    Medical Center
Davis, California

Robert E. Schmieg, Jr., M.D.
Fellow in Trauma Surgery
Louisville, Kentucky

Donald B. Schmit, M.D.
Resident in Anesthesia
University of Virginia
Charlottesville, Virginia

Paul Shin, B.A.
Medical Student
University of Virginia
Charlottesville, Virginia

Kimberly Sinclair, M.S.
Director, Thoracic-Cardiovascular
   Research Laboratory
University of Virginia
Charlottesville, Virginia

John Sperling, M.D.
Resident in General Surgery
Mayo Clinic
Rochester, Minnesota

Pierre Theodore, M.D.
Resident in General Surgery
The Johns Hopkins Hospital
Baltimore, Maryland

Steven D. Theis, M.D.
Chief Resident in General Surgery
Roanoke Memorial Hospital
Roanoke, Virginia

Michael Tjarksen, M.D.
Chief Resident in Orthopedic
   Surgery
The Johns Hopkins Hospital
Baltimore, Maryland

Jeffry Watson, M.D.
Resident in General Surgery
University of Texas
Dallas, Texas

Mark Watts, M.D.
Chief Resident in Neurosurgery
The Johns Hopkins Hospital
Baltimore, Maryland

Joseph Wells, M.D.
Resident in General Surgery
Parkland Memorial Hospital
Dallas, Texas

David White, M.D.
Resident in Surgery
Duke University
Durham, North Carolina

Kate Willcutts
Nutritionist
University of Virginia
Charlottesville, Virginia

Jonathan Winograd, M.D.
Senior Resident in General Surgery
The Johns Hopkins Hospital
Baltimore, Maryland

Disciaimer

This book is intended to be a study guide for the acquisition of basic surgical facts and should not be used to guide patient care.

Dedication

The General Surgery section of this book is dedicated to my father, Dr. Brian D. Blackbourne, and my wife, Patricia Stuart Blackbourne. Without both, inspiration would be only a concept.

Lorne H. Blackbourne, M.D.

The Subspecialty section of this book is dedicated to my parents and my wife for their love, guidance, and unending support.

Kirk J. Fleischer, M.D.

Foreword

Advanced Surgical Recall is a study aid for students and residents who have progressed past their introductory experiences in the discipline of surgery. In actuality, this group includes surgical residents, senior medical students, surgeons studying for their board exams, practicing surgeons, and even junior medical students who have progressed past the usual introductory materials. This book should also serve as a source of questions for teachers of surgery, particularly for the venerable activity of teaching rounds.

The best teachers usually are those individuals who have thought the most about how they themselves learned. The editors of *Advanced Surgical Recall* clearly are teachers who have given an enormous amount of thought to learning and teaching. They have used the principles of the Socratic method and of their own self-education techniques to develop this collection of questions. These two editors have a special knack for writing and editing these types of questions and study aids; through their impressive medical and surgical educational trajectories, they have made good grades, won teaching awards, and created a plethora of study aids.

This collection of questions and answers is useful to students of surgery, not only because it will help them learn the answers they need to know, but also because it will help them remember the questions. Knowing the right questions is, in my opinion, more important than knowing the answers, at least in real life. After all, the answers will change over time. The questions are timeless.

Curtis G. Tribble
Professor of Surgery
Division of Cardiothoracic Surgery
University of Virginia
Charlottesville, Virginia

Preface

We have tried in *Advanced Surgical Recall* to include information that surgical residents and students need for the wards, in-service examination, and boards. We have arranged the questions in the same format as those in *Surgical Recall* and have tried to put forward the information in the most rapid-fire way possible, emphasizing the basic sciences. This book is intended to be complementary to the basic surgical facts covered in *Surgical Recall* and, therefore, many basics are not covered to avoid redundancy. We welcome your comments and suggestions to make future editions more concise, complete, and useful. To reach our goals for this book, we have recruited surgical residents and medical students from several institutions. This diversity is the strength of this book.

Lorne H. Blackbourne, M.D.
University of Virginia

Kirk J. Fleischer, M.D.
Johns Hopkins University

Contents

SECTION III
SUBSPECIALTY SURGERY

Section I

Introduction and Background Surgical Information

1

Introduction

Lorne H. Blackbourne, MD

HOW ADULTS LEARN

Learning is accomplished through **motivation, repetition,** and **association**. **Motivation** must come from within, and most surgical residents are obviously motivated to learn surgery. **Repetition** is obtained by reading, rereading, and studying information until it is mastered. **Association** is obtained by connecting information that has already been mastered to some new knowledge, such as remembering the anatomic order of the trauma neck zones 3,2,1 in conjunction with the Le Fort fractures 3,2,1.

HOW TO STUDY

Always read about your patient's disease while you are taking care of him or her. This habit serves two purposes: you will **associate** the information to the patient for life, and your increased knowledge base will improve the quality of care for that patient.

WHAT TO STUDY

For the surgical resident, the study of surgery is a varied and onerous task that covers basic science, diseases, and surgical anatomy and technique. Regular reading in one of the "big three" surgical texts (Greenfield, Sabiston, or Schwartz) and regular review and study of technique in a surgical atlas/anatomy book are essential. It is a good idea to keep files of pertinent scientific papers, and *Selected Readings in General Surgery* from the university of Texas at Dallas is a great start for your files. An excellent primer for the intensive care unit is *The ICU Book* by Marino, et al. O'Leary's book, *The Physiologic Basis of Surgery*, is a useful text for covering the basic sciences of surgical disease. Moore's book on trauma is another book that has been effectively used by many surgery residents. Every surgery resident must be familiar with the ACLS^R protocols and **must** take the ATLS^R course. Other classics include Cope's *Acute Abdomen* and Pestana's *IVF*. A recent study by Wade and Kaminski (1995) showed that residents who engage in **self-study,** read text early on, study selected readings, take a review course (if they are especially at risk of failing), and SESAP do the best on the Boards.

Many residents write down questions to themselves during rounds or conferences and look up the answers later.

USING THIS BOOK

After completion of the surgical basics in *Surgical Recall*, your attention should be focused on this book. The answers on the right should be reviewed until mastered. This book is designed to foster the acquisition of surgical information and will not help you gain experience in test taking; this skill can be learned from other books.

NURSES

Treat nurses with respect and professional courtesy at all times; they often know more than you in any given situation. If your relationship is based on mutual respect, it is also less likely that they will call you at 3 A.M. asking for Tylenol^R.

SLEEP DEPRIVATION

The best offense to combat sleep deprivation is to be in good physical shape and to be motivated. Staying up for 48 hours is no different than participating in a ultramarathon. Many residents find benefit from caffeine, orange juice, hot showers, brushing their teeth, doing push-ups, running steps, yelling, changing their socks, or listening to loud music. Studies have shown that sleep deprivation is mainly a mental problem and that physical abilities remain intact until extreme deprivation of sleep occurs. Try not to sit down, because sitting is conducive to falling asleep quickly. Overall, it is an attitude: "I am hardcore and I need no sleep!"

INTERNSHIP

THE PERFECT INTERN

1. Says only "Yes sir," "No sir," or "My fault, sir" and " Yes ma'am," "No ma'am," or "My fault ma'am"
2. Is always honest
3. Is a team player
4. Has a "can do" attitude
5. Always brushes teeth before rounds
6. Is the first to arrive and the last to leave clinic
7. Is always clean
8. Always makes the upper-level residents look good
9. Teaches the students
10. Does not scut the students too much
11. Knows more about the patients than anyone else
12. Is a physician and not only a scribe
13. Is never late
14. Never complains
15. Is never hungry, thirsty, or tired

16. Is always enthusiastic
17. Follows the chain of command

Here are some thoughts for interns to live by:
1. **"They can hurt you but they can't stop the clock."**
   Internship only lasts for 12 months.
2. **"Never trust your brain."**
   Write everything down, do not trust anything to memory, and check off your chores when completed.
3. **"Load the boat."**
   Inform your superiors when a patient is not doing well or if you have any questions. That way, if your patient's condition worsens (a proverbial sinking ship), you have **loaded** the ship with your superiors and they will go down with you.
4. **"NEVER LIE."**
   Simply: honesty is the best policy

INSERVICE EXAMINATION

You only have 6 months after graduation from medical school to prepare for your first inservice examination. The best way to prepare for your first exam is to read a mini-text, such as the **Lawrence** text.

LIVING WITH MISTAKES

You will make mistakes, and many times these mistakes will harm your patients. Mistakes are forgivable if you **are doing your absolute best.** Do not make mistakes that result from laziness.

There is a saying in surgery: "You cannot hurt yourself by getting out of bed." After a mistake is made and you have determined that you were doing your absolute best, you must then **forgive and remember.** That is, forgive yourself for the mistake, but always remember the mistake and try to learn something from it.

TEACHING SURGERY TO YOUR FELLOW RESIDENTS

It is a sad fact that at many teaching hospitals, surgery is approached with a "let's get the work done" attitude and without much instruction. Try these ideas:
1. Let the junior resident know as early as possible which cases he or she will be handling so they can review the anatomy and a surgical atlas.
2. Try a "chalk talk" and review the anatomy, procedure, and potential complications with the junior resident using a chalk board or a drawing pad.
3. Teach the junior resident preoperative imaging of the procedure and the potential complications and their treatment (preoperative imagery means running through the procedure in your head).
4. It is often said that you have not really performed a procedure until you have performed it yourself. For junior residents, the next best thing to

performing a procedure himself or herself is for the senior resident at every step of the way to say: "Now that you have completed this dissection, tell me what the next step is and how you are going to do it."

TEACHING STUDENTS

The real secret to teaching students is **just to do it!** The great student teachers are the ones who spend the most time teaching and who keep things as simple as possible.

LAB: TO DO OR NOT TO DO

Lab time can prepare you for a career in academic surgery, or it can convince you that you are not interested in research as a career goal. It will also help you to learn to read a scientific paper. Most experts say that you need at least two years in the lab to accomplish something, which is true if you know you want to do academic surgery and will need to know the statistics, how to set up a lab, and so forth. But if you are not sure you want to do research for the rest of your life, or if you are certain that you do not want to, or if you want to write several papers to enhance your chances at that million dollar fellowship, then one year in a **well-established lab** is usually sufficient.

FELLOWSHIPS

Most fellowships (e.g., plastics, vascular, cardiac, pediatric surgery, trauma/ ICU, transplant) are applied for during the fourth year of the general surgery residency. To maximize your chances for a fellowship, it is best to have an influential mentor who can write a good letter (or make an important phone call) for you and it is imperative to have some research papers to separate you from the pack. Your inservice scores will also be considered.

APPLYING FOR FELLOWSHIPS

Ask your residency advisor and your mentor about the number of programs you should apply to and interview for, and when and how to get the applications (as soon as you decide on the specialty).

RECOVERY ROOM PROTOCOL

Several things need to be done before you can eat some food, so the acronym F.O.O.D.D. is helpful:
  Family: Talk to the patient's family
  Operative note: Write in the chart
  Orders
  Dictate the procedure
  Doctor: Call the primary/referring doctor

DEALING WITH ACHES AND PAINS IN THE OR

Many residents find that taking NSAIDs before and after long cases helps decrease muscle strains. Others do sit-ups to strengthen abdominal muscles and reduce backache, or use the OSHA back support belts. Support hose can lessen foot edema and the pain associated with venous LE incompetence associated with long periods of standing.

AVOIDING MALPRACTICE

1. Do the right thing.
2. Talk to your patients and their families.
3. Be nice to your patients and their families.
4. **Document everything!**

HEIRARCHY AMONG SURGICAL RESIDENTS

There should be a free flow of suggestions and ideas regarding patient care among all surgical residents (including interns), but the decisions follow a concrete chain of command.

FOURTH YEAR MEDICAL STUDENT REQUIRED READING LIST

The fourth year of medical school for future surgery residents allows for some reading that you will never be able to do again. The following books should be read during your fourth year:
1. *Fluids and Electrolytes in the Surgical Patient.* Carlos Pestana
2. *House Officer's Guide to ICU Care.* John Elefteriades, Alexander Geha, and Lawrence Cohen.
3. *Cope's Early Diagnosis of the Acute Abdomen.* William Silen.
4. *A.T.L.S.*[R] Manual
5. *A.C.L.S.*[R] Manual
6. *Principles of Surgical Technique.* Gary Wing and Norman Rich.

READING FOR THE BOARDS

Many residents find the preparation courses and audiotapes useful for preparing for the boards. Cameron's *Current Surgical Therapy,* and Norton and Eiseman's *Surgical Decision Making* are also extremely valuable resources in preparing for the oral and written boards.

SURGICAL ABBREVIATIONS

RHIP   Rank has its privileges

WWDWWC   Wound was dry when we closed

ATFQ   Answer the first question

FIDO   Forget it; drive on

AMF YOYO   Adios my friend; you're on your own

OBTAINING A GENERAL SURGERY RESIDENCY

Lorne H. Blackbourne, MD
Donald B. Schmit, MD

THE FOURTH YEAR

Fourth Year Electives

Fourth year electives should be enjoyable, but they should also prepare you for internship. The following steps are recommended
Acting internship in general surgery
ICU rotation
Research (early)
Anatomy review
Radiology
Trauma rotation (go to a busy center like Cook County Hospital in Chicago or Maryland's Shock Trauma)
Pediatric surgery
Time off for board review

Research in the Fourth Year

A research elective is highly recommended in the fourth year. It will provide a real working relationship with an attending research mentor, build your curriculum vitae (CV), and give you some idea of whether or not you will want to pursue research during and after your residency. Research often separates you from the crowd of excellent medical student applicants. Take your elective in research early during your fourth year, so that you will have time to write one or two papers to add to your CV. It will also give you an opportunity to pursue a clinical study (chart review) while doing subsequent rotations. **Ask** your attending mentor if you can help write a review article or book chapter.

Extracurricular Activities in the Fourth Year

In addition to research and writing articles or book chapters, you can undertake other activities, such as helping to instruct an animal surgical techniques lab, assisting in a laparoscopic course (i.e., driving the camera), tutoring first or second year students, or participating in class government. Any of these activities will help to separate you from the pack.

Board Examinations

Take the board examinations in the fall and get them out of the way! If you take the boards in the spring, it may give the impression that you are trying to hide your scores.

THE INTERVIEW PROCESS

Overview
1. Choose an advisor
2. Obtain letters of recommendation, dean's letter, and official transcript; prepare CV and personal statement
3. Request applications (in writing)
4. Fill out applications
5. Wait for interview requests
6. Schedule interviews
7. Go to interviews
8. Rank list
9. Match day

Official Transcript

In most cases, the dean will submit your official transcript and dean's letter after your application is received. You should send an unofficial photocopy of your grades and board scores with your application. This will hasten the arrival of interview acceptance letters, and thus will allow you to maximize your scheduling and economize your trips. Otherwise, your interview invitations may be delayed until the dean's letter arrives with your transcript.

CV

Your CV represents the activities of your life and should include the following data:
Date
Name
Address (school and home)
Social Security number
Facsimile
Family information
Education
Military experience
Honors
Positions held
Organizations
Publications
Presentations
Book chapters
Review articles

Sample CV

CURRICULUM VITAE
August 1996

John Cushing
University of Virginia Medical Center
School of Medicine, Box 1145
Charlottesville, Virginia 22909

Home: 2234 Oxford Road
Charlottesville, Va 22909

Phone: Home (804) 983-1111
       School (804) 924-1212 (and have paged)

Facsimile: (804) 983-1111

SSN: 225-11-1111

Born: October 28, 1969
     Santa Barbara, California

Family: Married Patricia Stuart, July 11, 1984

Education:
    Washington-Lee High School, Lexington, Virginia
    University of Virginia, Charlottesville, Virginia
        Bachelor of Arts, May 1991 (Biology)
    University of Virginia School of Medicine, Charlottesville, Virginia
        Doctor of Medicine, expected May 1997

Military:
    Captain, Medical Corps, United States Army Reserve, 1991–present

Additional Postgraduate Education:
    American Heart Association Advanced Cardiac Life Support, 1996
    Microsurgical Course, Department of Plastic Surgery, University of
        Virginia, 1996
    Combat Casualty Care Course, 1995

Honors:
    Alpha Omega Alpha

Positions Held:
    Research Assistant, Department of Internal Medicine, University of
        Virginia, 1994
    Assistant Instructor, Surgical Techniques Lab, University of Virginia, 1996

Professional Membership:
    American Medical Association

Book Chapters:
    Surgical Nutrition in Blackbourne LH., SURGICAL RECALL, first ed,
        Williams & Wilkins, Baltimore, 1994.

Publications:
    Kocher H, Cushing J. A New surgical approach to the posterior pancreas.
        Ann Surg;110(3):248-254, 1995.

Personal Statement

The personal statement is difficult to write! You should include the following information:
1. Why you want to go into surgery
2. Why you are confident you will do a great job in your residency program (remember: confident, not arrogant)
3. Future plans (e.g., research, world missionary work, etc.)

The personal statement is often a focal point in the interview, so be comfortable and familiar with the thoughts expressed in your statement. Each person's statement is different and you need to create yours de novo to assure that it reflects you and your attributes.

What to Look for in a General Surgery Residency Program
1. Are the residents happy? (most important)
2. Number of cases
3. Call schedule
4. Pay/benefits
5. Parking
6. Area/crime/housing
7. Number of fellows to share cases with
8. Potential for Veterans Administration experience
9. Rotations
10. Moonlighting opportunity
11. Lab research opportunity
12. Vacations
13. What are the graduates doing now? (e.g., fellowships, academics, private practice, etc.)

Where to Apply

Ask your advisor, other attendings, your chairman, and residents at your school. You should apply to a full range of programs (very competitive to less competitive).

Interviews on a Low Budget

Some thoughts on minimizing costs while on the interview trail:
Drive
Stay with friends, family, medical school alumni (your dean's office should have a list)
Schedule multiple interviews in the same area (i.e., fly in, rent a car)

The Interview Day

Some suggestions:
Wear the traditional dark interview suit (men and women). This is not the time to make a fashion statement. Why stand out? Let your record do that!

Always **smile** when first introduced to the interviewer (actual studies have shown that this is very important!).

Firm handshake

Eye contact

Sit up straight.

Be polite to **everyone**.

Write thank you letters when you get home.

Questions You Might Be Asked

This is a list of **actual** questions that have been asked during general surgery interviews:

Personal

Tell me about yourself.

Tell me about your family.

How do you stay in good physical shape?

What do you do in your spare time?

What do you read?

What is the last nonmedical book you read?

Clinical

A 65-year-old man comes into the ER with right upper quadrant pain. How are you going to work him up?

How do you work up a pulmonary embolus?

How many mEq of sodium are in normal saline?

What situations will keep an enterocutaneous fistula open?

So, how is Dr. X, Y, or Z in Charlottesville?

Ethical/political

Okay, I have a situation for you. You are doing a laparotomy for bowel obstruction and you find a lap pad from a previous lap, but there is no association between the pad and the obstruction. Would you tell the patient? Would you tell the previous surgeon? If you were the previous surgeon who left the lap pad and were informed of your mistake by the subsequent surgeon, would you talk to the patient? What would you say?

Your attending tells you to schedule a patient for procedure A. You have been reading and discover that procedure B is more effective, in addition to having lower morbidity and mortality rates. You inform the attending, but he is adamantly in favor of procedure A. How do you handle the situation?

Academic

Tell me where you went to undergraduate college.

Do you think the college you went to had anything to do with your preclinical grades?

Why did you take Swedish as an undergraduate?

How do you study?

How do you feel about dog labs?

If you could change something about medical school, what would it be?

What is the funniest thing that happened to you during medical school?

Did any patient frustrate you during your surgery clerkship?

During your clinical years, did anything make you uncomfortable?

Tell me about your most interesting patient as a medical student, and tell me what you learned from that case.

Did you do a pediatric surgery rotation? If so, tell me about your most interesting pediatric surgery patient.

To which medical journals do you subscribe? What was the last article you read?

What electives are you taking in the fourth year?

Tell me about your grades in medical school. What were your undergraduate grades like?

Why did you get X (grade) in X (course/clerkship/elective)?

Why didn't you get a PhD?

What were your board scores? What was your overall percentage?

Did you tell the house staff on services other than surgery that you wanted to be a surgeon?

Why did you waive your right to read your letters of recommendation?

Explain this sentence in your personal statement.

Research

Tell me about your research. (Be prepared to answer some fairly in-depth questions regarding your research. This includes basic science questions, clinical applicability, specifics of experiment design, depth of literature review, and occasional pimping. Understand your research thoroughly!)

How did you find the time to do your research?

Do you plan to take time off as a resident to do research?

When do you think it is best to take time off for research?

How do you feel about animal research?

What is it about research that you like and what keeps you motivated?

What percentage of your time as an attending do you plan to spend on research?

What does academic medicine mean to you?

What does it mean to you to be an academic surgeon, researcner, or to have your own lab? Why is research important to you?

So, I see you have done some rat surgery. Can you tell me the name of the first abdominal muscle layer in the rat?

Residency

Do you have any questions? (Do not ask attendings questions that should be reserved for residents; for example, "what is your call schedule like?" or "does your program have any weaknesses?")

In our program you have to decide now if you want to do general surgery or
cardiac surgery, so what will it be? (It's essential to know about the program
beforehand.)

What do you like about our program? Why did you apply here?

What do you like and dislike about our program?

How did you find out about this program?

Why did you choose an academic program over a community program?

Where else have you applied? What programs have you liked?

Are you interested in staying at UVA? What have they told you?

Why didn't you apply to Duke?

Are we your first choice?

What do I have to say to make you come here? (Remember: talk is cheap)

What would you change about our interview process?

What are you looking for in a general surgery program?

If you could design your ultimate residency program, what would it include?
What would you look for in faculty members?

What if you do not match?

What do you think are the advantages and disadvantages of being on call every
third or every fourth night?

What do you think about being on call every other night?

Do you think you will be able to pursue your outside interests as a resident?

What is the worst thing a resident can do?

If you were on my service in June, what clinical weakness of yours would I
have to be concerned about?

As an intern, what do you see as your role in teaching medical students?

How do you work with nurses?

How many hours of sleep do you need a night?

How do you know when you're overworked?

Soul-searching

What makes you a better applicant than the other 20 students we are inter-
viewing today?

What makes you different from all those other applicants? Why should I pick
you to be one of our residents?

Why should we want you in our program?

What makes you believe that you will be a good surgeon?

What skill do you possess that will make you a good surgeon?

Do you think that you have leadership potential?

Do you think that surgeons are egotistical or arrogant? Is that a good or bad
trait and why?

If you could describe the ideal surgeon (and resident) in two adjectives, what
would they be?

Why do you like general surgery?

When did you become interested in surgery?

So, why do you want to be a surgeon?

Are you sure you can give 100% to general surgery?

So, why are you interested in academic surgery?

Why do you like cardiac surgery?

So, why not medicine?

Okay, tomorrow you lose your left hand. What would you do then?

What are your weaknesses?

What is your greatest strength/weakness (pick only one for each)? Why is that a strength/weakness?

What do you consider your greatest accomplishment outside of medical school the past three years?

What was the most memorable moment of your life outside of your academic career?

What aspect of your life are you most pleased about?

What aspect of your life are you most displeased about?

Who are your role models?

Who has had the greatest impact on you during your lifetime?

What are your two favorite books and why?

Which two books would you bring to a deserted island?

What book would you recommend to a historic figure being brought to the twentieth century?

What do you think is the greatest problem in society today?

If you could invite any two famous people (living or dead) to a private dinner party, who would they be? Why?

If you could visit any time and place in history for a day, when and where would it be? Why?

The crystal ball

What do you see yourself doing in ten/fifteen/twenty years?

How do you think you will be able to balance clinical practice, teaching, research, and family?

What is the greatest challenge to general surgery in the next five years?

What do you think about the future of general surgery, and what do you say to people who feel it's a dying field?

Making Your Rank List

You should list at least ten programs you are interested in (unless you are a blue-chip superstar). General surgery residency is becoming more and more competitive and you should list very competitive programs and not so competitive programs. You should list them in the order you really like them, because the computer will not hurt you for ranking a long shot first! Remember to write to the directors of the programs you list prior to their rank day to reiterate your interest.

GOOD LUCK!

2

Surgical History

David B. Musante, BS
Scott London, BA

What is the oldest document concerning surgery?

Smith papyrus. Although found in 1862, it has been dated to approximately 1600 B.C.

Who was Imhotep?

He wrote the first treatise on surgery in 2700 B.C. His status and reputation as a surgeon made him a god to his people.

Did early Egyptian surgery stress the ideals of socialized medicine?

No. It stressed specialization, as well as hygiene and personal cleanliness. There was even a position as "keeper of the royal anus." This overspecialization undoubtedly contributed to the decline in medical standards over the last 1000 years of the Egyptian empire.

What is the Code of Hammurabi?

Written in Mesopotamia in approximately 2000 B.C., it included guidelines for the proper conduct among healers. For example, it stated that if a man should die at the hands of a surgeon, then the surgeon shall have his hands cut off.

What document begins: "I swear by Apollo the Healer, by Aesculapius, Hygieia, and Panacea ..."?

The Oath of Hippocrates. Hippocrates, who was born on the Greek island of Cos in 460 B.C., is considered the "father of medicine." His Hippocratic Corpus defines medicine and surgery as a systematic science.

Who was the founder of anatomy?

Herophilus, of the Alexandrian school of surgery

Who was St. Agatha?

This nun is the most famous of all the surgical saints. Her breasts were ordered to be removed by a Roman governor because she snubbed his amorous advances. She is considered the patron of breast diseases.

Who was Galen?

He is considered the most influential figure in medicine, second only to Hippocrates. His career spanned from surgeon to gladiator Marcus Aurelius' personal physician.

Who promoted the ancient Greek concept of disease as an imbalance of four humors—phlegm, blood, yellow bile, and black bile?

The second century Greek anatomist Galen, whose theories were not challenged until the sixteenth century, promoted this concept. This doctrine was first developed around 400 B.C. by Polybos, son-in-law of Hippocrates. It described the four humors as cholera, phlegma, melancholia, and haima.

Although he made many great contributions to medicine, why is Galen remembered for stalling medical progress for centuries?

Because autopsies were forbidden in second century Rome, Galen was forced to base virtually all of his studies of anatomy and physiology (such as the two-chambered heart) on the dissection of animals.

Who was responsible for disproving the misconceptions propagated by Galen?

In 1543, Andreas Vesalius, at the age of 29, released his epoch-making study on human anatomy, leading to an academic battle with virtually the entire medical world. His work was so accurate that it can still be used to teach anatomy today.

Where and when was the first legitimate degree for physicians established?

Salerno, in western Europe, in 1000 A.D. The program combined medicine and surgery.

How were surgeons perceived in the Middles Ages?

They were not highly regarded and, unlike physicians, were not on the faculty of the universities.

How are physicians and surgeons in England addressed?

Because of the disdain for surgeons stemming from medieval times, the tradition of addressing physicians as "Doctor" and surgeons as "Mister" still exists today.

Where did the term barber–surgeons originate?

In Paris around 1300, licensed or "long robe surgeons," in an attempt to distinguish themselves from other surgical practitioners, introduced "short robe" or barber–surgeons. These surgeons were relegated to shaving the crown of patients and performing prophylactic phlebotomies, a custom of the time. Over the centuries, these two sects vied for influence.

How many anatomic drawings of the human body did Leonardo Da Vinci render?

779

Who is credited with the first accurate anatomic description of the human cardiovascular system?

Harvey (1578–1657)

Who is widely considered to be the father of experimental surgery?

Hunter (1728–1793), who was born in Scotland

Who was Dominique-Jean-Larrey?

Napoleon's surgeon. He was responsible for the first ambulance and Larrey's point (subxiphoid).

What three structures are named after Sir Astley Cooper (1768–1841)?

Fascia cremasterica Cooperi, ligamentum Cooperi, and the "ligaments" that support the mammary glands

Who was William Beaumont?

The American Army doctor who studied the gastric physiology of his patient, Alexis St. Martin, who formed a gastrocutaneous fistula from a musket wound in 1822.

Who performed the first surgery under anesthesia and what operation was it?

In 1846, at the Mass General Hospital, William Morton, a dentist, extracted a tooth after the patient, John Warren, inhaled ether.

Who is responsible for the "germ theory"?

Pasteur (1822–1895)

Who is considered the "father of aseptic surgery"?

Lister (1827–1912)

With what did Lister "disinfect" wounds, hands, and instruments?

Carbolic acid

Who performed the first successful gastrectomy?

Billroth (1829–1894). He also developed the Billroth I and II.

Who performed the first successful end-to-end vascular anastomosis?

Carrel (1873–1944), a Frenchman. His technique made transplantation a technical possibility.

Who is credited with the first cholecystectomy?

Langenbuch, in 1882. The patient was subjected to 5 days of preliminary enemas, but smoked a cigar the day after surgery, got up on the twelfth day, and went home 6 weeks later.

When and where did McBurney describe the point named after him?

In 1889, at the Roosevelt Hospital in New York

Who is credited with starting the routine use of sterile surgical gloves during operations?

Halsted, in 1890. His head nurse, Caroline Hampton, complained about dermatitis caused by surgical chemicals. His solution "won her hand," literally!

What role in surgery did Goodyear Rubber Company play?

It manufactured the first thin rubber gloves with gauntlets for Halsted.

On whom did Halsted perform his first gallbladder operation?

His mother, in 1882. He was a pioneer in gallbladder disease research and the first professor of surgery at Johns Hopkins.

Who was the first American to use the radiograph for surgical purposes?

In 1896, Burry used Roentgen's recent invention to localize and remove buckshot from a patient's hand.

Describe the first human radiograph performed by Roentgen.

It was a film of his wife's left hand, clearly showing bones and her wedding ring.

Who declared that "an operation on the heart would be a prostitution of surgery."

Billroth

The peustow procedure is actually a procedure described by whom?

Parrington. Peustow described placing the pancreas into the lumen of the small bowel.

What disease did Trousseau, of Trousseau syndrome, die of?

Pancreatic cancer

Why was Kocher's (1841–1917) surgical career marked by triumph as well as tragedy?

He perfected the total thyroidectomy by 1898, reducing operative mortality from 13% to 0.5%, but to his horror, produced scores of cretinous and myxedematous patients. He swore thereafter never to remove a complete thyroid again.

Who was Harvey Cushing?

A neurosurgeon who trained at Johns Hopkins. Cushing (1869–1939) was responsible for advances in neurosurgery, ICP, and pituitary disease (Cushing triad).

Why did Cushing insist upon complete silence in the OR?

To minimize droplet infection of wounds. This theory was gaining increasing acceptance because of the work by Flugge in approximately 1897. He proved that although masks protected against wound infection, they offered little protection if the surgeon was bearded.

Who is considered the "father of the modern residency system" in surgery?

A German named von Langenbeck (1810–1887), who trained Billroth

Who established the first surgical residency program in America?

Halsted, at Johns Hopkins Hospital

Who discovered the barium swallow?

Cannon, whose initial experiments involved "persuading" a goose to swallow a metal ball and following its path with the recently discovered radiograph.

What eponym is Le Fort associated with?	The Le Fort fractures were named for him, for experiments he conducted in 1900 in which he dropped cannonballs onto skulls.
Who performed the first successful human portacaval anastomosis?	Vidal, in 1903
Who is known as the "father of pancreatic surgical treatment"?	Allen Oldfather Whipple (1881–1963; Whipple triad), not to be confused with George Whipple, of small intestinal disease fame. The two men were unrelated.
Who set the standard of requiring complete physical examinations of all patients and started the first of many large clinics staffed with experts from various fields?	The Mayo Brothers. They built their famous clinic in Rochester, Minnesota, in 1910.
Who was Sister Mary Joseph?	The Mayos' nurse. She noticed the paraumbilical adenopathy associated with advanced gastric cancer.
Was Bovie an MD?	No, he was a PhD in physics. He developed the electrocautery in Boston in the 1920s.
What neurosurgeon operated on Ruth Penfield's brain tumor?	Her brother, Wilder Penfield, in 1928. Famous for his detailed mapping of the cerebral cortex, he removed a huge, malignant frontal lobe tumor from his sister under local anesthesia.
Who discovered penicillin?	Fleming, a surgeon, in 1928
What surgeon performed the first human cardiac catheterization?	Forssmann (1904–1979), in 1929 in Berlin, passed a tube through an arm vein into his own heart while watching it on a fluoroscope screen!

Who developed the first iron lung?

Sauerbruch (1875–1951), built the first air-tight, low-pressure cage with gloves built into the wall. He was first to operate on an open thorax without killing the patient from lung collapse. He is recognized as the "father of thoracic surgery."

Who is credited with developing the heart—lung machine (extracorporeal circulation)?

Gibbon (1903–1973) first used his device in 1953, after devoting his entire surgical career to the project.

Who performed the first carotid endarterectomy?

DeBakey, in 1953

Who performed the first saphenous vein coronary artery bypass grafting?

Sabiston, in 1963

Who performed the first successful human renal transplantation?

Murray, in 1954, using a donor kidney from an identical twin

Who performed the first unsuccessful human liver transplantation?

Starzl, in 1963

Who performed the first successful human liver transplantation?

Starzl, in 1967

In what field did Starzl earn his PhD?

Neuroanatomy

Who performed the first artificial heart valve surgery?

Starr, in 1960

Who was the first to administer total parenteral nutrition (TPN)?

Rhoades, in 1968

Who performed the first vascular anastomosis?

Carrel, in 1902

Who performed the first heart–lung transplantation?	Reitz, in 1982
Who performed the first abdominal aortic aneurysm/ aneurysmectomy?	Dubost, in 1951
Who performed the first successful human heart transplantation?	Barnard, in South Africa in 1967
Who performed the first successful human lung transplantation?	Hardy, in 1963
Who performed the first successful human pancreas transplantation?	Lillehei and Najarian, in 1966 at the University of Minnesota
Who performed the first human laparoscopic cholecystectomy?	Mouret in Lyon, France, in 1987
Who was the only surgeon to win the Pulitzer Prize?	Cushing, for *Biography of Osler*
How many surgeons have won the Nobel prize?	Nine:

1. Theodor Kocher (1909, for work on the thyroid gland)
2. Alexis Carrel (1912, for work on vascular suture and transplantation of blood vessels and organs)
3. Sir Frederick Grant Banting (1923, for discovery of insulin)
4. Werner Theodor Otto Forssman (1956, for discoveries concerning heart catheterization)
5. Charles Brenton Huggins (1966, for discoveries concerning hormonal treatment of prostate cancer)
6. Allvar Gullstrand (1911, for work in dioptrics)
7. Robert Barany (1914, for work on the vestibular apparatus)
8. Walter Rudolph Hess (1949, for discovery of the functional

organization of the inner brain as a coordinator of the activities of the internal organs)
9. Joseph E. Murray (1990, for pioneering work in human organ transplantation)

3

Drains

Lorne H. Blackbourne, MD

DRAINS

What are the possible complications of intraperitoneal drains?

Erosion into the bowel or vessel, enterocutaneous fistula, infection, breakdown of anastomosis, bowel obstruction, and hernia

What is an open drain?

A drain with open ends, such as a Penrose drain

What is a closed drain?

A closed external-end drain, such as a Jackson-Pratt (JP) drain

Which drainage system, open or closed, is associated with an increased rate of infection?

An open system, such as a Penrose drain

Is it possible to drain the free peritoneal cavity?

No

Should a drain ever be brought out of the body through a suture line?

No. It should be brought out through a separate incision.

How does a sump drain work?

It is a tube with two lumens; the first lumen has suction and the second allows air in that is sucked out by the first lumen, creating a circuit.

What is the maximum recommended rate of pleural effusion drainage?

It should not exceed 1 L over the first 30 minutes of drainage, because an increased rate could result in acute pulmonary edema caused by rapid lung re-expansion

Have prophylactic oral antibiotics been shown to help prevent drain tract infections after mastectomies?

Yes. Although controversial, antibiotics may help prevent closed-drain tract infections after mastectomy according to research by Touran and Frost (1990).

How long after placement are peritoneal drains completely surrounded by omentum?

≈48 hours

What is the main disadvantage of passive open drains (e.g., Penrose)?

Retrograde migration of bacteria, causing infection

Is a drain needed after an routine appendectomy?

No, according to current data

Are routine drains needed after a ruptured appendix?

In most cases drains are used (although the issue is controversial).

Is a drain needed after a cholecystectomy?

No, according to current data

Is a drain needed after an acute rectal perforation?

Yes. Presacral closed drains (JPs) are necessary, along with diverting colostomy and closure if the perforation is intraperitoneal or easily closed.

How important is wide drainage after debridement in cases of pancreatic abscess?

Very important

What is "marsupialization" for a pancreatic abscess?

It is the practice of packing the wound open with kerlex or other gauze pads, creating a wound "pouch," following debridement of the pancreas.

Are perineal drains indicated after closure of the perineum following an abdominoperineal resection (APR)?

Yes, closed drainage of the perineum is indicated after primary closure.

Are drains needed after minor pancreatic or duodenal trauma?

Yes, drains are indicated in most cases.

In liver trauma, what factors indicate the use of a closed drain?

1. Bile leak
2. Severe liver injury (class 4 or 5)

Is a drain needed after a trauma splenectomy?

No, according to current data

Does a drain after splenectomy lower or increase the intra-abdominal infection rate after a GI tract injury (concomitant)?

It actually increases the risk (especially after a colon injury); thus, concomitant GI tract injury is a relative contraindication for postsplenectomy drainage

What was the JP drain initially developed for?

For postoperative subdural hematoma drainage

What is the real purpose of chest tubes?

They facilitate decompression and drainage and allow apposition of the visceral and parietal pleura.

What percentage of all pulmonary injuries can be treated definitively with a chest tube?

Approximately 85%

In most cases, where should the chest tube be positioned?

Posteriorly into the apex

How can a chest x-ray show if the last hole on the chest tube is in the pleural cavity?

The last hole is cut through the radiopaque line in the chest tube and is seen as a break in the line on chest x-ray. The break in the line must be within the pleural cavity.

What is the chest tube "hooked-up" to?

A Pleuravac® (three-chambered box)

Name the three chambers of the Pleuravac®.

1. Collection chamber
2. Water seal
3. Suction control

How is a chest tube placed on water seal?

By removing suction. A tension pneumothorax (PTX) cannot form, because the one-way valve allows release of air buildup.

Should a chest tube ever be clamped off?

No, except to "run the system" momentarily

What does "run the system" mean?

To determine wheteher an air leak originates in the pleural cavity (i.e., visceral hole) or in the tubing. **Momentarily** occlude the chest tube, and if air is still leaking, it is from the tubing and not the chest.

What signals the presence of an air leak?

When the water seal chamber is on suction, bubbles through the water seal fluid signal a large air leak (into the chest tube). If no air leak is evident on suction, the suction should be removed and the patient should be asked to cough. If air bubbles through the water seal, a small air leak is present.

What is the usual method of removing a chest tube placed for a PTX?

1. Suction until the PTX resolves and the air leak is gone
2. Water seal for 24 hours
3. Remove the chest tube if no PTX or air leak is evident after 24 hours of water seal

How quickly will a small, stable PTX absorb?

Approximately 1% a day; therefore, 10% by volume will absorb in 10 days

How should a chest tube be removed?

1. Cut the stitch
2. Ask the patient to exhale
3. Rapidly remove the tube (split second), and replace with petroleum jelly-coated gauze covered by 4 × 4 tape
4. Obtain a chest x-ray

What treatment is indicated for an extraperitoneal bladder injury?

Drainage of the bladder (with a Foley catheter), in most cases

When the ureter is injured along with a duodenal and/ or pancreatic injury, what other urinary drain is needed in addition to a ureteral stent?

A nephrostomy tube

How long should a biliary T-tube be left in place?

Probably for at least 3 weeks, although data are not definitive

Currently, which method of draining intraperitoneal abscesses is most often used?

Percutaneous catheter placement, under the guidance of computed tomography (CT) or ultrasound

What are the relative contraindications for percutaneous drainage of an intraperitoneal abscess?

1. No safe route to the collection
2. Multiple septations
3. Multiple small abscesses
4. Phlegmon undefined collection
5. Contrast allergy (for CT guidance)
6. Coagulopathy

What is the purpose of a catheter contrast study prior to removal of a percutaneous catheter placed for abscess drainage?

To rule out an enteric abscess cavity fistula

How often is percutaneous transhepatic cholangiography (PTC) successful with dilated ducts? With nondilated ducts?

Approximately 90% successful with dilated biliary ducts and 75% successful with nondilated ducts

4

Surgical Anatomy

Lorne H. Blackbourne, MD

THYROID

Name the thyroid lobe appendage that courses toward the hyoid bone from approximately the area of the thyroid isthmus?	The pyramidal lobe
What percentage of patients have a pyramidal lobe?	Approximately 50%
What does the pyramidal lobe represent?	It is a distal remnant of the thyroglossal duct, from its descent from the foramen cecum on the tongue.
Name the lymph node group located around the pyramidal thyroid lobe?	The delphian lymph node group
What is the thyroid isthmus?	The midline border between the left and right thyroid lobes
Which ligament connects the thyroid to the trachea?	The ligament of Berry
Which nerve travels with the superior thyroid artery approximately 15% of the time?	The superior laryngeal nerve
What is the common course of the left recurrent laryngeal nerve?	It loops around the aorta at the level of the ligamenta arteriosum, and then extends up, posterior to the inferior thyroid artery.

What is the common course of the right recurrent laryngeal nerve?	It branches off of the vagus nerve, loops around the right subclavian artery, and courses posterior to the inferior thyroid artery.
Which vein does the middle thyroid vein drain into?	The internal jugular vein
Which vein does the inferior thyroid vein drain into?	The innominate vein, in most cases
What is the IMA (not I.M.A.) artery?	A small inferior artery that extends to the thyroid from the aorta or innominate artery
What percentage of patients have an IMA artery?	Approximately 3%
Name the most posterior extension of the lateral thyroid lobes	The tubercle of Zuckerkandl
During a thyroidectomy, should the inferior thyroid artery be transected as close to its origin as possible?	No. The parathyroids receive their blood supply from the inferior thyroid arteries; thus, the inferior thyroid artery should be transected as close to the thyroid as possible.

PARATHYROID

How many parathyroids are there?	Usually four: two superior and two inferior
What percentage of patients has five parathyroid glands?	Approximately 5%
What is the usual position of the superior parathyroid glands?	Posterior, laterally behind the thyroid gland, above the inferior thyroid artery
What is the usual position of the inferior parathyroid glands?	Posterior, laterally behind the thyroid, below the inferior thyroid artery

What is the most common location for an "extra" gland?

The thyroid gland

What is the embryologic origin of the superior parathyroid glands?

The fourth pharyngeal pouch

What is the embryologic origin of the inferior parathyroid glands?

The third pharyngeal pouch (counterintuitive)

From where do the parathyroid glands receive their blood supply?

From the inferior thyroid artery

What percentage of patients have all four parathyroid glands supplied exclusively by the inferior thyroid arteries?

Approximately 80%

NECK

Which nerve runs in front of the carotid artery at the level of the angle of the mandible?

The facial nerve (CN VII)

Which nerve runs in between the carotid artery and the jugular vein?

The vagus nerve (CN X)

Which nerve crosses in front of the carotid artery at 1–2 cm above the bifurcation?

The hypoglossal nerve (CN XII)

What clinical findings are associated with a damaged hypoglossal nerve?

The tongue deviates to the side of injury (the wheelbarrow phenomenon).

Which vein is located in front of the carotid artery at approximately the level of the bifurcation?

The facial vein

Which artery does the superior thyroid artery branch off of?

The external carotid artery (it is the first branch off of this artery)

Define the following trauma neck zones:

Zone III

The skull base to the angle of mandible

Zone II

The angle of mandible to the cricoid cartilage

Zone I

The cricoid cartilage down to the clavicles

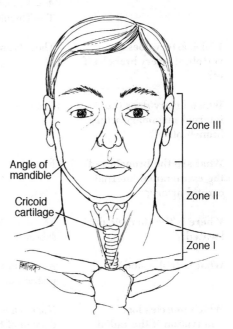

Angle of mandible

Cricoid cartilage

Zone III

Zone II

Zone I

Which structure separates the anterior from the posterior neck triangle?

The posterior border of the sternocleidomastoid muscle

How can you remember the order of the neck trauma zones?

They are in the same anatomic order as the Le Fort fractures: III, II, I

Which muscle is between the subclavian vein and subclavian artery?

The **anterior** scalene muscle

Which nerve runs along the anterior border of the anterior scalene muscle?

The phrenic nerve (transection of this nerve = paralyzed diaphragm)

What are the branches of the thyrocervical trunk?

1. Inferior thyroid artery
2. Ascending cervical artery (off of the inferior thyroid artery)
3. Transverse cervical artery
4. Suprascapular artery

How can you remember the branches of the thyrocervical trunk?

By the acronym S.T.A.T.:
S = Suprascapular artery
T = Transverse cervical artery
A = Ascending cervical artery
T = Thyroid artery (inferior)

Which artery does the vertebral artery branch off of?

The subclavian artery, bilaterally

Which artery does the internal mammary artery branch off of?

The subclavian artery, bilaterally

What are the branches of the extracranial internal carotid artery?

None

Where is the thoracic duct located?

The thoracic duct empties into the left subclavian vein.

What is Irish's node?

A node in the left axilla (associated with gastric cancer)

Which muscles lose innervation if the radial nerve is cut at the forearm?

None. Only sensory innervation to the dorsum of the hand is lost

What is a Langer's arch found in the axilla?

An accessory slip of the latissimus dorsi muscle traversing the axilla A congenital variant

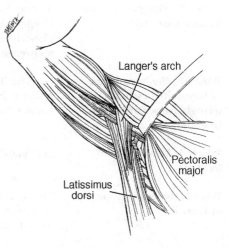

Where does the subclavian artery turn into the axillary artery?

At the lateral border of the first rib

Where does the axillary artery become the brachial artery?

At the inferior border of the teres **major** muscle

What are the clinical signs of a cut long thoracic nerve during an axillary dissection?

Loss of innervation to the serratus anterior muscle, resulting in a winged scapula

What is the usual distance from the skin at the right internal jugular vein to the pulmonary artery wedge?

50 + 5 cm

What is the usual distance from the skin at the right subclavian vein to the pulmonary artery wedge?

45 + 5 cm

What is the usual distance from the skin at the left subclavian vein to the pulmonary wedge?

55 + 5 cm

ABDOMEN

What are the boundaries of Petit's triangle (inferior lumbar triangle)?	Posterior boundary: Latissimus dorsi Anterior boundary: External oblique Inferior boundary: Iliac crest Floor: Internal oblique and the transversus abdominis muscle
What are the boundaries of Grynfeltt-Lesshaft's triangle (superior lumbar triangle)?	Superior: Twelfth rib Anterior: Internal oblique Floor: Quadratus lumborum
Where is Larrey's point located?	Subxiphoid
What is the criminal nerve of Grassi?	The small posterior branches of the vagus nerve occasionally missed during a truncal vagotomy.
What are the veins of Sappey?	The diaphragm veins that drain into the liver
What is Sappey's line?	A line drawn around the abdomen at approximately L2. It is thought that lymph drainage above Sappey's line goes to the axilla and below the line to the groin nodes.
What is the node of Lund?	The cystic node found in the triangle of Calot (also known as Calot's node)
What is the Hartmann's pouch?	The gallbladder infundibulum
What are the small ducts that drain bile directly into the gallbladder called?	The ducts of Luschka
What is the main pancreatic duct?	The duct of Wirsung
What is another name for the supreme artery of Kirk?	The dorsal pancreatic artery
What is another name for the small pancreatic duct?	The duct of Santorini (think: Santorini = Small)

What three structures comprise the triangle of Calot?

1. Cystic duct
2. Common hepatic duct
3. Lower edge of the liver

Identify the segments of the liver (French system).

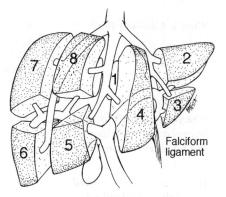

Falciform ligament

What is the rationale behind the segmental anatomy?

1. Most local and distant metastasis to the liver follow the portal venous system.
2. The segmental anatomy is based on the portal and venous systems of the liver.

How many segments are there?

Eight

What is Segment 1?

The caudate lobe (remember, the **caudate** lobe is **caudal** to the quadrate lobe)

What is the overall arrangement of the segments in the liver?

Clockwise, starting at Segment 1

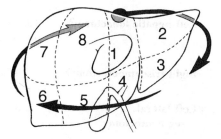

What is Segment 4?

Quadrate (named so because it has four sides)

Which segment is long and often subdivided into parts A and B?

Segment 4

Which segments are divided by the falciform ligament?	It divides Segments 2 and 3 from Segment 4.
What is Cantlie's line?	An imaginary line drawn from the left of the inferior vena cava (IVC) through the liver, just left of the gallbladder fossa (separates the left from the right lobes of the liver)
Which segment is located between Cantlie's line and the falciform ligament?	Segment 4
Which segment is located above the gallbladder?	Segment 5
Which structure lies within Cantlie's line?	The middle hepatic vein
Which segments are separated by Cantlie's line?	Segment 4 is separated from Segments 5 and 8
Which segments are resected in the following operative procedures:	
Right hepatic lobectomy?	5,6,7,8
Left hepatic lobectomy?	2,3,4 (classically, Segment 1 is not removed)
Right trisegmentectomy?	1,4,5,6,7,8
Left lateral segmentectomy?	2,3
What is the vein of Mayo?	The vein often seen during a pyloromyotomy for pyloric stenosis over the pylorus
What is the angle of His?	The gastroesophageal angle

**Define the different types
of gastric ulcers.**

Type I

An ulcer in the body of the stomach proximal to the incisura and not near the gastroesophageal junction—most are on a lesser curvature

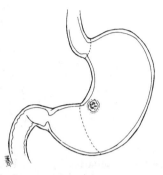

Type II

A type I ulcer and a duodenal ulcer (think: type II = 2 ulcers)

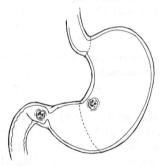

Type III

An ulcer in the pyloric or prepyloric area (think: type III = prepyloric, or 3 = pre)

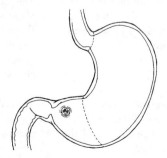

Type IV	An ulcer near the gastroesophageal junction (think: 4 near the "door" to the stomach)

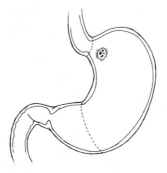

What are the boundaries of the gastrinoma triangle?	1. Third portion of the duodenum 2. Porta hepatis 3. Neck of pancreas
What is the meandering artery of Gonzalez?	A proximal collateral arterial arcade of the colon that shadows and is proximal and medial to the marginal artery
What is the advantage of a midline abdominal incision?	1. Wide exposure of peritoneal cavity 2. No major vessel, nerve, or muscle is cut
What is the significance of an arcuate line in the abdominal closure of a midline incision?	Below the arcuate line, all three abdominal wall muscle fascias form the anterior rectus sheath fascia. Above the line, the transversus and half of the internal oblique fascia form a posterior rectus sheath fascia.
What are the major structural differences between the jejunum and the ileum?	The jejunum has long vasa rectae, large plicae circulares, and a thicker wall. The Ileum has short vasa rectae, small plicae circulares, and a thinner wall (think: Ileum = Inferior vasa rectae, plicae circulares, and wall).
What are the major anatomic differences between the colon and the small bowel?	The colon has taenia coli, haustra, and appendices epiploicae (fat appendages), whereas the small intestine is smooth.

Where is the white line of Hilton located?	Between the external and internal anal sphincters
What is the space of Riolan?	The avascular area in the mesentery to the left of the middle colic artery
What are Jackson's veils?	Peritoneal folds across the ascending colon, from the cecum to the right flexure
What are Treves' folds?	Avascular ileocecal peritoneal folds (Treves was also the benefactor of the "Elephant Man")
How long on average is the:	
Anus?	3–3.5 cm
Rectum?	Approximately 12 cm
Define the amount of peritoneal covering of the rectum by thirds.	
Proximal third	Total peritoneal covering
Middle third	Anterior surface covered by peritoneum
Distal third	No peritoneal covering
What is Sudeck's point?	The watershed between the superior hemorrhoidal artery and the middle hemorrhoidal artery
What is Griffith's point?	The watershed area between the midgut and the hindgut blood supply to the colon—the area between the proximal two-thirds and the distal third of the transverse colon
What is the white line of Toldt?	The lateral peritoneal attachment of the colon

Identify the zones of the retroperitoneum.

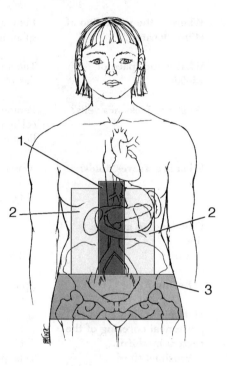

What is the space of Retzius?

The preperitoneal space between the pubis bone and the bladder

What is Denonvilliers' fascia?

The fascia between the rectum and the vagina or prostate

What is in Alcock's canal?

1. Internal pudendal artery and vein
2. Pudendal nerve branch (penile or clitoral branch)

What is Mackenrodt's ligament?

The cardinal ligament of the uterus

Define the boundaries of the femoral triangle.

1. Poupart's ligament
2. Sartorius
3. Adductor longus (acronym PSA)

Where does the external iliac artery become the femoral artery?

At the inguinal ligament (Poupart's ligament)

Where does the superficial femoral artery become the popliteal artery?	At the adductor hiatus, where the superior femoral artery leaves the adductor canal and turns into the popliteal fossa
What is another name for the adductor canal?	Hunter's canal
What is the node of Cloquet?	A node in the femoral triangle
What is another name for the femoral triangle?	Scarpa's triangle

GI Embryology

What are the most common sites for heterotopic pancreatic tissue?	The stomach, small intestine, and Meckel's diverticulum
How much does the stomach rotate during development?	90° clockwise; thus, the left vagus is anterior
How much does the midgut rotate during development?	270° counterclockwise around the superior mesenteric artery, when viewed anteroposteriorly
What is the embryonic origin of a Meckel's diverticulum?	The vitelline duct
To which adult organs does the foregut give rise?	The lungs, esophagus, stomach and duodenum (up to the ampulla of Vater). The pancreas, liver, bile ducts, and gallbladder are formed from outbuds of the duodenum.
To which adult organs does the midgut give rise?	The duodenum (distal to the ampulla of Vater), small bowel, and large colon (to the distal third of the transverse colon)
To which adult organs does the hindgut give rise?	The distal third of the transverse colon to the anal canal
Which pancreatic bud is connected to the bile duct?	The ventral pancreatic bud

Which pancreatic bud migrates to fuse with another bud?	The ventral bud migrates posteriorly to the left to fuse with the dorsal bud.
What does the ventral pancreatic bud form in the adult pancreas?	The uncinate process and the inferior aspect of the pancreatic head
What does the dorsal pancreatic bud form?	The superior aspect of the pancreatic head, and the body and tail of the pancreas
The small accessory pancreatic duct of Santorini forms from which pancreatic bud?	From the dorsal bud. The main duct of Wirsung forms from the entire ventral pancreatic duct that fuses with the distal pancreatic duct of the dorsal bud.
What abnormality arises if the ventral pancreatic bud migrates posteriorly and anteriorly to fuse with the dorsal pancreatic bud?	Annular pancreas
What abnormality arises with the persistence of the process vaginalis?	An indirect hernia

INGUINAL HERNIA ANATOMY

Which structures are located on the floor of the inguinal canal?	The transversalis and the "conjoint" tendon, inferiorly
Which nerve runs in and is posterior to the spermatic cord?	The genital branch of the genitofemoral nerve
What comprises Hesselbach's triangle?	1. Epigastric vessels 2. Inguinal ligament 3. Lateral border of the rectus sheath
What type of hernia goes through Hesselbach's triangle?	A direct hernia caused by a weak abdominal floor (rare in children)
Which side is affected more commonly?	The **right** (Approximately a 60%:40% ratio)

From which abdominal muscle layer is the cremaster muscle derived?	The internal oblique
From which abdominal muscle layer is the inguinal ligament (Poupart's ligament) derived?	The external oblique
Which nerves travel with the spermatic cord?	The ilioinguinal (on top of the cord) and the genital branch of the genitofemoral nerve (within the cord, posterior and medial in position)
What is in the spermatic cord?	1. Cremasteric muscle fibers (5) 2. Vas deferens 3. Testicular artery 4. Testicular pampiniform venous plexus 5. Genital branch of the genitofemoral nerve
From which abdominal muscle aponeurosis is the inguinal ligament derived?	The external oblique aponeurosis
Define a "true" conjoint tendon?	The internal oblique aponeurosis joined with the transversus abdominis aponeurosis
What percentage of patients have a "true" conjoint tendon?	Less than 5%
What do surgeons mistake for the conjoint tendon?	The transversus abdominis aponeurosis **alone,** attaching to the pubis
What is Cooper's ligament?	The thick periosteum of the superior ramus of the pubis bone
What is the hernia sac made of?	Primarily of peritoneum, or a patent procesus vaginalis
Name the fossa between the testicle and the epididymis?	The fossa of Geraldi

What attaches the testicle to the scrotum?	The gubernaculum
Name the remnant of the processus vaginalis around the testicle?	The tunica vaginalis
What could a yellow–orange tissue on the spermatic cord/testicle that is not fat be?	An adrenal rest
What is the most common organ in an inguinal hernia sac in men?	The small intestine
What is the most common organ in an inguinal hernia sac in women?	The ovary/fallopian tube
Instead of the vas, what is located in the inguinal canal in women?	The round ligament
In the inguinal canal, where is the indirect hernia sac located in relation to the other structures?	Anteromedially
What is a "cord lipoma"?	Preperitoneal fat on the cord structures (pushed in by the hernia sac)—these masses are not real lipomas, and should be removed surgically, if feasible
Within the spermatic cord, are the vessels or is the vas medial?	The vas is medial to the testicular vessels.
What is a small outpouching of testicular tissue off of the testicle?	A testicular appendage (appendix testes), which should be removed with electrocautery
How many compartments are in the lower leg?	Four

Name these compartments?

Anterior, lateral, deep posterior, and superficial posterior

What nerve can be injured during lateral lower leg fasciotomy?

The superficial peroneal nerve, which runs in the anterior aspect of the lateral compartment, can be injured, resulting in an inverted foot and loss of sensation of the dorsum of the foot and toes.

Identify the bones and compartments of the lower leg.

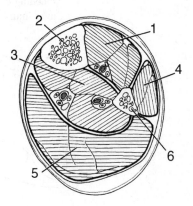

1. Anterior compartment
2. Tibia
3. Deep posterior compartment
4. Lateral compartment
5. Superficial compartment
6. Fibula

5

Surgical Manuevers

Lorne H. Blackbourne, MD

What is the Pringle manuever?

Occlusion of the porta hepatitis to decrease blood flow to the liver to slow bleeding during repair of a traumatic liver injury

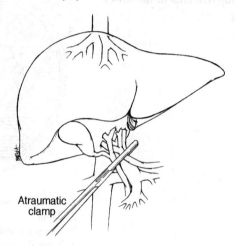

Atraumatic clamp

What is the Kocher maneuver?

The dissection of the lateral peritoneal attachments of the duodenum to allow inspection of the duodenum, pancreas, and other retroperitoneal structures

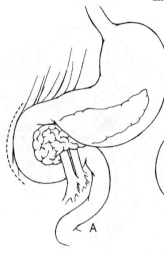
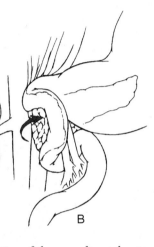

What is the Cattel maneuver?

Mobillization of the ascending colon to the midline. If combined with a Kocher maneuver, this maneuver will expose the vena cava (think: Cattel = Kocher = right sided)

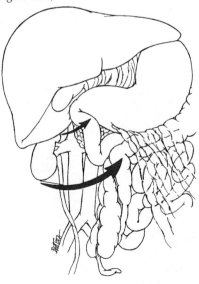

What is the Mattox maneuver?

Mobilization of the descending colon to the midline. This maneuver will expose the abdominal aorta.

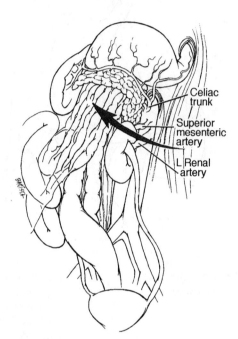

6

Power Review of Surgical Physiology

Lorne H. Blackbourne, MD

HORMONAL PHYSIOLOGY

ALDOSTERONE

What is its source?

The adrenal gland cortex and zona glomerulosa (think: glomerulosa = kidney; glomerulus as the kidney is the site of aldosterone action)

What stimulates its release?

1. Low sodium levels
2. High potassium levels
3. Angiotensin II
4. Adrenocorticotropic hormone (ACTH)
5. Neural stimulation mediated by decreased stretch in the carotid and aortic arteries and the left atrium

How does it act?

It increases sodium absorption from the distal tubules, potassium secretion, and hydrogen ion secretion.

What is the effect of aldosterone-mediated sodium retention?

It causes volume expansion and an increase in blood pressure.

RENIN

What is it?

An enzyme

What is its source?

The juxtaglomerular cells of the kidney

What stimulates its release?	1. Decreased pressure in the afferent renal arterioles 2. High potassium levels 3. Low sodium levels sensed by the macula densa of the kidney between the afferent and efferent renal arterioles
What inhibits its release?	Low potassium levels
How does it act?	It converts angiotensinogen to angiotensin I.

ANGIOTENSINOGEN

What is its source?	The liver
What converts it to angiotensin I?	Renin (from the kidney)
What converts angiotensin I to angiotensin II?	A converting enzyme in the lung
Describe the actions of angiotensinogen?	It has none.

ANGIOTENSIN II

What is its source?	It is converted from angiotensin I in the lung.
How does it act?	1. Potent vasoconstrictor 2. Stimulates release of aldosterone
How does an angiotensin-converting enzyme (ACE) inhibitor act?	It inhibits the conversion of lung enzymatic conversion of angiotensin I to angiotensin II and, thus, inhibits vasoconstriction and volume expansion from aldosterone-mediated sodium retention.

ANTIDIURETIC HORMONE (ADH)

What is another name for ADH?	Vasopressin

What is its source?	The **posterior** pituitary gland
What stimulates its release?	Hyperosmolarity, pain, ADH, stretch receptors in the carotid, aorta, and left atrium.
What inhibits its release?	Hypo-osmolarity
How does it act?	At the level of the renal tubules, ADH results in a concentrated urine formation, and fluid retention (the absence of ADH results in a dilute urine).
What is the effect of surgical stress and anesthesia on ADH release?	Surgical stress and anesthesia result in release of ADH.

PARATHYROID HORMONE (PTH)

What is its source?	The parathyroid gland
What are the major targets of PTH?	1. Osteoclasts 2. Kidney
What is the second messenger of the PTH effects?	Cyclic adenosine monophosphate (cAMP)
How does PTH act?	1. Increases clearance of phosphate (and, thus, less calcium phosphate complexes that would decrease serum calcium levels) 2. Stimulates osteocyte release of calcium 3. Activates enzymes of the most active vitamin D metabolite calcitriol in the kidney
What are the indirect effects of PTH?	PTH indirectly (via vitamin D effects) increases the GI-tract active duodenal absorption of calcium via an increase in the calcium-binding protein.
Where is calcium absorbed?	By active absorption in the duodenum and passive absorption in the jejunum

What is the effect of hypomagnesemia on PTH secretion?	Severely low magnesium results in inhibited secretion of PTH and, thus, must replete magnesium for normal calcium homeostasis.

VITAMIN D

Is vitamin D fat or water soluble?	Fat soluble
Name two sources of vitamin D?	1. Vitamin D_2 (ergocalciferol) from milk, etc. 2. Vitamin D_3 (cholecalciferol) from ultraviolet light absorbed by the skin
What is the site of hydroxylation of vitamin D_3?	The liver, where it is hydroxylated to calcifediol
What is the most potent active form of vitamin D?	Calcitriol
Where is calcitriol formed?	In the kidney, from stimulation of enzyme that is activated by PTH
What are the major targets of calcitriol?	1. Bone 2. Intestine
How does calcitriol act?	**Bone:** Increases osteoclast activity and releases phosphate and calcium from bone **Intestines:** Increases calcium-binding protein and the active absorption of calcium; also, increases absorption of phosphate and magnesium

CALCITONIN

What is its source?	Thyroid C cells (parafollicular cells)
What stimulates its secretion?	Low calcium levels
What inhibits its release?	High calcium levels

How does it act?	1. Inhibits osteoclast resorption of bone and resultant calcium release into the circulation 2. Increases elimination of phosphate
In which type of carcinoma is release of calcitonin increased?	Medullary thyroid carcinoma releases calcitonin.
What test stimulates release of calcitonin in malignancy?	Pentagastrin or calcium infusion results in an increased release of calcitonin in medullary thyroid carcinoma.
Medullary thyroid carcinoma is associated with which type of multiple endocrine neoplasia (MEN)?	MEN-II

THYROID

Name the active hormones?	1. Calcitonin 2. T_3 3. T_4
What is the most active thyroid hormone?	T_3
What are the precursors of T_3 and T_4?	Tyrosine and iodine
Name the two iodinized tyrosine residues?	1. Monoiodotyrosine (MIT) 2. Diiodotyrosine (DIT)
What couples to form T_3?	Monoiodotyrosine and a diiodotyrosine residue = T_3 (think: 1 + 2 = T_3)
What couples to form T_4?	Diiodotyrosine and a diiodotyrosine = T_4 (**think: 2 + 2 = T_4**)
What does the abbreviation TSH stand for?	Thyroid-stimulating hormone
What is the source of TSH?	The **anterior** pituitary gland

How does TSH act?

1. Stimulates absorption of iodine
2. Stimulates release of T_3 and T_4

What stimulates TSH release?

Thyroid-releasing hormone (TRH)

What is the source of TRH?

It is made in the hypothalamus and transported to the anterior pituitary gland.

What inhibits TSH release?

Thyroid hormones T_3 and T_4 (negative feedback)

Do T_3 or T_4 levels effect the secretion of TRH?

No

What is thyroglobulin?

A glycoprotein that contains the tyrosine residues (MIT and DIT) held in the thyroid follicular colloid

How can T_4 become T_3?

Approximately 75% of T_4 is converted to T_3 or reverse T_3 by peripheral conversion.

What is reverse T_3?

It is derived from T_4 and has very little, if any, potency.

What is the effect of thyroid hormones?

They increase oxygen and protein metabolism, fat breakdown, sensitivity to sympathetic nervous input, and red blood cell (RBC) production.

What binds thyroid hormone?

1. Albumin
2. Thyronine-binding protein
3. Thyroxine-binding protein

Are the thyroid hormones active if bound to a protein?

No

What is the Wolff-Chaikoff effect?

Excess iodine results in decreased thyroid hormone production.

How does propylthiouracil (PTU) work?

1. Inhibits peripheral conversion of T_4 to T_3
2. Blocks coupling of MIT to DIT
3. Inhibits the processing of iodine

CORTISOL

What is its source?	The adrenal gland cortex (think: **Cort**isol = **Cort**ex)
What stimulates cortisol production?	1. **ACTH** (adrenocorticotropic hormone) 2. **CRF** (corticotropin-releasing factor)
When does the nadir of cortisol production occur?	At night
When does the zenith of cortisol production occur?	In the morning

GROWTH HORMONE

What is its source?	The **anterior** pituitary gland
The effects of growth hormones on growth are mediated by which polypeptide insulin-like factors?	Somatomedins
Where are somatomedins synthesized?	In the liver
Define the effect of growth hormone on the following processes:	
Amino acid uptake	Increases
Protein synthesis	Increases
Protein catabolism	Decreases
Mobilization of fat as fuel	Increases
Glucose levels?	Increase
What stimulates growth hormone release?	Growth hormone—releasing hormone (GH–RH), stress, low blood glucose and protein, physical exercise

What inhibits growth hormone release?	Somatostatin
Which five hormones are secreted by the anterior pituitary gland?	1. Growth hormone 2. ACTH 3. TSH 4. Prolactin 5. Luteinizing hormone 6. Follicle-stimulating hormone (FSH)
Which hormones are secreted by the posterior pituitary gland?	Only two: vasopressin and oxytocin

GI PHYSIOLOGY

What is bilirubin conjugated to?	Glucuronic acid, by glucuronic transferase
Name the two primary bile acids?	Cholate and chenodeoxycholate
Name the two secondary bile acids?	Lithocholate and deoxycholate
What makes the secondary bile acids?	Bacteria
What is conjugated to the bile acids?	Glycine or taurine
What is a bile salt?	Conjugated bile acid at neutral pH results in an ionic salt and, thus, a bile salt.
What is in bile?	Cholesterol, lecithin, bile acids, bilirubin (bile pigments)
What does bile do?	It emulsifies fats.
What is the enterohepatic circulation?	The circulation of bile acids from the liver to the gut and back to the liver
Where are most of the bile acids absorbed?	In the terminal ileum

How many times is the entire bile acid pool circulated during a typical meal?	Two times
What stimulates emptying of the gallbladder?	1. Cholecystokinin 2. Vagal input
What inhibits emptying of the gallbladder?	1. Somatostatin 2. Sympathetics (it is impossible to flee and digest food at the same time) 3. Vasoactive intestinal peptide (VIP)
Which part of the large colon contains most of the H_2O-absorptive properties?	The ascending colon
Name the products of the following stomach cells: **Parietal cells**	1. Hydrochloric acid (HCl) 2. Intrinsic factor
Chief cells	Pepsinogen (think: "a peppy chief")
G cells	Gastrin (found in the antrum)
D cells	Somatostatin
Mucous neck cells	1. Bicarbonate 2. Mucus
Enterochromaffin cells	Serotonin

CHOLECYSTOKININ

What is its source?	Duodenal mucosal cells
What stimulates its release?	Fat, protein, amino acids, HCl
What inhibits its release?	Trypsin and chymotrypsin
How does it act?	1. Triggers gallbladder emptying 2. Opens ampulla of Vater 3. Slows gastric emptying 4. Stimulates pancreatic acinar-cell growth and release of exocrine products 5. Increases bowel motility

SECRETIN

What is its source?	Duodenal cells (specifically, the argyrophil S cells)
What stimulates its release?	1. Low pH (less than 4.5) 2. Fat in the duodenum
What inhibits its release?	High pH in the duodenum
How does it act?	1. Stimulates release of pancreatic bicarbonate enzymes 2. Triggers bile/bicarbonate release 3. Decreases lower esophageal sphincter tone (LES) 4. Decreases gastric emptying

GASTRIN

What is its source?	Gastric antrum G-cells
What stimulates its release?	1. Stomach peptides/amino acids 2. Vagal input 3. Calcium
What inhibits its release?	1. Low pH (less than 3.0) 2. Somatostatin
How does it act?	1. Triggers release of HCl from parietal cells 2. Has a trophic effect on mucosa of the stomach and small intestine

SOMATOSTATIN

What is its source?	D cells in the pancreas
What stimulates its release?	Food
How does it act?	It globally inhibits
Which hormone has been shown to be a marker for pancreatic tumors?	Pancreatic polypeptide

WOUND HEALING

Name the phases of wound healing?	1. Inflammation 2. Epithelialization 3. Fibroplasia 4. Contraction
What is the duration of the following phases: **Inflammation**	24 hours
Epithelialization	48 hours
Fibroplasia	72 hours to 4 weeks
Wound contraction	More than 5 days
Describe the actions that occur in each of the following phases: **Inflammation**	Vasoconstriction, followed by vasodilation and capillary leak
Epithelialization	Epithelial coverage of wound
Fibroplasia	Fibroblasts and accumulation of collagen, elastin, and reticulin
Wound contraction	Myofibroblasts contract the wound
What is the maximum contraction of a wound in mm/day?	Less than 0.75 mm/day
What factors inhibit wound healing?	1. Anemia 2. Malnutrition 3. Steroids 4. Cancer 5. Radiation 6. Hypoxia
What factors prolong the inflammatory phase of wound healing?	1. Bacteria 2. Foreign bodies
Which type of wound contracts better, circular or square?	A square wound contracts much better.

Define the following types of wounds:

Clean

No entry into the GI, respiratory, or GU tract (e.g., inguinal hernia treatment)

Clean contaminated

Entry into the GU, GI, or respiratory tract, but no obvious infection or spillage of succus, etc.

Contaminated

Entry into the GI, GU, or respiratory tract with infection or spillage

Dirty

Entry into pus (e.g., abscess)

Give the rate of infection for each wound classification:

Clean

Less than 5%

Clean contaminated

Less than 10%

Contaminated

Less than 15%

Dirty

25% to 40%

Which vitamin can reverse the effects of steroids on wound healing?

Vitamin A

What causes a keloid?

Hypertrophy of collagen synthesis

When a keloid is excised, should the entire mass be removed?

Although counterintuitive, a thin circumference of keloid should be left in the excision bed to inhibit collagen oversynthesis in the normal dermis.

VASCULAR PHYSIOLOGY

What is the systemic vascular resistance?

Using Ohms law

$$(\text{Resistance}) = \frac{\text{Pressure } \Delta}{\text{Flow}}$$

$(\Delta = \text{Difference})$

$$\frac{\text{BP--CVP}}{\text{CO}} \times 80$$

(In which BP = mean blood pressure, CVP = central venous pressure, and CO = cardiac output)

What does the abbreviation EDRF stand for?	Endothelial-derived relaxing factor
What is EDRF believed to be?	Nitric oxide
What is the effect of nitric oxide?	Vasodilation by the underlying smooth muscle
What is the precursor to nitric oxide?	L-arginine
What is the effect of nitric oxide on platelet aggregation?	It inhibits aggregation.
According to leading theories, what factors contribute to atherosclerosis?	1. Intimal injury/platelet aggregation 2. Growth factors/chemoattractants 3. Intimal proliferation, followed by smooth muscle proliferation
What are the most common sites where atherosclerosis forms?	1. Bifurcations (internal carotid) 2. Arterial fixation (Hunter's canal)
Define the following terms: **Bernoulli's principle**	The velocity of blood flow increases at an area of stenosis (think: thumb over the end of a hose to increase velocity of the water; also, **bern**oulli = **burn** rubber at area of narrowing).
Poiseuille's law	Resistance of a tube of fluid to flow is proportional to the length of the tube and inversely related to the radius of the tube (thus, a short 14-gauge IV has much less resistance than a long triple-lumen catheter).

CARDIAC PHYSIOLOGY

What is the formula for cardiac output?	**CO = HR × SV** (In which HR = heart rate and SV = stroke volume)

What is the formula for ejection fraction (EF)?

$$EF = \frac{SV}{EDV}$$

(EDV = end-diastolic volume)

When does the majority of coronary blood flow occur?

Approximately two thirds of coronary blood flow takes place during diastole.

In what part of the body does blood have the lowest O_2 saturation?

In the coronary sinus

What is the definition of DO_2?

Oxygen delivery:
$CO \times Hgb \times O_2$ saturation (thus, DO_2 can be increased by increasing Hgb or O_2 saturations, or CO)

How does a balloon pump work?

1. Balloon up during diastole to increase back flow into the coronary arteries
2. Balloon down during systole, resulting in a decreased afterload

Where on the EKG does the balloon pump inflate?

Around the T wave (think: **T** = **T**umor)

Where on the EKG does the balloon pump deflate?

Around the R wave (think: **R** = **R**egress or **R**educe)

RESPIRATORY SYSTEM

Define the spirometry waves.

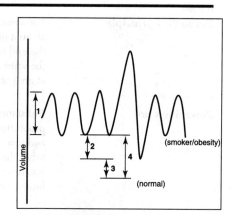

1. Tidal volume
2. Expiratory reserve volume
3. Residual volume
4. Functional residual capacity

Which cells produce surfactant?	Type II pneumocytes
What is the normal volume of intrapleural fluid?	Approximately 15 cc
What is the formula for pulmonary vascular resistance (PVR)?	$$PVR = \frac{PA - PCWP}{CO} \times 80$$ (PA = mean pulmonary artery pressure; PCWP = pulmonary capillary wedge pressure)

PROSTAGLANDINS, ETC.

Which enzyme is responsible for thromboxane formation?	Cyclooxygenase
What are the four main products of arachidonic acid?	1. Thromboxane 2. Prostacyclin (PGI_2) 3. Prostaglandins 4. Leukotrienes
Which enzymes are responsible for thromboxane?	1. Cyclooxygenase 2. Thromboxane synthetase
Which enzymes are responsible for prostacyclin?	1. Cyclooxygenase 2. Prostacyclin synthetase
Which enzyme catalyzes the biosynthesis of leukotrienes from arachidonic acid?	Lipoxygenase (think: **L**ipoxygenase = **L**eukotriene)
Which enzyme is responsible for prostaglandin synthesis?	Cyclooxygenase
What is the major source of thromboxane?	Platelets
What is the major source of prostacyclin?	Endothelial cells

Is thromboxane a vasodilator or vasoconstrictor?

A vasoconstrictor

Is prostacyclin a vasodilator or vasoconstrictor?

A vasodilator

What is the effect of prostacyclin on platelet function?

It inhibits platelet aggregation

What is the effect of thromboxane on platelet function?

It promotes platelet aggregation

How can you remember the function of thromboxane versus prostacyclin?

Thromboxane = thrombosis and thus causes vasoconstriction and platelet aggregation. Prosta**cyclin = cycling of platelets** and thus causes platelet cycling by inhibiting thrombosis by vasodilation and inhibition of platelet aggregation.

What is PGI_2?

Another name for prostacyclin

What effect does leukotriene B_4 have on interleukin-1 (IL-1) production?

It increases the production of IL-1.

What effect does prostaglandin $E_2(PGE_2)$ have on IL-1 production?

It decreases the production of IL-1.

Define the effect of PGE_2 on the following processes:
Production of gastric acid

Inhibits

Platelet aggregation

Inhibits

Tumor cell proliferation

Inhibits

Define the effect of PGE$_2$ on each of the following tissues:

Vascular smooth muscle   Dilates

Nonvascular smooth muscle   Contracts

What is used to keep a patent ductus arteriosus open?   PGE$_1$

What is used to close a patent ductus arteriosus?   Indomethacin, which inhibits prostaglandin synthesis

How do nonsteroidal anti-inflammatory drugs (NSAIDs) cause renal damage?   By inhibiting the prostaglandins that are responsible for renal artery vasodilation

What effect does furosemide have on prostaglandins?   It stimulates prostaglandin synthesis. NSAIDs can therefore inhibit its effects.

7

Renal Facts

David Musante, BS
Oliver Binns, MD

What is the anatomic relationship between the renal artery, renal vein, and renal pelvis?	Anterior to posterior: Vein, artery, and pelvis
What is the approximate size and weight of the adult kidney?	Length: ≈3 lumbar vertebrae Width: ½ the length Weight: 150 gm
How many nephrons are in each kidney?	≈10^6
Which ribs are anterior to the kidneys?	Superior left pole: 11 and 12 Superior right pole: 12
What is the anatomic nutcracker and what is its clinical significance?	Origin of the superior mesenteric artery (SMA) courses over the left renal vein and the third part of the duodenum; compression of the vein may cause abdominal pain and hematuria.
What is the approximate glomerular filtration rate (GFR) of the normal kidney?	120 ml/min (men) 100 ml/min (women) ≈160 L/day
What is the average urine output per day?	≈2 L/day
What is the approximate rate of renal blood flow?	1100 ml/min—approximately 20% of cardiac output
What is the approximate rate of renal plasma flow?	600 ml/min; therefore, the normal filtration fraction (FF) is 20%

What structures form the glomerular filter?

It is composed of three layers: the capillary endothelium, the basement membrane, and the podocyte foot processes

Name three factors of a molecule that decrease its ability to be filtered at the glomerular basement membrane (GBM)

1. Increased size ($\approx$MW)
2. Negative charge
3. Binding to plasma proteins

The GBM offers no obstacle at a molecular weight below what measurement?

7000 MW

Normal GBM is virtually impenetrable above what MW?

70,0000 MW (the approximate MW of albumin)

Can hemoglobin pass through the normal GBM?

Yes. In intravascular hemolysis it can cause tubular dysfunction (68,000 MW).

Name the five basic regions of the nephron?

1. Bowman's capsule
2. Proximal tubule
3. Loop of Henle—thin descending/thick ascending limb
4. Distal tubule
5. Collecting duct

Where does most water reabsorption occur?

80% of filtrate is reabsorbed in the proximal tubule.

Where does reabsorption of Na+, K+, amino acids, glucose, and phosphate occur?

They are all primarily reabsorbed in the proximal tubule.

Where does secretion of ammonia and K+, and acidification of urine occur?

In the distal tubule

Describe the mechanism of action of aldosterone.

It stimulates Na^+ resorption and K^+ and H^+ secretion, primarily in the distal tubule (Na+ and H_2O retention).

Describe the mechanism of action of ADH?

It promotes free water resorption, primarily in the collection duct.

Describe the mechanism of action for each of the following drugs:
1. Mannitol

1. Proximal tubule: not reabsorbable, causing osmotic diuresis

2. Furosemide

2. Thick ascending limb: inhibits Na^+/K^+/$2Cl^-$ co-transport resorption

3. Hydrochlorothiazide (HCTZ)

3. Distal tubule: inhibits Na^+/Cl^- antiport

4. Spironolactone

4. Distal tubule: inhibits aldosterone

What is the maximum urine specific gravity (sg) attainable by the adult kidney?

1.035 sg

What is the maximum urine osmolarity attainable by the adult kidney?

1400 mOsm/L (serum = 280 mOsm/L)

What is the minimum urine sg attainable by the adult kidney?

Approximately 1.003 sg (1.000 sg is water)

What is the approximate sg at which the kidney does the least amount of work?

1.010 sg

Why is the previous question true?

Because 1.010 sg corresponds to approximately 280 mOsm/L—the osmolarity of plasma

What is the normal range of urine pH?

5–8

How can the excretion of a weak acid be promoted?

By alkalinizing the urine (acidifying for a weak base and vice versa for promoting reabsorption)

Which ketone is detected with standard dipsticks?

Most standard dipsticks detect only acetoacetate, not β-hydroxybutyrate.

Which pathologic protein may give a false negative reading on a dipstick test?

Bence-Jones proteins (the acid precipitation test must be used)

What situations may give a false positive urine protein reading on a dipstick test?

Cases of highly concentrated urine, gross hematuria, and pH greater than 8

Which protein cross reacts with hemoglobin on urine dipstick?

Myoglobin

What measurement defines the upper limit of normal for daily urine protein excretion?

150 mg/24 hr

What amount of proteinuria is detectable by standard dipstick?

Generally, greater than 300 mg/24 hr, but it depends on urine concentration

What is meant by "microalbuminuria"?

Urinary albumin secretion less than 300 mg/24 hr, just below the sensitivity of a dipstick

What amount of proteinuria is present in nephrotic syndrome?

Greater than 3.5 g/24 hr/1.73 m^2

Renal vein obstruction can cause which type of urine abnormality?

Massive proteinuria

What is the normal range of red blood cells (RBCs) in urine?

0–5 HPF

What is the normal range of white blood cells (WBCs) in urine?

0–10 HPF

What is the general rule of thumb for determining the location of hematuria?

Dysmorphic RBCs: glomerular process
Isomorphic RBCs: nonglomerular process (best seen by phase contrast microscopy)

Are hyaline casts pathologic?

No, they are normal urinary constituents, which are increased in fever and after administration of loop diuretics.

What is the significance of granular casts?

They are formed by tubular epithelial cells and associated with tubular (ATN) and interstitial damage.

What is the significance of RBC casts?

They are most often caused by glomerular nephritis, but can also be present in acute interstitial nephritis, diabetic nephropathy, renal embolism, and renal vein thrombosis.

What is the significance of WBC casts?

They are most often caused by pyelonephritis, but can also be present in acute glomerular nephritis.

What can cause a false negative nitrite reading on a dipstick test?

Non-nitrate reducing organisms (many non-*Enterobacteriaceae* species), frequent voiding, high sg, pH less than 6, large vitamin C intake, or urobilinogen

What can cause a false negative leukocyte esterase reading on a dipstick test?

High sg, glycosuria, large vitamin C intake, or urobilinogen

What are the possible nonrenal causes of elevated serum blood urea nitrogen (BUN)?

Dehydration, catabolic states, high protein diet, reabsorption of hemorrhaged blood, and ureterocolic anastomosis

What does "azotemia" mean?

Excess of urea and other nitrogenous waste in blood

What does "oliguria" mean?

Urine excretion less than 0.5 ml/kg/hr, or approximately 500 ml/24 hr; generally, the level below which the daily osmolar load cannot be excreted

What does the term "acute renal failure" (ARF) indicate about urine output?

Nothing; it is possible to have oliguric or nonoliguric renal failure

Which type has the better prognoisis?	Nonoliguric
What is meant by "anuria"?	Urine excretion less than 100 ml/24 hr
What is believed to be the cause of nonoliguric (or polyuric) ARF?	Preservation of some GFR in the presence of tubular dysfunction
What causes the diuresis phenomenon during recovery from ARF?	1. High filtered urea concentration causes osmotic diuresis 2. Tubular insensitivity to aldosterone and ADH 3. Loss of medullary concentration gradient
Compare urea clearance with creatinine clearance.	Urea clearance is approximately two thirds creatinine clearance; therefore, BUN levels rise before Cr and fall after Cr during the onset and resolution of ARF.
Serum creatinine is an indirect measure of what renal process?	Glomerular filtration
How quickly does serum creatinine rise following the onset of ARF?	Only approximately 1.0 mg/dl/day, depending on the rate of production
What significance does this increase have for drug dosing in ARF?	Serum creatinine cannot be used to accurately estimate dosage adjustments until a new steady state has been reached.
What are the three classic forms of ARF?	Prerenal, renal, postrenal
Name the most common prerenal cause?	Kidney hypoperfusion, all types of shock, renal artery occlusion, ACE inhibitors in a setting of bilateral renal artery stenosis, hypovolemia
Name the most common postrenal causes?	Mechanical obstruction (bilateral, unless the patient has one kidney or marked renal insufficiency prior to insult)

Which initial screening studies detect the cause of oliguric ARF?

X-ray of the kidneys, ureter, and upper bladder (KUB) and ultrasound rule out obstruction; hydronephrosis should also be looked for.

Does glomerular filtration stop on the affected side in unilateral obstruction?

No, a small amount of filtration continues, but is completely reabsorbed by tubules.

What are the most common indications for intravenous pyelogram (IVP)?

Hematuria, renal colic, renal trauma, renal or pelvic surgery preparation (risky in the setting of ARF)

What are the contraindications to IVP?

Pregnancy, iodine allergy, previous adverse reaction, diabetes mellitus with renal insufficiency, iodine-labeled radio-isotope administration with thyroid disease

How is the urine Na$^+$ useful in the work-up of ARF?

Pre-renal azotemia: Na$^+$ generally <20 mEq/L
Renal azotemia: Na$^+$, generally > 30 mEq/L because of tubular dysfunction and ensuing inability to reabsorb Na+

Name one drawback of this method?

Urine Na$^+$ levels are affected by diuretic use.

What other urine component is useful in ARF?

Urea, the level of which is unaffected by diuretics (high urine urea—prerenal azotemia)

How long does it take a normal person to excrete an oral water load?

Urine flow increases within 30 minutes and excess fluid is lost within 3 hours.

How is urine osmolarity helpful in ARF?

Prerenal: >400 mOsm/L
Renal: <400 mOsm/L, because of tubular inability to concentrate urine

What classic urine abnormality is present in interstitial nephritis?

Eosinophilia

What are the most commonly encountered nephrotoxins?

Antibiotics (aminoglycosides, β-lactams, amphotericin B), NSAIDs, ACE inhibitors, radiocontrast dyes

What is the most common cause of ARF?

Acute tubular necrosis (ATN), frequently postoperative

What are the most common emergent problems encountered in ARF?

Hyperkalemia, severe uremia, severe acidosis, coagulation defects, respiratory failure, severe hypertension

What are the indications for dialysis?

Acidosis, **e**lectrolytes (hyperkalemia), **i**nflammation (uremic pericarditis), fluid **o**verload/drug **o**verdose, **u**remic encephalopathy (think: **AEIOU**)

What are the three dialysis modalities?

Hemodialysis, peritoneal dialysis, chronic arteriovenous hemofiltration with or without dialysis

What are the most common coagulation defects in ARF?

DIC, platelet dysfunction

What is the most common cause of death associated with ARF?

Infection

What is the usual recovery time for ARF?

A few days to 3–4 weeks

What percentage of patients have persistent GFR or tubular dysfunction following recovery from ARF?

Up to 10%

What is the mortality rate following ARF alone?

10%

Define ARF

An abrupt decrease in renal function severe enough to result in retention of nitrogenous waste (i.e., creatinine and BUN)

What is the most common cause of ARF in hospitalized patients?

Volume depletion (i.e., pre-renal)

What is the most common intrinsic renal cause of ARF?

Acute tubular necrosis (ATN)

How is ATN diagnosed?

By exclusion of pre-renal and post-renal causes first, followed by differentiation from other intrinsic renal causes (i.e., acute interstitial nephritis or glomerulonephritis)

What are the causes of ATN?

Ischemia, nephrotoxins sepsis, and myoglobin

What are the classic signs of acute interstitial nephritis?

1. Fever
2. Rash
3. Arthralgias

What is the single best test for differentiating prerenal from renal ARF?

Fractional excretion of sodium (FENa)

What is the fractional excretion of sodium FENa?

A quantitative expression of renal sodium retention:

$$\frac{(U/P)\ Na}{(U/P)\ Cr} \times 100$$

What is the value of FENa for prerenal ARF?

Less than 1%

What is the value of FENa for renal ARF?

Greater than 2%

How is uremic platelet dysfunction treated?

DDAVP

How is myoglobinuria treated?

1. Alkalinize urine with a bicarbonate IV
2. Mannitol diuresis
3. IV hydration

8

Blood and Blood Products

Lorne H. Blackbourne, MD

What are the signs of blood transfusion anaphylaxis?

Bronchospasm, hypotension, and urticaria

What is the appropriate treatment for anaphylaxis?

The mainstay of acute treatment includes administration of epinephrine, diphenhydramine, and fluids, as well as increasing or decreasing intubation as required. Steroids may be useful if symptoms persist. And of course, stop the transfusion!

What is the most common cause of transfusion hemolysis?

ABO incompatibility (resulting from clerical error, in most cases)

What is the appropriate treatment for transfusion hemolysis?

Administration of fluid and an osmotic diuretic, to protect the kidneys

Which blood components are most likely to trigger a febrile reaction in a blood transfusion?

WBCs

Which blood component is the most common source of bacterial infection in a transfusion?

Platelets, because they are stored at room temperature and staphylococci or streptococci from the donor's skin may be incubated

What percentage of a unit of packed RBCs can be hemolyzed in the first 24 hours after transfusion?

Up to 25%!

What medication can alleviate platelet dysfunction caused by uremia, aspirin use, or following cardiopulmonary bypass (CPB)?	DDAVP
Which molecules are responsible for platelet aggregation?	Adenosine diphosphate (ADP), thromboxane, and serotonin
Which enzyme is responsible for thromboxane formation?	Cyclooxygenase
What are the two main products of arachidonic acid?	1. Thromboxane 2. Prostacyclin (PGI_2)
Which enzymes are responsible for thromboxane?	1. Cyclooxygenase 2. Thromboxane synthetase
Which enzymes are responsible for prostacyclin?	1. Cyclooxygenase 2. Prostacyclin synthetase
What is the major source of thromboxane?	Platelets
What is the major source of prostacyclin?	Endothelial cells
Is thromboxane a vasodilator or vasoconstrictor?	A vasoconstrictor
Is prostacyclin a vasodilator or vasoconstrictor?	A vasodilator
What is the effect of prostacyclin on platelet function?	It inhibits platelet aggregation

How can you remember the function of thromboxane compared with that of prostacyclin?

Thromboxane = thrombosis, and thus causes vasoconstriction and platelet aggregation. Prostacyclin = **cycling of platelets,** and thus causes platelet cycling by inhibiting thrombosis through vasodilation and inhibition of platelet aggregation.

What is the function of platelet-derived growth factor?

It is released from platelets and causes growth and migration of fibroblasts and smooth muscle cells.

What do fibroblasts make?

Collagen

How does von Willebrand factor (vWF) work?

It binds the platelet to subendothelial collagen.

How does DDAVP work?

It causes release of vWF and procoagulant factor VII:C from tissue stores.

When should IV calcium be administered following a massive blood transfusion?

Most experts believe that calcium should be infused after 10 units of packed RBCs because of the citrate (a calcium binder).

Which contains more ionized calcium, calcium chloride or calcium gluconate?

Calcium chloride has three times as much ionized calcium as calcium gluconate.

What is the dreaded complication of peripheral infusion of IV calcium?

Infiltration of IV calcium can cause skin and sub-Q tissue necrosis. Calcium chloride is more dangerous peripherally than calcium gluconate because it contains a higher amount of ionized calcium.

Do packed RBCs have any clotting factors?

No

Name the most common causes of thrombocytopenia?

Heparin-induced antiplatelet antibodies, H_2 blockers, PA catheters, sepsis, disseminated intravascular coagulation (DIC)

How and when should postsplenectomy thrombocytosis be treated?

With aspirin when platelet count is greater than 1,000,000/μl

What percentage of patients receiving IV heparin develop antiplatelet antibodies?

Up to 10%!

What does the abbreviation HIT stand for?

Heparin-induced thrombocytopenia

How should HIT be treated?

By stopping the administration of heparin (Note: always follow platelet counts in patients receiving heparin)

Can heparin prolong the prothrombin time (PT), as well as the partial thromboplastin time (PTT)?

At very high doses, the PT can also be prolonged with heparin.

How does heparin work?

It activates antithrombin III.

What side effect is associated with prolonged heparin infusion (>2 months)?

Osteoporosis

What disorder may inhibit heparin anticoagulation in a patient?

Antithrombin III deficiency

What are the most common causes of platelet dysfunction?

Aspirin, uremia, CPB, and von Willebrand disease. (Aspirin administration should be stopped 7 days before surgery.)

At what level of thrombocytopenia is spontaneous hemorrhage expected?

Platelet count less than 20,000/μl

When should platelets be administered?

1. Platelet count less than 20,000/μl
2. Hemorrhage/surgery and platelet count less than 50,000/μl
3. Massive blood transfusion

Which drug can help platelet function in uremic or CPB platelet dysfunction?

DDAVP

What percentage is widely accepted (on rounds) as the optimal hematocrit?

Approximately 30% (maximum O_2 delivery and decreased viscosity)

What is the ideal hematocrit in a patient with a history of heart disease or stroke?

Approximately 30%

What factors can cause the oxyhemoglobin dissociation curve to shift to the right?

Acidosis, elevated 2,3-diphosphoglycerate (2,3-DPG), fever, elevated pCo_2

Give the normal life span for each of the following blood components:
RBCs

120 days

Platelets

7 to 10 days

Polymorphonuclear neutrophil leukocytes (PMNs)

1 day

What are the possible side effects of blood transfusion?

HIV, hepatitis B and C, adult respiratory distress syndrome (ARDS), fever, and anaphylaxis

Which test measures the extrinsic clotting system, the PT or the PTT?

The PT (think: pet = extrinsic)

Which test measures the effect of heparin on the clotting system, the PT or the PTT?

The PTT (often reported by the lab as the "heparin PTT")

Which enzyme activates factor XII?

Kallikrein (think: Kall = XII = 12)

What is another name for factor XII?

Hageman factor

What substance binds platelets to each other?

Fibrinogen (vWF binds platelets to collagen)

What substance binds platelets to vWF?

Platelet glycoprotein Ib (GPIb) (think: GPIb = Grab Platelet)

What is Bernard-Soulier syndrome?

A bleeding disorder caused by decreased levels of GPIb, factor V, and factor IX

What is Glanzmann thromboasthenia?

A defect in platelet aggregation caused by the absence of GPIIb and GP IIIa, which bind platelets to fibrinogen and thus to each other

What lab findings are associated with hemolysis?

Increased **indirect** bilirubin, normal direct bilirubin, decreased hematocrit, decreased haptoglobin

What disorder (other than hemolysis) can cause decreased haptoglobin levels?

Liver disease. Haptoglobin, which is synthesized by the liver, is increased in inflammatory reactions (i.e., acute phase reactant).

What is the function of haptoglobin?

It binds hemoglobin and then is cleared by macrophages.

Which enzyme causes fibrinolysis?

Plasmin

What substance activates plasmin?

Tissue plasminogen activator (TPA) activates plasmin from plasminogen.

Which test measures the effect of warfarin, the PT or the PTT?

The PT

What does the international normalized ratio (INR) represent?

The ratio of "normal" PT and the patient's PT. INR helps standardize the difference between labs. (The ratio should be between 2 and 3 in most cases that require warfarin anticoagulation.)

How does ε-aminocaproic acid (ε-ACA) work?

ε-ACA is an antifibrinolytic that inhibits plasminogen-to-plasmin conversion, thereby inhibiting fibrinolysis by plasmin.

How does aprotinin work?
1. Inhibits fibrinolysis by inhibiting plasmin and kallikrein
2. Promotes platelet adhesion receptors

What does the abbreviation ACT stand for?
Activated clotting time

What is ACT?
A widely used measure to assess heparin anticoagulation in the OR

What is an abnormal ACT?
Greater than 120 seconds

Is hetastarch an anticoagulant?
Yes; if more than 1500 cc are infused, it is associated with dilution of coagulation factors and inhibits factor VIII.

What type of medications increase the breakdown of warfarin?
Medications that increase cytochrome P-450 liver microsomal enzyme metabolism (e.g., barbiturates, carbamazepine)

How does warfarin work?
It inhibits vitamin K–dependent factors (II, VII, IX, X)

Which factor is deficient in hemophilia A?
Factor VIII

How can you remember the clotting factor for hemophilia A?
Think: **Eigh**t sounds like "A"

What is the appropriate treatment for hemophilia A prior to a major operation?
Factor VIII infusion to levels equal to normal levels

Which coagulation study is elevated with hemophilia A?
The PTT

How can you remember which coagulation study is affected by the hemophilias?
There are **two** major types of hemophilia and **two** "t"s in **PTT**

Which factor is deficient in hemophilia B?	Factor IX
What is the appropriate preoperative treatment for hemophilia B?	Factor IX infusion (to 20% of normal level for minor operations and 50% for major operations)
How can you remember which factors are deficient in hemophilia A and hemophilia B?	Alphabetically and chronologically: A before B and VIII before IX. Hemophilia A is factor VIII and hemophilia B is factor IX.
What is Christmas disease?	Hemophilia B
What is hemophilia C?	A deficiency of factor XI
What percentage of patients with hemophilia develop antifactor-8 or -9 antibodies?	Approximately 15%. These patients are a major challenge operatively.
Which type of hemophilia is more common in the United States?	Hemophilia A is four times more common than other types of hemophilia.
How are hemophilia A and B inherited?	They are sex-linked recessive.
What is von Willebrand disease?	A deficiency of von Willebrand factor (vWF) and factor VIII:C
Where does vWF come from?	Endothelial cells
How is von Willebrand disease inherited?	Autosomal dominant
Which medication can increase levels of vWF?	Depending on the subtype of von Willebrand disease, DDAVP can increase the levels of vWF (i.e., useful in type I, possibly useful in type IIA, useless in type III, and contraindicated in type IIB and "pseudo von Willebrand disease").
Which hemostatic parameter is increased in von Willebrand disease?	Bleeding time

Which blood product has the highest concentration of vWF?

Cryoprecipitate has a higher concentration than FFP.

What is lupus anticoagulant?

An antibody associated with systemic lupus erythematosus (SLE), procainamide, phenothiazine, hydralazine, quinidine, and HIV infection. It can prolong the PTT in vitro, but **does not inhibit hemostasis in vivo,** and can in fact cause thrombotic problems.

What is the effect of aspirin on platelet function?

Irreversible inhibition of platelet function for the life of the platelet (approximately 10 days) by inhibiting cyclooxygenase and, thus, ADP-mediated aggregation

Which medication may help platelet function in patients who take aspirin?

DDAVP

What effect does uremia have on platelets?

It inhibits platelet function

How should uremic platelet dysfunction be treated?

With dialysis and/or DDAVP

What can cause a coagulopathy in brain-injured patients?

Brain thromboplastin

What are the main inhibitors in coagulation regulation?

Antithrombin, protein C, and protein S

What does antithrombin do?

It binds factors (heparin accelerates this process)

What does protein C do?

1. Inhibits factors V and VIII
2. Possibly releases tissue plasminogen activator (TPA)

What does protein S do?

It stimulates and enhances the effects of protein C

How should protein C deficiency in the acute thrombotic setting be treated?

Although counterintuitive, FFP is the best source of protein C and heparin, and should be supplemented with antithrombin III, as needed. (Consult a hematologist.)

If a patient has a deficiency in protein C, S, or antithrombin III, what is the effect on the coagulation system?

A hypercoagulable state

Which renal disease is associated with a hypercoagulable state?

Nephrotic syndrome with the wasting of proteins, including proteins C and S

What is the effect of hypothermia on clotting?

It inhibits both the clotting factors and platelet function.

Does double gloving lower the incidence of finger blood soilage in the OR?

Yes (so do it!)

On average, how many HIV particles are transmitted on a solid bloody needle through one glove? Two gloves?

One glove = 10 HIV particles per puncture
Two gloves = 1 HIV particle per puncture!

9   Surgical Medications

Pierre Theodore, MD
Lorne H. Blackbourne, MD

POWER REVIEW

**Define the mechanism of
action for each of the
following medications.**

Aminoglycosides	Inhibit 30S ribosome
Penicillins	β-Lactam inhibits synthesis of bacterial cell walls
Vancomycin	No one really knows, but it destroys bacterial cell walls
Quinolones	Inhibit DNA gyrase
Clindamycin	Inhibits 50S bacterial ribosome subunit
H$_2$ blockers	Inhibit H$_2$ receptors
Promethazine	An antinausea agent; affects medullary chemoreceptor trigger zone
Haloperidol	Competitive blocker of postsynaptic dopamine receptors in the brain (contraindicated in patients with Parkinson disease)
Metoclopramide	Dopamine blocker in the stomach
Omeprazole	Proton pump inhibitor; **blocks the H$^+$—K$^+$—ATPase of the parietal cell in the stomach**
Sucralfate	Binds ulcer craters

Misoprostol

Prostaglandin analog for gastric cytoprotection

Cyclosporine

Inhibits IL-2

FK-506

Inhibits secretion and blocks IL-2 receptors

Papaverine

Mesenteric vasodilator

Bacitracin

Inhibits bacterial cell walls, mostly gram-positive coverage; used for peritoneal irrigation because it causes severe nephrotoxicity if given systemically

Digoxin

Inhibits the Na^+—K^+—ATPase, which leads to an increase in intracellular Ca^+ (+ inotrope and—chromotrope)

Imipenem

Binds with penicillin-binding proteins and disrupts cell wall

Cilastatin

Inhibits renal excretion of imipenem

Warfarin

Inhibits vitamin K–dependent clotting factors II, VII, IX, X (think: 2 + 7 = 9 . . . and 10)

Heparin

Activates antithrombin III

Streptozocin

Selective uptake and death of pancreatic β-cells

Cisapride

Causes acetylcholine release from the GI plexi, resulting in increased GI motility

Tamoxifen

Competitive estrogen-receptor blocker

Sulfasalazine

Cleaved into two compounds: 5-aminosalicylate (5-ASA) and sulfapyridine (which is absorbed); the 5-ASA stays in the gut and most likely wreaks havoc with the arachidonic pathways

Metronidazole

Breaks up DNA

GENERAL PHARMACOLOGY

Name the four major routes by which drug molecules move from sites of administration to sites of action.	1. Aqueous diffusion—across capillary pores (drugs with molecular weights of 20,000–30,000 D) 2. Lipid diffusion—across the lipid membrane by a concentration gradient 3. Facilitated diffusion (e.g., amino acids across the blood–brain barrier) 4. Pinocytosis—engulfing of extracellular material into membrane vesicles
In the human body, what are the volumes of body weight in cc/kg for each of the following fluids: Total body water?	600 cc/kg
Extracellular water?	200 cc/kg
Blood?	80 cc/kg
Plasma?	50 cc/kg
What are the most important factors in determining the distribution of a drug?	Protein binding, blood flow, membrane permeation, and tissue solubility
What are the two mechanisms for renal clearance of a drug?	1. Glomerular filtration 2. Tubular secretion
What is the chief role of cytochrome P-450 in the clearance of drugs?	Oxidation of drugs
What is the effect of the conjugation of a drug with glucuronic acid?	The greater the extent of protein binding, the less the glomerular filtration of the drug. Nutritional status and albumin concentrations can be important determinants of a drug's activity.
What effect does the enterohepatic cycle have on the elimination of drugs?	Drugs secreted by the biliary system can be resorbed from the intestine and reappear in the vascular compartment in an unchanged and bioactive form.

| What formula provides an estimate of the creatinine clearance? | Cr Cl = [(140-age)/serum Cr] × weight (kg)/72 × (0.85) (for women) |

| What are the principle locations of the nicotinic receptor? | 1. Muscle cell end plate of the neuromuscular junction
2. Peripheral autonomic system
3. Central nervous system |

| What is the main endogenous inhibitory neurotransmitter of the central nervous system? | γ-Aminobutyric acid (GABA) |

| Which secondary receptor is activated by β-adrenergic, H_2, and D_1 receptor subtypes? | cAMP |

| Through which secondary messengers do α-1-adrenergic and muscarinic receptors act? | IP_3 and 1,2-diacylglycerol (DAG), leading to the release of intracellular stores of Ca^{2+} |

| What is the therapeutic index and how is it calculated? | The therapeutic index is an estimate of the margin of safety of a pharmacologic agent. It is equal to the dose producing toxic effects in 50% of patients (LD_{50}) divided by the dose that is therapeutic in 50% of patients (ED_{50}). |

CARDIOVASCULAR MEDICATIONS

| What is the American Heart Association definition of hypertension? | Prolonged arterial blood pressure in excess of 140/90 mmHg |

| What are the four major means of controlling blood pressure? | 1. Decrease the force or rate of myocardial contraction
2. Decrease the blood volume
3. Relax the smooth muscle
4. Decrease the sympathetic outflow |

| What methods of reducing blood pressure are clinically available? | 1. Diuresis
2. Direct vasodilation
3. Sympatholytic agents
4. Agents that block the renin angiotensin axis (ACE inhibitors) |

Which classic causes of hypertension are surgically correctable?

1. Pheochromocytoma
2. Renovascular hypertension
3. Conn syndrome (aldosterone-secreting tumor)
4. Cushing syndrome
5. Coarctation of the aorta

What are the major complications of long-standing hypertension?

Atherosclerosis, aortic aneurysms, stroke, hypertensive renal disease, retinopathy, left ventricular hypertrophy, and increased myocardial demand

In the postoperative patient, what are the most likely causes of hypertensive crisis?

Sympathetic discharge (pain, anxiety), fluid shifts and fluid retention in response to increases in vasopressin and aldosterone, and inadequate preoperative control of hypertension

Name the conditions that require rapid reduction in blood pressure.

Postoperative management of pheochromocytoma; hypertensive-related encephalopathy; refractory hypertension of pregnancy; acute left ventricular failure with evidence of excessive afterload; aortic dissection; and intracranial hemorrhage

To a great extent, the toxicity of nitroprusside is caused by the buildup of which toxin?

Cyanide, leading to metabolic acidosis, hypotension, and arrhythmia

What is the treatment of choice for the toxic accumulation of cyanide following the administration of sodium nitroprusside?

Hydroxocobalamin, which forms a nontoxic cyanocobalamin, and discontinuation of the drug

What common drugs raise digoxin levels?

Quinidine, amiodarone, verapamil, erythromycin, tetracycline, diphenoxylate hydrochloride-atropine sulfate. Antibiotics that induce changes in GI flora may result in changes in digoxin levels. Digitalized patients that have antibiotics added to their medical regimen should be closely monitored to assure steady digoxin levels.

A 62-year-old woman with a history of congestive heart failure undergoes a partial gastrectomy and Billroth II for a gastric outlet obstruction. Is she likely to require a change in her digoxin dosing?

No. Although digoxin levels may be diminished in certain malabsorption states, neither Billroth I nor II is associated with a decrease in serum digoxin levels.

What is the proposed mechanism of action for the cardiac glycosides?

Inhibition of the Na^+—K^+—ATPase results in the collection of intracellular Na^+, leading to increases in intracellular Ca^{2+} as calcium is displaced from the sarcoplasmic reticulum.

What are the common ECG effects that occur with the use of the cardiac glycosides?

P-R interval prolongation, shortening of the Q-T interval, S-T segment depression, T-wave anomalies

How is blood pressure affected by IV glycoside administration, compared with oral administration?

IV glycosides are more likely to cause an acute rise in blood pressure from direct vasoconstrictive effects than orally administered glycosides.

What is the effect of toxic doses of digoxin on coronary blood flow?

Toxic digoxin levels may cause coronary vasoconstriction and reduction in coronary blood flow.

When should serum digoxin levels be drawn to assess the serum peaks?

The question is controversial, but typically the best estimate of serum concentration can be obtained 2 to 2.5 hours after injection or 8 hours after oral administration.

What are the common manifestations of digoxin toxicity?

Nausea and vomiting; visual field defects (i.e., seeing a yellow tint on white objects), depression, varying degrees of A-V block; conduction defects; and accelerated junctional rhythm

What type of patient with atrial fibrillation should never receive digoxin?

A patient with an associated pre-excitation syndrome, because the digoxin can facilitate passage of the atrial impulse through the aberrant pathway, leading to serious tachyarrhythmias

What is the effect of digoxin on ventricular ectopy and ventricular refractory period?	It tends to increase ectopy and decrease refractory period.

ANTIBIOTIC PROPHYLAXIS IN SURGERY

When is the proper time to administer prophylactic antibiotics in surgery?	Prior to performing the procedure to assure adequate serum levels at the **time of incision**
In routine surgery, has multiple drug dosing proved more effective than single perioperative antibiotic administration in reducing the risk of infection?	No
Do prophylactic antibiotics have a protective effect during chest tube insertion?	Although evidence is sketchy, antibiotics have been shown to prevent empyemas following chest tube insertion for blood, chyle, pus, and fluid.
What factors increase the risk of infection following gastroduodenal surgery?	Decreased gastric acidity Prolonged ileus Obstruction Hemorrhage Gastric ulcer Malignancy Prolonged use of H_2 blockers
In surgery of the colon, prophylactic antibiotics must be used to protect against which types of organisms?	Facultative gram-negative organisms and anaerobes
What advantage does cefoxitin offer over cefazolin?	Better coverage against anaerobes
Should third generation cephalosporins be used in the prophylaxis of surgery?	No. They are not effective against staphylococci and their indiscriminate use may contribute to the problem of antibiotic resistance.

How often do patients taking antibiotic medications develop diarrhea?	In 5% to 20% of cases
How often is antibiotic-associated diarrhea caused by *C. difficile*	1:1000 cases
What are the most frequent antibiotics implicated in antibiotic-associated colitis?	Ampicillin, clindamycin, and third-generation cephalosporins—although effectively all antibiotics have been implicated in this complication. The aminoglycosides are seldom associated with this disease.

ANTICOAGULATION

Does warfarin cross the placental "barrier"?	Yes; it is therefore contraindicated in pregnant women.
What is the routine timing of warfarin administration for a patient who is scheduled for elective surgery?	Warfarin should be stopped 48 to 72 hours prior to surgery, and heparin should be titrated to therapeutic levels. Heparin should be discontinued 4 to 8 hours prior to surgery, and resumed 12 hours after the procedure. Warfarin can be resumed 2 to 3 days postoperatively. Heparin is discontinued once the INR or PT has returned to the therapeutic range.

GI MEDICATIONS

What is the correct dosage of polyethylene glycol—electrolyte solution?	2 to 4 L, administered orally
How long after administration does catharsis occur?	1 to 3 hours
What is the correct dosage of metoclopramide?	10 mg, four times daily

What are its possible side effects?	Sedation and acute dystonia; it can also cause severe hypertension in patients treated with monamine oxidase inhibitors.
What substances are associated with reflux symptoms?	EtOH, chocolate, caffeine, nicotine, theophylline, diazepam, Ca^{2+}-blocking agents, meperidine hydrochloride, β-agonists, α-agonists, contraceptives
During what surgical procedures can unabsorbed bile acid to lead to diarrhea?	During resection of the terminal ileum, after cholecystectomy, and after vagotomy
What medical treatment is often effective in such cases?	4 g cholestyramine, three times daily
What risk is associated with over-the-counter antidiarrheals in chronic inflammatory bowel disease?	Precipitation of toxic megacolon
Have chronic steroids been definitively demonstrated to prevent acute episodes of inflammatory bowel disease?	There is no evidence that chronic steroids are beneficial in the majority of cases; however, prednisone (40–60 mg/day) reduces the severity of acute illness.
Which NSAID is the cornerstone of chronic management of inflammatory bowel disease?	Sulfasalazine (2 g daily)
What are the most common medications used to treat irritable bowel disease?	Corticosteroids, metronidazole (0.4 g, twice daily), sulfasalazine
Is there an urgent need to operate on a patient who presents with vomiting, abdominal pain, and radiologic evidence of toxic megacolon?	Toxic megacolon and perforation are dreaded complications of inflammatory bowel disease, and the mortality rate for patients who experience perforation before colectomy is nearly 50%. Furthermore, the colon may become atonic, leading to increases in stool output and giving the false impression of

clinical improvement. These patients are best managed by urgent resection of the colon if no improvement with medical management.

Is medical therapy warranted for asymptomatic gallstones?

The national cooperative gallstone study showed that treatment with chenodeoxycholic acid led to the dissolution of cholelithiasis in only 14% of cases following 2 years of therapy and cannot be recommended in the routine therapy of asymptomatic gallstones. Furthermore, two-thirds of patients that have asymptomatic cholelithiasis will not develop symptoms.

What common medications are thought to cause pancreatitis?

Azathioprine, furosemide, sulfonamide, valproic acid, tetracyclines, thiazides

What medications can be used to stabilize patients with upper GI hemorrhages caused by esophageal varices?

Vasopressin, somatostatin

What drug should be on hand during the use of vasopressin?

A nitrate preparation should be available, because vasopressin will often precipitate the onset of angina pectoris or MI.

What is the effect of metoclopramide on dopamine actions within the central nervous system?

It is a dopamine **antagonist**

How does metoclopramide stimulate gastric motility?

It facilitates the release of postganglionic stores of acetylcholine and sensitizes the gastric smooth muscle to muscarinic stimulation.

What is the mechanism of action of cisapride?

It is similar to metoclopramide in that it stimulates the release of acetylcholine; however, it does not have an antidopaminergic effect.

**Give the mechanism of
action for the following
antiemetic agents:**

Antihistamines

Block the peripheral stimulation of
emetic centers (most effective in inner
ear dysfunction-associated nausea)

Benzodiazepines

Prevent central cortical-induced
vomiting

Cannabinoids

Unknown (appear to act on the central
nervous system)

Domperidone

Centrally inhibits stimulation of the
chemoreceptor trigger zone, and
stimulates gastric emptying

**Phenothiazines (e.g.,
promethazine)**

Inhibits dopamine transmission at the
chemoreceptor trigger zone

TOXICOLOGY/OVERDOSAGE

**What dose of naloxone
should be given to an
obtunded patient with
suspected narcotic
overdose?**

IV adminiatration of 0.4 to 2.0 mg

**Will the cessation of
smoking two weeks prior
to surgery significantly
lower the risk of
pulmonary complications
in a patient who has
smoked for 20 years?**

Yes

ENDOCRINE MEDICATIONS

**What is the most common
cause of adrenal
insufficiency in surgical
patients?**

Suppression of the hypothalamic—
pituitary—adrenal axis by therapeutic
steroid administration.

**How long after the
discontinuation of chronic
steroid use is a patient at
risk for adrenal
insufficiency?**

Up to 1 year

What is the treatment of choice for acute adrenal insufficiency?	100 mg of hydrocortisone, every 8 hours
What are the medical options in the treatment of diabetes insipidus?	Free access to water DDAVP (0.1 to 0.4 ml via nasal spray, twice daily) Pitressin (IM administration of 5 to 10 U every 24 to 48 hours) Chlorpropamide (100 to 500 mg—can cause hypoglycemia at higher doses)
What are the two most common causes of hypercalcemia?	Malignancy and hyperparathyroidism
What are the medical regimens for prompt treatment of hypercalcemia?	Forced saline diuresis Mithramycin (IV administration of 25 μg/kg daily as required) Etidronate (7.5 mg/kg daily) Glucocorticoids (50 mg prednisone in divided doses)—steroids tend to have a limited effect in hypercalcemia secondary to primary hyperparathyroidism Calcitonin
What are the principal risks of hypocalcemia?	Tetany, laryngospasm, cardiac dysrhythmia, seizures
What is the treatment for low Ca^{2+}?	A combination of Ca^{2+} (1–2 gm/day) and vitamin D (100,000 U/day). Acute or life-threatening hypocalcemia requires treatment with IV administration of 10% calcium gluconate.
What associated electrolyte abnormality must be corrected to assure a normocalcemic state?	Hypomagnesemia

CHEMOTHERAPEUTICS

Of what antineoplastic agent is azathioprine an analog?	6-Mercaptopurine

ANESTHETICS

What causes the drop in blood pressure associated with halothane?

Direct depression of cardiac contractility and a decrease in peripheral resistance. Additionally, halothane commonly causes bradycardia.

What adverse reaction in the central nervous system has been associated with enflurane?

Seizures and epileptiform activity on EEG

What is the principle advantage of propofol as an agent of anesthesia induction or for ICU sedation?

Rapid onset after infusion and short (8 minute) recovery time. It is limited by its potential for causing hypotension

Why is it significant that local anesthetic agents exhibit frequency and use dependency?

The probability of nerve conduction blockage is greater in repetitively discharging nerves. The more rapidly and recently the nerve blockage discharged, the more likely the block.

What is the order of susceptibility to local anesthetic agents of the various sensory or motor modalities?

Pain→temperature→soft touch→movement (in order of susceptibility to lidocaine)

What is the chief mechanism of action of the local anesthetics?

Diminution of the Na^+ influx associated with depolarization of neurons, increase in the action potential threshold, and decrease in the action potential currents

What are the signs of central nervous system toxicity associated with excess dosages of lidocaine?

Tinnitus, nervousness, tremor, anxiety, and seizures

Does the practice of withdrawal of the syringe plunger prior to the instillation of local anesthetic agents guarantee that the drug has not been inadvertently delivered intravascularly?

No

What are the relative lengths of duration of lidocaine, procaine, tetracaine, and bupivacaine?

Bupivicaine→tetracaine→lidocaine→procaine (decreasing lengths of duration)

Which of the common local anesthetics has been found useful in transcutaneous use?

Benzocaine. Many of these agents (e.g., cocaine, tetracaine, proparacaine) are useful in local anesthesia across mucus membranes.

What is the mechanism of action of the drug dantrolene in the management of patients with malignant hyperthermia?

Interruption of the sarcoplasmic reticulum's excitation–contraction coupling in skeletal muscle via inhibition of the release of intracellular stores of Ca^{2+}

SEDATIVES AND CNS MEDICATIONS

What is theorized as the mechanism of decreased respiration during the administration of opioid analgesics?

Suppression of the CO_2 drive to increase ventilation

What is the effect of supplemental O_2 therapy on patients who are heavily medicated with opioids?

Rapid increase in supplemental O_2 can abolish the hypoxic drive to respire and result in respiratory arrest.

Which receptors along the pain–analgesia pathways of the brain are affected by the analgesic properties of morphine?

κ- and μ-receptors

What is the effect of antipsychotic medications on the seizure threshold?

Extrapyramidal side effects, acute dystonia, acouesthesia, hypotension, seizure

What is the initial treatment for an adult in prolonged seizure?

Establish and maintain an airway, obtain large-bore IV access, administration of IV diazepam in 2 mg doses up to a total dose of 10 mg, administration of **dilantin at a dose not to exceed 50 mg/min** (alternative treatment— lorazepam as an initial fast-acting antiepilepsy drug and phenobarbital for more prolonged seizures)

| In patients with Parkinson disease, why is dopamine administered in the form of levodopa? | Because other forms of dopamine cannot pass the blood–brain barrier |

NSAIDs

From which membrane lipid does aspirin, a widely used NSAID, inhibit the formation of prostaglandin?	Arachidonic acid
Why is it significant that as much as 90% of acetylsalicylic acid (ASA) travels in blood bound to albumin?	Aspirin may displace other naturally occurring or therapeutic compounds that show significant protein binding (warfarin, phenobarbital, penicillin, thyroxine)
Inhibition of which prostaglandin is thought to be responsible for the effect of ASA on platelets?	Thromboxane A_2
What are the early signs of salicylate poisoning?	Tinnitus, decrease in auditory acuity, headache, sweating, nausea, vomiting, hyperventilation
What are the three main mechanisms by which NSAIDs result in gastrointestinal adverse reactions?	Inhibition of PGE_2 results in decreased intestinal motility, promotion of gastric HCl secretion, and diminished mucosal barrier within the gastric lumen.
What is the chief condition that results in NSAID-related renal damage?	Hypovolemia and hyperreninemia in the setting of pre-existing renal disease

MISCELLANEOUS

| In which section of the small bowel is iron best absorbed? | In the duodenum and proximal jejunum |
| How long would it take to replenish depleted stores of iron with typical iron therapy (200–400 mg/day of elemental Fe)? | 3 to 6 months |

What is the objective indicator of adequate replenishment of Fe in the profoundly Fe-deficient patient?

A brisk reticulocytosis

What drugs are associated with a disulfiram effect when taken with alcohol? What is the disulfiram effect?

Chloramphenicol, oral hypoglycemics, moxalactam antibiotics, **metronidazole,** quinacrine, and some cephalosporins are associated with a disulfiram effect when taken with alcohol. Disulfiram inhibits the enzyme responsible for eliminating the aldehyde by-products of alcohol metabolism. In the presence of accumulation of acetaldehyde, peripheral vasodilation occurs and a reflex sympathetic discharge is activated. The result is flushing, palpitations, nausea, vomiting, perspiration, and abdominal pain.

Is the disulfiram ethanol response a threat to hemodynamic stability?

Rarely. Disulfiram has the added effect of interference with the synthesis of norepinephrine, which can blunt the sympathetic response to peripheral vasodilation and, in individuals with insufficient cardiac reserve, may result in cardiovascular collapse.

Is there a specific therapy for disulfiram-related cardiovascular collapse?

4-Methylpyrazole is an antagonist of alcohol dehydrogenase and may limit the conversion of EtOH into acetaldehyde.

What is the mechanism of action of allopurinol?

It is a competitive inhibitor of xanthine oxidase.

At which receptor does atropine block ACH?

At the muscarinic receptor

Which nebulized medication is contraindicated in patients allergic to sulfa?

Acetylcysteine, which contains sulfa

Who should not receive cephalosporins?

Patients with a history of anaphylaxis, swelling/edema, or hives after receiving penicillin, because cross reactivity occurs in approximately 8% of cases

Give the relative potency of the following substances, with cortisol as 1.0:	
Hydrocortisone	1.0
Prednisone	4.0
Prednisolone	4.0
Methylprednisolone	5.0
Dexamethasone	30.0
How can you remember the relative potency of prednisone compared with cortisol?	Think: **Pred**nisone = **Fred**nisone = **F**our times the potency
Which substance has more mineralocorticoid effects, hydrocortisone or methylprednisolone?	Hydrocortisone; therefore, methylprednisolone may be preferred for patients on fluid restriction
Which drug is used to treat refractory hiccups?	Thorazine
Does acetaminophen affect platelet function?	No
Which common medications can cause thrombocytopenia?	Heparin, H_2 blockers
Which medications increase the metabolism of warfarin?	Any drugs that increase the cytochrome P-450 microsomal enzyme system in the liver (e.g., barbiturates)
What type of patient should avoid β-blockers?	Patients with asthma or reactive airway disease, because β-blockers can cause bronchospasm (albuterol is a β-agonist), and **patients taking a calcium channel blocker**
What are the major side effects of imipenem?	Seizures

Which electrolyte will cause muscle/skin necrosis if infused subcutaneously (i.e., IV infiltration)?

Calcium

When a patient does not respond to a dose of furosemide, should the dose be repeated? Increased? Decreased?

The dose should be **doubled** if the patient does not respond to the initial dose.

Why can shortness of breath be alleviated more quickly than diuresis in patients with congestive heart failure who are being treated with furosemide?

Because furosemide is a venodilator and thus increases the venous capacitance quicker than the diuresis

Which medication is used to treat promethazine-induced dystonia?

IV administration of diphenhydramine hydrochloride

How does cisapride work?

It increases acetylcholine release from myenteric nerve cells (Auerbach plexus) and increases enteric smooth-muscle contraction.

What are its effects?

1. Increases esophageal peristalsis
2. Increases lower esophageal sphincter (LES) tone
3. Increases gastric emptying

In what cases is it indicated?

In cases of GE reflux (heartburn)

How is theophylline administered intravenously?

It is not; there is no IV form of theophylline. IV aminophylline should be given, instead.

What long-term side effect is thought to be associated with estrogen therapy?

Breast/endometrial cancer

What are the benefits of long-term estrogen therapy?

Decreased incidence of coronary disease and osteoporosis

What substance must be avoided by patients taking metronidazole?	Alcohol
What is the antidote for acetaminophen overdose?	Acetylcysteine
What drug is used to treat malignant hyperthermia?	Dantrolene
What drug is used to treat a Brown recluse spider bite?	Dapsone
Which electrolyte is inotropic?	Calcium

10

Preoperative Evaluation

Lorne H. Blackbourne, MD

What are the Goldman criteria for cardiac risk in patients undergoing noncardiac surgery?

Aortic stenosis, MI within 6 months, jugular venous distension (JVD), S3 gallop, ectopy, poor medical condition, emergency surgery, thoracic or intraperitoneal procedure, age greater than 70 years, nonsinus rhythm

Give the points by Goldman Criteria for each of the following factors (more points, more risk):

Poor medical condition	3
S3 gallop or JVD	11
Ectopy or nonsinus rhythm	7
Greater than 5 premature ventricular contractions (PVCs)	7
MI within 6 months	10
Aortic stenosis	3
Emergency surgery	4
Intraperitoneal or thoracic surgery	3
Age greater than 70 years	5

Define poor medical condition.	Bedridden, abnormal blood gas (PO_2 < 60/ pCO_2 > 50), abnormal electrolytes (K^+ < 3.0, HCO < 20), renal dysfunction (BUN > 50/ creatinine > 3.0), chronic liver disease
What is the mortality rate for patients who have less than 5 points according to the Goldman criteria?	0.2%
What is the mortality rate for patients who have more than 26 points according to the Goldman criteria?	50%
Is cardiac risk for noncardiac surgery increased in patients with uncomplicated isolated hypertension?	Usually not
Historically, what is one of the strongest predictors of a major cardiac postoperative complication in patients undergoing noncardiac surgery?	The inability to exercise
Name the physical findings that identify the risk of perioperative congestive heart failure (CHF)?	The third heart sound and JVD in a patient with a history of CHF indicate high risk for postoperative CHF.
What heart valvular disease is associated with the highest risk for postoperative cardiac complications?	Aortic stenosis
Why?	With aortic stenosis, the heart responds poorly to fluid shifts.
What are the signs and symptoms of aortic stenosis?	Systolic ejection murmur, angina, syncope, CHF (think: **a**ortic **s**tenosis **c**omplications = **a**ngina, **s**yncope, **c**ongestive heart failure)

What noncardiac surgeries are associated with the highest rates of perioperative cardiac complications?

Operations on the aorta, followed by operations on the peripheral vascular system (because of associated CAD)

Are the duration of the operation and anesthesia independent risk factors for a perioperative cardiac complication?

No (but remember, duration is correlated with a higher wound infection rate)

Name the risk factors for perioperative cardiac complications after noncardiac surgery.

1. MI (especially less than 6 months prior to surgery)
2. Angina
3. Pulmonary edema (especially in the week prior to surgery)
4. Critical aortic stenosis
5. PVCs (> 5/min) or nonsinus rhythm
6. Age greater than 70 years
7. Vascular surgery (especially on the aorta)
8. Emergency operation
9. Overall poor medical condition

Is spinal or epidural anesthesia safer than inhalational anesthetics in patients with CAD?

No; although counterintuitive, the associated loss of vascular resistance associated with these modes of anesthesia have failed to allow significantly lower rates of perioperative cardiac events.

Which inhalational anesthetic has the highest degree of cardiac depression?

Halothane, which can lead to direct cardiac depression coupled with peripheral vascular dilatation, without the normal compensatory tachycardia

What are the contraindications for epidural and spinal anesthesia?

1. Hypertrophic obstructive cardiomyopathy
2. Cyanotic congenital heart disease (because of loss of vascular tone and increase in venous capacitance)

11

Common Ward Emergencies: Diagnosis and Treatment

Jeffry Watson, MD
Joseph Wells, MD

RESPIRATORY DISTRESS

What are the symptoms of excessive work of breathing?

Respiratory rate greater than 30/minute, use of accessory muscles of respiration, tachycardia, widened paradoxical pulse, diaphoresis, and distressed facial expression

What diagnostic tests are indicated?

1. Arterial blood gas (ABG)
2. Chest x-ray
3. Electrocardiogram (EKG)

What is the differential diagnosis?

1. Pneumothorax
2. Pulmonary edema
3. Pulmonary embolus
4. Pneumonia
5. Aspiration
6. Mucus plugging

What are the indications for initiating mechanical ventilatory support?

1. Progressive refractory hypoxemia ($PaO_2 < 50$ mmHg, despite supplemental O_2)
2. Progressive respiratory acidosis ($PaCO_2 > 50$ mmHg, pH < 7.30)
3. Excessive work of breathing
4. Protection of airway patency
5. Prevention of aspiration

Under what circumstances is intubation indicated to protect airway patency or prevent aspiration?

1. Depressed consciousness (especially with no cough on nasotrachael [NT] suctioning)
2. Facial or neck trauma
3. Infectious, infiltrative, or malignant disease of the upper airway

Name the different types of emergent intubation?

1. NT
2. Orotracheal, with or without rapid sequence induction
3. Surgical (tracheotomy or cricothyroidotomy)

When is NT intubation contraindicated?

In patients with apnea

What are the relative contraindications to NT intubation?

1. Midface fractures
2. Bleeding disorders
3. Elevated ICP

What are the disadvantages of NT intubation?

1. If a smaller tube is used, suctioning and weaning may be difficult.
2. Increased risk of sinusitis

What is rapid sequence intubation (RSI)?

Administration of sedative and/or analgesic agents in concert with paralyzing agents to facilitate orotracheal intubation

What are the advantages of RSI?

1. Minimizes patient discomfort
2. Minimizes muscular resistance
3. Causes less increase in ICP

What is the key disadvantage of RSI?

It may necessitate a surgical airway if intubation fails, and effective ventilation with a bag valve mask is impossible.

What are the steps in RSI?

1. Preoxygenation
2. Sedative and or analgesic administration (midazolam 0.1 mg/kg IV)
3. Cricoid pressure (Sellick maneuver) with administration of succinylcholine (1 mg/kg IV)
4. Positioning of patient's head and intubation
5. Verification of tube position (auscultation, chest x-ray, end-tidal CO_2)

When is cricothyroidotomy indicated?

In cases of failed endotracheal intubation

PULMONARY EDEMA

What are the symptoms?	Dyspnea, cough productive of frothy sputum, tachypnea, rales, and cyanosis
What diagnostic tests are indicated?	Chest x-ray, ABG
What are the differential diagnoses?	1. Volume overload (massive transfusions, plasma expanders) 2. ARDS (sepsis, trauma, aspiration) 3. Left ventricular failure (myocardial infarction) 4. Pulmonary embolus 5. Pneumothorax
What are the early anatomic findings?	Accumulation of perivascular fluid, thickening of capillary and alveolar walls
What are Kerley B lines?	On chest x-ray, linear densities oriented perpendicularly to the pleura and resulting from increased pulmonary venous pressure/lymphatic edema
What is cephalization?	On chest x-ray, increased pulmonary vascular markings superiorly, resulting from increased pulmonary venous pressure
What is the appropriate treatment?	1. Oxygen 2. Furosemide (diuresis) 3. Continuous positive airway pressure, positive end-expiratory pressure (PEEP) if the patient is mechanically ventilated 4. Treatment of underlying cause
In chronic heart failure, why does furosemide work before diuresis?	It causes systemic venous dilatation and a subsequent decrease in preload.

ASPIRATION

What is aspiration pneumonitis?	An acute condition caused by aspiration of acidic gastric contents into the airway, resulting in an intense inflammatory response with atelectasis, pulmonary edema, and hemorrhage.

What is aspiration pneumonia?

A bacterial infection that develops gradually after gastric or oropharyngeal contamination. It may occur after pneumonitis.

What is the eponym for aspiration pneumonitis?

Mendelson syndrome

What are the associated risk factors?

Decreased level of consciousness, head trauma, oral intake within 6 hours of anesthesia, bowel obstruction, esophageal reflux disorder, obesity, and supine position

What are the symptoms?

Acutely, symptoms include dyspnea, cyanosis, tachypnea, rales, and bronchospasm. Obstruction of bronchi by larger particles can result in severe hypoxia and cardiac arrest. Fever, egophony, and sputum production may occur later as bacterial pneumonia sets in.

What are the associated x-ray findings?

Within hours, diffuse infiltrates similar in appearance to pulmonary edema are evident. Over days, necrosis can result in multiple small cavitations and abscess formation. Bacterial infection often shows consolidation of lower lobes.

What is the appropriate treatment?

Immediate pharyngeal or endotracheal suctioning is indicated. Bronchoscopy may be necessary to remove larger particles. Intubation and mechanical ventilation may be needed if respiratory status and blood gases so indicate. Broad antimicrobial therapy should be initiated to limit the deleterious effects of subsequent pneumonia. NGT to decompress the stomach is also necessary.

What preventive measures can be taken?

Nothing by mouth for at least 6 hours prior to anesthesia, cricoid pressure prior to intubation, elevation of the head of the bed

WHEEZING

What are the differential diagnoses?	1. Acute bronchospasm 2. Pneumonia/ bronchitis 3. Allergic reaction 4. Fluid overload 5. Aspiration
How should bronchospasm be treated?	1. Aggressive endotracheal or NT suctioning 2. Nebulized metaproterenol/albuterol 3. Aminophylline IV for refractory bronchospasm 4. Mechanical ventilation as necessary 5. Epinephrine

MUCUS PLUGGING

What are the symptoms?	Increasing respiratory distress, especially hypoxia
What is the mechanism of hypoxia?	Plugging of airways results in a ventilation/perfusion mismatch.
What diagnostic test is indicated?	Chest x-ray, which can identify a newly collapsed segment or lobe
What are the differential diagnoses?	1. Pneumonia 2. Pulmonary Embolus 3. Aspiration
What is the appropriate treatment?	Bronchoscopy to remove the plug

PNEUMOTHORAX

What factors predispose patients to spontaneous pneumothorax?	Eighty percent are tall, thin, young males with no history of pulmonary disease. Chronic obstructive pulmonary disease (COPD) patients are also susceptible ("Bleb" disease).
What are the symptoms?	Chest pain, dyspnea, decreased breath sounds on the involved side, and tachycardia; **be aware that healthy young patients can be almost completely asymptomatic at rest**

What are the symptoms of tension pneumothorax?	JVD, hypotension, and deviated trachea, shortness of breath
How should a tension pneumothorax be decompressed prior to chest tube placement?	With a large-bore needle through the second intercostal space, at the midclavicular line
Why are postoperative patients at risk for pneumothorax?	1. Positive pressure ventilation 2. Central line placement
Is a chest tube indicated in all cases of pneumothorax, regardless of size?	No. In cases with less than 50% lung collapse or less than 3 cm separation from the chest wall, many patients may be observed without tube thoracostomy (always give supplemental O_2). Obviously, if the patient shows signs of respiratory distress with decreased breath sounds, a chest tube is required.
What percentage of a pneumothorax is absorbed per day?	1% (10 days for a 10% pneumothorax)
Where should the chest tube be inserted?	At the midaxillary line, at the level of the nipple (≈ fourth intercostal space [ICS])
What is a potential danger of rapid reexpansion after chest tube insertion?	Pulmonary edema

PULMONARY EMBOLISM

What is the incidence in elderly patients after operative repair of hip fractures?	10%; therefore, maintain a high degree of suspicion for such patients
What is the prognosis for patients who have experienced pulmonary embolism?	Ten percent die within one hour. Of the remaining 90%, one-third are diagnosed and treated, with an 8% mortality rate observed. Two-thirds are not diagnosed, of which 30% die.

What are the symptoms?	Dyspnea, tachypnea, chest pain, hemoptysis, mental status changes, splinting, and accentuated second heart sound
What are the associated chest x-ray findings in most cases?	The chest film is usually normal. Westermark sign (cone-shaped area of decreased vascular markings) is insensitive.
What ECG changes occur?	Ten to twenty percent of patients may have S-T segment depression in leads III, V1, V3, and V4.
What urgent treatment is indicated?	1. Place the patient on a 100% oxygen mask 2. Check the arterial blood gas (ABG) 3. Administer heparin in a bolus injection of 10,000 U, followed by 1000 U/hr
Which ventilation/ perfusion (V/Q) scan readings are helpful and which are not helpful?	High probability scans in the appropriate setting may be relied upon to initiate treatment. Intermediate or indeterminate scans require arteriogram.
When is embolectomy indicated?	Upon documenting massive pulmonary artery occlusion on angiogram; thrombolytic therapy is also a treatment option

TRACHEOSTOMY

Describe the mechanism of tracheoesophageal fistula formation?	Pressure necrosis by tracheostomy tube in apposition to NGT
What are the symptoms?	1. Marked increase in tracheal secretions 2. Gastric distention 3. Hypoxia
What diagnostic test is indicated?	Bronchoscopy
What is the appropriate treatment?	Surgical repair

Describe the mechanism of tracheoinnominate artery fistula formation?	Pressure necrosis by tracheostomy tube against the innominate artery
What symptom is associated with the disorder?	Tracheal bleeding (ranging from minor to exsanguinating)
What nonemergent diagnostic test is indicated?	Bronchoscopy
What is the Utley maneuver?	Direct digital innominate artery pressure through the tracheostomy stoma, with or without orotracheal intubation, to control massive bleeding
What else can be done to control massive bleeding?	Hyperinflation of the tracheal cuff
What is the appropriate treatment?	Surgical repair

CARDIOVASCULAR COMPLICATIONS

ARRHYTHMIAS

What diagnostic tests are indicated?	EKG, chest x-ray, ABG, serum electrolytes
What are the associated risk factors?	1. Pneumothorax 2. Pneumonia 3. Electrolyte disturbances 4. Myocardial ischemia
What is the most common postoperative arrhythmia?	Supraventricular tachycardia (SVT)
What EKG findings are associated with SVT?	Heart rate greater than 100 BPM, narrow QRS morphology
What treatment is appropriate if the patient's condition is unstable?	Cardioversion
At what energy level?	100 j

What is the appropriate treatment if the patient's condition is stable?	Adenosine, verapamil, or procainamide
What EKG findings are associated with atrial flutter?	1. Atrial activity at 250 to 350/min 2. Sawtooth pattern 3. Constant ventricular response with narrow QRS
What is the appropriate treatment if the patient's condition is unstable?	Cardioversion
What is the appropriate treatment if the patient's condition is stable?	Digoxin, diltiazem
What EKG findings are associated with atrial fibrillation?	1. Undulating baseline without P waves 2. Irregular ventricular response
What are the symptoms?	Palpitations, dyspnea, and angina pectoris
What is the appropriate treatment if the patient's condition is unstable?	Cardioversion, with or without a class I antiarrhythmic (e.g., quinidine)
What EKG findings are associated with ventricular tachycardia (VT)?	1. Wide QRS tachycardia 2. Independent atrial activity
What is the most common underlying heart disease associated with VT?	Coronary artery disease
What are the common metabolic precipitants of VT?	1. Hypokalemia 2. Hypomagnesemia
What are the common pharmacologic precipitants?	1. Quinidine 2. Procainamide
Which subtype of VT occurs with the previously mentioned precipitants?	Torsade de pointes

What is the appropriate treatment if the patient's condition is unstable?	Cardioversion
What is the appropriate treatment if the patient's condition is stable?	Lidocaine
What is the usual dosage?	100 mg bolus administration, followed by 2 mg/min drip

BRADYCARDIA

What diagnostic tests are indicated?	1. EKG 2. Chest x-ray 3. ABG
When should bradycardia be treated?	If the heart rate is less than 60 and the patient is symptomatic (hypotension, congestive heart failure, chest pain, dyspnea, and decreased level of consciousness)
What is considered the first-line medical therapy?	Atropine 0.5 to 1.0 mg IV every 3 to 5 minutes
Why may an atropine dose of less than 0.5 mg be dangerous?	It may cause a paradoxical **worsening of the bradycardia** via blockade of M_1 receptors on postganglionic parasympathetic neurons.
What are the indications for temporary transcutaneous pacing?	Second degree (non-Wenckebach) A-V block, third degree A-V block
What electrolyte changes are known to cause bradycardia?	Hypocalcemia causes increased Q-T interval; hypokalemia can result in digoxin toxicity in such patients.

CARDIAC ARREST

If an unresponsive patient is found to have no pulse, what action should be taken next?	Establish an airway, bag ventilate, perform CPR until a defibrillator/monitor arrives, then assess for VTs while continuing CPR.

How is asystole managed?	1. Intubate 2. Confirm bilateral breath sounds (pneumothorax is possible in postoperative patients) 3. Place an IV line 4. Administer epinephrine 1 mg IV push every 3 to 5 minutes 5. Administer atropine 1 mg IV every 3 to 5 minutes, up to total of 3 mg 6. Begin transcutaneous pacing (if available) 7. Check electrolytes (K^+)
When should lifesaving measures be discontinued?	After the patient has been intubated and received an initial round of the medications previously listed, yet remains in asystole with no reversible causes
What are the indications for open cardiac massage?	1. Cardiac arrest with penetrating chest trauma 2. Anatomic deformity precluding adequate chest compressions 3. Arrest from severe hypothermia 4. Arrest from ruptured aortic aneurysm 5. Cardiac tamponade

CHEST PAIN

What immediate questions should the patient be asked (assuming he or she is responsive)?	The location, nature, and severity of pain, activity at onset, history of coronary artery disease, and other symptoms
What life-threatening causes can be responsible for chest pain?	Myocardial ischemia, tension pneumothorax, aortic dissection, and pulmonary embolism
What is the appropriate initial treatment?	1. Oxygen face mask 2. Chest x-ray (**stat**) 3. ABG 4. EKG (**stat**) 5. Three doses of sublingual nitroglycerin 0.4 mg every 5 minutes (as required)

How should hypertension with ripping, tearing substernal pain be treated?

With sodium nitroprusside, esmolol, or labetalol to decrease systolic blood pressure (SBP) to less than 110 mmHg, while awaiting CT with contrast or aortogram to rule out aortic dissection

What steps should be taken if a patient has evidence of persistent myocardial ischemia on EKG?

1. Sublingual nitroglycerin 0.4 mg every 5 minutes
2. Oxygen 4 liters nasal cannula
3. If pain persists, IV nitroglycerine 10 meq/min, titrated to pain
4. If ectopy is evident on EKG, lidocaine 75 to 100 mg IV bolus, infused at a rate of 2 mg/min
5. Aspirin (**stat**)
6. Morphine IV
7. β-Blocker if heart rate is greater than 90
8. Cardiac enzyme tests, ABG, EKG, chest x-ray, serum electrolytes
9. ICU monitoring

DEEP VENOUS THROMBOSIS (DVT)

According to Virchow, what are the three factors that predispose patients to DVT?

1. Stasis
2. Endothelial injury
3. Hypercoagulability

Name the other factors associated with DVT occurrence.

Obesity, pregnancy, aging, oral contraceptive use, previous DVT, pneumoperitoneum, laparoscopy, cancer, CHF

Name the clinical entities associated with hypercoagulability.

Malignancy, oral contraceptive use, recent trauma, sepsis, recent major surgery, vasculitides, congestive heart failure, polycythemia vera

What are the symptoms?

Classic features include calf swelling and tenderness, positive Homan sign, and low grade fever (37.5–38.5 degrees centigrade). **Keep in mind that only 50% of patients with DVT by venography have any clinical signs.**

What is *phlegmasia alba dolens*?

"White pain," characterized by pain, profound pitting edema, and blanching of the leg; these symptoms are indicative of a large clot in the deep veins of the pelvis or thigh (which may also impede arterial inflow)

Define *phlegmasia cerulea dolens*?

Painful, edematous leg with loss of sensory and motor function, indicative of cessation of arterial flow caused by profound venous congestion; gangrene will set in quickly if flow is not reestablished

How is DVT best diagnosed?

Venography is the **gold standard,** but is both expensive and invasive. Doppler sonography, though operator dependent, has been shown to have 90% sensitivity and specificity at detecting large clots.

What is the appropriate initial treatment?

1. Bed rest with the foot of the bed elevated slightly
2. 10,000 U bolus IV heparin, followed by continuous infusion at 10 U/kg/hr, titrated to PTT at twice the normal level for 7 to 10 days
3. Warfarin for 3 months

What is the appropriate prophylaxis?

1. Pneumatic compression stocking (sequential compression device [SCD])
2. Subcutaneous heparin 5,000 U twice daily (must be given preoperatively if it is the sole prophylaxis)
3. Early postoperative ambulation

FAT EMBOLISM

In which settings are fat embolisms more likely to occur?

After long bone fractures, total joint replacements, closed CPR, burns, and liposuction

What are the symptoms?

Dyspnea; tachypnea **petechial rash** over the neck, axillae, skin folds (60% of patients); and mental status changes exacerbated by progressive hypoxemia, fever, and tachycardia

What are the components of Bergman triad?

1. Dyspnea
2. Confusion
3. Petechial hemorrhages

When does fat embolism usually occur in relation to the injury or procedure?

48 to 72 hours later

What are the associated x-ray findings?

Bilateral fluffy infiltrates identical to ARDS

Acutely, what is the appropriate treatment?

1. 100% oxygen facemask
2. Intubation if PaO_2 levels are less than 60 mmHg
3. PEEP
4. Reduce any long bone fracture

PULSELESS EXTREMITY

What are the symptoms of lost blood supply to an extremity?

As with compartment syndrome, pain, pallor, paresthesias, pulselessness, paralysis, and pain on passive extension

Aside from compartment syndrome, what are the two etiologic categories to be considered when pulses are lost?

Embolus versus acute main thrombosis

Which of the two represents a greater threat to limb viability?

Acute arterial embolic occlusion is more threatening, because collateral vessels have had no chance to form.

What findings are suggestive of an embolus?

1. Arrhythmias (three-fourths of emboli are associated with atrial fibrillation)
2. Myocardial infarction (beware of "silent" infarcts; it may be ideal to rule out MI in all patients who are not experiencing atrial fibrillation)
3. Valve disease
4. Normal pulses in contralateral limb
5. Absence of other predisposing factors (peripheral vascular disease, atherosclerosis)

What findings are suggestive of thrombosis?	1. History of peripheral vascular disease or claudication 2. Diminished pulses proximally or in the other limb 3. Predisposing factors (peripheral vascular disease, atherosclerosis)
What immediate steps should be taken?	1. Initiate anticoagulation with IV heparin bolus of 10,000 U, followed by continuous infusion at a rate of 1000 to 2000 U/hr. This treatment is crucial in preventing proximal and distal thrombus propagation. 2. Preoperative orders: CBC Serum electrolytes BUN and creatinine Coagulation parameters Type and cross 2 U of packed RBCs chest film 3. If the level of the embolus is obvious, there may be no need for arteriogram and the patient may be able to go directly to surgery; otherwise, arteriogram is necessary.
What additional action should be taken if the patient is known to have prosthetic material in the limb?	Administration of IV antibiotics, because infected grafts have an increased risk of thrombosis
After pulses have been restored, what levels should be closely monitored?	Pulses, to monitor for reocclusion; potassium and urine myoglobin, in case of reperfusion syndrome; and compartment pressures, for compartment syndrome

COMPARTMENT SYNDROME

What is it?	A condition in which circulation and function of tissues in a closed space are compromised because of increased pressure in that space

What are the common precipitants?	Tight, compressive cast or dressings; crushing injuries; burns; supracondylar humerus fractures; status posttibial nailing; vascular injury; and electrical injury
What are the symptoms?	The five Ps: Pain upon passive stretching, pulselessness, pallor, paresthesias, and paralysis
Which of these symptoms are early findings?	Pain and paraesthesias
Irreversible ischemia and tissue death tend to occur after what duration of vascular compromise?	After approximately 6 hours
When does myoglobinuria reach its peak?	Approximately 3 hours after perfusion has been restored
What is the appropriate treatment for myoglobinuria?	1. Maintain a brisk urine output, using mannitol if necessary 2. Administer sodium bicarbonate to alkalinize the urine, which may decrease the likelihood of precipitation
How is compartment syndrome treated?	First, remove any compressive dressings (an 85% decrease in intracompartmental pressure is possible from removal of a cast alone). If symptoms persist, immediate fasciotomy of the involved compartment is indicated.
What is the most common cause of orthopedic malpractice cases?	Missed compartment syndrome

ACUTE RENAL FAILURE

PRERENAL

What are the symptoms?	Tachycardia, hypotension, poor skin turgor, dry mucous membranes, abdominal distention, and fever

What are the differential diagnoses?	Hemorrhage, inadequate fluids, sepsis, third space losses, congestive heart failure, neoplastic syndrome, and renal artery occlusion
What laboratory findings are suggestive of prerenal failure?	Bun/Cr greater than 20:1 Urinary Na less than 20 mmol/day FENa less than 1
What is the initial treatment for prerenal failure?	Treat the underlying conditions and administer bolus fluids

POSTRENAL

What is the initial step in evaluating suspected postrenal failure?	1. Placement of a Foley catheter, or irrigation of an existing catheter with 50 ml normal saline 2. Ultrasound to check for renal calyx dilatation
What are the differential diagnoses?	Prostatic hypertrophy, ureter obstruction (calculi, tumor, blood clot, trauma), prolonged effect of anesthesia (spinal or epidural)
What are the associated physical examination findings?	Blood at urethral meatus, prostatic enlargement on rectal exam, suprapubic tenderness to percussion, bladder enlargement

INTRINSIC RENAL

When evaluating the oliguric patient, what is the best way of confirming that the problem lies within the kidneys?	By exclusion, because prerenal and postrenal pathology can usually quickly be ruled out based on physical findings and the previously mentioned labs.
Although the list can be extensive, name the most common differential diagnoses.	1. **ATN** from shock, sepsis, or myoglobinuria (most common cause in postoperative patients) 2. Acute interstitial nephrosis from penicillins, NSAIDs, hypercalcemia

What is the appropriate initial management?	1. Monitor volume status closely (central venous pressures are helpful) 2. Limit or remove supplemental potassium 3. Try to increase urine output with titrating doses of furosemide or bumetanide drip 4. Administer mannitol or low-dose dopamine 5. Discontinue any potentially nephrotoxic drugs
What are the most common surgical nephrotoxic drugs?	Gentamicin, amphotericin B

HYPOTENSION AND SHOCK

Name the four etiologic categories of shock.	1. Hemorrhagic 2. Cardiogenic 3. Neurogenic 4. Septic
Which ward patients are more prone to hypovolemic shock?	1. Post-trauma patients 2. Postoperative patients bleeding internally or through drains 3. Patients who received inadequate intraoperative fluids 4. Patients with GI bleeds or ulcers 5. Patients with ongoing fluid losses through burns or third-space losses
What physical findings are associated with hypovolemic shock (early and late)?	**Early:** Anxiety, tachycardia, decreased urine output, narrowed pulse pressure, cool skin, decreased capillary refill **Late:** Profound anxiety, confusion, or altered consciousness; pulse rate greater than 120 BPM, decreased blood pressure; cold, ashen skin; severely diminished urine output; tachypnea; and decreased capillary refill
Can a patient be hypertensive and hypovolemic?	Yes, secondary to increased sympathetic tone

In hemorrhagic shock, what happens to pulse pressure as volume losses continue?

Pulse pressure initially narrows as increased sympathetic tone **increases** the **diastolic pressure.** Systolic pressure eventually decreases as compensatory mechanisms are overwhelmed.

Under what circumstances can a patient can be in hypovolemic shock with normal or decreased heart rate?

1. Neurogenic shock
2. β-Blocker therapy

What is the initial treatment for acute hemorrhagic shock?

Blood and balanced salt solution (such as lactated Ringer's) along with treatment of underlying cause

What percentage of isotonic crystalloid will be intravascular 2 hours after infusion in a postoperative patient?

20% to 30%

Are colloid solutions routinely as effective as crystalloid?

No. Colloid has shown no resuscitative benefit over crystalloid in patient outcome, it is merely more expensive and does not allow replenishment of extracellular volume as effectively as crystalloid.

What is the best bedside parameter in assessing tissue perfusion?

Urinary output

What physical examination findings are suggestive of cardiogenic shock?

Jugular venous distention, pulmonary rales, muffled heart sounds, new murmurs, and friction rub

What is the appropriate treatment for cardiogenic shock?

Alleviate any obvious mechanical causes of pump failure (e.g., tension pneumothorax, tamponade); otherwise, cardiac output must be maximized.
Treat any identified arrhythmias.
Begin careful crystalloid volume infusion (Swan-Ganz monitoring is helpful in avoiding volume overload).
Inotropic agents, such as dobutamine, may be required to augment cardiac output.
Begin afterload reduction.

Name the guiding principles in the treatment of septic shock.

1. Begin with volume resuscitation using crystalloid.
2. Because of various cardiac, pulmonary, and circulatory derangements associated with sepsis, placement of arterial and pulmonary artery catheters may be helpful.
3. Dopamine may be helpful if fluids fail to restore perfusion pressure.
4. Search meticulously for underlying causes and treat accordingly.

What are the hemodynamic parameters associated with neurogenic shock.

Hypotension or decreased perfusion with normocardia or bradycardia

What is the most likely cause of hypotension in a patient with an isolated closed head injury?

Never assume that it is caused by the head injury. Always search for another source.

BLEEDING

What is the appropriate initial management of an acute drop in hematocrit?

1. Assess hemodynamic status
2. Resuscitate/stabilize
3. Type and crossmatch, transfuse as necessary
4. Search for potential sources of blood loss, especially ongoing losses that may necessitate operative intervention.

UPPER GI BLEEDING

What are the symptoms?

1. Hematemesis (blood or coffee grounds), usually specific for upper gastrointestinal (UGI) bleed
2. Melena or hematochezia, if bleeding is brisk
3. Hemodynamic instability

What are the most common etiologies?

1. Peptic ulcer disease
2. Esophagitis
3. Gastritis
4. Varices
5. Mallory-Weiss tear
6. Vascular anomalies
7. Aortoenteric fistula
8. Neoplasms

What diagnostic tests are indicated?	Endoscopy is sensitive and specific, but bleeding may be too brisk for adequate visualization. In such cases, labeled RBC scans and arteriography are the procedures of choice.

LOWER GI BLEEDING

What are the symptoms?	1. Usually hematochezia, however, a slow bleed from a proximal lower GI site may present as melena 2. Hemodynamic instability
What are the most common etiologies?	1. Diverticulosis 2. Vascular anomalies 3. Ischemic bowel 4. Inflammatory bowel disease 5. Neoplasms 6. Meckel diverticulum 7. Aortoenteric fistula 8. Hemorrhoids
What diagnostic tests are indicated?	1. NGT to rule out an upper gastrointestinal source 2. Anoscopy or proctosigmoidoscopy may demonstrate rectosigmoid sources 3. Colonoscopy 4. Labeled RBC scan 5. Arteriography

THROMBOCYTOPENIA

What number of platelets is necessary for hemostasis?	60,000 platelets/mm^3
What is the most reliable test of platelet function?	Template bleeding time
What are the differential diagnoses?	1. Massive transfusion 2. Heparin induced 3. Idiopathic thrombocytopenic purpura (ITP), thrombotic thrombocytopenic purpura (TTP), or SLE 4. Splenic sequestration, as in sarcoidosis, Gaucher disease, lymphoma, or portal hypertension 5. Leukemia 6. Uremia

What is the incidence of heparin-induced thrombocytopenia?	0.6%
Through what mechanism does it act?	It is immune mediated
When do the low counts occur?	4 to 15 days after initiation of therapy in those receiving heparin for the first time
What are the indications for platelet transfusion in nondestructive thrombocytopenia?	1. Platelets less than 20,000/μl in nonbleeding patients 2. Platelets less than 50,000/μl in preoperative patients 3. Platelets less than 50,000/μl in bleeding patients
What is a platelet pack?	The platelets from 1 U blood
How much should one pack raise the platelet count?	6,000/μl
What is the volume of a platelet pack?	50 ml

TRANSFUSION REACTIONS

What are the symptoms of hemolytic transfusion reaction?	Pain at infusion site, fever, chills, nausea, hypotension, abnormal bleeding, lumbar pain, constricting chest pain, eventual progression to shock and ARF
What conditions might occur in anesthetized or comatose patients?	Abnormal bleeding and persistent hypotension
What is the most common cause of hemolytic transfusion reaction?	Clerical error, resulting in the patient receiving mismatched blood
What is the appropriate initial treatment?	1. Immediately stop the transfusion. 2. Send the remaining blood and a sample of the patient's blood to the lab for crossmatching. 3. Send a urinalysis for hemoglobin. 4. Force diuresis with 20 gm mannitol or 40 mg furosemide with 2 L Ringer's lactate and 50 meq sodium bicarbonate to alkalinize the urine.

What are the symptoms of allergic transfusion reaction?	Urticaria, itching, bronchospasm, and anaphylaxis
What is the usual treatment for allergic reactions?	Antihistamines, epinephrine

ENDOCRINE EMERGENCIES

DIABETIC KETOACIDOSIS

Who is at risk?	Type I patients, following cessation of insulin therapy or stress that renders an insulin dose inadequate
What are the possible precipitants?	Traumatic injury, infection, MI, surgery
What is the pathogenesis?	The ratios of **glucagon,** GH, catecholamines, and cortisol to insulin increase, causing unrestrained glycogenolysis, gluconeogenesis, and ketogenesis.
What are the symptoms?	Vomiting, polyuria, thirst, weakness, altered mental status, abdominal pain, orthostasis, and hyperventilation
What diagnostic laboratory results are found?	1. Hyperglycemia 2. Ketoacidosis 3. Pseudohyponatremia 4. Elevated serum potassium 5. Urine ketones
What is the appropriate treatment?	1. Administration of insulin and glucose to maintain serum glucose levels between 200 and 300 mg/dl 2. Administration of isotonic saline until hypovolemia is corrected, then one-half NS 3. Administration of potassium in fluids when levels are less than 4.5 meq/l 4. Administration of phosphorus, as needed 5. Administration of bicarbonate when diabetic ketoacidosis (DKA) is accompanied by shock, when pH is less than 7.1, or with the presence of severe hyperkalemia

| **What are the possible complications?** | 1. Shock caused by hypovolemia or acidosis
2. Vascular thrombosis
3. Cerebral edema
4. Hypokalemia
5. Hypophosphatemia |

THYROID STORM

What are the precipitants?	Surgery, infection, or trauma in an already thyrotoxic patient
What are the symptoms?	High fever, tachycardia, and altered mental status
What is the appropriate treatment?	1. Supportive therapy (O_2 fluids, fever reduction) 2. Propranolol 3. PTU, iodide 4. Hydrocortisone
What is the mortality rate?	10% to 20%

PHEOCHROMOCYTOMA

| **What are the symptoms?** | 1. Episodic hypertension
2. Palpitations
3. Headache
4. Diaphoresis |
| **What is the appropriate emergent treatment?** | 1. Phentolamine/fluids
2. Propranolol |

SEIZURES

| **Define status epilepticus.** | Continuous seizure activity beyond 30 minutes, or at least two sequential seizures without full recovery of consciousness |
| **What actions should be taken when a patient experiences a seizure?** | Use the ABCs of life support:
1. Administer oxygen by nasal cannula or mask
2. Position head for optimal airway patency, intubate if necessary
3. Monitor ECG
4. Establish IV access and order appropriate laboratory tests
5. NGT to decompress the stomach and decrease the chance of massive aspiration |

What laboratory tests should be ordered immediately?

Electrolytes, antiepileptic drug levels (if applicable), ABG, hemogram, urinalysis, **low bicarbonate associated with seizures** secondary to local areas of anaerobic metabolism

How is suspected hypoglycemia best treated?

By administration of 100 mg of IV thiamine, followed by 50 ml of 50% glucose IV push

In what situations and at what dosages should benzodiazepines be given?

Diazepam 0.2 mg/kg at 5 mg/min
Lorazepam 0.1 mg/kg at 2 mg/min
Repeat at 5 minutes if the patient is still having a seizure

What medications should follow benzodiazepines?

Phenytoin at 50 mg/min to a maximum of 30 mg/kg. If the patient is still having a seizure, general anesthesia should be considered.

What is the potential danger of phenytoin administration in patients with known cardiac conduction problems?

It can cause arrhythmias.

When an IV line cannot be established, how should medications be given?

Per rectum

Name the five most common precipitants of status epilepticus in adults.

1. Cerebrovascular phenomena
2. Medication changes
3. Anoxia
4. Alcohol or drugs
5. Metabolic/electrolyte imbalances

Name the five most common causes in children.

1. Fever/infection
2. Medication changes
3. Idiopathic origin
4. Metabolic origin
5. Congenital origin

Who should be placed on chronic antiepileptic therapy?

Patients whose seizures are caused by structural brain lesions or patients with known epilepsy

HYPERTENSION

Name four common causes of postoperative hypertension (HTN).	1. **Pain** 2. Hypoxia 3. Fluid overload 4. Preoperative HTN
Define malignant hypertension.	Sustained diastolic blood pressure greater than 130 mmHg
Name some of the symptoms and findings in a patient experiencing a hypertensive crisis.	Headache, nausea, vomiting, visual changes, papilledema, loss of consciousness, and convulsions
What is the best agent for lowering blood pressure in a patient experiencing a hypertensive crisis?	Sodium nitroprusside or labetalol
Name some situations in which blood pressure should be tightly regulated.	Patients with a history of coronary artery disease, cerebral bleeds, or possible dissecting aortic aneurysm, or patients who have undergone vascular repairs

DIGOXIN TOXICITY

What are the symptoms?	1. Fatigue, visual disturbances, anorexia 2. Bradyarrhythmias (second- or third-degree AV block) 3. Tachyarrhythmias (VT or ventricular fibrillation [VF]) 4. Hypokalemia
What is the frequency?	2% to 5% of the hospitalized patients on digoxin
What is the emergent treatment for life-threatening toxicity?	Digoxin-specific antibody fragments

ANAPHYLAXIS

What is it?	An acute allergic response mediated by IgE-stimulating release histamine, leukotrienes, kinins, and prostaglandins from mast cells and basophils

What are the precipitants?	1. Drugs 2. Transfusions 3. Contrast agents 4. Insect stings 5. Foods
What are the symptoms?	Pruritus, urticaria, angioedema, laryngeal edema, laryngeal spasm, bronchospasm, and vascular collapse
What is the appropriate treatment?	1. Airway control 2. Epinephrine 0.5 mg (5 ml of 1:10,000 solution) IV, repeat as needed 3. Oxygen 4. Fluids to maintain blood pressure 5. Steroids for prolonged reactions 6. Diphenhydramine

NARCOTIC OVERDOSE

What are the symptoms?	CNS depression, respiratory depression, hypotension, miosis
What is the appropriate treatment?	Naloxone hydrochloride
At what dose?	0.4 to 0.8 mg IV, repeated as needed

BENZODIAZEPINE OVERDOSE

What are the symptoms?	**Respiratory depression,** incoordination, ataxia, confusion, blurred vision, and stupor
What is the appropriate treatment?	Flumazenil
At what dose?	0.2 mg IV, repeated as needed

ALCOHOL WITHDRAWAL

What are the symptoms after 6 to 8 hours?	Tremulousness and irritability
At 8 to 12 hours?	Hallucinosis (usually auditory)
At 12 to 24 hours?	Generalized withdrawal seizures

At 3 to 4 days?	Delirium tremens: confusion, delusions, hallucinations, tremor, agitation, autonomic overactivity (dilated pupils, fever, tachycardia, diaphoresis)
How is it treated?	1. Supportive therapy: fluids, thiamine, folate 2. Chlordiazepoxide (titrate to desired effect and taper)

DELIRIUM

Describe delirium.	A patient is disoriented to person, place, or time with fluctuating levels of consciousness. Hallucinations, which are usually visual, may also occur.
What is the usual perioperative timing of onset?	Onset occurs at approximately three days postoperative, although it can obviously occur at anytime, depending on the patient and the circumstances.
What is the treatment approach?	1. Check electrolytes, CBC, urinalysis, and O_2 saturation to that assure mental status changes are not caused by a simple organic cause. 2. If the patient is not frankly psychotic or agitated, reassurance may be all that is needed. 3. If restlessness continues, sedate the patient with haloperidol 2 to 5 mg IM every 4 to 6 hours as required, IV
When is a CT scan indicated?	If the condition persists with no identifiable systemic cause or with focal findings of any type

EPISTAXIS

What is the most common site of epistaxis?	In the inferior portion of the nasal septum in Kiesselbach triangle (90% of bleeds occur here)
Define Kiesselbach triangle?	A plexus of vessels in the anteroinferior part of the septum

What is the appropriate treatment of bleeds at this site?

Simple pressure and a topical vasoconstrictor

What is the appropriate treatment for a patient bleeding from the posterior nasal cavity?

1. Patients can swallow a great deal of blood while bleeding from this site; begin by assessing their overall volume status and assuring that they are not in shock.
2. The bleed can be obstructed with an inflated Foley balloon or with a nasal pack constructed with gauze and 2-0 silk that is pulled retrograde through the mouth up into the posterior nasopharynx, and removed 4 days later. Give prophylactic antibiotics to prevent sinusitis and otitis media from developing (consult ENT).

What is the usual relationship between hypertension and epistaxis?

When they occur together, hypertension is often the result of patient anxiety. Rarely is it the cause of the bleed, but an ongoing bleed may persist until pressure is lowered.

12

Fluids and Electrolytes

Jeffry Watson, MD
Joseph Wells, MD

ELECTROLYTE DISTURBANCES

HYPONATREMIA

When is aggressive treatment indicated?	Acute symptomatic hyponatremia when Na is less than 120 meq/l and plasma osmolality is low
What are the symptoms?	Nausea, malaise, lethargy, seizures, mental status changes, and coma
What causes these symptoms?	Cerebral edema
What groups of patients are at greatest risk?	1. Women with postoperative hyponatremia 2. Patients with psychogenic polydipsia 3. Elderly women on thiazide or loop diuretics 4. Postoperative patients who have been over-resuscitated
What is the appropriate emergent treatment?	Furosemide in conjunction with normal saline (NS) or, rarely, hypertonic saline to increase serum Na 10 to 12 meq; thereafter, fluid restriction
What risk is associated with treatment?	If treatment is too rapid, central pontine myelinolysis (CPM) or osmotic cerebral demyelinating syndrome may result.
Which patients are at greatest risk of CPM?	1. Patients with preexisting alcoholism or malnutrition 2. Patients with a rate of correction greater than 2.5 meq/l/hr or greater than 20 meq/l/day

What is the most common cause of mild postoperative hyponatremia?	Fluid overload

HYPERNATREMIA

What symptoms are present when Na is greater than 160 meq/l?	Irritability, ataxia, anorexia, and cramping
What symptoms are present when Na is greater than 180 meq/l?	Confusion, stupor, seizure, and coma
What is the appropriate treatment?	1. Correction of volume deficit, if present 2. Replacement of water deficit with D5W 3. Treatment of underlying cause
What is the rate of correction?	One-half of the water deficit in the first 24 hours, with a rate of sodium decrease not greater than 1 meq/l/hour; correction of the remaining water deficit should occur over next 1 to 2 days
What is the risk of overly rapid correction?	Cerebral edema and resultant neurologic dysfunction (lethargy, seizures)

HYPOKALEMIA

What is the normal daily potassium requirement?	40 to 60 meq/day
Why is the serum potassium level important in patients taking digoxin?	Because digoxin and potassium compete for the same receptors, making these patients vulnerable to sequelae of digoxin toxicity when serum potassium levels are low
What are the most common causes of low potassium in the surgical patient?	Vomiting, diarrhea, nasogastric suction, loop diuretics, and deficient oral intake

What acid—base disturbance causes decreased serum potassium levels?

Alkalosis. As hydrogen ions leave the cells to lower extracellular pH, potassium ions enter the cells, thereby lowering the extracellular potassium. Remember that bicarbonate is a treatment for hyperkalemia.

What symptoms are associated with hypokalemia?

Ileus, weakness, nausea, vomiting

What EKG changes occur with hypokalemia?

1. U-waves greater than 1 mm in height and larger than the T-waves
2. S-T depression
3. T-wave flattening and inversion

What other electrolyte imbalances often occur with hypokalemia?

Hypocalcemia, hypomagnesemia

How is potassium replaced emergently?

Suggested maximum infusion rate is 20 meq/hour via CVL, and 10 meq/hour peripherally

HYPERKALEMIA

What situations call for emergent reduction of serum potassium levels?

Patients with serum potassium greater than 7 mmol/L or EKG changes

What is the most serious complication of hyperkalemia?

Life-threatening arrhythmia

What EKG changes are associated with the disorder?

1. Peaked T-waves
2. Flat P-waves
3. Increased P-R interval
4. Widened QRS interval with eventual progression to sine wave pattern

In addition to vital signs, which bedside parameter should immediately be checked?

Urine output, because renal failure results in rapidly increasing potassium levels

What is pseudohyperkalemia?	Artificially elevated potassium levels caused by hemolysis or by a tourniquet left in place too long on the arm before collection of a blood sample

How is potassium emergently reduced?

1. Hypertonic glucose infusion and insulin administration (causes potassium to merely shift from extracellular space into cells)
2. Administration of kayexalate resin 20 g four times daily to induce passage of loose stools, orally or by enema
3. In renal failure, hemodialysis may be required
4. Administration of bicarbonate to alkalinize
5. Calcium, administered in cardioprotective IV form
6. Furosemide (wastes K^+)

HYPOCALCEMIA

What is the most dangerous consequence of severe hypocalcemia?

Laryngeal spasm may occur at very low levels.

What are the symptoms?

Peripheral paresthesias, Chvostek sign, Trousseau sign, tetany, seizures, and mental status changes

Give the formula for corrected total calcium level.

0.8 (Normal albumin – observed albumin) + observed calcium

What is the most accurate measure of calcium?

Ionized calcium

How is severe hypocalcemia treated?

With administration of 200 mg elemental calcium, as either calcium gluconate or calcium chloride

What is the most dreaded complication of peripheral IV infusion of calcium?

Infiltration causes skin necrosis (CaCl is worse than Ca-gluconate)

HYPERCALCEMIA

What levels of serum calcium warrant emergent therapy?	13 to 15 mmol/L, or any patient with symptoms
What are the symptoms?	Nausea, vomiting, mental status changes, delirium, polyuria, polydipsia, and constipation
What is the appropriate treatment for severe (symptomatic) hypercalcemia?	Increase IV fluids to maintain a urine output of 80 to 100 cc/hour. Furosemide may be given to maintain vigorous diuresis, taking care to replete potassium and magnesium.

MISCELLANEOUS

Which IV fluid may precipitate a panic attack in patients who suffer from this condition?	Lactated Ringer's
Which colloid can lower serum calcium and free ionized calcium levels?	Albumin
Is hetastarch an anticoagulant?	At infusions greater than 1500 cc, this colloid solution has been shown to dilute clotting factors, as well as inhibiting factor VIII moieties.
What is the best colloid solution?	Blood
In postoperative patients, how much of 1 L isotonic IV fluid (normal saline or lactated Ringer's) remains intravascularly after several hours?	Only approximately 200 to 300 cc! (Thus, the "three for one rule" of the ATLS manual)
In the postoperative patient, how much of 1 L albumin will remain intravascularly after 2 hours?	Approximately 500 cc

Which electrolytes are most important to the cardiac system?

Calcium, potassium, and magnesium (potassium and magnesium are particularly important in reducing arrhythmias in patients receiving digoxin)

What is the formula for mEq of bicarbonate infusion in metabolic acidosis?

$$\frac{1/3 \times \text{wt/kg} \times \text{base deficit}}{2}$$

13

Deep Venous Thrombosis and Pulmonary Embolus

Lorne H. Blackbourne, MD

What is DVT?

Thrombosis of the deep veins of the leg (**d**eep **v**enous **t**hrombosis)

What is the classic syndrome of DVT?

1. Homan sign
2. Edema
3. Calf pain
4. Venous distention

What percentage of patients with DVT have the classic syndrome of DVT?

Only approximately 33%

What is Homan sign?

Pain on manual dorsiflexion of the foot

What are the differential diagnoses of DVT?

1. Baker cyst
2. Muscle/bone problems
3. Impaired lymphatic or venous flow without thrombosis

What is a Baker cyst?

An inflamed popliteal cyst

What invasive test confirms diagnosis of DVT?

Contrast phlebography

What noninvasive procedures test for DVT?

1. Real-time ultrasound
2. Impedance plethysmography
3. CT, especially pelvic thrombi

What is the most sensitive test of real-time ultrasound?

Failure of the vein to be compressed, thus revealing an intramural thrombus

What is the incidence of DVT in general surgery patients with no prophylaxis for DVT?

Approximately 25%!

What are the risk factors for DVT?

Advanced age; vein trauma; surgery, especially major procedures and orthopedic procedures; bed rest; pregnancy; previous history of DVT; malignancy; hypercoagulable states; oral contraceptive use; CHF; obesity; MI; stroke; bone fracture; varicose veins; male sex; nephrotic syndrome; lupus anticoagulant; dysfibrinogenemia; long operations (>2 hours); laparoscopy with pneumoperitoneum

Why is total hip replacement risky for DVT?

1. Trauma to veins
2. Bed rest
3. Heat from cement

What preventive measures are effective against DVT?

Sub-Q heparin, warfarin, calf/thigh compression devices

When should sub-Q heparin be started?

Preoperatively

What is the main relative contraindication of compression devices?

Arterial insufficiency of the lower extremity

What invasive mechanical measure can protect a patient from pulmonary embolism (PE)?

Intracaval Kimray-Greenfield filter

What are the indications for a cava filter?

The issue is controversial, but generally, recurrent PE, failure of conservative measures, multitrauma, brain bleed, and cor pulmonale from multiple PE

What is the source of PE with a functioning filter in place?

Via the ovarian vein, upper extremities, right heart, or small clots through the filter

What is the standard treatment for DVT?

1. 5 to 7 days of IV heparin infusion
2. Warfarin for 3 months

What is the goal of warfarin therapy in terms of INR?

Achieving an INR of 2 to 3

What is the role of surgical venous thrombectomy?

It should be reserved for patients with acute iliac/femoral venous occlusion resulting in hindered arterial supply to the leg, causing the leg to be threatened (phlegmasia alba dolens or phlegmasia cerulea dolens).

What is the major risk of sub-Q heparin in the postoperative patient?

Wound hematoma

What is the risk of heparin-induced thrombocytopenia with sub-Q heparin?

Almost none

What is the site of DVT thrombus nidus?

The valve sinus of the vein

What kind of filter should be used in patients with large IVCs?

A bird's nest filter is often used for the "megacava."

What are the most common signs of PE?

Tachypnea and dyspnea

What are the most common EKG findings associated with PE?

Nonspecific S-T segment changes or T-wave changes

What lab test is sensitive, but not specific, for a PE?

Elevated D-dimer

What is the gold standard diagnostic test for PE?

Pulmonary angiogram

When is a V-Q scan helpful in the diagnosis of PE?

"High probability" scans **and** high clinical suspicion are accurate.

What is the standard treatment for mild PE?

IV heparin for 5 to 7 days, followed by long-term warfarin therapy

What are the options for more severe PE?	1. Standard heparin therapy 2. Thrombolytic treatment (urokinase) 3. Catheter pulmonary embolectomy using cup suction
What are the options for severe hypotensive PE?	1. Operative embolectomy 2. Partial cardiopulmonary bypass followed by operative embolectomy
What is the mortality rate for patients with operative embolectomy?	At least 40%

14

Surgical Nutrition

Kate Willcutts, MS, RD, CNSD
Carol Bognar, RN, MSN, CNSN

ASSESSMENT

What is an easy way to do a nutritional assessment?

Subjective Global Assessment (SGA)

What is the SGA?

A method of assessing nutritional status based on clinical criteria

What clinical criteria are used in the SGA?

1. Weight loss in the previous 6 months
2. Recent dietary intake compared with usual intake
3. Presence of anorexia, nausea, vomiting, or diarrhea that persisted more than 2 weeks
4. Functional capacity or energy level
5. Metabolic demands of underlying disease
6. Physical exam: loss of subcutaneous fat, muscle wasting, ankle edema, sacral edema, ascites

Which criteria are the most important?

Weight loss, poor dietary intake, loss of subcutaneous fat, and muscle wasting

How much weight loss is considered significant?

10% unintentional weight loss in 6 months, 7% unintentional weight loss in 3 months, 5% unintentional weight loss in 1 month

How is ideal body weight (IBW) calculated?

Men: 106 lbs for 5'0" plus 6 lbs for each inch over 5'0"
Women: 100 lbs for 5'0" plus 5 lbs for each inch over 5'0" (± 10% depending on frame size)

What laboratory values are used for assessing nutritional status?

Serum proteins, which may reflect visceral protein stores (albumin, prealbumin, transferrin)

Why are laboratory values often poor indicators of nutritional status?

Many factors other than nutrition can effect serum protein levels

What conditions or treatments can increase serum albumin?

Dehydration, marasmus, blood transfusions, IV albumin

What conditions or treatments can decrease serum albumin?

Overhydration, ascites, hepatic failure, inflammation, infection, stress, burns, cancer, trauma, postoperative state, bedrest, corticosteroid use, kwashiorkor

What is the half-life of albumin?

Approximately 3 weeks

Is albumin a good indicator of the adequacy of nutrition support?

No

When is albumin potentially a good indicator of nutritional status?

On admission or on an outpatient basis in patients who are not dehydrated or marasmic

What conditions or treatments can increase serum prealbumin?

Renal failure, corticosteroid use

What conditions can decrease serum prealbumin?

Acute catabolic state, postsurgical (5 days), liver disease, infection, stress, inflammation

What is the half-life of prealbumin?

Approximately 2 days

What conditions increase transferrin?

Iron deficiency, dehydration, hepatitis, chronic blood loss, chronic renal failure

What conditions decrease transferrin?

Pernicious anemia, overhydration, iron overload, chronic infection, acute catabolic state

What is the half-life of transferrin?	8 to 10 days
Are single measurements sufficient or are serial measurements more accurate?	Serial measurements better reflect nutritional adequacy.
Which factor is more important in assessing nutritional status on admission: percent of IBW, percent of weight loss, or level of serum albumin?	Percent of weight loss
Which patients need nutrition support and when should it be started?	1. Malnourished patients need it as soon as possible 2. Well-nourished patients in hypermetabolic states who are not expected to take adequate oral nutrition for at least 5 days; nutrition should be started immediately 3. Previously well-nourished patients who have been without nutrition 5 to 7 days and are not expected to take adequate oral nutrition; nutrition should be started as early as possible
How many calories should be given to most patients?	25 to 35 kcals/kg/day
What are the average caloric needs of paraplegics?	25 kcals/kg/day
What are the average caloric needs of quadriplegics?	23 kcals/kg/day
What is the Harris-Benedict equation?	An equation for calculating basal energy expenditure (BEE) in kcals/day
What is the Harris-Benedict equation for men?	$66 + (13.7 \times \text{wt/kg}) + (5 \times \text{ht/cm}) - (6.8 \times \text{age})$

What is the Harris-Benedict equation for women?	655 + (9.6 × wt/kg) + (1.7 × ht/cm)—(4.7 × age)
What body weight should be used in the equations for underweight patients?	Actual weight
What body weight should be used for overweight patients?	An adjusted weight if the patient is more than 120% of IBW (if the extra weight is not muscle)
Why is an adjusted weight used?	Fat is not as metabolically active as muscle.
How is adjusted body weight calculated?	[(Actual weight—IBW) × 0.25] + IBW
What are the stress factors?	Factors to multiply times the BEE to account for different degrees of stress Low stress × 1.2 Moderate stress × 1.2–1.3 Severe stress × 1.3–1.5 Burns up to × 2.0 (depends on surface area burned)
What are some conditions that increase metabolic rate?	Fever and sepsis; activity; burn; head injury; trauma; surgery; and overfeeding
What are some conditions that decrease metabolic rate?	Sedation, paralyzation, β-blockers, sleep, and underfeeding or starvation
What is indirect calorimetry?	By measuring oxygen consumed and carbon dioxide produced, an indirect calorimeter (or metabolic cart) extrapolates 24-hour resting energy expenditure and measures respiratory quotient.
What are some conditions that warrant indirect calorimetry?	Failure to wean from vent; severe sepsis; multitrauma; morbid obesity; burns and/or large nonhealing wounds; and paralysis

How are actual energy needs calculated using the REE from the metabolic cart study?

Multiply REE × 100% to 120% to account for energy expended during daily activities.

What is respiratory quotient (RQ)?

$RQ = VCO_2/VO_2$

What does an RQ of less than 0.7 indicate?

Starvation or underfeeding (ketosis)

What does an RQ of 0.7 indicate?

The majority of substrate oxidized is fat

What does an RQ of 0.8 to 0.85 indicate?

A balanced mixture of substrates are oxidized

What does an RQ of 1.0 indicate?

The majority of substrate oxidized is carbohydrate

What does an RQ of greater than 1.0 indicate?

Lipogenesis or overfeeding

What are the adverse effects of overfeeding?

Increased CO_2 production, increased lipogenesis and fatty liver, slower recovery, impaired immune response

What is refeeding syndrome?

Intracellular movement of potassium, magnesium, and phosphorus, as well as sodium and fluid retention associated with administration of glucose in poorly nourished patients. Refeeding syndrome is potentially fatal.

Who is at risk for refeeding syndrome?

Patients with chronic alcoholism, patients who have experienced prolonged fasting, prolonged IV hydration without nutrition, and/or chronic malnutrition

How can refeeding syndrome be prevented?

Correct serum electrolyte abnormalities prior to starting nutrition support. Feeding should be started slowly. Some sources recommend starting with 20 kcals/kg/d. Monitor electrolytes daily and replace as needed.

When does refeeding syndrome manifest?	A day or two after starting parenteral nutrition and about 5 to 7 days after starting enteral nutrition
How many calories are in a gram of protein?	4
How much protein do healthy individuals need?	0.8 to 1.0 gm/kg/d
How much protein is recommended in mild stress?	1.0 to 1.2 gm/kg/d
How much protein is recommended in moderate stress?	1.3 to 1.5 gm/kg/d
How much protein is recommended in severe stress?	1.5 to 2.5 gm/kg/d
How much protein is recommended in liver disease?	1.0 to 1.5 gm/kg/d depending on tolerance
What is the protein restriction in hepatic encephalopathy?	0.8 gm/kg/d
How much protein should be given to renal failure patients?	It depends on their degree of stress and the type of dialysis, if any.
How much protein should be given to patients on hemodialysis?	Stressed—1.0 to 1.5 gm pro/kg/d Unstressed—1.0 to 1.3 gm pro/kg/d
How much protein should be given to patients on continuous arteriovenous hemofiltration (CAVH) or continuous arteriovenous hemodialysis (CAVHD)?	1.0 to 1.5 gm pro/kg/d; greater than 1.5 gm pro/kg/d for repletion
What is nitrogen balance?	The difference between the amount of nitrogen ingested and the amount excreted.

What does a positive nitrogen balance indicate?

More protein ingested than excreted, indicating net anabolism

What does a negative nitrogen balance indicate?

More protein is excreted than ingested, indicating net catabolism

What is the nitrogen balance goal?

In critical illness, equilibrium is the goal. Positive nitrogen balance is more likely during recovery.

What is measured for a nitrogen balance?

Urine that is collected over 12 or 24 hours.

What is the equation for converting grams nitrogen to grams protein?

Protein is 16% nitrogen; nitrogen (gm) × 6.25 = protein (gm)

What is the equation for estimating the amount of protein output?

(Grams urinary nitrogen per 24 hrs + 2–4) × 6.25

How many calories are in carbohydrates?

IV dextrose = 3.4 kcal/gm
Other carbohydrates = 4 kcal/gm

How much carbohydrate do patients need?

A minimum of 100 grams/day for the brain and RBCs

What is the maximum recommended amount of carbohydrate?

Stressed patients cannot metabolize more than 5 mg carb/kg/min. More carbohydrate may be incompletely oxidized.

How many calories are in fat?

Fat = 9 kcal/gm
10% lipid = 1.1 kcal/ml
20% lipid = 2 kcal/ml

What is the minimum amount of fat required?

To prevent essential fatty acid deficiency (EFAD), at least 3% to 5% of calories as fat are needed.

How much should patients receive?

Limit to 25% to 40% of total calories

Is there danger in giving too much fat?

Yes. Theoretically, too much fat can have adverse effects on immunity and gas exchange, and can increase the risk of sepsis.

How can the adverse effects of fat be avoided?	Keep serum triglycerides less than 350 mg/dl Most complications are associated with rates greater than 0.10 gm/kg/hr Some sources recommend 30 to 60 mg/kg/hr
Should lipids be given continuously or intermittently?	Continuous lipid infusion promotes improved triglyceride clearance. Administer continuously over more than 10 hours.
What are the goals for nutrition support?	1. Meet caloric requirement without overfeeding. 2. Use appropriate route and method 3. Use appropriate substrate mixture 4. Facilitate recovery, wound healing, and tissue repair

ROUTE

Which route is better?	Enteral nutrition is more physiologic, cheaper, carries less risk of infection, and helps maintain the integrity of the gut mucosa.
What are two nutrition support mottos?	If the gut works, use it. Use it or lose it.
When is the enteral route indicated?	When nutrient needs cannot be met by mouth and the gut works
When is the parenteral route indicated?	Inability to provide sufficient nutrients enterally Short gut/severe malabsorption Intractable vomiting or diarrhea Severe pancreatitis Bowel obstruction Prolonged ileus, high output enterocutaneous fistula Lack of enteral access
When should both routes be used?	Low rates of enteral nutrition may be sufficient to prevent gut mucosa atrophy; therefore, if full nutrition cannot be delivered enterally, a combination of both routes is recommended.

ENTERAL

How early is "early" enough for the benefits of enteral nutrition?	Ideally, within the first 24 to 48 hrs after injury or surgery. Studies in burn patients show reduced hypermetabolic response, lower infection rate, improved nitrogen balance, and decreased length of hospital stay when nutrition support is started within hours of the injury. Benefits of early enteral feeding seem to be gone by 4 to 5 days after injury or surgery.

Enteral Feeding After Surgery

How long is the typical postoperative ileus?	Gastric: 24 to 48 hrs Small bowel: 12 to 24 hrs Colon: 48 to 72 hrs
Are bowel sounds or flatus necessary?	No, normal small bowel motility is possible without bowel sounds. Most critically ill patients have small bowel function despite gastric and colonic ileus.
What else should be considered prior to starting enteral nutrition?	Consider adequacy of blood flow to the GI tract. Hemodynamic stability may be required prior to starting nutrition. Consider the potential for leaking anastomoses.
Does diluting-tube feeding improve tolerance?	No, most tube feeding formulas are isotonic, therefore they do not require dilution. The hypertonic formulas are well tolerated when the initial flow rate is low. Diluting formulas may reduce absorption by making the formula hypotonic, and are therefore not recommended.
How quickly can the rate of tube feeding be advanced?	Start with 10 to 20 cc/hr. Advance as quickly as tolerated over 24 to 72 hrs.
What are signs of possible intolerance to enteral feedings?	Nausea, vomiting, abdominal distention, pain, diarrhea, high gastric residuals

What is diarrhea?

Greater than 250 grams of liquid stool/ day

Does tube feeding cause diarrhea?

Occasionally

What are the possible causes of diarrhea in tube fed patients?

Hyperosmolar medications, including sorbitol-containing elixirs, KCl, and magnesium

Stool softeners/ cathartics

Infection—viral or bacterial or bacterial toxins

Bacterial overgrowth from broad-spectrum antibiotics

Microvilli atrophy caused by a prolonged period without enteral nutrition

Switching medications from IV route to enteral route at the same time tube feeding is started

Impaction

Does a fiber-containing formula decrease diarrhea?

It depends on the type of fiber in the formula. Pectin and other soluble fibers decrease diarrhea. Insoluble or bulk fibers increase stool viscosity, but have not been shown to reduce diarrhea. Currently, most fiber-containing formulas contain mostly insoluble fiber. Some newer products contain a combination of the two types of fiber.

What level of gastric residuals is too high?

There is no clear data yet to indicate what level is safe; however, the typical textbook quoted amount of 150 cc, or twice the flow rate, is considered too low by many clinicians. To assess gastric emptying, also check abdominal distention and presence of bowel sounds.

Are gastric residuals the best way to monitor tube feeding tolerance?

No, they are just one way.

What is an elemental formula?

A formula in which all of the protein is in the form of amino acids (usually low fat)

Is an elemental formula ever needed?

Probably not. Compared with polypeptide (intact protein) formulas, elemental formulas are associated with poorer nutritional parameters, more bacterial translocation, more microvilli atrophy, poorer wound healing, and reduced survival.

What is a semi-elemental formula?

The protein consists of a combination of at least two of the following substances: amino acids, peptides, and intact protein.

When might a semi-elemental formula be needed?

When the digestive system is working well, formulas made from 100% intact protein are the best choice; however, some studies indicate that formulas with small peptides are better absorbed when the digestive system is impaired, as in pancreatic insufficiency, after prolonged periods without enteral nutrition, or in patients with short gut

What are options for tube-feeding schedules?

1. **Continuous:** Most critically ill patients should receive nutrients in a slow, controlled manner. Patients with jejunal feedings should receive continuous feedings to minimize complications.
2. **Nocturnal:** Patients transitioning to oral diet or who are able to meet some of their needs orally, may benefit from nighttime feedings.
3. **Intermittent:** This method involves delivery of a prescribed volume of formula over 30–60 minutes every 3 to 4 hours and is generally tolerated by stable patients with gastric access.
4. **Bolus:** Not generally recommended in the acute care setting, but may be tolerated by patients requiring chronic feedings into the stomach.

PARENTERAL

What effect does TPN have on liver enzymes?

AST (SGOT) and ALT (SGPT) may peak 10 to 15 days after starting TPN, then slowly decrease. Levels may rise to approximately two to three times the normal amount. Alkaline phosphatase may also rise after starting TPN. Not all patients receiving TPN have elevated liver enzymes.

Can TPN cause hepatic steatosis?

Fatty infiltration is possible, but it resolves rapidly after stopping TPN.

Can TPN cause cholestasis?

Gallbladder sludge formation is possible, probably because of a lack of enteral feeding rather than the TPN. Cholestasis resolves after enteral feeding is started.

How quickly can TPN be tapered off?

The rate should be decreased by half for 2 hours, then discontinued. Check capillary blood glucose one hour after discontinuing TPN. A slower taper may be indicated in patients requiring insulin.

What is "3-in-1"?

A mixture of amino acids, dextrose, and lipid in one bag. Also called total nutrient admixture (TNA).

Enteral Access

What is one of the largest obstacles to the provision of enteral nutrition?

Lack of enteral access

What is the most common feeding route for short-term tube feeding?

Nasoenteric feeding tube

Should patients be fed into the stomach or the small intestine?

It depends; if the stomach is functioning, there is no gastric outlet obstruction, and the patient is not at risk for aspiration, gastric feeding can be attempted. Otherwise, postpyloric feedings are usually recommended.

Does small-bowel feeding reduce the risk of aspiration?

The issue is controversial and results of the studies are ambiguous. Most studies are flawed in design. The distinction between aspiration of oropharyngeal secretions and gastric contents should be considered.

How can placement of transpyloric feeding be accomplished?

At the bedside, under fluoroscopy, endoscopically, or in the operating room

What medications may facilitate feeding-tube migration transpylorically?

Metoclopramide, erythromycin

When should patients receive long-term feeding tubes?

When feeding is needed for more than 4 weeks

When should a patient receive a surgically placed feeding tube enterostomy?

When long-term feeding is required, abdominal surgery is performed, and endoscopic tube placement is not possible, or when a known complication of the operation (such as anastomotic leak) will prevent oral intake for a lengthy period after surgery

What is the most common method of long-term feeding into the stomach?

Percutaneous endoscopic gastrostomy (PEG)

Can a PEG be used for jejunal feedings?

Yes, if a jejunal extension is added

What complications are related to nasoenteric feeding tubes?

Pulmonary intubation
Tube clogging
Nasal mucosal ulceration
Esophagitis
Pulmonary aspiration

What complications are associated with endoscopic feeding—tube placement?

Intraperitoneal placement, stomal leakage, and tube clogging

What complications are associated with surgical gastrostomies or jejunostomies?

Fistula
Stomal leakage
Wound infection
Wound dehiscence
Small bowel volvulus
Bowel perforation

What can be done to avoid tube clogging?

1. Do not mix medications with tube-feeding formulas
2. Order routine water flushes
3. Do not use tube for medication delivery, if possible

Parenteral Access

What routes are used for delivery of parenteral nutrition?

Central, peripheral, peripherally inserted central (PICC), or midline catheter

Why are long term catheters or ports preferable for patients requiring home TPN?

Long-term catheters are tunneled under the skin and therefore have a lower incidence of infection. Access ports are also inserted under the skin (e.g., Groshong, Hickman, port-a-cath)

What complications are associated with central access?

The most serious complication is catheter-related sepsis; other complications include pneumothorax, catheter migration, catheter occlusion, venous thrombosis.

What is the disadvantage of peripheral parenteral nutrition?

Higher flow rate is required to reduce osmolarity, and peripheral veins do not tolerate parenteral nutrition for very long.

DISEASE SPECIFICS

Are IV lipids safe to use during pancreatitis?

Intravenous lipids are considered safe when the patient's serum triglycerides are less than 350 to 400 mg/dl, indicating adequate clearance of triglycerides. IV lipids do not stimulate pancreatic activity.

Can a patient with pancreatitis be fed enterally?

Bowel rest and nasogastric suctioning are traditional methods of managing pancreatitis. Patients with pancreatitis have been safely fed enterally when fed into the proximal jejunum and given pancreatic enzymes. If enteral feeding is not tolerated, as evidenced by abdominal pain, abdominal distention, nausea, and vomiting, parenteral nutrition should be used.

Should high branched-chain amino acid formulas be used?

The effectiveness and role of high branched chain amino acid (low aromatic amino acid) enteral and parenteral formulas is controversial. These formulas are expensive. Many clinicians opt not to use the formulas until more convincing clinical studies are published. Others believe that if conventional medical therapy of lactulose and/or neomycin fails to prevent encephalopathy, specialty branched chain amino acid mixtures should be used.

Why would high branched chain amino acid solutions be beneficial in liver disease?

The theory is that normalizing the serum amino acid balance in liver failure patients will reduce encephalopathy.

Should specialty amino acid solutions be used for renal failure?

Specialty solutions for renal failure contain high levels of essential amino acids. They are expensive and have not been shown to be efficacious.

Should patients with enterocutaneous fistulas be fed enterally?

Yes, if possible. If fistula output is greater than 500 cc/d and the feeding tube tip cannot be placed distal to the fistula, feed parenterally. If fistula output is less than 500 cc/d and/or the feeding tube tip can be placed distally, attempt enteral feedings and monitor for an increase in fistula output.

Will a high fat-to-carbohydrate ratio improve pulmonary function?

Controlled trials have shown numerically significant differences in CO_2 production with increased percentage of calories from fat; however, these differences were not clinically significant.

Supplementation of which nutrients is associated with improved wound healing?

Vitamins C, A, and zinc

What is "immunonutrition"?

Nutrition fortified with nucleotides, arginine, omega-3 fatty acids and glutamine to augment immune function.

What is glutamine?	An amino acid thought to be conditionally essential after injury and in critical illness.
What are two roles of glutamine?	1. Important fuel for the small-bowel enterocytes. It slows mucosal atrophy when given intravenously 2. Required for lymphocyte and macrophage production
Is glutamine in TPN?	No; free glutamine is unstable in TPN. Glutamine peptides are stable and are being tested for potential commercial use.
Is glutamine in tube feedings?	Yes, all tube feedings contain glutamine either in free form, in a peptide, or in an intact protein. The optimal amount for humans is not yet known.

MISCELLANEOUS

What issues need to be addressed for patients going home with nutrition support?	1. Financial coverage 2. Appropriate access 3. Education and ability of patient and caregiver 4. Appropriate regimen to promote mobility and enhance the quality of life (i.e., nocturnal delivery, if possible)
What are the signs of each of the following deficiencies:	
Vitamin A?	Poor wound healing
Vitamin B$_{12}$/folate?	Megaloblastic anemia
Biotin?	Skin rash, neuromuscular signs, EKG changes
Vitamin C?	Poor wound healing
Vitamin K?	Decrease in the vitamin K—dependent clotting factors (II, VII, IX, and X)

Chromium?   Diabetic state, especially in patients with
                              adult onset diabetes mellitus (ADOM)

Selenium?   Anergy, cardiomyopathy

Zinc?   Poor wound healing, alopecia,
                              dermatitis, ↓ taste

Fatty acid?   Dry, flaky skin; alopecia;
                              thrombocytopenia

15

Operative Pearls

Lorne H. Blackbourne, M.D.

What must be in place prior to doing a diagnostic peritoneal lavage (DPL) for trauma?

1. Foley catheter
2. NGT (or OGT)

Where must the catheter be placed for a DPL with a pelvic fracture?

Supraumbilical position (pelvic hematoma tracks up the medial umbilical ligaments); even with a supraumbilical approach, there is up to a 20% false positive rate!

What are the pearls of successfully placing a subclavian central line?

1. Place towels below scapulae transversely or between the scapulae
2. Place patient in the Trendelenburg position (think: headdownenburg)
3. Keep the needle flat
4. Go for the left subclavian, if all things are equal
5. Always have one hand on the wire at all times and **never** let go
6. Always go on the side of a chest tube
7. Always get a chest x-ray after the procedure or before trying the other side

What are the pearls for maximizing the placement of an NGT?

1. Flex the head (chin to chest)
2. Apply mild topical anesthetic (cetacaine spray, etc)
3. Apply lubrication
4. Have the patient drink water

What will help open the pylorus and stop the contractions of the stomach/duodenum during an EGD?

IV glucagon

What will help retain contrast dye during a biliary cholangiogram?	IV morphine
Can the suprarenal IVC ever be ligated?	No; a mortality rate of approximately 100% is associated with such attempts.
Can the infrarenal IVC be ligated?	Yes, but with a morbidity rate of approximately 50%
Should the spleen bed be drained after a splenectomy for an isolated spleen injury?	No; a higher abscess rate is associated with drainage.
What factor indicates use of a closed drain after a trauma splenectomy?	Possible injury to the pancreas
Which veins must be ligated during a warren distal splenorenal shunt for esophageal varices?	1. Coronary vein (left gastric vein) 2. Right epiploic vein 3. Left gonadal vein
If a 12 French Foley catheter cannot be inserted into the bladder, what should be tried next?	1. Larger Foley catheter 2. Lidocaine jelly to anesthetize the urethra 3. Coude catheter
During a inguinal hernia repair, the suture needle goes through the femoral vein or artery. What should be done?	Remove the suture and hold pressure; do not tie the suture down!
How should an anal fistula that goes above the anal sphincters be treated?	Seton, which will allow subsequent tightening and scarring down of the sphincter muscles
What is the minimal margin size for resection of a colon cancer?	3 cm
How low can the cancer be for a low anterior resection?	Approximately 8 cm from the anal verge

What action should be taken if the fascial stitch for placement of a hasson laparoscopy trocar goes through a loop of bowel?	The stitch should not be pulled out. The fascial incision should be enlarged and the loop of bowel should be pulled up through the incision. The stitch and the damage should then be examined.
How should a through-and-through penetrating injury to the IVC be fixed?	Enlarge the anterior defect, fix the posterior defect, and then close the anterior defect
What test should be performed after a tracheostomy?	A chest x-ray
After the mesoappendix is stapled off during a lap appy, the appendiceal artery continues to pump blood. What should be done?	A metallic clip (as used for lap choles) must be applied or a suture must be placed
How should the skin be closed after a grossly contaminated abdominal case?	It should be left open and closed by secondary intention or delayed primary closure.
How should a vas injury be repaired during a procedure to correct an inguinal hernia?	A urologist should be called in to perform an end-to-end repair (unless the patient is elderly).
How should an ilioinguinal nerve transection be repaired during a procedure to correct an inguinal hernia ?	A metallic clip should be applied to prevent neuroma formation.
What can help identify the ureters during a difficult pelvic dissection (e.g., postradiation)?	Ureteral stents placed by a urologist
What can help identify an occult ureteral injury?	IV indigo carmine (collects in urine and will most likely be seen in operative field with ureteral injury)

What is a newly described way to treat an isolated intercostal penetrating injury?	1. Chest tube 2. Placement of a Foley catheter into a penetrating wound; blow up the balloon and the pull until the intercostal artery injury reaches tamponade; place a Kelly clamp at skin to hold in tamponade position!
What is a Kraske procedure?	Trans coccygeal resection of a low rectal mass (coccyx is removed)
What is a Grillo patch?	A **pleural** wrap of an esophageal injury repair
What is the major difference between a Nissen and a Belsey Mark IV fundoplication?	Nissen has a 360 degree wrap (usually through the abdomen) Belsey Mark IV has a 240 to 270 degree wrap (through the thorax)
Why do some surgeons "bowel prep" for gastric cancer surgery?	In case of the unexpected gastrocolonic fistula
Prior to prepping a patient, what mental checklist should be reviewed?	Position Antibiotics? Clip hair? SCD boots? NGT? Foley? Special equipment ready and available? Fluoroscopy needed?
What postoperative checklist should be reviewed?	Several things need to be done before you can eat some food, so the acronym F.O.O.D.D. is helpful: **F** Family—talk to the patient's family **O** Operative note—write on the chart **O** Orders **D** Dictate the procedure **D** Doctor—call the primary/referring doctor
What are the intraoperative signs of Crohn disease?	1. Creeping mesenteric fat 2. Thickened mesentery 3. Thickened bowel wall 4. Serositis 5. Abscess/fistulae/strictures

Should a frozen section be taken to rule out microscopic disease at the margins prior to an anastomosis after a small bowel resection for Crohn disease?

NO; microscopic disease at an anastomosis does not have any effect on the rate of anastomotic healing. (1 cm of grossly normal bowel is needed for margins with Crohn disease)

A stable patient has a chest-penetrating wound in the box formed by the clavicles, nipples, and costal margins. How should this patient be evaluated for cardiac injury?

Subxiphoid pericardial window

What is the strongest layer of bowel for an anastomosis?

The **submucosa** (not the serosa)

What condition contraindicates a hemorrhoidectomy?

Crohn disease

LAPAROSCOPY PEARLS

What MUST you do when you use the Argon laser during laparoscopy?

Open a trocar vent; otherwise, there will be a build up of intraabdominal pressure that may result in a CO_2 embolus.

What is the appropriate treatment for bladder veress needle puncture?

Postoperative Foley drainage

What is the appropriate treatment for trocar bladder injury?

Closing by suture and placement of Foley drainage

How can placement of a trocar through an epigastric vessel be avoided?

Transilluminate the abdominal wall and identify the vessels

How can a bleeding trocar site be fixed?

1. Inserting of a Keith needle into the peritoneal cavity, out the abdomen, under the vessel, and tying over a bolster
2. Cutting down and tying off the vessel
3. Inserting of a Foley catheter through the trocar site; pressure should be held with outward traction

16

Surgical Radiology

Lorne H. Blackbourne, MD

Define the following abbreviations:

AXR	Abdominal x-ray
CXR	Chest x-ray
U/S	Ultrasound
ERCP	Endoscopic retrograde cholangiopancreatography
BE	Barium enema
UGI	Upper gastrointestinal contrast study
A-gram	Angiogram
PTX	Pneumothorax
Prior to reading any x-ray study, what must be checked?	Patient's name and the date

ABDOMEN

What percentage of kidney stones are radiopaque?

90%

What percentage of gallstones are radiopaque?

≈ 10% to 20%

What percentage of radiopaque fecaliths are present in appendicitis?

5%

What signs of abdominal pathology are visible on AXR?

Loss of fat stripe, loss of psoas shadow, sentinel loops, cut-off sign, and air—fluid levels

What is the "parrot's beak" or "bird's beak" sign?

Evidence of sigmoid volvulus on barium enema; evidence of achalasia on barium swallow

What are the differential diagnoses of retroperitoneal calcification?

Pancreatitis, abdominal aortic aneurysm, generalized aortic calcification, kidney stone, renal-cell carcinoma, renal artery aneurysm (phleboliths, if seen in the pelvis)

What are the differential diagnoses of free peritoneal air?

Intraabdominal viscus perforation, status post laparotomy, status post needle biopsy, status post paracentesis (or, rarely, from the female reproductive tract, such as after water skiing).

What is the best position for the detection of free peritoneal air?

Upright CXR; with free air, **both** sides of the bowel wall can be seen and as little as 1 cc of air can be detected.

What is the best position if the patient cannot stand or sit up?

Left lateral decubitus, because it prevents confusion with gastric air bubbles and air tracks up over the liver

What is the significance of an air—fluid level?

Seen in obstruction or ileus on an upright x-ray, the intraluminal bowel diameter increases, allowing for separation of fluid and gas.

What is meant by a "cut-off sign"?

Seen in obstruction, bowel distention and air—fluid level are "cut off" from the normal bowel.

What are sentinal loops?

Distention and/or air—fluid levels near a site of abdominal inflammation (e.g., seen in the right lower quadrant with appendicitis)

What is loss of the psoas shadow?

Loss of the clearly defined borders of the psoas muscle on AXR, signifying inflammation or ascites

What is loss of the peritoneal fat stripe (preperitoneal fat stripe)?

Loss of the lateral peritoneal/preperitoneal fat interface (implies inflammation)

What is pneumatosis intestinalis?

Air in the bowel wall

What is the "string" sign?

On a contrast study of the GI tract, an area of stricture or stenosis that shows up as a narrow line of contrast, giving the appearance of a "string"

What is "thumbprinting"?

An edematous colon mucosa that looks like thumb impressions on AXR

What study must be done prior to using a NGT or nasoduodenal feeding tube?

A low chest/high abdominal film to confirm placement of the tube in the GI tract and not in the lung (i.e., feed the lung = death)

What evidence of acute appendicitis can be visible on AXR?

(Most x-rays appear normal)
1. Fecalith (appendolith)
2. Sentinel loops (right lower quadrant dilated small-bowel loops)
3. Scoliosis (convex away from right lower quadrant) because of pain and splinting
4. Psoas shadow obliteration
5. Loss of preperitoneal fat stripe
6. Free air from appendiceal perforation (very rare)

What signs of acute pancreatitis are visible on AXR?

1. Sentinel loops
2. Colon cut-off sign
3. Dilated duodenum

What signs of chronic pancreatitis are visible on AXR?

Pancreatic calcifications

Which kidney stones are radiolucent on AXR?

Uric acid (**uric** = **u**nseen)

What is the 3,6,9 rule of AXRs?

A rough rule of thumb: The normal small bowel should be less than **3** cm in diameter, the normal transverse colon should be less than **6** cm in diameter, the normal cecum should be less than **9** cm in diameter.

What is Chiladidee's sign on AXR?

Air in the colon **above** the liver, simulating free air

What signs of small bowel obstruction are visible on AXR?

1. Distended loops of the bowel
2. Air fluid levels
3. String of beads
4. Step-ladder appearance of distended small bowels
5. Paucity of gas in the colon

What is the "step-ladder" appearance on AXR associated with small bowel obstruction?

Dilated small-bowel loops lining up on top of each other from the right lower quadrant to the left upper quadrant

What AXR finding is associated with a diffuse ileus?

Distended loops throughout, with gas in the small bowel **and** colon

What is the "string of beads" on AXR?

Seen with small bowel obstruction; small air bubbles (beads) trapped and separated by the plicae circulares, giving the appearance of a string of beads

What is the source of gas with small bowel obstruction?

Swallowed air

Should barium or water-soluble contrast be used in an upper gastrointestinal series for a patient with small-bowel obstruction?

Barium (the water soluble contrast will just get diluted out)

What is the most common cause of calcifications above the kidney?

Adrenal calcifications (make sure they are not pancreatic calcifications)

Can there be free air after a PEG procedure?

Yes

What is a "lead pipe" on BE?

Seen on BE with chronic ulcerative colitis owing to haustral obliteration and smooth narrowing of the colon; the contrast looks like a smooth lead pipe

What are "collar button" ulcers on BE?

Asymptomatic deep ulcers associated with Crohn disease

What is an "apple core" lesion on air contrast BE?

A circumferential lesion of the colon (a vast majority owing to colon cancer)

What do aphthous ulcers look like on BE?

Punctate ulcers with a "lucent halo" of surrounding edema

What is the gold standard test for DVT?

Lower extremity venogram

What is the gold standard test for a pulmonary embolus?

Pulmonary artery A-gram

What is the "double bubble" sign?

Seen on AXR with duodenal obstruction, a duodenal bubble in addition to the gastric bubble

What is a "Meckel's scan"?

A nuclear medicine scan for ectopic Meckel's gastric mucosa

What test is used for localizing a pheochromocytoma?

A metaiodobenzylguanide (MIBG) scan (a norepinephrine analog)

What diagnostic study is used to evaluate rectal cancer invasion preoperatively?

A transrectal U/S

What diagnostic studies are used to localize the parathyroid glands with hyperparathyroidism?

1. U/S
2. MRI
3. Sestamibi scintigraphy
(CT and thallium—technetium scans are losing favor)

What radiologic studies should be considered for a patient in the ICU with a fever of unknown origin?

1. CXR (to rule out pneumonia)
2. Sinus films/CT (to rule out sinusitis)
3. LE U/S, doppler, venogram (to rule out DVT)
4. Abdominal CT (to rule out abscess)
5. Gallbladder U/S (to check for acalculus cholecystitis)

What is the initial study of choice for evaluation of the gallbladder and bile ducts?

U/S

What is the major limitation of U/S?

It is operator dependent

What are some signs of acute cholecystitis that are evident on U/S?

1. Positive sonographic Murphy's sign (pain upon pushing U/S probe directly over the gallbladder)
2. Thickened gallbladder wall (nl < 3 mm)
3. Pericholecystic fluid
4. Gallstones (supportive data)
5. Distended gallbladder

What is the diameter of a dilated common bile duct (CBD)?

It is generally believed to be greater than 10 mm if the gallbladder is present, but the real number is closer to 7 mm or greater (it is commonly accepted that if the gallbladder has been removed, an additional 2 mm can be added because of the loss of the gallbladder capacitance)

How often can U/S detect cholelithiasis?

More than 98% of the time!

How often can U/S detect choledolithiasis?

Only about 1/3 of the time!

How often can U/S detect the cause of biliary obstruction?

Only about 50% of the time!

Define distal versus proximal biliary obstruction.

Proximal bile ducts are near the liver, the distal bile duct is near the duodenum (think of blood flow: proximal arteries are near the heart and blood flows distally, just as proximal bile ducts are near the liver and bile flows distally to the duodenum).

What diagnostic test is often used after U/S to evaluate the ductal anatomy in proximal ductal obstruction?

PTC maps proximal extent of the ductal involvement to assess anastomotic potential, provides cytology brushings, and allows stent placement for bile drainage, operative palpation, and anastomotic stenting.

| What diagnostic test is often used after U/S to evaluate the ductal anatomy in distal ductal obstruction? | ERCP allows direct visualization of the ampulla of Vater, allows for cytologic brushings, stent placement, and dye study of the distal and, usually, proximal extent of duct involvement. |

TRAUMA RADIOLOGY

What CXR findings can provide evidence of traumatic aortic injury?	Widened mediastinum Apical pleural capping Pleural fluid Loss of aortic knob Inferior displacement of left main bronchus Nasogastric tube displaced to the right Tracheal deviation Large hemothorax
Is an isolated sternal fracture a risk factor for aortic injury in patients involved in automobile accidents?	No; if the shoulder belt is worn, it might even be a protective injury!
What is the most common finding of aortic injury visible on CXR?	Widened mediastinum (anteroposterior is most sensitive)
What can be missed on an anteroposterior CXR in trauma?	Anterior pneumothorax
What radiologic test may be indicated for an unstable patient with a pelvic fracture and negative suprapubic diagnostic peritoneal lavage (DPL)?	A pelvic A-gram and, possibly, therapeutic embolization
What study must be performed prior to placement of a Foley catheter when a urethral injury is suspected?	Retrograde urethrogram (RUG)

What are the common "trauma triple" x-rays taken in the ER?	1. Lateral **c-spine** 2. Anteroposterior **chest** 3. Anteroposterior **pelvis**
What views must be taken to evaluate the bony c-spine in trauma?	1. Anteroposterior 2. Lateral 3. Odontoid
What percentage of all c-spine bony injuries can be seen on a lateral c-spine film that scans down to T1?	Approximately 80%
What x-rays are used to evaluate for ligamentous c-spine injuries?	Lateral flexion and extension c-spine films
What is the role of abdominal/pelvic CT in blunt trauma?	To evaluate the abdomen and pelvis in the **stable** patient
What is the significance of hepatic periportal blood tracking on abdominal CT after blunt trauma?	It has no effect on conservative (nonoperative) management after blunt trauma (ARCH SURG 1996;131:255.)
In addition to the abdomen, what must be scanned to evaluate the peritoneal cavity in blunt trauma?	The pelvis
What subtle abdominal CT findings are associated with pancreatic injury after blunt trauma?	Thickened left anterior perirenal fascia and edema of peripancreatic fat
What abdominal CT findings are associated with small-bowel injury?	Free air, contrast extravasation, mesenteric infiltration, sentinel clot sign, and thickened bowel wall
What is the sentinel clot sign on abdominal CT?	A blood clot in the mesentery associated with small-bowel injury

What is the most common direction of pancreatic fracture after blunt trauma?	Perpendicular to the pancreatic duct
What major injuries does abdominal/pelvic CT miss?	Small bowel injury Diaphragm injury
What injury does DPL miss?	Retroperitoneal injuries that are contained by the overlying peritoneal covering (e.g., kidney fracture)
How long should it take for a 10% pneumothorax to reabsorb without a chest tube?	A pneumothorax reabsorbs approximately 1% of the measured PTX volume per day; therefore, a 10% pneumothorax should reabsorb in 10 days.
How long after a laparotomy can free air be seen on AXR?	Approximately one week
What is the study of choice to evaluate for head trauma?	**Unenhanced** head CT (blood "lights up")
Define the head CT findings associated with the following conditions: Epidural hematoma	Blood in a **biconcave** or **lens** (lenticular) configuration caused by restriction by the underlying dura mater
Subdural hematoma	Blood in a **crescent shape** conforming to the contour of the brain
Subarachnoid hemorrhage	A layer of blood over the brain cortex with blood collecting in the cisterns at the base of the brain
Increased cranial pressure	1. Effacement of the ventricles 2. Flattening of the brain sulci 3. Loss of the gray-white matter interface 4. Loss of cisterns
What is the best test for brain shear injury?	MRI

What is the falx sign?	Seen with subarachnoid hemorrhage as blood tracts along the falx, it results in a "thickened" falx on unenhanced head CT.

CHEST

How many lung lobes are on the right?	Three
How many lung lobes are on the left?	Two
The lingula is part of which lobe?	The left upper lobe
What is the normal heart size?	The transverse heart diameter is normally less than half of the transverse diameter of the chest.
What are the signs of fluid overload on chest x-ray?	1. Large heart 2. Cephalization (distended large vessels in upper lung fields) 3. Pulmonary edema 4. Kerley B lines 5. Pleural effusion
What are Kerley B lines?	Horizontal straight (not curly) lines seen on chest x-ray in the peripheral lung fields caused by lymphatic edema with fluid overload (e.g., congestive heart failure)
What x-ray indicates whether a pleural effusion is free or loculated?	An ipsilateral lateral decubitus CXR; free fluid will "layer out"
If an endotracheal tube is placed down too far, which bronchus will it most likely be in?	The right mainstem bronchus
How much pleural fluid can be hidden by the diaphragm on an anteroposterior upright CXR?	Classically, up to 500 cc can be hidden, but will appear on a lateral CXR and can be identified as free fluid if it layers out on ipsilateral decubitus CXR.

What is the optimal position of a central line tip?

In the superior vena cava

What is the optimal position of endotracheal tube on CXR?

Above the carina, below or at the clavicles

What is the optimal position of Swan-Ganz catheter tip?

The tip should not be past the right heart border

What x-ray must be taken after a tracheostomy is performed?

CXR (to rule out PTX)

What x-ray must be taken after placement of a central line?

CXR (for line placement and to rule out PTX)

What x-ray must be taken after a bronchoscopy?

CXR (to rule out PTX, collapsed lobe)

What x-ray must be taken after placement of a Swan-Ganz catheter?

CXR (for line placement and to rule out PTX)

How can you tell if all the holes in a chest tube are in the pleural cavity on CXR?

The last hole on the chest tube goes through the radiopaque line on the chest tube (seen as a break in the radiopaque line on CXR, indicating placement in the chest)

17 Surgical Infectious Diseases

Lee Butterfield, MD

BACKGROUND AND GENERAL INFORMATION

What impact did antiseptic techniques have on elective operations?

Infection rate dropped from greater than 90% to less than 10%

Define surgical infection.

Infections that require operative treatment **or** result from operative treatment (Schwartz, 146)

What are the major differences between pathogens causing surgical infections and those causing "medical" infections?

In surgical infections, pathogens are usually opportunistic, mixed (aerobes and anaerobes), and originate from the patient's endogenous flora.

How much does a postoperative infection increase the cost of a single hospital stay?

It doubles the cost.

What is the cost of caring for postoperative wound infections in the United States?

Greater than $3 billion

What percentage of postsurgical infections develop after discharge?

More than 50%

By how much is the incidence of infection reduced through simple monitoring of surgical-specific infections with feedback to the surgeon?

50%

What reduction in blood transmission does double gloving afford from a solid suture needle stick?

40 nl with one glove to 2 nl of blood transmission with 2 gloves! (25 guage solid needle)

What are the most sensitive tests for detecting infection and determining location?

History and physical examination

What sign leads to the diagnosis of a postsurgical wound infection?

A discharge of purulent material from the wound

Within what time period do postsurgical infections occur?

Within 30 days postoperative

The development of a surgical infection depends upon what four factors?

1) Microbial pathogenicity
2) Host defenses
3) Local environment
4) Surgical technique

What is generally accepted as the number of contaminating bacteria that must be present to establish a clinical infection in a noncompromised host?

10^5

What are some patient factors that contribute to the development of infection?

Advanced age
Decreased blood flow to surgical incision (vascular occlusive states, hypovolemic shock, vasopressors, vasoconstricion)
Reduced vascular reactivity (uremia, advanced age, steroids)
Cancer, trauma, diabetes, obesity, malnutrition, acquired and inherited immunodeficiency, immunosuppression

What is the most common cause of acquired immunologic deficiencies leading to serious infections in surgical patients?

Malnutrition

True or false: Most surgical infections occur in patients with intact host defenses?

False; most are the result of damaged host defenses

Where is epithelium multilayered?

In the nasopharynx, oral cavity, esophagus, and GU tract

Where is epithelium single layered?

In the tracheobronchial tree, GI tract, and eye

Name some local wound factors that increase the potential for wound infections.

Presence of foreign bodies (including sutures)
Lack of accurate approximation of tissues
Strangulation of tissues with too tight sutures
Presence of dead tissue, hematomas, or seromas

How do fluid collections and edema increase the likelihood of infection?

They act as culture media and inhibit phagocytosis and WBC migration.

What is the best method for preventing fluid collection and infection when a large, potentially dead space occurs in an operative wound that may be contaminated?

Closed suction drainage (never use a Penrose drain for any wound that is not already infected)

When does a central line culture mandate a new central line at another site?

Most experts believe that greater than 15 CFU mandates a new central line site.

What are some important factors in preventing wound infection?

Preoperative clipping (not shaving)
Vigilance for breaks in a-septic technique
Therapeutic levels of antiobiotics during the operation
Limited use of electrocautery
Continuous suture closure, whenever possible
Monofilament sutures, whenever possible
Oxygen delivery (increased postoperative)
Surveillance of wound infection

By what percentage does hair removal by shaving increase the infection rate when compared with removal by clippers or no removal at all?	100%
How many viable staphylococci are necessary to produce a clinical infection when injected subcutaneously into normal tissue?	Greater than 10^5
How many are necessary when introduced on a piece of silk suture material?	Less than 100; therefore, never use silk in contaminated wounds
When a wound has been heavily contaminated, how should the fascia be closed?	With running sutures
What is the proper closure for heavily contaminated wounds or wounds in which all of the foreign bodies or devitalized tissues cannot be satisfactorily removed?	**Delayed** primary closure
When can delayed primary closure be initiated and why?	After 5 days, because the number of phagocytic cells at the wound edges, as well as capillary budding, reaches a peak at about 5 days.
What are the infection rates for each of the following types of wounds:	
Clean?	Less than 1.5%
Clean-contaminated?	Less than 3%
Contaminated?	Less than 5%

What is a clean surgical wound?

Nontraumatic; no break in technique; respiratory, alimentary, or GU tract are not entered

What is a clean-contaminated surgical wound?

GI or respiratory tract entered without significant spillage; oropharynx, vagina, or noninfected GU or biliary tract entered; minor break in technique

What is a contaminated surgical wound?

Major break in technique; traumatic; gross spillage from GI tract; entrance into GU or biliary tracts in presence of infected urine or bile

In multiple organ failure, what is the classic sequence of organ system failure?

Pulmonary, renal, GI, hematopoitic, hepatic, CNS, cardiovascular

ANTIBIOTICS

Generally, how long should antibiotics be administered for surgical infections?

Until the patient demonstrates obvious clinical improvement with a normal temperature for at least 48 hours

When do preoperative IV antibiotics need to be in the body?

Within 2 hours **before** the incision

What clincal signs of improvement are expected in surgical patients with infection?

Improved mental status
Return of bowel function
Spontaneous diuresis

What are the four major groups of β-lactam antibiotics?

Penicillins, cephalosporins, carbapenems, and monobactams

How do β-lactam antibiotics work?

They bind to one of several penicillin-binding proteins (PBP) and interfere with bacterial cell-wall synthesis.

Which bacteria is Penicillin G effective against?

Streptococcus organisms, except
    Enterococcus
Neisseria, except lactamase-producing
    gonococcus
Treponema pallidum, Bacillus anthracis

What are the differences between Penicillan G, Penicillan V, procaine, and benzathine Penicillan G?

Penicillan G—IV administration
Penicillan V—oral administration
Procaine—maximum blood levels reached in 3 to 4 hours
Benzathine—slowly released at low levels for several weeks

What are the four β-lactamase inhibitor/β-lactam combinations currently in use?

Amoxacillin-clavulanic acid
Ticarcillin-clavulanic acid
Ampicillin-sulbactam
Piperacillin-sulbactam

What are the two major antistaphylococcal penicillins in use today?

Oxacillin and nafcillin

What types of bacteria are antistaphylococcal penicillins ineffective against?

Gram-negative rods
Anaerobes
Decreased activity against streptococcal species

What are the four extended-spectrum penicillins?

Carbenicillin, ticarcillin, mezlocillin, piperacillin

Which two extended-spectrum penicillins have increased activity against *Pseudomonas*, *Acinetobacter*, and *Serratia*?

Mezlocillin and piperacillin

What are two potentially serious side effects of carbenicillin and ticarcillin?

1) High sodium load
2) Inhibition of platelet aggregation

Which penicillin has significant antianaerobic activity?

Ticarcillin, especially when combined with clavulanic acid

Which bacteria do first generation cephalosporins have good activity against?

Methicillin-susceptible staphylococci
Streptococcus organisms

Which cephalosporins are effective against *Enterococcus*?

None; in fact, some evidence suggests that they encourage enterococcal overgrowth

Which first generation cephalosporin has the longest half life, how long, and why is this information important?	Cefazolin, 8 hours, maintains more reliable serum and tissue levels when used for **prophylaxis**
Compared with first generation cephalosporins, what type of spectrum do second generation cephalosporins have?	Expanded gram-negative activity
Can second generation cephalosporins be used for empiric treatment of hospital-acquired gram-negative rod infection?	No, they are only effective against community-acquired gram-negative rod infections with known susceptibility patterns
Which cephalosprins have good anaerobic activity?	Second generation cephalosporins: cefoxitin and cefotetan
Which has a longer half-life, cefoxitin or cefotetan?	Cefotetan
What is the potentially serious side effect unique to cefotetan?	Prolonged PT
What antibiotic is associated with gallbladder sludge and cholestatic jaundice?	Ceftriaxone
Which bacteria do third generation cephalosporins have increased activity against?	Gram-negative rods
What do third generation cephalosporins sacrifice for increased gram-negative rod coverage?	Activity against *Staphylococcus* and *Streptococcus* Anaerobic coverage
Which third generation cephalosporins have increased activity against *Pseudomonas*, *Acinetobacter*, and *Serratia*?	Cefoperozone and ceftazidime

What is the only β-lactam antibiotic that does not crossreact in patients who are allergic to penicillins or cephalosporins and what class is it in?

Aztreonam, monobactam

What type of bacteria is aztreonam effective against?

Gram-negative, including most *Pseudomonas* organisms

What type of bacteria is aztreonam ineffective against?

Gram-positive cocci
Anaerobes

What is the representative drug of the carbapenem class of β-lactams?

Imipenem

What are the five exceptions to imipenem's broad coverage [hint: MEXIP]?

Methicillin-resistant *Staphylococcus aureus* (MRSA)
Enterococcus
Xanthomonas maltophila
Indole plus strains of *Proteus*
Pseudomonas cepacia

Do susceptible strains of *Pseudomonas* develop resistance to imipenem during treatment as readily as they do to other β-lactams?

Yes

What other drug is imipenem always combined with and why?

Cilistatin (enzyme inhibitor), because it prevents hydrolysis of the active form of the drug in the kidneys

What side effect of imipenem is important to remember?

It is associated with a significantly higher incidence of **seizures**.

What is the mechanism of action of trimethoprim-sulfamethoxazole?

Trimethoprim is a structural analog of folic acid and competes with dihydrofolic acid for the binding site of dihydrofolate reductase. Sulfamethoxazole is an analog of para-aminobenzoic acid (PABA), which is required for the synthesis of folic acid.

What are the major side effects of trimethoprim-sulfamethoxazole?

Allergic reactions (rash, fever, photosensitivity), kernicterus (infants), renal damage (secondary to toxic nephrosis or allergic nephritis), hemolysis in G6PD-deficient patients, Steven-Johnson syndrome (erythema multiforme)

What is the mechanism of action of quinolones?

They inhibit DNA gyrase, thus inhibiting DNA replication.

Are quinolones effective against gram-negative rods? Pseudomonas? Gram-positive cocci? MRSA?

Yes (effective against all)

What are the two most commonly used quinolones?

Norfloxacin and ciprofloxacin

Why is norfloxacin limited in its scope of utility?

It reaches therapeutic levels best in urine.

What is the mechanism of action of aminoglycosides?

They inhibit protein translation by blocking the initiation complex.

What types of bacteria are aminoglycosides effective against?

Aerobic and facultative gram-negative rods
Gram-positive cocci (possibly)
Synergistic with penicillin or vancomycin for *Enterococcus*

What types of bacteria are aminoglycosides ineffective against?

Anaerobes or facultatives in an anaerobic environment

Which aminoglycoside is most active against *Enterococcus* and *Serratia?*

Gentamicin

Which aminoglycoside is most active against *Pseudomonas?*

Tobramycin

Which aminoglycoside can often be used against gentamycin- and tobramycin-resistant organisms?	Amikacin
Are aminoglycosides effective against anaerobes?	No
Why is aminoglycoside dosing difficult?	Because they distribute in interstitial fluid that tends to vary considerably with disease and is greatly enlarged in patients with life-threatening infection
What factor determines the dosing of aminoglycosides?	Serum levels
Is it more common to find toxic levels or inadequate levels of aminoglycosides?	Inadequate levels
What ratio of therapeutic to toxic levels is associated with aminoglycosides?	2:3
What are the major toxicities of aminoglycosides?	Nephrotoxicity and ototoxicity (eighth cranial nerve)
Which aminoglycoside may have somewhat less nephrotoxicity clinically?	Tobramycin
Which component of cranial nerve VIII do aminoglycosides affect, auditory or vestibular?	Both
Which three antibiotics offer the most complete activity against anaerobes?	Chloramphenicol (CAM) Clindamycin Metronidazole
What is mechanism of action of CAM?	Interruption of translation elongation (bacteriostatic)

What side effects are associated with CAM?

Gray baby syndrome, reversible bone marrow suppression, aplastic anemia

Why is CAM seldomly used?

Because of the potential for bone marrow toxicity

What guidelines are recommended for the use of CAM?

1) Restrict use to life-threatening infections in which the drug of choice cannot be used and CAM is clearly a superior alternative.
2) Avoid prolonged usage and repeated exposure.
3) Differential leukocyte counts should be taken 2 to 3 times weekly and therapy should be discontinued if leukopenia occurs.

What is the mechanism of action of clindamycin?

Static, similar to that of CAM and erythromycin

How much more likely is clindamycin to cause C. difficile colitis than other antibiotics?

It is not more likely; *C. difficile colitis* can be caused by any antibiotic (except vancomycin and metronidazole), and there is no difference in frequency between the various antibiotics

Why is clindamycin never used alone empirically?

Although effective against anaerobes and gram-positive cocci, it completely lacks activity against gram-negative rods (aerobic and facultative)

Which of the three anaerobic antibiotics possesses the most complete anaerobic coverage?

Metronidazole

What is the mechanism of metronidazole?

It interrupts the bacterial electron transport process

Is metronidazole effective against any aerobic or facultative pathogens?

No (neither gram-negative nor gram-positive)

Is metronidazole combined with an aminoglycoside effective in the treatment of gram-positive cocci mixed aerobic/anaerobic infections?

No

Name two side effects of metronidazole (one short term and one long term).

Short term—disulfiram (antabuse)-like reaction with alcohol
Long term—peripheral neuropathy

What class of antibiotic is erythromycin and when is it often used in the surgical setting?

Macrolide
Used orally in combination with oral neomycin for reduction of bacteria in the bowel lumen prior to surgery of the colon

What is the mechanism of action of erythromycin?

Bacteriostatic—binds to 50s ribosomal unit and inhibits protein synthesis (Lynch, 29)

What are the other two commonly used macrolides?

Clarithromycin and azithromycin

Does oral erythromycin affect anaerobic bacteria in the large bowel?

Yes; it reaches high enough levels to markedly suppress anaerobic growth

What other organisms is erythromycin effective against?

Gram-positive cocci (for penicillin-allergic patients)
Neisseria (for penicillin-allergic patients)
Mycoplasma
Chlamydia
Legionella (IV)
Rickettsia
Campylobacter jejuni

What are the major side effects of erythromycin (PO and IV)?

PO—nausea
IV—cholestasis

What type of antibiotic is vancomycin?

A glycopeptide

What is the mechanism of action of vancomycin?

Cell-wall inhibitor; inhibits the transfer of subunits to peptidoglycan by binding to D-alanine residues of penta-peptide moiety

What general class of organisms is vancomycin effective against, and what three specific pathogens is it most commonly used to treat?

Gram-positive cocci:
1. MRSA
2. *Enterococcus*
3. *C. difficile*

Name four side effects of vancomycin.

1) Hypertension (during infusion)
2) Histamine release (Redman syndrome; during infusion)
3) Nephrotoxicity
4) Ototoxicity

What are the symptoms of Redman syndrome?

Flushing, tachycardia, hypotension

What is the mechanism of action of amphotericin B?

Complexes with fungal sterols (predominantly ergosterol) in plasma membrane, alters membrane permeability

What are the adverse effects of amphotericin B?

Fever, hypotension, chills
Dose-dependent nephrotoxicity (in up to 80% of patients)
Progressive, reversible anemia
Potassium wasting

What is the dosage range and dosing interval of amphotericin B?

IV administration of .25 to 1 mg/kg daily, depending on the type of infection and renal functioning

What cumulative dose of amphotericin B should not be exceeded?

None; treat until either the infection is cleared or renal function becomes seriously compromised

What electrolyte problem is associated with amphotericin administration?

Hypokalemia

What is major use of flucytosine?

It is used with amphotericin B for cryptococcal infection and systemic candidiasis.

What is the major use of ketoconazole?

It is used as a fungistatic in patients who are not severely ill or immunocompromised (e.g., blastomycosis, esophageal candidiasis, coccidioidomycosis, histoplasmosis, paracoccidioidomycosis).

What are the side effects of ketoconazole?

Anorexia, nausea, vomiting, impotence
H_2 blockers decrease bioavailability
Increases coumadin and cyclosporin levels
Increases dilantin toxicities

What is major use of fluconazole?

Oropharyngeal and esophageal candidiasis, lifetime maintenance of AIDS patients with cryptococcosis to help prevent relapse of cryptococcosis meningitis

What are the four major drugs used in treatment of TB? Which are static and which are cidal?

Isoniazid (INH)—cidal
Rifampin—cidal
Pyrazinamide—cidal
Ethambutol—static

What are the current treatment recommendations for noncomplicated, disseminated, and drug-resistant TB?

INH plus rifampin for 9 months, pyrazinamide for the first 2 months
INH plus rifampin plus ethambutol for 9 months, pyrazinamide for the first 2 months
INH plus rifampin plus pyrazinamide plus for 9 to 12 months

What is the mechanism of action of INH?

Bacteriocidal against actively growing tubercle bacilli; inhibits synthesis of mycolic acids

What vitamin must be given with INH?

Pyidoxine (B_6)

What are the major side effects of INH, what is the frequency of these effects, and what population is at increased risk?

Hepatotoxicity
10% to 20% of patients develop subclinical evidence, as indicated by increased aspartate aminotransferase (AST) and bilirubin
Rare in patients under 20; significant in patients over 50; concern begins at age 35

What is the mechanism of action of rifampin?	Bacteriocidal; binds to the β-subunit of bacterial RNA polymerase
When is rifampin used alone in the treatment of TB and why?	Never, because of rapid development of resistance
In what other situations is rifampin commonly used?	Prophylaxis for *H. influenza* in exposed pediatric populations Prophylaxis for patients exposed to *N. meningitidis* Prophylaxis for certain types of endocarditis In combination with IV erythromycin for severe *Legionella*
What are the major side effects of rifampin?	GI disturbances Allergic reactions Hepatotoxicity Orange coloration of tears, urine, sweat, saliva, and feces
What are the major side effects of pyrazinamide?	Hepatotoxicity Hyperuricemia
What is the major side effect of ethambutol?	Retrobulbar neuritis
What agents is acyclovir effective against?	Herpes simplex virus 1, herpes simplex virus 2, varicella-zoster virus, Epstein-Barr virus, CMV
Is acyclovir effective in the treatment of HSV-caused encephalitis?	Yes
Is acyclovir an effective cure of genital herpes (HSV-2)?	No, it only relieves symptoms, it does not cure the disease
How does acyclovir work?	It inhibits HSV-DNA polymerase, causing chain termination
What is ganciclovir used for?	Life and sight-threatening CMV infection

Is ganciclovir effective against HSV-1 and HSV-2?

Yes, it is effective against both, but is not used often because of toxicities

What are the adverse effects of ganciclovir?

Bone marrow suppression
CNS toxicities (e.g., headache, psychosis, seizures, coma)

Are prophylactic antibiotics indicated for a patient undergoing a clean surgical procedure?

No

When are prophylactic antibiotics recommended (hint: DOG-COP-HAVE-CAB)?

Debridement cannot be performed
Orthopedic situations (e.g., open fractures, penetrating joint injuries, joint prosthesis)
Gross bacterial contamination is known to have occurred
Clean-contaminated operation
Oropharyngeal cavity is entered in continuity with neck dissection
Penetrating injuries of the hollow intra-abdominal viscus
Hysterectomy (abdominal or vaginal)
Amputation of extremity with impaired blood supply
Valvular heart damage is present
Emergency operation with pre-existing or recently active infection
Clostridial-prone injuries (e.g., devitalized muscle, heavy contamination, impaired blood supply)
Accidental wounds with heavy contamination and tissue damage, or those in which surgical therapy is unavoidably delayed
Bowel surgery (e.g., large and small bowel resection and anastomosis)

When is prophylactic antibiotic therapy ineffective?

When continuing contamination is apt to occur (BICUT):
Burns or other open wounds
Immunologically deficient patients or those receiving immunosuppressive therapy
Central indwelling venous lines
Urinary catheters (indwelling)
Tracheostomies or tracheal intubation to prevent pulmonary infections

What oral antibiotics are generally used as preparation for colon surgery and why?

Neomycin and erythromycin, because they are nonabsorbable and have some anaerobic activity

What other IV antibiotics can be used for large bowel preparation and when should they be administered?

Cefoxitin, cefotetan, and gentamycin plus clindamycin; they should be given immediately before, during, and after an operation

What are the most popular antibiotics for topical irrigation?

Kanamycin, first generation cephalosporins, bacitracin

What are some problems associated with the indiscriminate or blind use of antibiotics?

Secondary or superinfections with antibiotic-resistant strains
Hypersensitivity reactions
Postponement of indicated surgical treatment
Development of antibiotic resistant strains

What is a superinfection?

A new infection that develops during antibiotic treatment for the original infection

What percentage of hospitalized patients receiving antibiotics develop superinfections?

2% to 10%

What are the two best preventions against superinfections?

1) Limiting the dose and duration of antibiotic treatment
2) Being alert to the possibility of superinfections

What is the most common type of superinfection to occur after therapy for intra-abdominal infections?

Respiratory tract infection

Besides respiratory tract infections, what other superinfection is relatively common?

Antibiotic-associated colitis

What is the etiology of antibiotic-associated colitis?	*C. difficile*
Which antibiotics are known to cause antibiotic-associated colitis?	All except vancomycin and metronidazole
What is the most important aspect of treating antibiotic-associated colitis?	Suspecting it
Name three ways of diagnosing antibiotic-associated colitis.	1) Endoscopy 2) Stool assay for toxin 3) Stool culture to recover *C. difficile*
How is antibiotic-associated colitis treated?	1) Supportive therapy with fluid and electrolytes 2) Withdrawal of offending antibiotic if possible 3) Oral vancomycin or metronidazole
In treating *C. difficile colitis*, which antibiotic is the drug of choice and why?	Metronidazole (PO), because of decreased cost compared with vancomycin and decreased likelihood of patient becoming infected with vancomycin-resistant *Enterococcus* (VRE)

SPECIFIC MICRO-ORGANISMS

What are the most common organisms recovered in nosocomial bacteremia?	Coagulase-negative *Staphylococcus*
Can coagulase-negative *Staphylococcus* cause serious disease?	Yes
What types of patients are especially susceptible to coagulase-negative staphylococcal infections?	Those compromised by trauma, extensive surgical procedures, metabolic diseases, or invasive vascular devices

What are the most common types of infection caused by coagulase-negative *Staphylococcus*?

Endocarditis, prosthetic joint infections, vascular graft infections, postsurgical mediastinitis

What is the most common infection caused by coagulase-negative *Staphylococcus* and how is it usually treated?

Intravascular device-associated infection
Removal of device (seldom requires drug therapy)

What is the drug of choice for coagulase-negative staphylococcal infections and why?

Vancomycin, because the majority of coagulase-negative staphylococcal infections are methicillin-resistant

What is the most common pathogen associated with infections in wounds and incisions?

S. aureus

Is *S. aureus* coagulase-positive or coagulase-negative?

Coagulase-positive

Can any coagulase-positive *Staphylococcus* organisms be treated with penicillin?

No; it must be assumed that all coagulase-positive *Staphylococcus* organisms are resistant to penicillin and therefore should be treated by a penicillinase-resistant antibiotic

In which disease and patient population is methicillin-resistant *S. aureus* (MRSA) especially prominent?

Endocarditis associated with IV drug use

What is the drug of choice in the treatment of MRSA?

Vancomycin

Is MRSA more pathogenic than other staphylococci?

No, it is simply more difficult to treat secondary to antibiotic resistance

What are the four major types of clinically important streptococcal species?

β-hemolytic
α-hemolytic
S. pneumoniae
Enterococcus

Are all of the four previously mentioned groups of streptococci uniformly sensitive to penicillin G?

All except *Enterococcus*

From what sites are enterococci commonly recovered?

Intra-abdominal infections; however, they are rarely recovered alone

What is the role of enterococci in intra-abdominal infections?

Unknown, but in animal models they have been clearly shown to increase the virulence of other bacteria

In what two systems have enterococci been shown to clearly cause significant disease?

Urinary and biliary tracts

How are enterococcal infections usually treated?

Although no single antibiotic is reliably effective for eradicating deep-seeded infections or bacteremia, the most effective antibiotic combination is gentamycin combined with either ampicillin (or another advanced generation penicillin) or with vancomycin

What are the two most important clinically isolated species of enterococcus in humans leading to VRE?

E. faecalis
E. faecium

As of 1993, approximately what percentage of enterococci isolated from ICU patients were vancomycin resistant?

15%

Why is VRE such a problem?

Because most of these organisms are also resistant to penicillins and aminoglycosides (VRE is a misnomer; the organisms should be called multiple drug—resistant enterococci)

What is teicoplanin?

A glycopeptide antibiotic related to vancomycin

Is teicoplanin more or less effective against enterococci than vancomycin?

More effective

How have VRE been treated traditionally?

Synergistically with high level aminoglycosides and cell-wall active agents (β-lactams and glycopeptides)

For urinary tract infections with VRE, what drug is often effective and why?

Nitrofurantoin, because it reaches therapeutic levels only in urine

What family of gram-negative rods is most commonly associated with surgical infection and how is it metabolically classified?

Enterobacteriaceae
Facultative anaerobes

Name the three "easy" to treat genera within Enterobacteriaceae in terms of sensitivity to a broad variety of antibiotics.

Escherichia
Proteus
Klebsiella (think: **EPK—E**asy **P**ests to **K**ill)

Name the four "hard" to treat genera within Enterobacteriaceae in terms of having the greatest intrinsic antibiotic resistance.

Serratia
Enterobacter
Morganella
Providencia (think: **SEMP,** as in Semper Fi, marines, and tough to kill)

Which genera within Enterobacteriaceae ("easy" or "hard") are more commonly found in hospital-acquired and postoperative surgical infections?

"Hard"

What are the two most common obligate aerobic gram-negative rods found in surgical infections?

Pseudomonas
Acinetobacter

What types of infections are *Pseudomonas* and *Acinetobacter* most commonly associated with in surgical patients?

1) Hospital-associated pneumonia
2) Peritoneal cavity infections
3) Severe soft-tissue infections

Why can *Pseudomonas* and *Acinetobacter* be particularly difficult to treat?

They are often antibiotic resistant, even to the most specific and effective antibiotics, and therefore must be treated with combination antibiotics until in vitro susceptibility testing results are received. Combination drugs can even be continued after test results are received, because both genera tend to develop resistance to antibiotics during therapy.

Does treatment with two different antibiotics in *Pseudomonas* or *Acinetobacter* infections reduce the rate of development of resistance?

No, it simply provides a backup if the strains become resistant to one of the antibiotics

What broad class of bacteria are the most numerous inhabitants of the GI tract, including the mouth?

Anaerobes

What is the most common anaerobic isolate from surgical infections?

B. fragilis

What does the recovery of anaerobes from a soft tissue infection or from blood imply about the site of infection? Why?

They indicate that the site is a focus of dead tissue, because they only grow in settings with low oxidation—reduction potential that are incompatible with the survival of mammalian tissue.

What else does an anaerobic infection usually imply and why?

A defect in the anatomic integrity of the GI tract, because the GI tract is a predominant source of anaerobes

What do *Clostridium* organisms need for growth and invasion?

Despite an ability to survive while exposed to oxygen, they require an anaerobic environment for growth, invasion and elaboration of toxins.

What is the classic description of clostridia seen under a microscope with Gram stain?

Gram-positive, spore-forming rods

What would a Gram stain of clostridia recovered from a soft-tissue infection look like?

Gram-positive rods without spores, because in human infections clostridia do not form spores

What two anaerobes are notorious for being resistant to β-lactam antibiotics (hint: both are *Bacteroides*)?

B. fragilis
B. thetaiotaomicron

What are the most effective antibiotics against these species?

Metronidazole
Clindamycin
Imipenem
Ticarcillin-clavulanic acid
CAM

True or false: *Candida* organisms recovered from open wounds usually represent true invasion and infection?

False; usually only contamination

In what cases are *Candida* infections usually found in surgical patients?

As opportunistic invaders in patients with serious surgical infections who have received broad-spectrum antibiotic treatment that suppresses normal endogenous flora

What can be done to prevent these opportunistic *Candida* infections?

Judicious use of systemic broad-spectrum antibiotics
Prophylaxis with oral nystatin or ketoconazole when broad-spectrum antibiotics are required

Which three blood-borne viruses are especially of concern in surgical patients receiving blood transfusions?

HIV, HBV, HCV

Which type of bacteria is associated with colon cancer?	*Clostridium septicum*

POSTOPERATIVE FEVER

True or false: Fever in the first 3 days after an operation is most likely to have a noninfectious etiology?	True
What percentage of infected postoperative patients are afebrile?	Greater than 50%
What percentage of postoperative febrile patients are not infected?	Greater than 50%
What are the two most likely infectious causes of fever within the first 36 hours of an operation?	1) Injury to the bowel with intraperitoneal leak (characterized by hemodynamic changes, tachycardia, hypotension, decreased urine output, diffuse abdominal tenderness, increased fluid requirements) 2) Invasive soft-tissue infection beginning in the wound secondary to β-hemolytic streptococci or *Clostridium* (usually *C. perfringens*)
What is the most common nonsurgical infection in postoperative patients?	Urinary tract infection
What type of nosocomial infection is the leading cause of death in surgical patients?	Lower respiratory tract infection
What are some of the most common nonsurgical causes of postoperative infection and fever?	Urinary tract infections, respiratory tract infections, IV catheter–associated infections, atelectasis, DVT, and medications

After an abdominal operation, what is one of the common causes of lower lung—field atelectasis and/or pleural effusion?	Inflammatory process below the diaphragm

SOFT-TISSUE INFECTIONS

Name two pathogens in impetigo.	*S. pyogenes* and *S. aureus*
What is the appropriate treatment?	Penicillin/cloxacillin/dicloxacillin/first generation cephalosporins/macrolide
What is the most common pathogen in each of the following disorders: Bullous impetigo? Folliculitis? Furuncles? Carbuncles? What is the appropriate treatment for each?	**Pathogen:** S aureus (for all) **Treatment:** Penicillin/cloxacillin/ dicloxacillin/first generation cephalosporins/ macrolide (for all)/ drainage
What is the clinical difference between cellulitis and erysipelas?	Cellulitis usually has an indistinct border, whereas erysipelas has a sharp line of demarcation between the involved and the uninvolved skin.
What is the etiologic agent of erysipelas?	*S. pyogenes* (β-hemolytic)
What is the appropriate treatment of erysipelas?	Penicillin/first generation cephalosporins/ macrolide
What are the four characteristics of cellulitis?	Tenderness, edema, blanching erythema, local pain
What bacteria can cause cellulitis?	*S. pyogenes*, *S.aureus*, *S. pneumoniae*, other streptococci, *H. influenza*, aerobic and anaerobic gram-negative bacteria
What are the two most common pathogens in uncomplicated cellulitis?	*S. pyogenes* and *S. aureus*

What is the appropriate therapy?

Nafcillin/oxacillin/cloxacillin/dicloxacillin/ first generation cephalosporins/macrolide

What is an abscess?

It is an infection with a necrotic center without a blood supply, composed of dead and dying white cells, blood, plasma, and bacteria. It also has a semiliquid center surrounded by a vascularized zone of inflammatory tissue.

How does a subcutaneous abscess present clinically and is it differentiated from cellulitis?

It presents as localized swelling with inflammation and tenderness. Cellulitis is a soft-tissue infection with intact blood supply and viable tissue with acute inflammatory response (resolves with antibiotic therapy if given before tissue death occurs).

In what anatomic areas are abscesses notoriously difficult to diagnose?

Perirectal area, breast, posterior neck and upper back, and distal phalanx of the finger

What should always be considered when diagnosing a perirectal abscess?

Fistula

What percentage of perirectal abscesses will develop a fistula communicating with the anal crypt?

50%

What are the most common bacteria associated with perirectal abscesses?

Aerobic and anaerobic gram-negative

What are the most likely pathogens in abscesses of the head and neck, axilla, and below the waist?

Head and neck—*S. aureus,* often combined with streptococci
Axilla—gram-negative rods
Below the waist—mixed aerobic and anaerobic gram-negative flora

What is the most common cause of breast abscess?

S. aureus (occasionally gram-negative rods), often in nursing mothers

What is the most important means of preventing *Clostridium* infections?

Surgical debridement with removal of all devitalized tissue

What action is most important in diagnosing and treating any necrotizing soft-tissue infection (NSTI) ?

Operative exploration with definitive treatment

What are some of the earliest signs of a NSTI?

1) Rapid progression of a soft-tissue infection
2) Marked hemodynamic response to infection
3) Apparent cellulitis with ecchymosis, bullae, dermal gangrene, and crepitus

Why are NSTIs difficult to diagnose?

Absence of clear local boundaries or palpable limits
Relatively normal appearance of overlying skin (often)

What distinguishes NSTIs from "uncomplicated" soft tissue infections?

NSTIs are characterized by the absence of clear local boundaries or palpable limits. They are also marked by a layer of necrotic tissue that is not walled off, and the overlying skin has a relatively normal appearance.

What are the most common species of *Clostridium* found in infections?

C. perfringens
C. novyi
C. septicum

What is the most common and essentially only cause of a nonclostridial NSTI in which there has not been a prior injury or operation?

β-hemolytic streptococci (e.g., *S. pyogenes*)

What are the primary differences between a clostridial and nonclostridial NSTI?

A clostridial NSTI involves underlying muscle (e.g., clostridial myonecrosis or gas gangrene). A nonclostridial NSTI involves subcutaneous fascia (e.g., necrotizing fasciitis).

What are the most common causes of postoperative/postinjury NSTIs?

Mixed bacterial species (aerobic and anaerobic pathogens—gram-positive and gram-negative; similar spectrum to that seen in intra-abdominal infections)

What are the most common pathogens in dog/cat bites?

P. multocida, Staphylococcus (coagulase positive or negative), *Streptococcus, Bacteroides, Fusobacteria*

What is the appropriate therapy?

Amoxicillin-clavulanic acid/ampicillin-sulbactam

What are the most common pathogens in human bites?

Streptococcus, S. aureus, H. parainfluenza, K. pneumoniae, Eikenella corrodens, Bacteroides, Fusobacterium, anaerobic cocci

What is the appropriate therapy?

Amoxicillin-clavulanic acid; ampicillin-sulbactam

What else must be considered in the treatment of animal and human bites?

Tetanus prophylaxis

Does tetanus antitoxin effectively prevent infection with *C. tetani?*

No, it only inactivates the toxin that is produced as a result of the infection

Should a previously unimmunized patient receive tetanus toxoid, in addition to tetanus antitoxin?

Yes

What is a felon?

A purulent collection in the distal phalanx of the finger that causes intense pain and pressure in that compartment

What is a carbuncle?

A subcutaneous abscess, usually formed by a confluent infection of multiple contiguous hair follicles

Where are carbuncles usually found and what bacteria is the most common cause?

Posterior neck and upper back
S. aureus

What is lymphangitis and how does it present?	Inflammation of lymphatic channels in subcutaneous tissues Visible red streaks; may lead to lymphadenitis (inflammation of lymph nodes)

INTRA-ABDOMINAL INFECTIONS

What percentage of all primary laparotomies are followed by an operation for intra-abdominal infection?	2%
What percentage of all serious intra-abdominal infections occur postoperatively?	Approximately 50%
What are some of the systemic responses to intra-abdominal or retroperitoneal (RP) infection?	Fluid shifts (similar to those in burn patients), fever, tachycardia, hypotension, hypermetabolic response (catabolic response)
What types of intra-abdominal and RP infections do not require surgical intervention?	Pyelonephritis, salpingitis, amebic liver abscess, enteritis, spontaneous bacterial peritonitis, some cases of diverticulitis and cholangitis
What must the surgeon keep in mind even after promptly performing surgery and initiating the proper antibiotic regimen in a patient with a surgical intra-abdominal or RP infection?	There is significant likelihood that a change in antibiotics and/or re-operation may be necessary.
When a patient is diagnosed with an intra-abdominal infection, what does initial treatment consist of?	1) Cardiorespiratory support 2) Antibiotic therapy 3) Operative intervention

What three factors increase the risk of death or serious complication from intra-abdominal/RP infection?	1) Advanced age 2) Preexisting serious underlying disease 3) Malnutrition
How many bacterial species do most intra-abdominal infections yield?	Three to five different aerobic and anaerobic pathogens
In most cases, how long is it before responsible bacteria and their sensitivities are known?	**Bacteria:** at least 24 hours **Sensitivities:** 48 to 72 hours
What is the classic empiric antibiotic combination for initial treatment of intra-abdominal infection?	Ampicillin (broad spectrum), aminoglycosides (gram-negative coverage) plus clindamycin or metronidazole (anaerobic coverage)
For community acquired intra-abdominal infection in a patient who is not severely ill, which antibiotics are often employed initially? Why?	Cefoxitin or cefotetan, because they are effective against gram-positive, nonresistant gram-negative, and anaerobic organisms
When is the optimal time to obtain an abdominal CT to check for a postoperative intra-abdominal abscess?	7 to 10 days postoperative
Is electrocautery for midline abdominal incision associated with a higher wound infection rate?	No
What are some clinical symptoms of an abscess?	Persistent spiking fever, dull pain, anorexia, and weight loss
Why do abscesses enlarge?	Toxins and enzymes from bacteria, along with proteolytic enzymes from dying macrophages, liquefy abscess contents, thus increasing osmotic pressure and water content, and, consequently, pressure.

Do abscesses have a low or high potassium concentration versus serum K⁺?

High (up to 17 mmol)

Which is superior in the diagnosis of intra-abdominal abscess, CT or US?

CT

What do all intra-abdominal/RP abscesses require in terms of successful treatment?

Drainage (open or CT guided)

When is an intra-abdominal/RP abscess amenable to CT-guided drainage?

If it is single and there is a straight path through the abdominal wall that does not transgress the bowel

When a single subphrenic or subhepatic abscess is not amenable to CT-guided drainage, what is the next most desirable approach and why?

Drainage via an extra-peritoneal subcostal or posterior twelfth rib approach, because it does not expose the entire peritoneal cavity to the contents of the abscess

What is a RP phlegmon and how is it treated?

Also known as necrotizing cellulitis, this rare condition is usually associated with extravasation of infected urine. It requires extensive debridement, similar to that used to treat necrotizing fasciitis.

What are some alternative drainage approaches to certain pelvic abscesses besides transabdominal/ pelvic?

Transrectal or transvaginal drainage

When an abscess is drained, what role do antibiotics play?

They prevent bacterial infection in the tissue planes around the abscess.

When should antibiotic therapy be initiated in the treatment of an abscess?

Before percutaneous or operative drainage

What antibiotics should always be included in the treatment regimen for an abscess?	Metronidazole or another **anaerobic** drug
How long should antibiotics be given in the treatment of an abscess?	Until all signs of sepsis have resolved and the patient's appetite and sense of well being return
Is it necessary to continue antibiotic therapy until all drains are removed?	No
Why are antibiotics ineffective against abscesses?	They penetrate the abscess poorly and most bacteria in abscesses are not actively dividing
What is peritonitis?	Inflammation of the peritoneum
What is secondary peritonitis?	The presence of purulent exudate in the abdominal cavity from an enteric source
What is the most common form of acute intra-abdominal infection?	Peritonitis secondary to bowel perforation
What is implied if Gram stain of peritoneal fluid only shows gram-positive cocci? What if it only shows mixed flora? What if it only shows gram-negative rods?	**Gram-positive cocci**—likely primary spontaneous bacterial peritonitis (SBP) Mixed—likely bowel perforation Gram-negative rods—either primary or secondary peritonitis
What typically happens to WBC count in peritonitis?	Leukocytosis or leukopenia (because of recruitment of leukocytes to inflamed peritoneum)
Above and below what WBC count is mortality significantly increased in peritonitis?	Greater than 25,000 and less than 4,000
Why does polymicrobial peritonitis have a poor prognosis?	Mixed flora act synergistically (especially a combination of aerobes and anaerobes)

Why and how do aerobes and anaerobes work synergistically in peritonitis?

Aerobes increase virulence of anaerobes by decreasing redox potential and elaborating essential nutrients
Anaerobes increase virulence of aerobes by elaborating enzymes that destroy antibiotics

What is the relationship between mortality risk and total number of bacteria present in peritonitis?

Direct

What are the most common bacterial causes of polymicrobial peritonitis?

E. coli, Bacteroides, anaerobic and aerobic streptococci, Enterococcus, Clostridium

How much fluid can an increase in thickness of peritoneum of only 1 mm potentially sequester?

18 L

How is peritonitis in peritoneal dialysis patients diagnosed?

By one of the following three signs:
1) Positive culture from peritoneal fluid
2) Cloudy diasylate fluid
3) Clinical evidence

Which two organisms are most commonly found in patients with peritonitis secondary to CAPD and how often do these infections occur?

S. aureus and S. epidermidis
66% of patients

What are the three most common organisms found in CAPD patients with peritonitis and how are they treated?

Coagulase-negative staphylococci, S. aureus, enteric gram-negative rods
IP vancomycin plus gentamycin (may also require systemic therapy)

What is the initial treatment of dialysis-related peritonitis?

Antibiotics
Heparin in dialysate
Increased dwell time of dialysate fluid

What are the five relative indications for removal of a catheter in dialysis-related peritonitis?

1) Persistence of peritonitis after 4 to 5 days of therapy
2) Fungal or TB peritonitis
3) Fecal peritonitis
4) Pseudomonal peritonitis
5) Severe skin catheter–site infection

Which general age population is more likely to develop primary SBP?

Adults (no difference in incidence between genders)

Specifically, which two diseases in adults are most commonly associated with primary SBP?

Cirrhosis and systemic lupus

What other intra-abdominal pathology is present in most adults who develop primary SBP?

Ascites

Is primary SBP more likely to be polymicrobial or monomicrobial?

Monomicrobial

What is the order of frequency of etiologies of primary SBP among gram-negative rods, anaerobes, and gram-positive cocci?

Gram-negative rods—70%
Gram-positive cocci—20%
Anaerobes—10%

What is the most common bacterial cause of primary SBP (specific organism)?

E. coli

In children, which two organisms are the most common causes of primary SBP?

Hemolytic streptococcus
Pneumococcus

What two types of pre-existing infection are common in children who develop primary SBP?

Ear infection
Upper respiratory tract infection

What two underlying diseases in children are associated with increased incidence of primary SBP?

Nephrotic syndrome
Systemic lupus

True or false: The majority of children who develop primary SBP have ascites?

False

What diagnostic test confirms the diagnosis of primary SBP?	Peritoneal tap
What four tests/procedures should be done on peritoneal fluid?	1) PMN cell count 2) pH 3) Gram stain 4) Culture
Which of the previously listed tests is most sensitive and specific in making the diagnosis?	PMN cell count
What PMN cell count is considered positive for primary SBP?	250/mm^3
In primary SBP, is the pH of the ascitic fluid generally high or low?	Low
Of those cultures that come back positive in primary SBP, what fraction will contain bacteria evident on Gram stain?	1/3
How should primary SBP be treated?	With antibiotic therapy
Which bacteria are the most common pathogens in secondary peritonitis?	Enteric gram-negative rods, *B. fragilis, Bacteroides,* anaerobic cocci
What two other organisms must also be considered in secondary peritonitis?	*Enterococcus* and *Candida*
Which two antibiotics are notorious for producing symptoms mimicking peritonitis?	INH Erythromycin estolate
Fungal peritonitis most commonly occurs in which group of patients?	Those treated with continuous ambulatory peritoneal dialysis (CAPD)

Why is TB peritonitis of such concern again in this country?	Because of the increased prevalence of AIDS
What are the clinical manifestations of TB peritonitis?	Fever, anorexia, weakness, weight loss, mild ascites, dull and diffuse abdominal pain
What are the two phases of TB peritonitis and how are they characterized?	**Moist**—early onset, presence of fever, ascites, abdominal pain, and weakness **Dry**—late onset, no ascites present, formation of dense adhesions
What is present in the peritoneal fluid of patients with TB peritonitis?	Lymphocytes, tubercle bacilli (80% of the time if more than 1 L is taken), increased protein, less than 30 mg/dl glucose
Laparoscopically, how will TB peritonitis classically appear?	**Stalactite-like fibrinous masses** hanging from parietal peritoneum in the lower abdomen
How long must TB peritonitis be treated, and with how many anti-TB drugs?	Three drugs for 2 years
Typhoid perforation, though rare in the United States and Europe, is very common in third world nations. How is this type of perforation treated?	Surgical closure of the perforation, followed by antibiotic treatment with cefotaxime and metronidazole
What are the most common causes of pancreatic abscess?	Same as those of secondary peritonitis plus *S. aureus*
What is the appropriate therapy?	Third generation cephalosporins plus metronidazole Imipenem Cefoxitin/cefotetan plus gentamycin Ticarcillin-clavulanic acid plus gentamycin Surgical drainage

How must most pancreatic abscesses be approached and why?	Transabdominally, because they usually consist of diffusely infected, necrotic, peripancreatic RP tissue
True or false: Recovery of *Candida* from an established intra-abdominal abscess or from urine and sputum in an otherwise compromised patient may warrant therapy?	True
Intra-abdominal *Candida* infections are more commonly found following what intra-abdominal disease?	Severe pancreatitis
How are these intra-abdominal *Candida* infections treated (drug, dose, and length of treatment)?	Amphotericin B, 3 to 5 mg/kg over 10 to 14 days/débridement
What are the most common causes of liver abscess?	Same as those of secondary peritonitis and pancreatitis, but amebic abscess must also be considered
What is the appropriate therapy?	Same as for pancreatic abscess (antibiotics drainage), except for amebic abscess (usually no drainage; metronidazole instead)
What are the most common causes of splenic abscess?	*S. aureus, Streptococcus,* enteric gram-negative rods
What is the appropriate therapy?	Third generation cephalosporins/ imipenem
In what other condition does splenic abscess commonly occur?	Endocarditis
What bacteria can cause splenic abscess in patients with sickle cell anemia?	*Salmonella*

Infection with which micro-organism commonly mimics acute appendicitis?	*Yersinia enterocolitica*
What are the most common causes (infectious) of acute cholecystitis and cholangitis?	**Enteric gram-negative rods**, anaerobes (including *Bacteroides*), *Clostridium, Fusobacterium,* and *Enterococcus*
What is the appropriate therapy?	Third generation cephalosporins plus metronidazole Imipenem Ticarcillin-clavulanic acid Ampicillin-sulbactam Cefoxitin/cefotetan plus gentamycin
Which organisms are asplenic patients susceptible to and why?	*S. pneumoniae, H. influenza, N. meningitidis, N. gonorrhea,* some *E. coli,* and some *K. pneumonia* Encapsulated organisms
In a postsplenectomy patient, which vaccines should be administered?	They should receive pneumococcal polyvalent, *H. influenza* (type b), and meningococcal vaccines prior to or after splenectomy (best if given **before** splenectomy).

SPECIFIC INFECTIOUS CONDITIONS

What are the likely pathogens in acute sinusitis?	*S. pneumoniae, H. influenza*
What is the appropriate therapy?	Amoxicillin-clavulanic acid/second generation cephalosporins/trimethoprim-sulfamethoxazole/clarithromycin
What are the likely pathogens in chronic sinusitis?	*S. pneumoniae, H. influenza,* anaerobes, *S. aureus,* gram-negative rods
What is the appropriate therapy?	Amoxicillin-clavulanic acid/second generation cephalosporins plus metronidazole Surgical drainage (possibly)

Which population is at particular risk for otitis externa?	Patients with diabetes
What are the two most likely pathogens?	*S. aureus* and *P. aeruginosa*
What are the three most likely pathogens in otitis media/mastoiditis?	*S. pneumoniae, H. influenza, M. catarrhalis*
What is the appropriate therapy?	Amoxycillin-clavulanic acid/second generation cephalosporins
What are the two most likely pathogens in acute parotitis?	*S. aureus* and mumps virus
What is the appropriate therapy?	Nafcillin/oxacillin/vancomycin Expression of pus from the duct
What are the most likely pathogens in odontogenic infections?	Aerobic and anaerobic streptococci, *Fusobacterium, Bacteroides*
What is the appropriate therapy?	Amoxicillin-clavulanic acid/ampicillin-sulbactam/clindamycin/penicillin plus metronidazole Surgical drainage (possibly)
What are the three most common pathogens in suppurative thyroiditis?	*S. aureus, S. pyogenes, S. pneumoniae*
What is the appropriate therapy?	Nafcillin, oxacillin, or vancomycin
What are the likely pathogens in an acute exacerbation of chronic bronchitis?	*S. pneumoniae, H. influenza, M. catarrhalis, Mycoplasma pneumoniae, Chlamydia pneumoniae,* viruses
What is the appropriate therapy?	Amoxicillin-clavulanic acid/trimethoprim-sulfamethoxazole/second generation cephalosporins/clarithromycin/azithromycin

What are the most common pathogens in community-acquired pneumonia (CAP)?

S. pneumoniae, H. influenza, Legionella pneumophila, Mycoplasma pneumoniae, Chlamydia pneumoniae, S. aureus, influenza virus

What is the appropriate therapy?

Second generation cephalosporins/third generation cephalosporins/amoxycillin-clavulanic acid/erythromycin (for pneumonia)/amantadine (for influenza)

What are the clinical differences associated with atypical CAP?

Young patients, less acute disease, myalgias, headache

What pathogens cause atypical CAP?

M. pneumoniae, L. pneumoniae, C. pneumoniae

What is the appropriate therapy?

Erythromycin, clarithromycin, azithromycin

In addition to the normal CAP pathogens, what two other pathogens are of concern in a patient with cystic fibrosis who presents with pneumonia/bronchitis/bronchiectasis?

S. aureus and *P. aeruginosa*

What are the likely pathogens in community-acquired aspiration pneumonia?

P. melaninogenica, Bacteroides, Fusobacterium, aerobic and anaerobic streptococci

What is the appropriate therapy?

Clindamycin/cefoxitin/cefotetan/amoxicillin-clavulanic acid/ampicillin-sulbactam

What are the likely pathogens in nosocomial aspiration pneumonia?

Same as CAP plus enteric **gram-negative rods** and *S. aureus*

What is the appropriate therapy?

Imipenem/ticarcillin-clavulanic acid/
  ceftazidime plus clindamycin/
  clindamycin plus aztreonam/
  ciprofloxacin/gentamycin
If *Pseudomonas* organisms are present,
  gentamycin should be added

What are the likely pathogens in an empyema?	*S. aureus, S. pneumoniae, S. pyogenes*
What is the appropriate therapy?	Nafcillin, oxacillin, or vancomycin Drainage via chest tube (essential)
What are the likely pathogens in acute pyelonephritis?	*E. coli, Proteus, Klebsiella, Enterobacter, Enterococcus*
What is the appropriate therapy?	Third generation cephalosporins/ trimethoprim-sulfamethoxazole/ ampicillin-sulbactam/ciprofloxacin/ ofloxacin/piperacillin/ticarcillin/ ticarcillin-clavulanic acid Evaluation for obstruction
In addition to the previously mentioned pathogens associated with acute pyelonephritis, what other pathogen is associated with chronic pyelonephritis?	*P. aeruginosa*
How is it treated?	The same as acute pyelonephritis, plus gentamycin
What are the likely pathogens in cystitis and lower urinary tract infections?	*E. coli, S. saprophyticus, C. trachomata,* other enteric gram-negative rods, *Enterococcus*
What is the appropriate therapy?	Trimethoprim-sulfamethoxazole/ quinolones/amoxicillin-clavulanic acid/ first, second, or third generation cephalosporins/nitrofurantoin
What are the likely pathogens in prostatitis?	Enteric gram-negative rods, *N. gonorrhea, C. trachomata*
What is the appropriate therapy?	Ofloxacin/ciprofloxacin/trimethoprim- sulfamethoxazole Therapy is often necessary for 1 to 3 months

What are the likely pathogens in urethritis?	*N. gonorrhea, C. trachomata* (patient must be treated for both)
What is the appropriate therapy?	***N. gonorrhea***—ceftriaxone (500 mg IM) ***C. trachomata***—doxycycline (100 mg PO twice daily for 14 days)
What are the likely pathogens in epididymitis?	*N. gonorrhea* and *C. trachomata*, gram negative
What is the appropriate therapy?	Ceftriaxone (250 mg IM) plus doxycycline (100 mg PO twice daily for 10 days)
What are the likely pathogens in cervicitis?	*N. gonorrhea* and *C. trachomata*
What is the appropriate therapy?	Same as that of urethritis
What are the likely pathogens in pelvic inflammatory disease?	*N. gonorrhea, C. trachomata*, gram-negative rods, anaerobes
What else must be considered in a workup for pelvic inflammatory disease?	Retained IUD
What is the most common etiology of bacterial vaginosis?	*Gardnerella vaginalis*
What is the appropriate therapy?	Metronidazole (500 mg PO twice daily for 7 days) Clindamycin (intravaginal cream daily for 7 days) Metronidazole (intravaginal gel twice daily for 5 days)
Name three laboratory characteristics of bacterial vaginosis.	Positive amine odor test pH greater than 4.5 Clue cells
What are the three most likely body sources of sepsis?	Urinary tract, skin, gut

What are the likely pathogens in urinary sepsis?

Enteric gram-negative rods and *Enterococcus*

What is the appropriate therapy?

Third generation cephalosporins/ aztreonam/imipenem/ciprofloxacin/ ofloxacin/piperacillin/mezlocillin/ azlocillin/ticarcillin/ticarcillin- clavulanic acid
All of the above plus gentamycin

What are the likely pathogens in skin-source sepsis?

Staphylococcus and *streptococcus*

What is the appropriate therapy?

Nafcillin, oxacillin, cefazolin, or vancomycin

What are the likely pathogens in burn sepsis?

S. aureus, Enterobacter, S. pyogenes, E. faecalis, E. coli, P. aeruginosa

What are the likely pathogens in sepsis of gut source?

Enteric gram-negative rods, *B. fragilis,* anaerobic cocci

What are the likely pathogens in sepsis in a neutropenic patient?

Enteric gram-negative rods (including *Pseudomonas*), *Staphylococcus, S. viridans*

What is the appropriate therapy?

Ticarcillin/piperacillin/mezlocillin/ azlocillin/ticarcillin-clavulanic acid (all plus gentamycin)
Imipenem/ceftazidime
Vancomycin should be added if line sepsis is suspected or when resistant gram-positive cocci are suspected (Mandell, 52–53)

What are the four most common causes of acute inflammatory diarrhea (not C. difficile colitis)?

Campylobacter jejuni, Shigella, Salmonella, E. coli

What is the appropriate therapy?

Ciprofloxacin/ofloxacin/norfloxacin
Trimethoprim-sulfamethoxazole, with or without erythromycin

What clinical sign and laboratory sign indicate acute inflammatory diarrhea, as opposed to noninflammatory diarrhea?	Fever and fecal leukocytes
What are the most common pathogens in acute septic arthritis (children)?	S. aureus, H. influenza, Streptococcus, gram-negative rods
What is the appropriate therapy?	Third generation cephalosporins
What are the most common pathogens in acute septic arthritis (adults)?	S. aureus, N. gonorrhea, gram-negative rods
What is the appropriate therapy?	Third generation cephalosporins/ imipenem
What other disease must be considered in acute arthritis in both children and adults?	Lyme disease
What are the most common pathogens in diabetic foot infections?	Usually mixed (S. aureus, S. epidermidis, Streptococcus, gram-negative rods, anaerobes)
What is the appropriate therapy?	Cefoxitin/cefotetan, with or without gentamycin Imipenem Evaluation for bone involvement
What are the most common pathogens in acute hematogenous osteoarthritis?	S. aureus, gram-negative rods (Salmonella in sickle cell anemia)
What is the appropriate therapy?	Nafcillin/oxacillin/third generation cephalosporins

What are the most common pathogens in septic osteoarthritis secondary to contiguous spread of infection?	*S. aureus,* mixed with gram-negative rods and anaerobes
What is the appropriate therapy?	Nafcillin/oxacillin (both plus gentamycin and metronidazole) Third generation cephalosporins/ quinolone (both plus metronidazole)
What are the most common pathogens in osteoarthritis secondary to vascular insufficiency?	Mixed—especially *S. aureus, S. epidermidis, Streptococcus,* gram-negative rods, anaerobes
What is the appropriate therapy?	Cefoxitin/cefotetan (both plus gentamycin) Imipenem Ciprofloxacin/ofloxacin (both plus metronidazole)
Why does the presence of foreign material increase the potential for serious infectious complications?	It impairs local host defenses, especially PMN function
How should prosthetic device—associated infection be treated?	By removing the infected device
When a life-sustaining prosthetic device (e.g., cardiac valve) becomes infected, how should the infection be treated?	Intensive antibiotic therapy, followed by removal of the device with concurrent antibiotic treatment, and replacement with a new device, followed by prolonged antibiotic treatment

HIV AND THE SURGICAL PATIENT

Acute infection with HIV most commonly appears as what?	Flu-like or mononucleosis-like syndrome
When are HIV antibodies usually first able to be detected after infection?	6 to 8 weeks

How much time can elapse before antibodies become detectable in an HIV-infected patient?

Several years

How can a diagnosis of HIV infection be confirmed in a patient who is antibody negative?

By determining the presence of specific viral antigens or nucleic acids

What are the two currently employed methods of testing for HIV and how do they work?

1) **Enzyme linked immunosorbent assay (ELISA)**—detects the antibody to HIV
2) **Western blot**—demonstrates antibodies against envelope, core proteins, or a full array of HIV proteins (used to confirm a positive ELISA)

What are the three ways in which HIV infection may be transmitted?

1) Sexual contact with partners
2) Direct exposure to contaminated blood or blood products
3) Perinatal transmission

When is AZT prophylaxis recommended for health care workers exposed to HIV?

1) Massive exposure (injections or transfusions of infected blood)
2) Serious parenteral exposures (deep needle sticks)

What is the mechanism of action of AZT?

Inhibits viral reverse transcriptase and terminates chain growth

Does AZT prevent susceptible cells from de novo infection?

Yes, until the viral genome has been incorporated into the host cell's genome

What are some of the more common toxicities associated with AZT?

Granulocytopenia (50%)
Anemia
Headache, nausea, insomnia, myalgias, seizures, neurotoxicity

What are some of the major adverse drug interactions associated with AZT?

Increased bone marrow toxicity by amphotericin B, acetaminophen, aspirin, trimethoprim-sulfamethoxazole, probenecid
Increased neutropenia and hepatotoxicity with α-interferon

Which blood components have been known to transmit HIV?	1) Whole blood 2) PRBCs 3) FFP 4) Cryoprecipitate 5) Platelets 6) Pooled plasma products
What is the estimated risk of acquiring HIV per unit of blood transfused?	4–10:1,000,000
What is the risk of HIV transmission via organ transplantation?	≈1:100,000
Why is there still a risk of contracting HIV via blood products despite all of the current testing and screening procedures?	1) Technical error 2) Inability to detect infected individuals who have not yet developed anti-HIV antibodies
What is the most common esophageal lesion in HIV-infected individuals and what are the three most common causes?	Diffuse esophagitis *C. albicans,* herpesvirus, CMV
What are the symptoms of diffuse esophagitis and what condition is it usually confused with?	Dysphagia and retrosternal discomfort Reflux esophagitis
What empiric therapy is usually initiated for esophagitis?	Ketoconazole and acyclovir
What lesions related to HIV most commonly affect the stomach and duodenum?	Kaposi's sarcoma Non-Hodgkin lymphoma CMV
What is one of the most common cause of upper GI bleeding in HIV-infected individuals?	Kaposi's sarcoma lesions

What negatively affects the prognosis of Kaposi's sarcoma the most: lymph node involvement or visceral involvement?	Visceral involvement
What is the most common cause of stomach/duodenal perforation in HIV patients?	Local CMV infection
What percentage of HIV-infected patients have serologic evidence of previous hepatitis B infection?	95%
What are the most common etiologic agents cultured in HIV-associated acalculias cholecystitis (four Cs)?	*Cryptosporidium* CMV *Campylobacter* *Candida*
What other two biliary tract complications are common in HIV patients?	Papillary stenosis Sclerosing cholangitis
What are the two most common infectious etiologies of papillary stenosis and sclerosing cholangitis?	*Cryptosporidium* CMV
What are the two most common neoplasms affecting the small intestine of HIV patients?	Kaposi's sarcoma Non-Hodgkin lymphoma
What organisms can cause an inflammatory response in HIV patients in the terminal ileum that can often mimic regional enteritis or appendicitis?	*Yersinia* *Campylobacter* *Shigella* *Salmonella* *Mycobacterium avium intracellulare* (MAI)

What is the most common infectious agent causing colon lesions in HIV patients?

CMV

Why are anorectal lesions in AIDS patients treated as conservatively as possible?

Because AIDS patients heal extremely poorly after attempted surgical therapy

Do asymptomatic HIV-infected patients undergoing elective surgical procedures exhibit significantly more problems with wound healing and infection than their uninfected counterparts?

No

TOXIC SHOCK SYNDROME

What is it?

It is a syndrome of fever, hypotension, **skin rash,** and multiple organ failure (MOF). Other symptoms include diarrhea and headache.

What is it caused by?

Exotoxin from S. *aureus*

What are the associated risk factors?

Tampons, pelvic infection, and sinusitis (nasal packing)

18

Anesthesiology

Donald B. Schmit, MD

What is the American Society of Anesthesiologists (ASA) Physical Status Classification? What is its purpose?	It is a status rating (I–VI) assigned to each patient prior to receiving anesthesia. It allows for assessment of anesthetic outcome, but it is not meant to predict anesthetic risk and is independent of the surgery planned.
Describe the following ASA Physical Status categories:	
ASA I	A healthy patient
ASA II	A patient with mild to moderate systemic disease without significant impairment of activity
ASA III	A patient with moderate to severe systemic disease that limits activity
ASA IV	A patient with severe, life-threatening illness
ASA V	A patient who is critically ill and is not expected to live more than 24 hours
ASA VI	A transplant donor
What does the suffix "E" denote in ASA Physical Status rating?	Patients undergoing emergency surgery, regardless of the type of operation or their ASA classification (e.g., emergency appendectomy on an otherwise healthy, young patient: ASA IE)
What are the six indications for endotracheal intubation?	1. When a patent airway must be provided 2. When protection against aspiration is necessary 3. When it is necessary to control ventilation or provide positive pressure ventilation

4. When operative position is not supine
5. When the operative site is in or near the airway
6. When diseases affecting the upper airway are present

What is meant by a "rapid sequence induction"?

1. Preoxygenation (denitrogenation) of the lungs with 100% oxygen
2. Administration of an IV induction agent (thiopental, propofol, etomidate)
3. Administration of a rapidly acting muscle relaxant (succinylcholine, rocuronium)
4. Cricoid pressure
5. Intubation.

Note that cricoid pressure must be maintained until the endotracheal tube cuff is inflated and tracheal placement of the tube is confirmed (by auscultation and/or capnography).

What are the six indications for a rapid sequence induction?

Patients at risk for aspiration of gastric contents:
1. Recent meal/not NPO
2. Symptomatic hiatal hernia or gastroesophageal reflux
3. Delayed gastric emptying (i.e., diabetic gastroparesis)
4. Pregnancy
5. Clinically severe obesity
6. Bowel obstruction

Describe how intraoperative fluids are estimated in each of the following situations:

Deficits

Patients NPO from the night before surgery without IV fluids can be expected to be 500 to 1000 ml deficient (estimated as maintenance requirements times the number of hours NPO). Patients who have received a bowel prep can be expected to be 2 to 3 times more deficient than patients who have not.

Maintenance

Calculated according to the standard method: 60 ml/hr + 10 ml/kg/hr for every kg over 20 kg).

Third-space replacement — Fluids are administered at 4 to 8 ml/kg/hr, depending on the amount of tissue trauma involved (i.e., the expected amount of third spacing that might occur). 4 ml/kg/hr should be administered for superficial and distal extremity cases and up to 8 ml/kg/hr for intra-abdominal cases.

Ongoing losses — Urine is replaced 1:1. Blood is replaced 3:1 with crystalloid (or 1:1 with colloid or blood products).

MUSCLE RELAXANTS

What are the sedative or analgesic properties of neuromuscular blockers (NMB)? — None; patients are unable to move, but they can be fully aware of their surroundings.

What are the two classes of NMB?
1. Depolarizing
2. Nondepolarizing

What is the class, onset, and duration of succinylcholine (Sch)? — Depolarizing, onset less than 1 minute, duration 5 to 10 minutes (T = 3–5 minutes)

What is the primary indication for Sch? — Rapid muscle relaxation for endotracheal intubation or treatment of laryngospasm

What are the potential side effects of Sch?
1. Hypertension
2. Cardiac arrhythmias
3. Tachycardia
4. Bradycardia
5. Increased intracranial pressure
6. Hyperkalemia (usually a 0.5–1 mEq/L increase)
7. Prolonged paralysis (in patients with atypical plasma cholinesterase)
8. Malignant hyperthermia
9. Increased intraocular pressure

Which patients are at greatest risk for Sch-induced hyperkalemia (and for whom is the use of Sch contraindicated)?

Patients with:
1. Burns
2. Massive soft-tissue trauma
3. Spinal cord injury
4. Neurologic/neuromuscular disorders
5. Intraperitoneal sepsis
6. Renal failure (relative contraindication)

Is there a safe period for the use of Sch in acute spinal cord injury patients?

Yes, in the first 24 hours

What is malignant hyperthermia (MH)?

A genetic (autosomal-dominant with variable penetrance) skeletal muscle abnormality that results in a hypermetabolic state when triggered

What agents trigger MH?

SCh, volatile anesthetics

What are the manifestations of MH?

1. Trismus/masseter muscle spasm (considered to be premonitory of MH)
2. Hypercapnia (often the first sign to appear)
3. Tachycardia
4. Tachypnea
5. Temperature elevation (1–2° C every 5 minutes)
6. Hypertension
7. Cardiac dysrhythmias
8. Acidosis
9. Hypoxemia
10. Hyperkalemia
11. Skeletal muscle rigidity
12. Myoglobinuria (CPK > 20,000 within 12–24 hours)
13. DIC

What is the primary drug for treating MH?

Dantrolene

Name three long-acting nondepolarizing muscle relaxants (NDMR).

1. d-Tubocurarine (curare)
2. Pancuronium
3. Metocurine

Name three intermediate-acting NDMRs.

1. Atracurium
2. Vecuronium
3. Rocuronium

Name one (relatively) short-acting NDMR.

Mivacurium

Which NDMRs cause histamine release?

1. Curare
2. Metocurine
3. Atracurium

What is the principal hemodynamic effect of this histamine release?	Decreased blood pressure (and reflex tachycardia)
Which NDMR causes sympathetic nervous system stimulation?	Pancuronium
How is it manifested?	10% to 15% increase in heart rate and blood pressure
What is the advantage of rocuronium?	Rapid onset gives adequate muscle relaxation for rapid sequence intubation in patients with a contraindication to Sch.
What drugs are used to reverse NDMR?	Anticholinesterase drugs (neostigmine or edrophonium), which inhibit the breakdown of acetylcholine
What drugs must be combined with these reversal agents (and why)?	Anticholinergic drugs (glycopyrrolate or atropine) are used to counteract **systemic** cholinergic effects of the anticholinesterases.
What are the systemic cholinergic effects of anticholinesterases?	Vagotonic effects can cause severe bradycardia, as well as crampy abdominal pain and vomiting.

OPIATES

What opiates are commonly used in the OR and ICU?	Morphine and fentanyl; alfentanil and sufentanil are less commonly used
What are the primary therapeutic effects of the opiates?	Analgesia and sedation
What are their effects on respiratory drive?	Decreased respiratory drive is manifested primarily as **decreased respiratory rate** and secondarily as decreased tidal volume.
Which opiate causes the greatest histamine release?	Morphine

Which opiate is the best anxiolytic?	Morphine
What is the most commonly used narcotic antagonist?	Naloxone

BENZODIAZEPINES

What are the four commonly used benzodiazepines (BZD)?	Midazolam, diazepam, lorazepam, chlordiazepoxide; midazolam is practically the only BZD used for anesthesia
What are the clinical effects of BZDs?	Anxiolysis, hypnosis, amnesia, anticonvulsion, and skeletal muscle relaxation (note: no analgesic properties)
Which is the shortest acting BZD?	Midazolam (1.5–3.5 hours)
How are BZDs metabolized, and why is this important?	Hepatically; geriatric and liver failure patients are likely to have prolonged duration of action
What is the BZD antagonist?	Flumazenil

INTRAVENOUS ANESTHETICS

What is the purpose of IV induction agents?	Bolus infusion allows for achievement of rapid unconsciousness. Rapid onset allows the patient to avoid the "second stage" (excitability) of anesthesia. Brief, deep unconsciousness results in adequate conditions for laryngoscopy and tracheal intubation without patient recall (note: these agents have no analgesic properties)
Which three agents are most commonly used for induction?	Thiopental (pentothal), diprivan, and etomidate (methohexital, ketamine, and midazolam are less commonly used)

What are some advantages and disadvantages of thiopental?

It is inexpensive and predictable. It causes dose-dependent blood pressure decreases that can be especially dangerous in hypovolemic patients and in the elderly.

What is the advantage attributed to etomidate?

It produces little hemodynamic change and may be well suited for hemodynamically unstable patients (hypovolemic, frail, or elderly patients; patients with CAD).

What are the advantages of diprivan compared with benzodiazepines or barbiturates when used for sedation?

High lipid solubility allows for:
1. Rapid changes in the level of sedation (when administered by continuous infusion) by simply changing infusion rate
2. Rapid recovery (usually within 10–15 minutes) after a bolus dose or after infusion is stopped
3. Physical dependence does not seem to occur
4. Antiemetic properties (suggested by some studies)

What is the nutritional value of diprivan?

It is suspended in a carrier of 10% intralipids, providing 1.1 kCal per ml (as fat).

What are the CNS effects of ketamine?

It produces a state of "dissociative anesthesia," which is accompanied by amnesia and analgesia. Patients who receive large doses of ketamine can have hallucinations and unpleasant dreams.

What are the respiratory effects of ketamine?

Respiratory drive is largely preserved and laryngeal protective reflexes remain intact.

INHALATION ANESTHETICS

What does "minimum alveolar concentration (MAC)" mean?

It is the concentration of an inhalation agent (at 1 atm) at which 50% of patients do not move in response to surgical stimulation (similar to the ED_{50}).

What are the five most widely used inhalation anesthetics?

1. Nitrous oxide (gas)
2. Halothane
3. Sevoflurane
4. Isoflurane
5. Desflurane

What is the principal intraoperative risk of nitrous oxide?

Diffusion of nitrous oxide into closed gas spaces can cause complications related to the anatomic area involved. The doubling time of the volume of gas in closed or obstructed loops of bowel is about **3 to 4 hours**, whereas the doubling time for gas volume in a pneumothorax can be as little as **10 minutes**.

What does "diffusion hypoxia" mean?

At the cessation of nitrous oxide therapy, the nitrous oxide diffuses rapidly from blood into the alveolar space and can dilute the concentration of inspired oxygen, particularly if the patient is placed on room air. This hypoxia can be prevented by placing the patient on 100% oxygen for 3 to 5 minutes.

Which of the volatile inhalation agents is commonly used for mask (or inhalation) induction? Why?

Halothane, because of the volatile agents it has the least pungent odor and tends to be the least irritating to the respiratory tree

Which of the volatile inhalation agents is most commonly associated with cardiac dysrhythmias? Why?

Halothane, because it sensitizes the myocardium to endogenous (and exogenous) catecholamines

REGIONAL ANESTHESIA

What are the types of regional anesthesia?

Local (infiltration) or topical, peripheral nerve blocks (including ganglionic and plexus blocks), epidural, and spinal

What are the two most commonly used regional anesthetic agents?

Lidocaine and bupivacaine; other less commonly used agents include tetracaine, mepivacaine, procaine, 2-chloroprocaine, prilocaine, etidocaine, and ropivacaine

What are the signs of systemic toxicity from the injection of local anesthetics (in order of increasing toxicity)?

1. Lingular numbness
2. Visual and hearing disturbances
3. Sedation
4. Unconsciousness
5. Seizures
6. Respiratory depression
7. Cardiac arrhythmias
8. Cardiovascular collapse

What is the most common cause of toxic plasma levels of local anesthetics?

Inadvertent intravascular injection

Which local anesthetic is the most cardiotoxic?

Bupivicaine is approximately 16 times more cardiotoxic than lidocaine.

How does the addition of epinephrine alter the peak plasma levels of absorbed local anesthetics?

It decreases the peak level, presumably by causing local vasoconstriction and thus slowing absorption.

How does the addition of epinephrine affect the duration of local anesthetics?

It increases the duration, also presumably by local vasoconstricition.

In what cases is the addition of epinephrine to local anesthetics discouraged?

1. Uncontrolled hypertension
2. Cardiac arrhythmias
3. Unstable angina
4. Uteroplacental insufficiency
5. Local infiltration into tissues with poor or absent collateral blood flow (digits, ears, tip of nose, penis)
6. Regional IV anesthesia

What is a Bier block?

It is the technique of IV regional anesthesia that consists of inserting a small catheter in the affected extremity, exsanguinating the extremity using an Esmarch bandage, inflating a proximal tourniquet, and injecting lidocaine. It provides approximately 30 to 45 minutes of anesthesia for peripheral soft-tissue surgery.

Why are infected tissues difficult to anesthetize with the infiltration of local anesthetics?	Local tissue acidosis present in infected tissues tends to ionize the local anesthetics, preventing their spread and penetration into nerve sheaths.

SPINAL AND EPIDURAL ANESTHESIA

Which are the tissue layers in order from the skin to the spinal canal?

1. Skin
2. Supraspinous ligament
3. Interspinous ligament
4. Ligamentum flavum
5. Epidural space
6. Dura mater
7. Arachnoid mater

What are the contraindications to spinal and epidural anesthesia?

1. Lack of patient consent
2. Skin or soft-tissue infection at the puncture site
3. Uncorrected hypovolemia
4. Severe coagulation defects
5. Anatomic abnormalities
6. Sepsis

What are the complications associated with spinal anesthesia?

1. Hypotension
2. Spinal headache/postdural puncture headache (PDPH)
3. High spinal
4. Urinary retention
5. Nausea
6. Backache (usually caused by intraoperative positioning)
7. Neurologic impairment (including cauda equina syndrome, which is extremely rare)

What are the complications associated with epidural anesthesia?

1. Hypotension
2. Inadvertent spinal block
3. Inadvertent IV injection
4. Inadvertent dural puncture
5. PDPH
6. Epidural hematoma (rare)
7. Epidural abscess (rare)

What is a "high spinal"?

It is an excessively high level of spinal anesthesia resulting in respiratory depression. Symptoms range from difficulty breathing to apnea.

What are the risk factors for spinal headache/ PDPH?

1. Younger patients (< 50 years)
2. Gender (women > men, especially parturients)
3. Use of larger needles (22 ga versus 25 ga)

What are the characteristics of a PDPH?

Severe frontal or occipital headache that **worsens with sitting up**; with increasing severity, the headache becomes circumferential and can result in visual, auditory, or vestibular disturbances

What are the differential diagnoses of severe headache following epidural or spinal anesthesia?

1. PDPH
2. Caffeine withdrawal
3. Migraine headache
4. Meningitis
5. Cortical vein thrombosis
6. Intracranial hematoma

What is the appropriate treatment of PDPH?

1. Bed rest
2. Adequate hydration
3. Caffeine (IV)
4. Analgesics
5. Epidural blood patch (usually for headaches lasting longer than 24 hours)

What is an epidural blood patch?

It is a procedure used to treat a persistent or particularly severe PDPH. Ten to twenty ml of peripheral blood is drawn with careful sterile technique and injected into the epidural space at or near the level of the previous dural puncture. Relief occurs within 30 minutes (usually right away), and the success rate is 90% to 95%. A headache that persists despite two epidural blood patches raises serious concerns of an etiology other than PDPH.

What is a "saddle block"?

It is a low spinal anesthetic that affects primarily the perineum (i.e., the parts that would touch a saddle). A saddle block is performed using hyperbaric (heavier than CSF) anesthetic solutions with the patient sitting up to facilitate caudal spread of the anesthetic.

What is a caudal block?

It is an epidural block obtained by accessing the epidural space via the sacral hiatus. The epidural space can be cannulated or a single dose of anesthetic can be delivered through the needle.

In what patient population is the caudal block most popular?

Although this technique is feasible for both adults and children, pediatric patients receiving lower extremity, perineal, or lower abdominal surgery (e.g., inguinal herniorrhaphy) most commonly receive caudal blocks. A dose of 0.25% bupivacaine with epinephrine can provide 3 to 6 hours of analgesia. Because of body habitus, the sacral hiatus tends to be more easily located in children.

19

Cell Biology

Steven D. Thies, MD
Lorne H. Blackbourne, MD

List the major characteristics of prokaryotic cells.

Simplest cells
Few organelles
Lack nuclear membranes
(All bacteriae are prokaryotes)

List the major characteristics of eucaryotic cells.

Sophisticated cells
Specialized organelles
Distinct nucleus
(All animal cells are eucaryotes)

Describe the following phases of the mammalian cell cycle:

G_1

Slow biosynthesis (ploidy = 2n)

S

DNA synthesis (think: S = Synthesis)

G_2

Lag phase between DNA synthesis and mitosis (ploidy = 4n)

M

Mitosis (think: M = Mitosis)
Shortest phase
Cell division (two daughter cells, each 2n)

Describe the following organisms:

Gram-positive

Thick cell wall
Single-layer plasma membrane
Lacks mitochondria and a nuclear membrane

Gram-negative

Thin cell wall
Plasma membrane with inner and outer layers (outer = endotoxin)
Lacks mitochondria and a nuclear membrane

Fungus

Cell wall is structurally different than that of bacteria; has mitochondria and a nuclear membrane

Describe the function of the organelles listed as follows:

Smooth endoplasmic reticulum	Steroid and lipoprotein synthesis, detoxification, fatty-acid desaturation
Rough endoplasmic reticulum	Synthesis of proteins for export from cells
Free ribosomes	Synthesis of proteins for use within cells
Golgi apparatus	Protein modification prior to export
Lysosome	Proteolysis of cellular debris and exhausted organelles
Peroxisome	Enzymatic hydrolysis of fatty acids and amino acids; byproduct is toxic H_2O_2, which is reduced by catalase
Nucleus	Contains most of the cell's genetic material
Nucleolus	Also known as the nuclear organizing region, it synthesizes ribosomal RNA for export to cytoplasm.
Messenger RNA (mRNA)	Reads nuclear DNA to form the mRNA template; the template then moves to the cytoplasm for translation during protein synthesis
Ribosomal RNA (rRNA)	Site of mRNA interpretation during protein synthesis
Transfer RNA (tRNA)	Reads mRNA at the ribosome and delivers the appropriate amino acid for protein synthesis
Mitochondria	Site of cellular respiration and ATP production
What important biochemical reaction occurs in the mitochondrial matrix?	The Krebs cycle (citric acid cycle) generates NADH and $FADH_2$ to power the electron transport chain.
What is the electron transport chain?	A series of closely linked oxidative-phosphorylation reactions at the mitochondrial membrane that drives ATP production

What conditions inhibit the Krebs cycle (and therefore inhibit cellular respiration and ATP synthesis)?	Acidosis and excess pyruvate
What conditions inhibit the electron transport chain?	Hypoxia and cyanide poisoning; the clinical result is lactic acidosis

Describe the workings of the following second-messenger systems:

    cAMP — Generated by adenyl cyclase, it acts as an intracellular messenger by activating protein kinase A, which then activates target proteins.

    Phosphatidyl inositol phosphate (PIP) — Receptor activation leads to phosphorylase-C cleavage of PIP to IP_3 and DAG, both of which act as intracellular messengers.

    Calcium (Ca^{2+}) — Rapid increases in intracellular Ca^{2+} activate calmodulin, an intracellular protein that activates other cytoplasmic proteins.

Describe the location and/ or function of the following cell types:

Gastrointestinal
    Parietal cells — Fundus/body of stomach; produce HCl and intrinsic factor

    Chief cells — Fundus/body of stomach; produce pepsinogen

    Mucus neck cells — Fundus/body of stomach; produce mucus and HCO_3- to form a protective layer at the gastric mucosa

    G-cells — Antrum of stomach; produce gastrin in response to antral distention, vagal stimulation, and peptides; inhibited by pH less than 2.0

    S cells — Duodenum/jejunem; produce secretin in response to duodenal acidification

Kulchitsky cells
GI crypts/bronchial epithelium; progenitors of neuroendocrine tumors

Pulmonary
Type I pneumocytes
Alveolar epithelial cells responsible for gas exchange

Type II pneumocytes
Granular alveolar cell responsible for producing surfactant and new type I cells.

Pulmonary capillary endothelial cells
Convert angiotensin I to angiotensin II and degrade bradykinin

Endocrine
α-cells
Pancreas; produce glucagon; located at the periphery of the acinus; comprise 20% of the islet cell population

β-cells
Pancreas; produce insulin; located at the center of the acinus; comprise 70% of the islet cell population

δ-cells
Pancreas; produce somatostatin; located at the periphery of the acinus; comprise 5% of the islet cell population

PP-secreting cells
Pancreas; produce pancreatic polypeptide; located at the periphery of the acinus; comprise 5% of the islet cell population

Follicular cells
Thyroid; iodine uptake and T_3/T_4 production

C-cells
Thyroid, also known as parafollicular cells; produce calcitonin and are progenitors of medullary carcinoma of the thyroid

Immune system
B-cells
Lymphocytes responsible for humoral immunity (antibodies)

Plasma cells
Activated B-cells that produce antigen-specific immunoglobulins

T-cells
Lymphocytes responsible for cell-mediated immunity

Helper T cells (T_H)	Marked by the presence of CD_4 antigen; regulate all T-cell activity; produce IL-2 and IL-4; moderate interactions with other immune cells
Suppressor T cells (T_s)	Marked by the presence of CD_4 antigen; down-regulate T-cell activity and antibody production
Cytotoxic T cells (T_c)	CD_{8+}; lysis of foreign cells and neoplastic cells
NK cells	Lysis of neoplastic cells; become LAK cells in the presence of lymphokines
Macrophages	Antigen processing and presentation; produce IL-1, which stimulates T_H cells
Kupfer cells	Liver sinusoids; largest collection of macrophages in the body; responsible for clearance of antigens from the gut
Growth and Healing **Osteoblasts**	Produce bony matrix
Osteoclasts	Responsible for bone resorption and remodeling
Fibroblast	Collagen-producing cell line important in wound healing and remodeling
Myofibroblast	Specialized cell responsible for wound contraction; displays characteristics of both fibroblasts and smooth muscle
Vascular endothelial cells	Intimal cells; produce nitric oxide from L-arginine to mediate vasodilation

20

Tumor Biology

Jennifer Deblasi, MD
Lorne H. Blackbourne, MD
Gina Andrales, MD

Define the following terms:	
Aneuploidy	Abnormal amount of DNA
Malignant potential	The ability of a tumor to invade and metastasize
On average, how many cell doublings must take place for a cell to become a tumor of 1 cm³ in volume?	Approximately 30
What is flow cytometry?	Stained DNA passed through a laser beam to identify abnormal DNA of tumor cells
What is the duration of the cell cycle of tumors?	2 to 5 days
Name the tumors associated with the following oncogenes:	
C-myc	Breast and lung cancer
N-myc	Neuroblastoma (think: **N**-myc = **N**euroblastoma)
L-myc	Lung cancer (think: **L**-myc = **L**ung)
Erb B-2	Breast and ovarian cancer
K-ras	Pancreatic and colon cancer

How does radiation therapy work?	1. Breaks in DNA
	2. Forms free radicals that damage DNA and intracellular components

TUMOR MARKERS

Name the tumors often associated with the following tumor markers:

CEA	Colon cancer
AFP	Hepatoma
CA 19-9	Pancreatic cancer
CA 125	Ovarian cancer
β-HCG	Testicular cancer
PSA	Prostate cancer
CA 50	Pancreatic cancer
Neuron-specific enolase	Small-cell lung cancer
CA 15-3	Breast cancer
Ferritin	Hepatoma

MISCELLANEOUS TUMOR FACTS

Has the monitoring of postoperative CEA levels proved to prolong survival in colon cancer patients after resection?	No
What is the most common primary site with metastatic axillary lymph nodes in women?	Breast cancer
What is the most common malignant cause of axillary adenopathy?	Lymphoma

What is the most common site of sarcoma metastasis?	Lungs (via blood)
What is the most important factor in the prognosis of sarcomas?	Tumor grade
What are the Lynch tumors?	Familial colon cancer syndromes not associated with polyposis
How many types of Lynch syndrome have been identified?	Two
What is Lynch syndrome I?	Autosomal-dominant inheritance Early onset of colon cancer **Location of the tumor in the proximal colon** (think: Lynch 1 = 1 cancer)
What is Lynch syndrome II?	Colon cancer **and** Stomach cancer **and/or** Ovarian cancer **and/or** Endometrial cancer
Lynch syndrome colon cancer accounts for what percentage of all colon cancer?	Approximately 7%
In addition to prostate cancer, what other type of cancer must be ruled out in men with elevated PSA levels?	Breast cancer
Which bacteremia is associated with colon cancer?	*Clostridium septicum*
Which tumors are associated with left supraclavicular adenopathy?	GI tumors (the thoracic duct is right there!)

Why is meperidine contraindicated for long-term pain control in cancer patients?	Because of the buildup of **normeperidine,** a toxic metabolite that causes seizures and myoclonic movements

TUMOR STAGES

BREAST CANCER

Define the following stages:	
Stage 0	In situ carcinoma
Stage I	Tumor less than 2 cm
Stage IIA	Mobile ipsilateral axillary nodes with a tumor 2 cm or less **or** Tumor greater than 2 cm but not more than 5 cm without nodes
Stage IIB	Tumor greater than 2 cm but less than 5 cm **and** Mobile ipsilateral axillary nodes **or** Tumor greater than 5 cm without nodes
Stage IIIA	Tumor less than 5 cm **and** Fixed ipsilateral axillary nodes **or** Mobile or fixed ipsilateral axillary nodes with a tumor greater than 5 cm that does not involve the chest wall or skin
Stage IIIB	Tumor with direct extension to the chest wall or skin with fixed or mobile axillary nodes **or** Positive ipsilateral internal mammary nodes and any size tumor
Stage IV	Distant metastasis including **ipsilateral supraclavicular nodal spread**

COLORECTAL CANCER

Define the following stages according to Dukes' staging with Astler-Coller modification:	
Stage A	Tumor confined to the mucosa

Stage B	B1—invading the muscularis propria but not beyond B2—through the muscularis propria into the serosa
Stage C	Positive lymph nodes
Stage D	Distant metastasis (think: **D** = **D**istant)

CHEMOTHERAPEUTIC AGENTS

ALKYLATING AGENTS

What is the basic mechanism?	Alkylates susceptible to cell constituents, especially N^7 **of guanine**, leading to miscoding, strand breakage, and, most importantly, **cross-linkage of the DNA strands** so that they cannot replicate

NITROGEN MUSTARDS

Mechlorethamine

Which common lymphoma regimen is it a part of?	MOPP
What unique toxicity is it associated with?	The rapid cell kill achieved may lead to **hyperuricemia**, which can be prevented with **allopurinol.**
What other toxicities is it associated with?	Nausea and vomiting, leukopenia, and thrombocytopenia with a nadir at 2 to 3 weeks
In what cases is it often used?	Lymphomas, carcinomas of the lung, **mycosis fungoides** (topical application)

Cyclophosphamide (Cytoxan)

What are its pharmacologic actions?	Metabolized in the liver to yield the alkylator, **phosphoramide mustard**, and the toxin, **acrolein**
What unique toxicity is it associated with?	Hemorrhagic cystitis

How can this reaction be prevented?	Administration of sodium 2-mercaptoethanesulfonate (mesna) and large amounts of fluids
What other toxicities is it associated with?	Nausea and vomiting, alopecia, myelosuppression (dose-limiting), sterility

Ifosfamide

What are its pharmacologic actions?	An analog of cyclophosphamide, it is metabolized in the liver to yield active metabolites.
What toxicities is it associated with?	**Hemorrhagic cystitis** (again, can be prevented by administration of mensa), alopecia, nausea and vomiting, myelosuppression
In what cases is it often used?	Refractory testicular cancer, sarcomas, lymphomas, small-cell lung cancer

Melphalan

What toxicities is it associated with?	Myelosuppression and thrombocytopenia, iatrogenic leukemia, sterility, allergic hypersensitivity
In what cases is it often used?	Multiple myeloma, melanoma, carcinomas of the breast or ovaries

Chlorambucil

What toxicities is it associated with?	Potentially severe bone marrow depression, risk of iatrogenic leukemia
In what cases is it often used?	CLL, lymphomas, primary macroglobulinemia, multiple myeloma

NITROSOUREAS

What unique feature is associated with these agents?	They are lipophilic, and thus **enter the CSF.**

Carmustine (BCNU) / Lomustine (CCNU) / Semustine (Me-CCNU)

What toxicities are associated with these agents?	Nausea and vomiting, severe myelosuppression with a nadir at 35 days, severe thrombocytopenia with a nadir at 30 days, nephrotoxicity with a cumulative dose of 1.5 g/m^2, stomatitis, alopecia, carcinoma (possibly)
In what cases are they often used?	CNS tumors, multiple myeloma, melanoma, renal and small-cell lung cancer

Streptozocin

What unique toxicity is it associated with?	Insulin shock
What other toxicities is it associated with?	Nephrotoxicity, phlebitis, nausea and vomiting
In what cases is it often used?	**Insulinomas** (selectively destroys β-islet cells), carcinoid tumors
Notably, what toxicity is not associated with stretozocin?	Myelosuppression

OTHER ALKYLATING AGENTS

Busulfan

What unique toxicity is it associated with?	**Pulmonary fibrosis**, hyperpigmentation of intertriginous areas
What other toxicities is it associated with?	Myelosuppression (more granulotoxic than lymphotoxic), RBC toxicity at high doses, carcinoma, sterility
In what cases is it often used?	**Chronic** myelocytic leukemia (CML)

Dacarbazine

Can it enter the CSF?	Yes
What toxicities is it associated with?	Severe nausea and vomiting, myelosuppression, alopecia, flu-like syndrome

In what cases is it often used?	Malignant melanoma, lymphomas, sarcomas

Triethylenethiophosphoramide (Thio-TEPA)

What toxicities is it associated with?	Nausea and vomiting, anorexia, bone marrow depression
In what cases is it often used?	Carcinomas of the bladder, metastatic breast, or ovaries; intrathecal therapy for carcinomatous meningitis; intracavitary therapy for malignant effusions
What is the route of administration for bladder cancer?	Direct instillation

Cisplatin

What toxicity is it primarily associated with?	Cumulative **nephrotoxicity**, which may be prevented by administration of large amounts of fluid and diuresis
What other toxicities is it associated with?	Nausea and vomiting, **ototoxicity** (which can be prevented by administration of fosfomycin), immunosuppression, **peripheral neuropathy**, electrolyte abnormalities
Why is it sometimes used with x-ray therapy?	It sensitizes tissues and increases the cytotoxic effect of x-ray therapy.
What precaution must be taken when administering cisplatin?	Aluminum needles or cannulae should not be used, because aluminum will react with and inactivate the drug.
In what cases is it often used?	Cancers of the bladder, head and neck, metastatic ovaries/testicles, or thyroid; small-cell lung cancer; lymphomas

Carboplatin

How is it different from cisplatin?	Less reactive, delayed onset of action, less nephrotoxicity, ototoxicity, neurotoxicity, and nausea
In what cases is it often used?	Ovarian and small-cell lung cancers

ANTI-TUMOR ANTIBIOTICS

Describe their general mechanism of action?	These agents intercalate between DNA base pairs, decreasing DNA synthesis and mRNA transcription.

DACTINOMYCIN (ACTINOMYCIN D)

What toxicities is it associated with?	Nausea and vomiting, alopecia, myelosuppression, stomatitis
In what cases is it often used?	Pediatric solid tumors: Wilms tumor, rhabdomyosarcoma, Ewing sarcoma, choriocarcinoma

PLICAMYCIN (MITHRAMYCIN)

Why is this agent indicated for hypercalcemia?	Plicamycin has a selective effect on osteoclasts: it decreases their resorption of bone and the mobilization of Ca^{2+} stores.
What unique toxicity is it associated with?	**Hemorrhagic diathesis**, characterized by decreased platelet count and function, as well as decreased synthesis of clotting factors
What other toxicities is it associated with?	Nausea and vomiting, myelosuppression, nephrotoxicity, hepatotoxicity, hypocalcemia
In what cases is it often used?	Severe hypercalcemia, testicular carcinoma, trophoblastic neoplasms

DOXORUBICIN (ADRIAMYCIN)

What life-threatening toxicity is it associated with?	It can lead to cumulative dose-related severe **cardiomyopathy**, which can be fatal. Baseline multiple gated acquisition (MUGA) should be obtained prior to the onset of therapy and repeated at 400 mg/m^2 cumulative dose. The dose limit is 550 mg/m^2, or 400 mg/m^2 in patients who have had previous x-ray therapy to the chest or with pre-existing cardiac disease.

What increases the risk?	Chest irradiation, pre-existing cardiac disease, cyclophosphamide
What decreases the risk?	Continuous infusion
What startling side-effect is sometimes noted?	Red urine (**not** hematuria)
Indications?	Hodgkin disease, non-Hodgkin lymphoma, leukemia, sarcomas; small-cell cancer of the lung, head and neck, or ovaries/testicles

BLEOMYCIN

Describe its mechanism of action.	It does not simply intercalate, but binds DNA, creates free radicals, and causes single and double-strand scission.
What infamous toxicity is it associated with?	**Pulmonary fibrosis** (dose related; 1% of patients treated with bleomycin will die with this complication)
Notably, what toxicity is NOT associated with bleomycin?	Bone marrow suppression
Why?	Bleomycin is rapidly inactivated by aminopeptidase everywhere in the body except for the lungs and the skin.
In what cases is it often used?	Testicular cancer, lymphomas; squamous-cell cancer, especially in head, neck, and lungs

ANTIMETABOLITES

METHOTREXATE (MTX)

Describe its mechanism of action.	MTX is a folic acid analog that inhibits dihydrofolate reductase (DHFR), an enzyme that reduces dihydrofolate (FH_2) to tetrahydrofolate (FH_4). FH_4 is necessary for the one-carbon transfers that occur in the synthesis of purines, glycine, methionine, and thymidylate. Without it, DNA, RNA, and protein synthesis is impaired. The most important and lethal effect is the **inhibition of thymidylate synthesis.**

What is leucovorin "rescue"?

Leucovorin is **folinic acid.** It bypasses the need for FH_4 and thus alleviates the lethal inhibitory effects of MTX. Both leucovorin and MTX are **actively transported** into normal and tumor cells by the **same** mechanism; however, sometimes tumor cells develop resistance to MTX by decreasing transport. MTX can be forced into these cells by **passive diffusion at very high doses.** Subsequently, lower doses of leucovorin are given. Normal cells with intact transport systems take up the leucovorin and are rescued. The resistant tumor cells with decreased active transport do not take up leucovorin and die. (Kills bad, saves good!)

What toxicities are associated with MTX?

Bone marrow depression with pancytopenia, nausea and vomiting, GI mucositis, immunosuppression (sometimes used therapeutically), cirrhosis (rarely), neurotoxicity (with intrathecal administration)

What drug interactions may increase toxicity?

When MTX is used with highly protein-bound drugs such as acetylsalicylic acid, sulfonamides, and phenytoin, MTX may be displaced from proteins and reach higher serum levels.

In what cases is it often used?

ALL, non-Hodgkin lymphoma, osteogenic sarcomas, choriocarcinoma, bladder cancer, breast cancer, and squamous-cell cancer of the head and neck

MERCAPTOPURINE (6-MP) AND THIOGUANINE (6-TG)

Describe their mechanism of action.

These agents are purine analogues. They are converted to nucleotides (and thus activated) by hypoxanthine-guanine phosphoribosyl transferase (HGPRT). Then, through feedback and active inhibition at several sites and (in the case of 6-TG) incorporation into DNA molecules, they inhibit both de novo purine synthesis and interconversion of precursor molecules into dATP and dGTP, thus decreasing synthesis of DNA, RNA, and proteins.

What is the major metabolic difference between the two agents?

6-MP undergoes methylation and then oxidation via xanthine oxidase. Allopurinol inhibits xanthine oxidase; therefore, in patients taking allopurinol 6-MP, the dose must be decreased to avoid toxicity. 6-TG is not oxidized as part of its metabolism.

What toxicities are they associated with?

Nausea and vomiting, bone marrow depression, intrahepatic cholestasis at high doses (rare)

In what cases are they often used?

AML, ALL, CML

FLUOROURACIL (5-FU)

Describe its mechanism of action.

This agent is a fluorinated analog of the pyrimidine precursor **uracil**. Its active form, FdUMP, forms a covalent complex with FH_4 and thymidylate synthetase (TS), inhibiting TS and decreasing DNA synthesis.

How does it interact with leucovorin?

Leucovorin increases formation of TS–FdUMP complex, leading to an increase in cytotoxicity.

How does it interact with MTX?

MTX increases activation of 5-FU to FdUMP, but decreases formation of the TS–FdUMP complex because of a decrease in FH_4. MTX **followed** by 5-FU therefore results in an increased cytotoxic response.

What toxicities is it associated with?

Myelosuppression, nausea, GI mucositis, alopecia, neurotoxicity (rare)

In what cases is it often used?

GI tumors; cancer of the breast, ovaries, liver, bladder, pancreas; skin lesions (topical application)

HYDROXYUREA

Describe its mechanism of action.	Inhibits ribonucleotide reductase, blocking all production of deoxyribonucleotides and, thus, DNA
What toxicities is it associated with?	Nausea and vomiting, bone marrow depression
In what cases is it often used?	CML, melanoma, polycythemia, sickle cell anemia

INHIBITORS OF MICROTUBULE FUNCTION

VINCA ALKALOIDS

Name them.	Vincristine and vinblastine
From what source are they derived?	Periwinkle plant
Describe their mechanism of action.	These agents bind tubulin dimers, thus inhibiting tubule polymerization during mitosis (they are therefore M-phase specific).
What common toxicities are they associated with?	Nausea and vomiting, dose-limiting peripheral neurotoxicity (vincristine only), possible SIADH (both)
Which is less myelosuppressive?	Vincristine

PACLITAXEL (TAXOL)

From what source is it derived?	Bark of the yew tree, *Taxus brevifolia*
Describe its mechanism of action.	Promotes assembly of microtubules

ETOPOSIDE (VP-16)

From what source is it derived?	The may apple (mandrake)
Describe its mechanism of action.	Binds tubulin at same site as colchicine and inhibits topoisomerase II, causing double-strand breaks

OTHER AGENTS

MITOTANE

Describe its mechanism of action.	Destroys zona reticularis and zona fasciculata in the adrenal cortex
In what cases is it often used?	Inoperable adrenocortical cancer

L-ASPARAGINASE

Describe its mechanism of action.	Decreases asparagine concentrations; tumors with decreased asparagine synthase have decreased protein synthesis and death.
With which agent does it synergize?	Methotrexate
What toxicities is it associated with?	Nausea and vomiting, **hepatotoxicity**, anaphylaxis, pancreatitis, decreased synthesis of clotting factors, insulin, albumin, and PTH

PROCARBAZINE

Can it enter the CNS?	Yes
What toxicity is it sometimes associated with?	Oxidative damage in G6PD-deficient patients

TOPOTECAN

Describe its mechanism of action.	Topoisomerase I inhibitor

| In what cases is it often used? | Ovarian, lung, and childhood solid tumors |

GROWTH FACTORS

INTERLEUKIN-2 (IL-2)

From what source is it derived?	T cells, especially T_{h1} cells
Describe its mechanism of action.	Increases the number and cytotoxicity of T and NK cells
With what ingenious therapy has this agent been used?	Generating tumor-infiltrating lymphocytes (TIL) and lymphokine-activated killer cells (LAK) in vitro, which can be infused with lower doses of IL-2, thus decreasing systemic toxicity while retaining desired cytotoxic effect
What toxicities is it associated with?	Fever, hypotension, nausea and vomiting, fluid retention, shock, multi-organ toxicity
In what cases is it often used?	Renal cell cancer, melanoma

INTERFERON-α

From what source is it derived?	Macrophages and other leukocytes
Describe its mechanism of action.	It binds a cell surface receptor that induces dsRNA-dependent kinase, leading to phosphorylation of initiation factor 2 and, thus, inhibition of translation. Its anti-cancer action is caused by a decrease in oncogene expression.
What toxicities is it associated with?	Fever, myalgia, hypotension, multi-organ toxicity
In what cases is it often used?	CML, hairy cell leukemia, Kaposi's sarcoma

GRANULOCYTE COLONY-STIMULATING FACTOR (G-CSF)

What is its chemotherapeutic function?	Ameliorates chemotherapy-induced neutropenia
What dose-limiting toxicity is it associated with?	Sweet syndrome (also known as acute febrile neutropenic dermatosis)

HORMONES

TAMOXIFEN

Describe its mechanism of action.	Estrogen antagonist
In what cases is it often used?	Breast cancer
What long-term effect is it possibly associated with?	Endometrial cancer

COMMON THERAPEUTIC REGIMENS

Adrenocortical cancer	Mitotane
Breast cancer (adjuvant)	Cyclophosphamide/methotrexate/5-FU (CMF)
Colon cancer (adjuvant)	5-FU/levamisole
Colon cancer (metastatic)	5-FU/leucovorin
Hodgkin disease	Doxorubicin/bleomycin/vinblastine/ dacarbazine (ABVD), or mechlorethamine/vincristine/ procarbazine/prednisone (MOPP)
Ovarian cancer	Cisplatin (or carboplatin)/taxol
Testicular/germ-cell cancer	Cisplatin/etoposide/bleomycin (PEB)

MISCELLANEOUS FACTS

Which agents cross the CNS?	All nitrosoureas, hydroxyurea, etoposide, procarbazine, dacarbazine, 5-FU

Which agents are the least myelosuppressive?   Streptozocin, bleomycin, vincristine, mitotane, L-asparaginase

Which vitamin derivative treats promyelocytic leukemia (M3)?   Tretinoin (all trans-retinoic acid)

What type of cancer is IL-II approved to treat?   Renal cell cancer metastases

21

Biostatistics for the Unenlightened

Kimberly Shockey, MS

Define the following terms:

Mean

The **average** value of all data points

Mode

The **most common** numeric value of a set (e.g., in the set 2.3.4.4.4.5.6.7, 4 is the mode)

Median

The **middle value** within the ordered set

False positive

A data point that is reported as positive but is really negative

False negative

A data point that is reported as negative but is really positive

Distribution

A description of how the data look graphically (i.e., their shape)

Name some examples of common distributions.

Normal distribution, student's t distribution, chi-squared distribution, binomial distribution

Describe a normal distribution.

It is a bell-shaped curve that is symmetric around the middle.

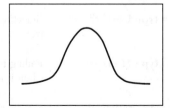

Describe a skewed distribution.	It is not symmetrical, but slanted to the right or left.

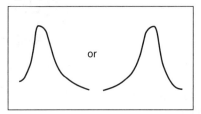

Describe a bimodal distribution	Two graphical peaks of the distribution (i.e., two modes)
Define the following terms:	
Sensitivity	$$\frac{\text{True positives}}{\text{True positives + false negatives}}$$
Specificity	$$\frac{\text{True negatives}}{\text{True negatives + false positives}}$$
Blind study	The patient is blind to the clinical intervention.
Double-blind study	The patient **and** the care providers are blind to the clinical intervention.
In statistical tests, what is the null hypothesis?	It is the hypothesis that states that there is no difference between the population value and the hypothesized value, or no difference between the groups being tested. The null hypothesis is often denoted H_o.
In statistical tests, what is the alternative hypothesis?	It is the outcome being tested (e.g., mean A is larger than mean B, or mean A is different from mean B).
What is a type I error?	Rejecting the null hypothesis when it is true
What is a type II error?	Failing to reject the null hypothesis when it is not true
Are incorrect statistical methods often cited in medical literature?	Yes; therefore you must be able to determine the validity of a study by how it was analyzed.

What is a parameter?

A value that describes a population of interest

What is a statistic?

A value that can be computed from a sample (or subset) of the population of interest

Is the statistic or the parameter usually known?

The statistic, but not the parameter, is usually known, because the population is often too large to measure precisely (think: **p** = **p**arameter and **p** = **p**opulation; **s** = **s**tatistic and **s** = **s**ample).

What does the variance of measure represent?

The spread of the data around the mean

Is a large or small variance desired?

Ideally, a small variance is desired (the data are more alike within the group).

What is the relationship between the variance and the standard deviation?

Standard deviation equals the square root of the variance.

How do you calculate the standard error of the mean?

It is the standard deviation divided by the square root of the sample size, n.

$$\frac{sd}{\sqrt{n}}$$

Why is the standard deviation used more frequently than the variance?

The variance is the square of the deviations from the mean of a sample; therefore, the units of measure are squared. The standard deviation is the square root of the variance; therefore, it is in the same units of measure as the mean and the data.

Why is the standard error of the mean (SEM) reported in medical literature more than the standard deviation?

The SEM compensates for the sample size in a study. It is the standard deviation divided by the square root of n, the sample size. It indicates the variability among means, whereas standard deviation represents the variation of an individual point.

Describe a quantitative variable.

It involves a set of continuous numbers as possible outcomes. Calculation of a mean gives a number that represents a particular factor (e.g., height, age).

Describe a categoric variable.

It is the number of objects or people in a particular classification or category (e.g., gender, race).

Define independent variables.

Two variables are independent if the outcome of one variable is in no way affected by the outcome of the other variable.

When is a proportion or percentage used as the variable of interest?

When the frequency of an occurrence is of interest

When can parametric tests be used on data analysis?

When it is assumed that the data represent a known distribution (i.e., the parameters that describe the population are known or can be estimated)

When are nonparametric tests used?

When it cannot be assumed that the data represent a known distribution (e.g., normal or Student's t-distribution). Nonparametric tests are often used on small data sets, because there is not enough data to determine what type of distribution they represent.

Can statistics be used properly on any study design?

No; if the study design has been improperly planned or executed, no amount of statistical expertise can salvage it.

What functions do statistics serve if the data have been collected properly?

They allow data to be collected and analyzed, trends to be summarized, and conclusions drawn, while still allowing for variability in the data.

How do you calculate the probability of an event occurring?

It is the number of outcomes that will give the event desired **divided by** the total number of outcomes possible.

When is a student's t-test the appropriate test to use on a sample?

If there are two independent groups and the variable is quantitative, then a t-test can be used to determine if there is a difference between the two groups, provided each of the samples represents a normal distribution. The t-test can also be used for a single sample test comparing the mean to a specified value (think: **t**-test = **t**wo groups).

Define a "before and after" or "paired" study.

The subjects are measured for a specific variable before the treatment is given. The same subjects are measured for the same variable after the treatment is given. (e.g., diet programs in which the individual's weight is measured before and after the diet is administered.)

What type of test should be used to determine a difference in a before and after study on the same subjects?

Because the same subjects are measured for both variables, the samples are **not** independent. A paired t-test must be used to determine a difference.

How is a paired t-test performed?

For each subject or pair of subjects, the difference is calculated for the two variables (e.g., weight before diet **minus** weight after diet). The difference is then analyzed using a one-sample t-test, to determine whether or not the differences are equal to zero.

When is the analysis of variance (ANOVA) method used?

When there are **more** than two groups to compare

What does ANOVA indicate?

Only whether or not there is a difference between the groups, not where the difference is located

If the ANOVA indicates that there is a difference between the groups, how can the location of the differences be determined?

Additional procedures called multiple (or post-hoc) comparisons must be performed. Most computers perform at least one method. Some common multiple comparison procedures include Tukey's Honestly Significant Difference (HSD), Bonferroni, Duncan's Multiple Range, Least Significant Difference (LSD), and Scheffe's.

When is the chi-squared test appropriate to use on a sample?

It is used when the variables measured are categorical. This also includes inferences that are made regarding proportions. The data are organized into an mxn table. The groups are listed as either the columns or the rows and the variables measured are listed as the other (row or column). The count of subjects is represented in the appropriate cells.

	Male	Female
Pass	11	9
Fail	8	6

What are the values obtained from the sample in the mxn table called?

The **observed** frequencies, because they were observed when collecting the sample (e.g., 11 for Male/Pass in Table 21-1)

What are the expected frequencies in an mxn table?

The values expected in each cell if no differences exist between the groups given the sample sizes observed (i.e., H_o is true)

How do you calculate an expected frequency?

It is calculated as the row total for that cell **multiplied by** the column total for that cell **divided by** the grand total of subjects in the study. Example: (from Table 21-1) for Male/Pass, E = (20)(19)/34 = 11.18

When should Fisher's Exact Test be used?

When the table is a 2 x 2 table and any of the **expected** frequencies are less than 2, or if more than half the expected frequencies are less than 5

When can a normal approximation be used to compare proportions?

Even though proportions are obtained from categoric variables, the normal approximation can be used instead of chi-squared when analyzing one or two variables. The only restrictions are that the sample size multiplied by the proportion, $n \times p$, and the sample size multiplied by 1 minus the proportion, $n(1-p)$, must be greater than 5.

What does the binomial distribution represent?

The probability that a specified outcome occurs in a given number of independent trials (e.g., the probability of heads when tossing a coin 50 times)

In what study designs is the binomial distribution appropriate?

If the outcomes are dichotomous (e.g., yes or no, positive or negative), then the binomial distribution can be used to analyze the data.

What distribution is used most frequently when determining the probability of rare events?

The Poisson distribution gives the probability that an outcome occurs a specified number of times when the number of trials is large and the probability of any one occurrence is small.

What is a major assumption that is made when using a student's t-test?

That the data represent a symmetric bell-shaped normal distribution

What are degrees of freedom?

Used in conjunction with the t-distribution, the chi-squared distribution, and so forth, they essentially represent the number of independent observations in a sample. Example: It is known that the sum of the angles in a triangle is 180. If you are told to choose the three angles, you can choose two of the angles freely, but the third is predetermined because of the condition that they must add up to 180. Therefore, you have 2 degrees of freedom. If you were told to choose four numbers with no restrictions, then there would be 4 degrees of freedom because you were free to choose any four numbers.

What does the p-value represent?

It is the probability of observing the value obtained or one more extreme given that the null hypothesis is true (i.e., more extreme meaning further from the "true" value). Another way to think of it is that the p-value is the probability that the result is caused by chance alone. For example, if a test is conducted to determine whether two means are equal and a p-value less than 0.05 is obtained, then the difference in the two means is considered too extreme to assume they are equal. The conclusion would be that the means are not equal in 95 of 100 cases.

What does it mean when variables are confounding?

It is not possible to determine which variable is causing the effect being studied.

What is the name of an inactive treatment in a study?

A placebo treatment

Is it unusual to observe an effect with a placebo?

No, people often show an improvement with a placebo if they were blinded to the treatment.

What does correlation measure?

Correlation measures the **linear** relationship between two variables. The correlation coefficient is denoted as r. It has values between +1 and -1; +1 indicates that all the data points lie on a straight line with a positive slope, and -1 indicates that all the data points lie on a straight line with a negative slope.

What is the sensitivity of a test?

It measures how well the test detects a disease.

How do you calculate the sensitivity?

It is the proportion of those with the disease who give a positive result.

What is the specificity of a test?

It measures how well the test detects the absence of a disease.

How do you calculate specificity?

It is the proportion of those **without** the disease who give a negative result.

Define predictive values.

A positive predictive value is the proportion of those with a positive result that do have the disease. A negative predictive value is the proportion of those with a negative result that do not have the disease.

How is the incidence of a disease defined?

It is the number of new cases that occur during a specified amount of time **divided by** the number of people at risk of developing the disease at the beginning of the time interval.

What is the relative risk of a disease?

It is a measure of the relative amount of disease occurring in different populations.

How do you calculate the relative risk?

Relative risk = (incidence of disease in exposed group) **divided by** (incidence of disease in the unexposed group).

What is the odds ratio as a measure of disease occurrence?

Odds ratio = (odds in favor of the disease in the exposed group) **divided by** (odds in favor of the disease in the unexposed group). The odds in favor of an event are the frequency with which an event occurs divided by the frequency with which it does not occur.

What is the Kaplan-Meier analysis used for?

It is a method of estimating the survival of subjects in a study. It is especially appropriate for studies involving a small number of patients.

What does the power of a test mean?

It is the probability of rejecting the null hypothesis when it is false or of accepting the alternative hypothesis when it is true. It is the probability of making the "correct" decision.

What test is often used to compare more than two groups when the sample sizes are small or the data do not follow a normal distribution?

The nonparametric Kruskal-Wallis test is used to compare more than two samples when the samples indicate extreme departures from normality. The test is based on the ranks of the data among the samples.

22

Spanish Every Surgery Resident Should Know

Lorne H. Blackbourne, MD

Translate the following phrases:

Hello	Hola (o la)
Good-bye	Adios
Please	Por favor
Sir	Señor
Ma'am	Señora
You	Tu
Where	Donde (dohn-day)
Is	Es (esta)
Pain	Dolor (dough-lore)
Worse	Peor
Better	Mejor (mehor)
Nauseated	Mareado or nau sea
Where is the pain?	Donde esta dolor?
Is the pain worse?	Es dolor peor?
Is the pain better?	Es dolor mejor?
Speak	Hablas
English	Ingles

23

GI Physiology and Hormones

Robert E. Schmieg, Jr., MD

GENERAL

What are the general functions of the gastrointestinal tract?

Movement of food from the mouth distally

Digestion and absorption of carbohydrates, fats, and proteins

Absorption of fluids, electrolytes, and vitamins

Elimination of waste products

Endocrine activity

Immunologic surveillance and defense

What are the histologic layers of the gastrointestinal tract?

Mucosa (epithelium, lamina propria, muscularis mucosae)

Submucosa

Muscularis externa (inner circular, outer longitudinal)

Serosa

What is the strongest structural layer?

Submucosa

Where are the intramural neural plexi located?

Meissner's—submucosal

Auerbach's—myenteric (between the circular and longitudinal layers)

Which neurotransmitters are associated with external innervation to the gut?

Acetylcholine (parasympathetic)

Norepinephrine (sympathetic)

What structures are associated with sympathetic innervation of the gut?

Cell bodies of postganglionic adrenergic neurons located in the prevertebral and paravertebral plexi (celiac, superior mesenteric, inferior mesenteric, hypogastric plexi)

What is the effect of sympathetic stimulation of the gut?

Inhibits motility
Causes vasoconstriction
Stimulates contraction of sphincters

What is the effect of parasympathetic stimulation of the gut?

Stimulates motility, secretion, and digestion

What is the origin of afferent signals from the gut?

Chemoreceptors and mechanoreceptors in mucosal and other layers

What are the major dietary sources of carbohydrates?

Starches from plants (e.g., amylose and amylopectin)
Lactose from milk
Fructose from fruits

What are the steps in carbohydrate digestion?

Mouth—salivary amylase
Stomach—amylase inactivated by acid
Intestines—pancreatic amylase
Intestinal brush border—oligosaccharidases (e.g., sucrase, lactase, maltase)

What are the products of starch digestion by amylase?

Amylase hydrolyzes the α-1,4-glycosidic linkages (except for the branching points), and results in maltose (gluc-gluc), maltotriose (gluc-gluc-gluc), and limit dextrins.

What occurs in the final digestion of starch?

Small oligosaccharides are broken down to monosaccharides in the intestinal brush border (epithelial cells). Brush border enzymes include disaccharidases, oligosaccharidases, and limit dextrinase. Monosaccharide products are glucose, galactose, and fructose.

Describe the digestion of lactose.

Lactose is (galactose-glucose) hydrolyzed by β-galactosidases in the intestinal brush border; these enzymes can be rate-limiting.

Describe the absorption of carbohydrate digestion products.

Monosaccharides undergo carrier-mediated transport by intestinal epithelial cells. Absorption is usually completed in the first 1.5 meters of the proximal small intestine. Absorption is driven mostly by NA gradient created by the Na-K-ATPase pump on the basolateral membrane of enterocytes. Glucose and galactose are absorbed by the Na^+-glucose cotransport system; fructose is absorbed by facilitated transport.

What is the route of carbohydrate products after absorption?

They are transported from epithelial cells across the basal membrane by the Na^+-independent system, which is monosaccharide-dependent. Monosaccharides travel via the portal vein to the liver, which metabolizes galactose and fructose to glucose or glycogen, as needed.

DIGESTION

What are the essential fatty acids?

Linoleic (18-carbon)
Linolenic (20-carbon)

Describe the digestion of lipids.

Start as fat droplets
Emulsification by bile salts and
    phosphatidylcholine to form micelles
    occurs in the duodenum
Lipids in micelles are hydrolyzed by
    pancreatic lipase, cholesterol esterase,
    and phospholipase A2.
Lipids in micelles diffuse across the
    luminal membrane of enterocytes.

What are micelles composed of?

Bile salts
Monoglycerides
Fatty acids
Phospholipids

What is the fate of lipid digestion products after absorption?

**Short- and medium-chain fatty
    acids**—directly passed into portal
    venous system
Long-chain fatty acids—reformed into
    triglycerides
Chylomicrons—formed in enterocytes;
    released into extracellular space by
    exocytosis across the basolateral
    membrane; travel into lacteals
    (intestinal lymphatics; empty into

systemic circulation through thoracic duct)

Lipoprotein lipase removes lipids from chylomicron and forms chylomicron remnants.

Chylomicron remnants are cleared by the liver.

What are chylomicrons composed of?

Core—triglycerides
Coat—phospholipids, cholesterol esters, and proteins

What are the types of lipoproteins and what function is each responsible for?

VLDL—transport of triglycerides from liver
IDL—formed in plasma by degradation of VLDL
LDL—formed in plasma from IDL; transports cholesterol esters to body tissues
HDL—transports cholesterol to liver

What are the essential amino acids?

Histidine
Isoleucine
Leucine
Lysine
Methionine
Phenylalanine
Threonine
Tryptophan
Valine
(think: HIS ISOlated Lover Lied; Mike Pushed THen TRipped VALerie)

Describe the digestion of proteins.

Stomach—denatured by acid; hydrolyzed by pepsin
Pancreas—secretes multiple endopeptidases and carboxypeptidases into the intestine; trypsin, chymotrypsin, and carboxypeptidase hydrolyze protein to small peptides and amino acids

Approximately half of protein digestion and absorption is completed in the duodenal intestinal brush border.

Dipeptides, tripeptides, and free amino acids are formed by the action of aminopeptidases and dipeptidases.

Describe the absorption of protein digestion products.	Enterocytes absorb dipeptides, tripeptides, and free amino acids. Dipeptidases and tripeptides are digested to free amino acids by cytosolic enzymes. Protein digestion and absorption are completed by the mid-jejunum.
What are the characteristics of pepsin?	Stored as inactive proenzyme (pepsinogen) in chief cells as zymogen granules Secreted from chief cells by exocytosis at apical surface Secretion stimulated by gastric acid and by stimulators of gastric acid secretion Acts upon approximately 20% of intragastric proteins Requires acidic environment for enzymatic action Permanently inactivated in neutral duodenal environment
What are the characteristics of enterokinase?	Secreted by duodenal mucosa Activates trypsinogen, chymotrypsinogen, and procarboxypeptidase
What are the characteristics of trypsin?	Secreted by pancreatic acinar cells Actives proenzyme trypsinogen In turn activates chymotrypsin, elastase, and carboxypeptidases A and B
What are the characteristics of chymotrypsin?	Secreted by pancreatic acinar cells Inactivates proenzyme chymotrypsinogen Activated by trypsin
What are the characteristics of carboxypeptidase?	Secreted by pancreatic acinar cells Inactivates proenzyme procarboxypeptidase Activated by trypsin

GASTROINTESTINAL MOTILITY

What types of myoelectric activity occur in the gut?	Slow waves (pacesetter potentials; electrical control activity) Oscillating resting potential of smooth muscle cells Spike activity (action potentials) Bursts of depolarization activity (correlate with mechanical contraction)

What are the characteristics of slow waves?	Different frequencies at different levels of the gut:
	    Stomach—3 cycles per minute
	    Duodenum—12 cycles per minute
	Frequency decreases from the duodenum to the ileum.

What are the characteristics of spike activity?	Occur at peaks of slow waves in bursts Increase phasic contractions of smooth muscle cells Summed from individual cells to produce mechanical contraction of bowel segment

GASTRIC ACID SECRETION

What three main agonists act on parietal cells to secrete acid?	Acetylcholine at muscarinic cholinergic receptors Histamine at H_2 receptors Gastrin at gastrin receptors (second messenger-phosphoinositide system)
What are the phases of gastric acid secretion?	Cephalic Gastric Intestinal
What stimulates the cephalic phase?	Thought, smell, taste, or the presence of food in the mouth (classic Pavlov experiments)
What are the pathways of the cephalic phase of acid secretion?	Telencephalon → nucleus tractus solitarius → dorsal motor nucleus → vagal muscarinic cholinergic efferent fibers → parietal cell (cholinergic receptors) → secrete acid Vagus nerve to G cells → secrete gastrin → to parietal cells (gastrin receptors) → secrete acid (chief cells also increase secretion of pepsinogen in cephalic phase)
What stimulates the gastric phase?	Gastric distention
What are the pathways of the gastric phase of acid secretion?	Local and vagovagal reflexes → G cells → gastrin → parietal cells (gastrin receptors) → secrete acid

Local and vagovagal reflexes → parietal cells (cholinergic receptors) → secrete acid

Gastric mast cells → histamine → parietal cells (histamine-2 receptors) → secrete acid

What inhibits the gastric phase?

Antral acidification

How is gastric secretion measured?

Basal acid output (BAO)—4 to 6 mEq/hr

Maximal acid output (MAO)—30 to 40 mEq/hr

Why are gastric acid secretion measurements important?

Achlorhydria can be diagnosed definitively.

ESOPHAGUS

What are the general functions of the esophagus?

Unidirectional passage of food bolus and ingested fluids into stomach

Describe the differences in esophageal wall muscle cells.

Upper esophageal striated muscle originates from the mesenchyme of caudal branchial arches; innervated by the vagal fibers

Lower esophageal smooth muscle originates from the splanchnic mesenchyme; innervated by the visceral nerve plexi from neural crest cells

Anatomically, where does the esophagus begin?

At the sixth cervical vertebra, as a continuation of the pharynx (landmarks: cricoid cartilage, transverse processes of C6)

Anatomically, where does the esophagus end?

GE junction at the T11 level

Name three points of anatomic narrowing of the esophagus.

1. Cricopharyngeus muscle (most common point of iatrogenic esophageal perforation)
2. Compression by left mainstem bronchus and aortic arch (located 24–26 cm from incisors, serves as a

landmark for identifying the location of endoluminal lesions on esophagoscopy)

3. LES at the diaphragmatic hiatus (average length of esophagus is 38–40 cm in men, 36–38 cm in women)

What supplies arterial blood to the esophagus?

Cervical—inferior thyroid artery
Proximal thoracic—branches from the bronchial artery
Distal thoracic—branches from the aorta
Abdominal—inferior phrenic artery and branches from the left gastric artery

Describe the path of venous return from the esophagus.

From the submucosal venous plexi into the periesophageal venous plexi into the esophageal veins, which drain by regions:
  Cervical—inferior thyroid vein
  Thoracic—bronchial, hemizygous, azygous vein
  Abdominal—left gastric vein (coronary vein)

Name the three phases of swallowing (glutition).

1. Voluntary propulsion of food bolus by the tongue and mouth muscles into the hypopharynx
2. Passage of food bolus into the upper esophageal sphincter region by automatic synchronized contractions of the pharyngeal constrictor muscles
3. Involuntary propulsion of food down the esophagus and into the stomach

What are the components of the upper esophageal sphincter (UES)?

1. Cricopharyngeus muscle
2. Posterior third of cricoid cartilage
3. Circular muscle fibers of upper esophagus

What are the physical characteristics of UES?

2.5 to 4 cm in length
Mean resting pressures of 20 to 60 mm Hg

What are the actions of UES?

Closed at rest
Open for swallowing, eructation, emesis, and gagging

What controls the UES?

Medulla and lower pons
Innervation of cricopharyngeus muscles
by right and left recurrent laryngeal
nerves from vagus nerves

What are the normal pressures in the body of the esophagus?

-2 to +2 mm Hg

Name three types of esophageal motility.

1. Primary peristalsis
2. Secondary peristalsis
3. Tertiary contractions

What are the characteristics of primary esophageal peristalsis?

Peristaltic contraction waves have
elevated pressures (40–80 mm Hg).
Each wave lasts 4 to 8 seconds.
Waves propagate distally at 1 to 5 cm/
sec.
Propagation is more rapid in the middle
of the esophagus than at either end.
Duration of pressure waves is inversely
proportional to propagation speed.

What controls primary esophageal peristalsis?

Modulated by afferent vagal impulses
Afferent vagal stimuli include bolus size,
consistency, pH.

What are the characteristics of secondary esophageal peristalsis?

Incomplete esophageal emptying causes
distention, which stimulates stripping
waves of esophageal contraction.
Inhibited by the initiation of primary
waves above the level of distention

What are the characteristics of tertiary esophageal contractions?

Nonperistaltic
Nonpropagated
More frequent in the distal esophagus

What controls tertiary esophageal contractions?

Probably local reflex loops from the
myenteric plexi

What are the most common sites of esophageal perforation?

Iatrogenic—level of cricopharyngeus
Boerhaave syndrome—left lateral wall
below T8

What factors contribute to LES competency?	Thickening of wall muscle fibers in cardia and distal esophagus Intraabdominal position of distal esophagus Acute angle between gastric fundus and distal esophagus
What is a major cause of pharyngoesophageal (Zenker's) diverticulum?	Lack of coordination of upper esophageal sphincter relaxation with food bolus passage

VAGUS

Describe the neuroanatomy of the vagus nerve (cranial nerve X).	Ninety percent of fibers are afferent (transmit from GI tract to CNS). Ten percent of fibers are efferent. Parasympathetic efferent fibers originate in the dorsal nucleus of the medulla. Pass to synapse with postsynaptic neurons in the gastric wall, myenteric, and submucous neural plexi Main neurotransmitter is acetylcholine
What is the course of the vagus nerve?	Left and right vagus descend with the esophagus as distinct trunks to the level of the tracheal bifurcation. Left vagus is anterior; right vagus is posterior. Left vagus divides into the anterior lesser curvature gastric branches and hepatic branches, which pass through the gastrohepatic ligament to the liver and biliary tract. Right vagus divides into the posterior lesser curvature gastric branches and a celiac vagal division.

STOMACH

What are the general functions of the stomach?	Temporary storage of ingested food Mechanical distention of stomach (compliance) Regulation of passage of gastric chyme into duodenum Preparation of ingested food for digestion in other parts of the GI tract Mechanical degradation of food particles Mixing of secretions and gastric chyme

Digestive enzyme (pepsinogen) secretion
Intrinsic factor secretion for absorption
of vitamin B_{12}
Initiation of digestion of proteins
Microbiologic barrier
Acid secretion

What digestion phases occur in the stomach?

Mostly mechanical
Minor protein digestion by acid and pepsin (approximately 20%)

What does the stomach absorb?

Water, alcohols, poisons (e.g., arsenic and cyanide)

What are the anatomic divisions of the stomach?

Cardia (adjacent to the GE junction)
Fundus (above and lateral to the cardia)
Corpus/body (between the fundus and antrum)
(Boundary between corpus and antrum line between incisura angularis on lesser curvature and point about one-fourth of the distance on the greater curvature from the pylorus to the GE junction)
Antrum
Pylorus

Describe the histology of the stomach mucosa.

Simple columnar epithelium
Surface mucous cells
Gastric pits (openings of gastric glands)

What cell types are present in the gastric mucosa?

Parietal cells (oxyntic; produce acid and intrinsic factor)
Chief cells (secrete pepsinogen)
G cells (columnar epithelium)
Mucous cells
Undifferentiated cells

Where are parietal cells located?

In the gastric body

What stimulates parietal cell action?

Histamine
Gastrin
Acetylcholine (vagal)

Where are chief cells located?

In the gastric body and fundus

What is the action of chief cells?	Release pepsinogen (think: a peppy chief; pepsinogen = chief cell)
What stimulates chief cell action?	Acetylcholine (vagal)
What is the location of G cells?	The gastric antrum
What is the action of G cells?	Secrete gastrin (think: **G** cell = **G**astrin)
What stimulates G cell action?	Acetylcholine (vagal) Gastric pH greater than 2.0 Histamine
What inhibits G cell action?	Gastric pH less than 2.0

Name the types, locations, and characteristics of gastric glands.	**Cardiac**—located in the gastric cardia
	  Usually branched
	  Short gastric pits
	  No parietal or chief cells
	Oxyntic—located in the fundus and body
	  Usually straight, sometimes branched
	  Composed of three regions: isthmus, neck, and base

What are the sources of arterial blood supply to the stomach?	1. Left gastric artery from the celiac axis 2. Right gastric artery from the hepatic artery 3. Right gastroepiploic artery from the gastroduodenal artery 4. Left gastroepiploic artery from the splenic artery 5. Short gastric artery from the splenic artery
Which networks supply gastric innervation?	**Efferent**—parasympathetic nerves from the vagi (CN-X); sympathetic nerves from T5 to T10 to the celiac plexus (synapse), which pass with blood vessels to stomach **Afferent**—parasympathetic vagal nerves to the dorsal nucleus of medulla; sympathetic nerves, which extend to the dorsal spinal roots

Which nerves sense gastric pain?	Afferent sympathetic nerves passing along arteries to dorsal spinal roots
Where is the fixation of the stomach located?	At the GE junction and at the retroperitoneal duodenum
What are the types of gastric volvulus?	**Organoaxial**—along the line between the GE junction and the duodenal bulb **Mesenteroaxial**—perpendicular to the previously described line

DUODENUM

What are the general functions of the duodenum?	Feedback control of gastric functions, especially acid secretion Neutralization of gastric acid
What are the sources of arterial blood supply to the duodenum?	**Duodenal bulb**—supraduodenal artery Branch from hepatic artery Gastroduodenal artery from hepatic artery Anterosuperior and posterosuperior pancreaticoduodenal arteries from gastroduodenal artery Anteroinferior and posteroinferior pancreaticoduodenal artery from superior mesenteric artery **Fourth portion of duodenum**—small branches from first jejunal branch of superior mesenteric artery

JEJUNUM AND ILEUM

What are the general functions of the jejunum and ileum?	Digestion of carbohydrates, fats, and proteins Absorption of carbohydrates, fats, proteins, electrolytes, vitamins, and fluid Microbial barrier function IgA motility Mixing of intestinal chyme Rapid passage of intestinal chyme to distal gastrointestinal tract Endocrine functions

What is the source of arterial blood supply to the jejunum and ileum?

Superior mesenteric artery—multiple jejunal and ileal branches as the superior mesenteric artery travels along the small bowel as the marginal artery and finally anastomoses with the ileal branch of ileocolic artery

What are the differences between the jejunal and ileal arteries?

Jejunum—short jejunal arcades with long end arteries
Ileum—small vasa recta

COLON

What are the general functions of the colon?

Absorption of fluids and nutrients
Temporary storage and slow distal propulsion of chyme

Describe the histology of the colon.

Four layers of colon wall (serosa, muscularis, circumferential circular smooth muscle layer, longitudinal muscle layer in three bands [taeniae])
Insertion aspect (begins at the base of the appendix; continues to the rectum; becomes the circumferential layer at the rectum)
Submucosa
Mucosa (columnar epithelium; flat; villi are absent)
Glands (crypts of Lieberkühn; open into colonic lumen mucous cells; columnar epithelium; some endocrine cells)

What are the sources of arterial blood supply to the colon?

Right—superior mesenteric artery, ileocolic artery, right colic artery, middle colic artery
Left—inferior mesenteric artery, middle colic artery, left colic artery

Name the arterial collaterals in the colon blood supply system.

Marginal artery of Drummond—series of arcades along the mesenteric border throughout the length of the colon
Arc of Riolan—short artery from the root of the superior mesenteric artery or one of its branches to the root of inferior mesenteric artery or one of its branches

What is the venous drainage of the colon?	**Right**—superior mesenteric vein **Left**—inferior mesenteric vein

Through what networks is the colon innervated?	Two intramural plexi:
	   Submucosal plexus (Meissner's plexus; innermost between the muscularis mucosa and the circular muscularis propria)
	   Myenteric plexus (Auerbach's plexus; outermost between the circular and the outer longitudinal muscle layers)

What are the major types of colon motility and how do they function?	Ring contractions:
	   Mix contents
	   Move contents (either antegrade or retrograde)
	   Enhance surface contact with contents
	 Left colon—sustained giant migrating contractions:
	   Propel stool toward rectum
	   Empty colon of luminal contents

What stimulates colonic motility?	Fatty acids, bile acids, undigested food particles, luminal distention, cholinergic stimulation
What is the function of the bacterial load of the colon?	Breakdown of carbohydrates to short-chain fatty acids, which can then be absorbed

APPENDIX

What are the possible variations of appendix location?	**65%**—low retrocecal, still intraperitoneal **30%**—tip at pelvic brim or in the pelvis **5%**—retroperitoneal behind the cecum or distal ileum
What landmarks are reliable in locating the appendix?	Locate the colon; follow the taeniae to the base of the cecum; the taeniae fuse together at the base of the appendix.

RECTUM AND ANUS

What are the general functions of the rectum and anus?	Storage and defecation

What is the source of arterial blood supply to the anal canal?

Superior two-thirds—superior rectal, inferior mesenteric, middle rectal, and internal iliac arteries (or branches thereof)
Inferior third—inferior rectal and internal iliac arteries

What is the venous drainage of the anal canal?

Superior two-thirds—superior rectal vein, inferior mesenteric vein
Inferior two-thirds—inferior rectal vein, internal pudendal vein, internal iliac vein

What is the lymphatic drainage of the anal canal?

Superior two-thirds—inferior mesenteric lymph nodes
Inferior third—superficial inguinal lymph nodes

Through what networks is the anal canal innervated?

Superior two-thirds—autonomics
Inferior third—inferior rectal nerve

PANCREAS

What are the general functions of the pancreas?

Exocrine—secretion of digestive enzymes, neutralization of gastric acid
Endocrine—glucose homeostasis

What is the source of arterial blood supply to the pancreas?

Head—anterosuperior and posterosuperior pancreaticoduodenal arteries, from the gastroduodenal artery; anteroinferior and posteroinferior pancreaticoduodenal arteries, from the superior mesenteric artery
Body and tail—Splenic artery; dorsal pancreatic artery (close to the celiac trunk); pancreatic magna (midportion of the pancreatic body); caudal pancreatic artery (pancreatic tail)

What anomalies can occur in the vascular supply to the head of pancreas?

The superior mesenteric artery may give rise to the common hepatic, right hepatic, or gastroduodenal arteries.

What does the abbreviation APUD stand for?

Amine precursor uptake decarboxylase cells

What are the modes of action of GI hormones?	**Endocrine**—released into the bloodstream **Paracrine**—released into intracelllular space **Autocrine**—released into intracellular space and acts on secreting cell (Many GI hormones also act as neurotransmitters)
What are the stress hormones?	Hormones that are elevated in stress states: epinephrine, cortisol, glucagon, and growth hormone
What are the characteristics of GI-hormone endocrine tumors?	Most arise in the pancreas, although they can occur throughout the gut. Usually caused by one hormone Elevation of multiple other GI hormone levels is often observed clinically.
What clinical syndromes are associated with GI-hormone endocrine tumors?	Gastrinoma (Zollinger-Ellison syndrome) Glucagonoma Verner-Morrison syndrome (watery diarrhea, hypokalemia, achlorhydria [WDHA]) Somatostatinoma insulinoma (carcinoid syndrome)

GLUCAGON

What is its general role?	Energy utilization
What is its source?	**α-islet cells of the pancreas**—pancreatic glucagon **Stomach**—gastric glucagon **Intestines**—enteroglucagon
In what forms does it exist?	Perproglucagon (180-amino acid peptide; contains glicentin, glucagon, and glucagon-like peptides 1 and 2 [GLP-1 and GLP-2]) Various tissue-specific forms come from different cleavage sites of perproglucagon: Pancreatic glucagon (29-amino acid peptide) Gastric glucagon Enteroglucagon

What stimulates its release?	Hypoglycemia Elevated serum amino acids (alanine, arginine) Cholinergic (neural stimulation; β-adrenergic; stimulate weakly) Gastic-inhibiting peptide (GIP; only in vitro, not in vivo) Gastrin-releasing peptide (GRP)
What inhibits its release?	Hyperglycemia Insulin Somatostatin α-adrenergic (neural stimulation) GLP-1 (feedback control)
What does it target?	Liver Adipose tissue
How does it act?	Increases hepatic glycogenolysis and gluconeogenesis (i.e., mobilizes glucose into the bloodstream) Increases lipolysis and ketogenesis
What other actions is it associated with?	Inhibits gastric acid secretion Causes relaxation and dilatation of the stomach and duodenum Increases intestinal motility and transit time Inhibits pancreatic secretion of water and bicarbonate
What are its clinical uses?	Decreases motility of the stomach and duodenum for endoscopy and radiography

SOMATOSTATIN

What are the signs of somatostatinoma of the pancreas?	Hypochlorhydria Impaired glucose tolerance Weight loss Steatorrhea Gallstones

GASTRIN

What is its general role?	Regulates **acid secretion** by gastric parietal cells

How does it act?	Stimulates parietal cells to secrete HCl and intrinsic factor Stimulates chief cells to secrete pepsinogen Increases gastric mucosal blood flow
What stimulates its release?	Small protein fragments and amino acids in the stomach Calcium in the stomach Alcohols in the stomach Antral distention pH greater than 3 Vagal stimulation
What inhibits its secretion?	Antral acidification (pH < 1.5 completely blocks)
What does it target?	Parietal cells in the stomach Chief cells in the stomach
What long-term action is it associated with?	Trophic effect on intestinal mucosal cells

GASTRIC INHIBITORY PEPTIDE (GIP)

By what other name is it known?	Glucose-dependent insulinotropic polypeptide (same acronym!)
What is its source?	K cells of the duodenal glands
What stimulates its release?	Duodenal amino acids Glucose Long-chain fatty acids Hyperglycemia
What does it target?	Pancreas islet cells Stomach
How does it act?	Enhances insulin release Inhibits gastric acid secretion

CHOLECYSTOKININ

What is its source?	I cells of the duodenum and proximal jejunum
What is its general role?	Aids in fat digestion by bile secretion

What does it target?	Gallbladder Pancreas Sphincter of Oddi
What stimulates its secretion?	Duodenal fat (long-chain fatty acids in micelles) Duodenal amino acids (especially tryptophan and phenylalanine = essential amino acids)
How does it act?	Gallbladder contraction Relaxation of the sphincter of Oddi Increase in pancreatic exocrine secretion (bicarbonate-rich pancreatic juice) Increased intestinal motility and transit time Decreased gastric emptying Trophic factor on pancreas and gallbladder mucosa

SECRETIN

What does it target?	Pancreas (main target) Stomach (minor target)
What stimulates its release?	Acid, fat, and bile salts in the duodenum
What inhibits its release?	Duodenal pH greater than 4
What are its major actions?	Increases bicarbonate secretion from the pancreas, with decreased Cl^- secretion Works in combination with cholecystokinin
What are its other actions?	Increases bile flow Decreases acid secretion from parietal cells Inhibits gastrin release stimulated by food Decreases gastric emptying
What is a "secretin stimulation test"?	Secretin significantly increases gastrin release and gastric acid production in patients with Zollinger-Ellison syndrome, but has no effect or decreases gastrin levels in healthy patients.

VASOACTIVE INTESTINAL POLYPEPTIDE

What is its source?

Diffuse pattern of cells throughout the gut and pancreas
Peripheral nerve fibers

What stimulates its release?

Intragastric fat
Vagal input

What are its effects?

Vasodilation
Smooth-muscle cell relaxation
General increase of water and electrolyte secretion by gut mucosal cells

PANCREATIC POLYPEPTIDE

What is its source?

Islet cells of the pancreas and of other tissues of the pancreas

What stimulates its release?

Food, vagal input, and other GI hormones (e.g., cholecystokinin)

How does it act?

Inhibits pancreatic water and bicarbonate secretion in postprandial state
Inhibits gallbladder contraction
May help regulate intestinal motility
Causes a change from fasting to digestive patterns

What is its clinical significance?

Tumor marker for pancreatic apudoma tumors

PEPTIDE YY

What is its source?

Cells in the distal ileum, colon, and rectum

What stimulates its release?

Intraluminal fat in the intestine

What does it target?

Stomach

How does it act?

Inhibits gastric emptying
Inhibits gastrin-stimulated acid secretion
Inhibits pancreatic exocrine secretion stimulated by cholecystokinin
May mediate the "ileal brake"

NEUROTENSIN

What is its source?   N cells in distal small intestine

**What stimulates its
release?**   Intraluminal fat

How does it act?   Inhibits gastric acid secretion
Inhibits intestinal motility
Stimulates pancreatic secretion of water
    and bicarbonate
Triggers mesenteric vasodilation

MOTILIN

What is its source?   Cells throughout the gut (highest
concentration is in the duodenum and
jejunum)

**What stimulates its
release?**   Duodenal acid and food
Vagal tone
Gastrin-releasing peptide

What inhibits its release?   Somatostatin
Secretin
Pancreatic polypeptide
Duodenal fat or mixed meal

How does it act?   Increases interdigestive gut motility
   (think: **M**otilin = **M**otility)
Initiates MMCs

**What is its clinical
significance?**   Erythromycin and other macrolodes may
stimulate gastric motility as motilin
receptor agonists.

BOMBESIN

What is its source?   Peptide isolated from the skin of a
European frog (*Bombina bombina*)

How does it act?   Stimulates release of most GI hormones
Increases motility
Increases secretion in the gut, pancreas,
   and stomach
(Similar in structure to gastrin-releasing
   peptide)

Section II

General Surgery

24

Acute Abdomen

Lorne H. Blackbourne, MD

"The general rule can be laid down that the majority of severe abdominal pains which ensue in patients who have been previously fairly well, and which last as long as 6 hours, are caused by conditions of surgical import."

Sir Zachary Cope
(1881–1974)

Define acute abdomen.	A condition of acute abdominal pain
Is an acute abdomen the same as a surgical abdomen?	No

What are the most likely diagnoses for the following types of abdominal pain:

Right upper quadrant?

Cholecystitis, hepatitis, peptic ulcer disease, perforated ulcer, pancreatitis, liver tumors, gastritis, hepatic abscess, choledocholithiasis, cholangitis, pyelonephritis, nephrolithiasis, appendicitis (especially during pregnancy), cancer (e.g., colon, liver, kidney), thoracic causes (e.g., PE, pleurisy/pneumonia, pericarditis, MI)

Left upper quadrant?

Peptic ulcer disease, perforated ulcer, gastritis, splenic disease or rupture, abscess, reflux, dissecting aortic aneurysm, thoracic causes (previously mentioned), pyelonephritis, nephrolithiasis, hiatal hernia (strangulated paraesophageal hernia), Boerhaave syndrome, Mallory-Weiss tear

Left lower quadrant?

Diverticulitis, sigmoid volvulus, perforated colon, colon cancer, urinary tract infection, small bowel obstruction, inflammatory bowel disease, nephrolithiasis, pyelonephritis, fluid

Right lower quadrant?

accumulation from aneurysm or perforation, referred hip pain, gynecologic causes

Same as left lower quadrant, especially **appendicitis;** also, mesenteric lymphadenitis, cecal diverticulitis, and Meckel's diverticulum

What are the differential diagnoses of gynecologic causes of lower quadrant pain?

Mittelschmerz, ovarian cyst, endometriosis, fibroids (with or without necrosis; found in approximately 20% of women less than 40 years old), ovarian torsion, pelvic inflammatory disease, ovarian tumor (e.g., Krukenberg tumor/ teratoma), ectopic pregnancy, adhesions in the pelvis, pregnancy, infection of the uterus following gynecologic procedures, threatened abortion, round ligament pain secondary to pregnancy

What is round ligament pain?

Lower quadrant pain secondary to stretching of the round ligament attached to the uterus (remember, the round ligament, instead of the spermatic cord, travels through the inguinal canal in women); may be confused with appendicitis in pregnancy

What are the symptoms of endometriosis?

Classic triad:
1. Dyschezia (painful defecation)
2. Dyspareunia (painful sexual intercourse)
3. Dysmenorrhea (painful menstruation)
Also, spotting, pain, and infertility

SIGNS OF ACUTE ABDOMEN

What is the Chandelier sign?

Extreme pain upon manual palpation of the cervix during bimanual exam; may be due to **any** cause of pelvic peritonitis (think: pain is so intense, the patient hits the ceiling and reaches for the chandelier)

What is Blumer's shelf?

Metastatic disease to the rectouterine (pouch of Douglas) or rectovesical pouch, creating a "shelf" that is palpable on rectal exam

What is Charcot's triad?

Occurs with cholangitis:
1. Fever (chills)
2. Jaundice
3. Right upper quadrant pain

What is Courvoisier's gallbladder?

An enlarged nontender gallbladder that occurs with obstruction of the common bile duct, most often associated with pancreatic cancer (note: not present with acute cholecystitis, because the gallbladder is scarred secondary to chronic cholelithiasis)

What is Cullen's sign?

Bluish discoloration of the periumbilical area caused by retroperitoneal hemorrhage tracking around to the anterior abdominal wall through fascial planes (i.e., in acute pancreatitis)

What is Kehr's sign?

Severe left shoulder pain, often with left upper quadrant pain in patients with splenic rupture (owing to referred diaphragmatic irritation)

What is McBurney's point?

One-third the distance from the anterior iliac spine to the umbilicus on a line connecting the two

What is McBurney's sign?

Tenderness at McBurney's point in patients with appendicitis

What is the Meckel's diverticulum "rule of 2s"?

Two percent of the population has a Meckel's diverticulum; 2% of those patients are symptomatic, and they occur 2 feet from the ileocecal valve.

What is mittelschmerz?

Lower quadrant pain caused by ovulation

What is Murphy's sign?

Pain in the right upper quadrant during inspiration, while palpating under the right costal margin; the patient cannot inspire deeply because it places an inflamed gallbladder under pressure (seen in acute cholecystitis).

What is obturator sign?   Pain upon internal rotation of the leg with the hip and knee flexed; occurs in patients with appendicitis/pelvic abscess

What is psoas sign?   Pain elicited by extending the hip with the knee in full extension, or downward pressure as the patient attempts to lift the thigh; occurs with appendicitis and psoas inflammation

What is Reynold's pentad?
1. Fever
2. Jaundice
3. Right upper quadrant pain
4. Mental status changes
5. Shock/sepsis

Charcot's triad plus 4 and 5
Occurs in patients with suppurative cholangitis

What is Rovsing's sign?   Palpation of the left lower quadrant that results in pain in the right lower quadrant; also, rebound in the left lower quadrant that causes rebound pain in the right lower quadrant

What is Markle's sign?   "JAR" abdominal tenderness, elicited by shaking the bed, foot, or pelvis; sign of peritoneal inflammation

What is Blumberg's sign?   Rebound tenderness

What should a work-up for a patient with acute abdominal pain involve?
History and physical examination
Labs
CBC with differential
β-hCG (for all women of childbearing age)
Amylase (possibly)
Liver function tests (possibly)
Type and screen
T. Bilirubin
Electrolytes
Coagulation
Urinalysis
X-rays (possibly; including upright chest or left lateral decubitus abdomen)
U/S, CT (possibly)

What must be included in every CBC in patients with an acute abdomen?	A differential
What test must every woman of childbearing age have?	A β-hCG
What additional tests must be given to every patient suspected of having ischemic bowel?	1. Blood gas 2. Lactic acid
What is the best x-ray to evaluate for ischemic bowel?	A-gram
What is the classic finding associated with ischemic bowel?	Pain out of proportion to exam
What is the best radiographic test to evaluate right upper quadrant pain?	Ultrasound
What is the best radiographic test to evaluate the viability of the pancreas?	Abdominal CT with IV contrast (a dead pancreas does not light up)
Can pyelonephritis be seen on abdominal CT?	Yes; it usually appears as a swollen bean
What intraabdominal conditions can result in death within minutes?	All involve massive bleeding: ectopic pregnancy with rupture, ruptured abdominal aortic aneurysm, aortic-enteric fistula, ruptured splenic aneurysm, splenic rupture (usually after mononucleosis, malaria, etc.), ruptured dissecting aorta into the abdomen (very rare), ruptured uterus (during pregnancy), ruptured liver hemangioma (most common benign tumor of the liver), ruptured subcapsular liver hematoma, abdominal trauma

PELVIC INFLAMMATORY DISEASE (PID)

How many women will get PID per year?	Approximately 1 million!
What are the associated signs/symptoms?	Bilateral lower quadrant abdominal pain, vaginal discharge, cervical motion tenderness, fever
What is the most common time in the menstrual cycle for PID to occur?	Usually the first half
What are the most common organisms responsible for PID?	1. *Neisseria gonorrhea* 2. *Chlamydia*
What long-term complications are associated with PID?	1. Pelvic pain 2. Ectopic pregnancy 3. Infertility
What percentage of women with PID will be infertile?	Approximately 8%
What are the signs/symptoms associated with gastroenteritis?	Vomiting is followed by abdominal pain, with or without diarrhea. Symptoms usually resolve in less than 12 hours.
What is the classic sequence of vomiting and abdominal pain in acute appendicitis?	Pain followed by vomiting, in most cases
What question is important to ask in the work-up of appendicitis?	"Are you hungry?" Anorexia is almost always present in acute appendicitis.
Other than the laparoscope or knife, what diagnostic measures are available in evaluating the appendix?	1. Pelvic ultrasound 2. Barium enema
What is the most common type of MI associated with abdominal pain, nausea, and vomiting?	Inferior MI

What are the differential diagnoses of thoracic causes of abdominal pain?

MI, pneumonia, PE, empyema, esophageal rupture, aortic aneurysm, pneumothorax, pericarditis

Name the possible unique cause of nonsurgical abdominal pain in the following scenarios:

African-American with a history of joint pain

Sickle cell crisis

Child who eats paint and has a history of recurrent right lower quadrant pain with no evidence of true right lower quadrant tenderness or peritoneal signs

Lead poisoning

Patient with abdominal pain and high porphobilinogen in the urine

Acute porphyria, usually in women 30 to 40 years old with a history of recurrent abdominal pain radiating to the back out of proportion to abdominal exam findings; fever; elevated WBC (often)

Patient on preoperative steroids

Addisonian crisis or acute adrenal insufficiency

Abdominal wall pain in a patient on warfarin

Rectus sheath hematoma

Patient with a DVT

PE

Patient with skin hyperesthesia in a dermatomal distribution

Herpes

Individual of Jewish or Armenian background with a history of recurrent epigastric abdominal pain; status post two negative exploratory laparotomies; fever to 39° C

Familial Mediterranean fever (autosomal recessive inheritance)

25

Hernias

David D. Graham, MD
Lorne H. Blackbourne, MD

BACKGROUND INFORMATION

What is the definition of a hernia?

It generally consists of a sac of peritoneum through a congenital or an acquired defect in the musculoaponeurotic structures of the abdominal wall.

What is the overall incidence of hernias in the United States?

Hernias occur in approximately 1%–5% of the general population.

What types of hernias make up this incidence?

The vast majority of hernias occur in the inguinal region; approximately 50% are indirect and 25% are direct. Ventral hernias comprise approximately 10% of hernias, femoral hernias approximately 5%, and umbilical hernias approximately 3%. Various rare types of hernias comprise the remaining 7%.

What is the male to female ratio?

Male:female = 9:1.

Name the layers of the abdominal wall.

Skin, subcutaneous fat, Scarpa's fascia, external oblique, internal oblique, transversus abdominis, transversalis fascia, and peritoneum

Define the following descriptive terms:
    Reducible

The ability to return the displaced organ or tissue/hernia contents to their usual anatomic site

Incarcerated	Swollen or fixed within the hernia sac (imprisoned), and may or may not cause intestinal obstruction (i.e., an irreducible hernia)
Strangulated	Incarcerated hernia with resulting ischemia, leading to signs and symptoms of ischemia and intestinal obstruction (i.c., **pain and vomiting**)
Complete	Hernia sac and its contents protrude all the way through the defect.
Incomplete	Defect present without the sac or its contents protruding completely through it

Define the following types of hernias:

Sliding	The hernia sac is partially formed by the wall of a viscus.
Littre's	Hernia involving a Meckel's diverticulum
Spigelian	Hernia through the linea semilunaris (or spigelian fascia); also known as a spontaneous lateral ventral hernia
Internal	Hernia into or involving the intra-abdominal structure
Obturator	Hernia through the obturator canal (more common in women than men)
Petit's	Hernia through Petit's triangle (rare)
Grynfeltt's	Hernia through Grynfeltt-Lesshaft triangle
Lumbar	Petit's hernia or Grynfeltt's hernia
Pantaloon	Hernia sac is both a direct **and** indirect hernia, straddling the inferior epigastric vessels and protruding through the floor of the canal, as well as the internal ring

Richter's   Incarcerated or strangulated hernia
                                involving only one wall of the bowel,
                                which can spontaneously reduce,
                                resulting in gangrenous bowel and
                                perforation within the abdomen without
                                signs of obstruction

Incisional   Hernia through an incisional site; most
                                common cause is **wound infection**

Ventral   Incisional hernia in the ventral
                                abdominal wall (note: obesity is
                                associated with recurrence)

Epigastric   Hernia through the linea alba above the
                                umbilicus

Umbilical   Hernia through the umbilical ring,
                                associated with ascites, pregnancy, and
                                obesity

Intraparietal   Hernia in which abdominal contents
                                migrate between the layers of the
                                abdominal wall

Properitoneal   Intraparietal hernia between the
                                peritoneum and the transversalis fascia

Cooper's   Hernia involving the femoral canal and
                                tracts into the scrotum or labia majus

Indirect inguinal   Inguinal hernia **lateral to** Hesselbach's
                                triangle

Direct inguinal   Inguinal hernia **within** Hesselbach's
                                triangle

Hiatal   Hernia through the esophageal hiatus

Velpeau's   Hernia through the Gimbernat's
                                ligament (also known as Laugier's or
                                lacunar ligament hernia)

Hesselbach's   Femoral hernia that passes **laterally** to
                                the femoral vessels

Sciatic	Hernia through the sacrosciatic foramen in the pelvis
Cloquet's	Femoral hernia that penetrates the pectineus muscle fascia (thigh muscle lateral to the adductor longus muscle)
Parastomal	Hernia through the same fascial opening created for a colostomy or ileostomy
Serafini's	Femoral hernia that travels **underneath** the femoral vessels

Diagnosis and Treatment

What is the epidemiology of inguinal hernias?	Inguinal hernias occur most often in men and are frequently right sided. Bilateral inguinal hernias also occur frequently.
What are some common causes of inguinal hernias, particularly abdominal direct inguinal hernias?	Increased pressure caused by sudden straining, heavy exercise, obesity, chronic cough, ascites, straining at stool, or pregnancy
What are the differential diagnoses of an inguinal hernia?	Lymphadenopathy, varicocele, undescended testicle, hematoma, soft-tissue sarcoma, and lipoma
Should inguinal hernias be repaired?	Inguinal hernias do not resolve spontaneously, but continue to enlarge and lead to serious complications; therefore, with only rare exceptions, these hernias should be corrected surgically in a timely fashion.
What serious complications can arise in an untreated inguinal hernia?	Incarceration, intestinal obstruction, and infarction of the bowel
What is the rate of incarceration of inguinal hernias?	Approximately 10%
What is the most common complication that arises after inguinal hernia repair?	Urinary retention

Which inguinal hernia repair involves merely a tightening up of the internal inguinal ring?

Marcy treatment

How often does a wound infection occur following inguinal hernia repair?

Approximately 2% of cases

How often is manual reduction successful?

Thirty percent to fifty percent of the time

What action should be taken if manual reduction is not successful?

Immediate operative repair is recommended to prevent complete strangulation and, ultimately, tissue gangrene.

What is the Bassini procedure?

A type of hernia repair, often used for direct inguinal hernias, involving approximation of the conjoined tendon and the transversalis fascia to the shelving edge of the inguinal (Poupart's) ligament

What is the McVay procedure?

A type of hernia repair in which the conjoined tendon of the internal oblique muscle and the rectus abdominis muscle is approximated to Cooper's ligament; this procedure usually requires a relaxing incision in the rectus sheath

What is the Canadian hernia repair?

Shouldice repair

What nerves may be injured during hernia repair and what are the sequelae?

The ilioinguinal nerve, causing anesthesia of the ipsilateral penis, scrotum, and medial thigh; and the iliohypogastric, causing anesthesia of the ipsilateral lower abdominal wall and inguinal region

What is a femoral hernia?

A groin hernia in which there is a protrusion of a peritoneal sac underneath the inguinal ligament between the lacunar ligament medially and the femoral vein laterally

Is there a particular risk associated with this type of hernia?

Yes; incarceration occurs in about 25% of patients with femoral hernias

How is a femoral hernia repaired?

The transversalis fascia must be approximated to Cooper's ligament in order to close the femoral triangle located beneath the inguinal ligament.

Can the inguinal ligament be divided in the case of an incarcerated femoral hernia?

Yes

What is the incidence of femoral hernias?

Femoral hernias account for approximately 5% of all hernias, and about a third of all hernias in women.

Do umbilical hernias occur in adults?

Yes. They are generally acquired lesions caused by any number of factors related to increased abdominal pressure, such as obesity, ascites, or pregnancy.

What causes a ventral hernia?

Most ventral hernias are the result of a previous surgical incision that has separated because of either poor wound healing, increased abdominal strain, or wound infection.

Generally speaking, how are ventral hernias treated?

Surgery is generally recommended and requires mobilization of tissues with primary closure. Large defects may require prosthetic material and have a higher recurrence rate than the low rate expected with smaller defects.

What are the two most common contents found in an epigastric hernia?

The falciform ligament and the omentum

In terms of hernia prevention, where is the ideal site for a colostomy?

Through the rectus muscle

What are the indications for repair of a parastomal hernia?

An unsatisfactory stoma requiring placement at another site, stricture or prolapse of the stoma, large size of the hernia, presence of a small fascial defect surrounding the hernia, incarceration or strangulation of the hernia, and cosmetic repair

With what type of hernia is a Richter's hernia commonly associated?

Richter's hernias constitute approximately 15% of all incarcerated hernias, and 80% to 90% of these are femoral hernias.

What is the Howship-Romberg sign?

Pain along the distribution of the obturator nerve, which supplies sensation to the upper medial aspect of the thigh (may be noted in patients with obturator hernias)

What is a cord lipoma?

Preperitoneal fat mass

Should the cord lipoma be removed?

Yes

What is the most popular repair for imbrication of the transverse aponeurosis?

Shouldice treatment

Which popular treatment involves the use of prosthetic material?

Lichtenstein treatment

HERNIA ANATOMY

Translate the following terms:

    Poupart's ligament

Inguinal ligament

    Cooper's ligament

Pectineal ligament

    Gimbernat's ligament

Lacunar ligament

    Colles' ligament

Reflected inguinal ligament

    Henle's ligament

Falx inguinalis (rectus sheath fibers that insert on the pectin pubis)

Hesselbach's ligament	Interfoveolar ligament (thickened transversalis fascia anterior to the epigastric vessels)
What is the first superficial fascia encountered upon abdominal groin incision?	Camper's (almost nonexistent)
What is the second superficial fascia encountered upon groin incision?	Scarpa's

MISCELLANEOUS HERNIA FACTS

What is the rarest type of hernia?	Sciatic
Who first described a sliding hernia?	Scarpa
Who first described "pants over vest" repair for umbilical hernias?	Mayo (most surgeons now repair the "umbo hold the mayo")
In what type of patient are infantile umbilical hernias most common?	African-American infants
Why can a reduced incarcerated abdominal wall hernia still progress to strangulation?	The hernia is out of the fascia defect but still in the hernia sac.
Which two types of hernias are not associated with early small bowel obstruction?	1. Richter's hernia 2. Littre's hernia

26

Laparoscopy

Stephen Bayne, MD
Lorne H. Blackbourne, MD

What is laparoscopy?

A means of viewing the peritoneal cavity with endoscopic technology for diagnostic and interventional purposes

When did therapeutic laparoscopy begin?

Gynecologists have been using the laparoscope for gynecologic procedures since 1976. The first appendix was removed in 1983. The first cholecystectomy was performed in 1987.

What are the common components of laparoscopy?

Scope 0° to 45°
Light source
CO_2 gas insufflator with pressure monitor
Television monitor(s)
Irrigation device
Electrocautery device
Veress needle, trocars, laparoscopic instruments, endo pouches, and so forth

What complications can occur with laparoscopy?

Trocar-site bleeding
Veress needle or trocar **injuries to the bowel,** bladder, vessels, or solid organs
Hypercarbia
Carbon dioxide infusion into the vascular system resulting in a CO_2 **embolus**
Increased rate of **DVT** secondary to pressure placed on the iliac veins by pneumoperitoneum
Respiratory compromise secondary to diaphragmatic compression
Burn injuries from cautery source or light
Hernias at the trocar site
Infection at the trocar site

Pneumothorax, pneumomediastinum, pneumoscrotum, and so forth
Increased incidence of hypothermia

How can laparoscopic complications be avoided?

Proper hemostatic technique
Careful attention to anatomic detail when placing the Veress needle or trocars
Continuous monitoring to allow early identification of hypercarbia

What measures should be taken to correct hypercarbia?

Decreasing the upper limit of the insufflator to 12 to 15 mm Hg, hyperventilation, and "blowing off" CO_2 through a trocar

How can DVT be prevented?

By placing pneumatic cuffs on all patients prior to pneumoperitoneum

Which trocar sites should be sutured?

Suturing of sites greater than 0.7 cm is recommended.

What is the appropriate treatment of CO_2 embolism?

CO_2 embolization occurs by direct Veress needle/trocar infusion of CO_2 into a vein or through open venous channels at a surgical site or at extremely high intraperitoneal pressures. Diagnosis starts by identifying the classic "mill wheel" murmur, tachycardia, jugular vein distension, and hypoxemia. The cause is CO_2 embolus to either the right heart or to the pulmonary vasculature, producing a functional obstruction. Therapy involves stopping the CO_2 infusion, releasing the pneumoperitoneum, and using Trendelenburg and left lateral decubitus positions. Also, hyperventilation should be followed by central venous access to manually extract the CO_2.

What are the advantages of laparoscopy?

Decreased postoperative pain
Decreased abdominal deformity
Decreased hospital stay (up to 50% can be performed on an outpatient basis)
Decreased ileus

Are common bile duct injuries more common with open or laparoscopic cholecystectomy?

They are two to four times more common with laparoscopic cholecystectomies.

Define the measures outlined by Crist and Gadacz that will help prevent common bile duct injuries during a laparoscopic cholecystectomy:

    Type of scope — 30°

    Fundus retraction — Firm cephalad

    Infundibulum retraction — Lateral retraction

    Gallbladder neck dissection — Complete identification and mobilization of the neck

    Junction of the gallbladder and cystic duct — Complete identification of the gallbladder and cystic duct junction

    Porta hepatis bleeding — No blind clips or electrocautery

    Unclear anatomy — Open

Why is electrocautery contraindicated for transection of tissue between clips?

Because of the potential for thermal injury to surrounding tissue and arcing of the current

What is the most common cause of common bile duct injury?

Mistaking the common bile duct for the cystic duct

Is there any evidence that routine intraoperative cholangiography decreases the risk of common bile duct injury?

No

Which laparoscopic instrument is responsible for the most visceral injuries?

The Veress needle

What action should be taken if a major vascular structure is injured by a cannula trocar?

Opening of the abdomen through a midline incision

What action should be taken if a major vessel is stuck with the Veress needle?

Removal of the needle; opening of the abdomen if vital signs are unstable, a large expanding retroperitoneal hematoma is present, or free intraperitoneal bleeding occurs; otherwise, close postoperative monitoring is recommended

How should a bleeding trocar site be repaired?

1. Insert a Keith needle into the peritoneal cavity and out the abdomen under the vessel and tie over a bolster
2. Insert a Foley catheter through the trocar site and hold pressure with outward traction
3. Cut down and tie off vessel

What is the incidence of intestinal injury by a Veress needle or trocar?

Approximately 1/1000

Which major laparoscopic complications can result in death?

Missed intestinal or major vessel injury

What four things must be in place before a laparoscopic procedure can be performed?

1. Foley catheter
2. OGt or nasogastric tube
3. Compression boots
4. IV antibiotics

What action should be taken if a Veress needle small bowel injury is suspected?

1. Remove the needle
2. Place a camera through a different site using the Hasson technique
3. Inspect the site and observe, if sealed
4. If a full-thickness laceration is present, sew shut laparoscopically or open

Should a trocar be removed from the abdomen if a small bowel injury is suspected and the patient's abdomen will be opened?

It should be left in place to help indicate the site of injury and to minimize the leak of succus.

What is the most common cause of bladder needle/ trocar injury in laparoscopy?

Failure to insert the Foley catheter

What are the signs of bladder injury?

Air bubbles in the Foley catheter
Hematuria
Visualized bladder mucosa

How should a bladder Veress needle puncture be treated?

Postoperative Foley drainage

How should a trocar bladder injury be treated?

Suturing and Foley drainage

What is the most common cause of a postoperative periumbilical trocar site urine leak?

Transection of a patent urachal sinus

How can placement of a trocar through an epigastric vessel be avoided?

Transillumination of the abdominal wall and identification of the vessels

What type of hernia often occurs postoperatively at the trocar site?

Richter's hernia

What types of patients have problems with the increase in pco_2 and acidemia associated with CO_2 peritoneal insufflation?

Those with cardiac problems (e.g., arrhythmias), chronic obstructive pulmonary disease (COPD), or sickle cell disease

What cardiac problem is associated with pneumoperitoneum and distention of the peritoneum?

Vagal stimulation and bradycardia

What complication is associated with a "mill wheel" murmur?

CO_2 embolus

What preventive measure might be required in patients with massive CO_2 subcutaneous emphysema?

Prolonged ventilation, to "blow off" the CO_2 stores from the body

Can the camera endoscope light cause small bowel injury?

Yes; the xenon light source can become quite hot and burn a hole in the bowel wall

What can prevent injuries caused by electrocautery?

1. Having the weapon on the TV monitor at all times
2. Using a high audible signal to indicate that the cautery is on
3. Using lowest possible current setting

What is the advantage of lasers over electrocautery?

Lasers have no advantage over electrocautery and actually have an increased expense, longer operating time, and less efficient hemostasis; in addition, they may be associated with more injuries to surrounding tissues. (Christ, p.265)

What is the "trapezoid of doom" associated with inguinal hernia laparoscopic repair?

The trapezoid lateral to the femoral vessels and below the iliopubic tract in which several nerves run; if a staple is placed in this region, a painful neuralgia may occur postoperatively

What nerves are located in the "trapezoid of doom"?

Femoral branch of the genitofemoral nerve, lateral cutaneous nerve of the thigh, femoral nerve

What problem is associated with laparoscopic colon cancer resection?

There have been numerous accounts of abdominal wall recurrence following laparoscopic procedures. The seeding occurs either by direct contact of the specimen or instruments, or via aerosolization of tumor cells by the CO_2, with implantation at the trocar sites.

Why is CO_2 used for pneumoperitoneum?

It is noncombustible.
It is soluble in blood, reducing the likelihood of gas embolization.
It is part of the buffering system.
In healthy patients, CO_2 infusion produces clinically insignificant changes in CO_2 homeostasis.

Which procedures are currently being performed with the laparoscope?

Exploratory laparoscopy
Cholecystectomy, with or without common bile duct exploration
Appendectomy
Hernia repair (inguinal/ventral)
Gastric fundoplication
Oophorectomy
Resection of the bowel
Diverting ostomies
Truncal/parietal cell vagotomy
Wedge resections and biopsies
Lymph node sampling
Adrenalectomy
Splenectomy
Nephrectomy

What is the Veress needle?

A spring-loaded needle that allows access to the peritoneal cavity and infusion of CO_2

How can the location of the Veress needle be verified?

By passive saline infusion; aspirate first
If the aspiration is negative, place saline passively into the hub of the needle. If the needle is placed correctly, exhalation will increase the negative intra-abdominal pressure and allow free flow of the saline into the peritoneal cavity.

What is the Hasson technique?

An open cutdown on fascia and peritoneum using direct vision to place the first trocar into the peritoneal cavity, followed by CO_2 infusion

What are the disadvantages of the Hasson technique?

Larger skin and fascial incision, possible air leak from fascia around the trocar

Which patients should receive the Hasson technique?

Those with a history of previous surgery or intra-abdominal infection

How can CO_2 embolus be prevented when using the laparoscopic argon laser coagulator?

With an open port, so that the intraperitoneal pressure does not build up

27

Amputations

Lorne H. Blackbourne, MD

Define the following terms:

BKA	Below the knee amputation
AKA	Above the knee amputation
Syme's amputation	Amputation of the foot

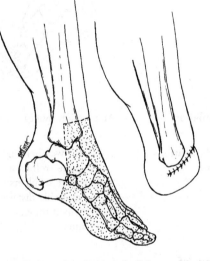

Ray amputation	Removal of the metatarsal head and digit of foot

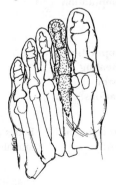

Transmetatarsal amputation	Foot amputation at the level of the metatarsals

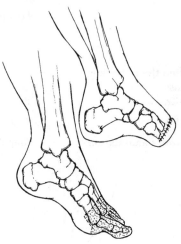

Hip disarticulation	Amputation by hip dislocation
What are the indications for amputation?	1. Gross overwhelming infection/ gangrene (refractory) 2. Rest pain or ulcers/infection without any graftable distal arteries 3. Malignant tumors 4. Trauma
What percentage of patients with claudication will receive an amputation in 5 yrs?	Only approximately 5%
Which type of amputation has the highest healing rate of all the lower extremity amputations?	AKA
What is the significance of a nonhealing AKA?	Bodes poorly; associated with a high mortality rate
What is the best amputation for a grossly infected limb?	Guillotine amputation with formal closure after infection clears

What is the best graft material after an infection clears?	Saphenous vein graft
Which flap—anterior or posterior—has the best blood supply for a BKA?	The posterior flap has more collaterals than the anterior flap because of the closer proximity to the popliteal artery
Should dog ears be removed from the skin closure?	No (controversial)
What is the best type of suture for apposing the muscle fascia layer of a BKA or an AKA?	Absorbable (i.e., Vicryl®)
Should electrocautery be used extensively during an amputation?	No; it is associated with a large necrotic tissue load and may cause infection/ischemia
What are the principles of operative technique for amputations?	1. Remove bone 2. Avoid tension on closure 3. Administer antibiotics 4. Avoid hematoma 5. Handle tissue with care 6. Do not separate skin from underlying fascia
What is the rate of operative mortality for an AKA or a BKA?	Approximately 10% to 15%
What is the most common cause of operative mortality in this group?	Heart attack/arrhythmia (accounts for 50%)
What is the mortality rate 3 years after an AKA or BKA?	Approximately 50%
Will a toe amputation heal in a patient with dry gangrene?	Usually not; therefore, do not perform an amputation until revascularization is completed
What percentage of patients with an AKA will walk independently?	Only about a third

What percentage of patients with a BKA will walk independently?	About two-thirds
In a BKA, how long should the fibula be in relation to the tibia?	Approximately 1 cm proximal to the tibia
What can help prevent post-BKA knee flexion contracture?	A knee immobilizer (or cast)
What bedside sign is used by many experienced surgeons to determine the level of amputation?	Warm skin
What is the best predictor of failure of a BKA to heal?	Absence of any palpable or dopplerable popliteal arterial pulsation; less than 70 mm Hg pressure
What toe pressure is thought to correlate with the failure of a transmetatarsal or toe amputation to heal?	Systolic toe pressures less than 45 mm Hg (the presence of a palpable pedal pulse correlates closely with the healing of a transmetatarsal amputation)
What systolic popliteal pressure is associated with healing of the stump?	Greater than 50 to 70 mm Hg by Doppler
What percentage of all BKAs will heal?	Approximately 80%
What type of patient has falsely elevated leg Doppler blood pressures?	Patients with diabetes and noncompressible calcified vessels

28

Trauma

Oliver Binns, MD
Lorne H. Blackbourne, MD
S. Duke Herrel, MD
John Sperling, MD

BACKGROUND INFORMATION

What are the "ABCs" of trauma?	**A**irway with cervical spine control **B**reathing **C**irculation **D**isability—brief neurologic exam **E**xposure
What is the currently accepted standard approach to the trauma patient?	The ATLS course of the American College of Surgeons
What are the two most common causes of immediate death from trauma?	**Head injury**—50% **Exsanguination**—35%

AIRWAY

What is the most common cause of upper airway obstruction?	Tongue
What must be protected when obtaining an airway?	Cervical spine
Approximately what percentage of unconscious patients with injuries above the level of the clavicles have cervical spine fractures?	Twenty percent

What is the initial maneuver to obtain an airway?	Chin lift or jaw thrust
What condition contraindicates a nasopharyngeal airway?	Midface trauma
If an airway cannot be obtained by endotracheal intubation, what other method is available?	Access via the cricothyroid membrane
Is visualizing C1-7 on x-ray an adequate view of the cervical spine?	No; T-1 must also be seen

BREATHING

What should be checked for on inspection?	Whether or not the patient is able to talk Whether or not there is air movement out of the patient's mouth Respiratory rate, rhythm, force, and volume Presence of an open wound in the chest Asymmetric chest expansion Prominent neck veins Presence of cyanosis
What should be checked for on auscultation?	Stridor or gurgling Breath sounds over lung fields
What should be checked for on percussion?	Hyperresonance or dullness to percussion
What should be checked for on palpation?	Subcutaneous emphysema, bony stability
What are the six thoracic causes of early death that must be recognized?	1. Tension pneumothorax 2. Cardiac tamponade 3. Open pneumothorax 4. Hemothorax 5. Flail chest 6. Airway obstruction

What is a tension pneumothorax?

It is the presence of air in the pleural space under pressure. Lung collapse and mediastinal shift interfere with expansion of the contralateral lung and compromise venous return to the heart. The condition is extremely dangerous and requires urgent action.

What are the associated signs and symptoms?

Tachypnea, contralateral tracheal deviation, hyperresonance, distended neck veins, dyspnea, and hypotension

What is the appropriate treatment?

Needle thoracentesis in the second intercostal space in the midclavicular line, followed by chest tube placement

What is cardiac tamponade?

Increased pressure in the pericardial sac, which interferes with the filling of the heart

What are the associated signs and symptoms?

Neck vein distention, hypotension, pallor, and distant heart sounds

What is the appropriate treatment?

Pericardiocentesis in the subxiphoid area

What is an open pneumothorax?

An open defect in the chest wall that results in inspiratory/expiratory efforts that move air across the defect

What is the appropriate treatment?

Intubation with positive pressure and closure of the opening in the chest wall; if the defect is small, occlusive dressing can be taped on three sides of the wound

What is a hemothorax?

Bleeding into the thoracic cavity with resultant loss of circulatory volume and decreased ventilation

What is the appropriate treatment?

Circulatory volume replacement and chest tube placement

What test must be performed after chest tube placement?

CXR, to ensure lung re-expansion, blood evacuation, and tube position

What is flail chest?	Multiple rib fractures in each rib, resulting in paradoxical respiration and subsequent hypoventilation
What is the appropriate treatment?	Intubation

CIRCULATION

What is the goal of circulation?	To ensure adequate tissue perfusion and control hemorrhage
What type of access is preferable?	Two 14- to 16-gauge percutaneous IV catheters
In an adult, what percentage of body weight is constituted by blood volume?	Seven percent
Is this percentage higher or lower in children?	Higher (8%–9%)
How much of a fluid bolus should be administered?	**Adults**—1 to 2 L **Children**—20 ml/kg
How should the results of a fluid challenge be monitored?	Vital signs, mental status, capillary refill, and urinary output; if the patient requires continued boluses, a site of continued volume loss should be sought

DISABILITY

What prognostic information does the Glasgow Coma Scale provide?	In addition to quantitating CNS dysfunction over time, the Glasgow Coma Scale provides prognostic information on the probability of future recovery.
What responses are tested?	Eye opening and motor/verbal response
What percentage of all spinal cord injuries are caused by automobile accidents?	Sixty percent

EXPOSURE

Why is exposure necessary?	To ensure that no sites of bleeding or injury are missed

SECONDARY SURVEY

When is the secondary survey begun?	Only after primary survey and resuscitation
What does the secondary survey entail?	A complete physical examination is performed. Additional procedures are also performed, and may include additional radiologic examination and peritoneal lavage.

HEAD AND NECK

With a diagnosed fracture of the parietal bone, what associated injury must be ruled out?	Epidural hematoma
What injury must be ruled out with trauma to the midface?	Cervical spine fracture
How should bleeding from the scalp greater than 100 ml/min be controlled?	Rapid closure with monofilament suture; wound can be reclosed at a later time

GUNSHOT WOUNDS

What is a semiautomatic versus an automatic rifle?	A semiautomatic shoots one bullet for each pull of the trigger, whereas an automatic repeatedly fires bullets while the trigger is held down ("machine gun").
What is an automatic handgun?	A misnomer; an automatic handgun is actually a semiautomatic handgun
What is a magnum versus a nonmagnum?	A magnum has a larger amount of gunpowder to propel it.
What is a hollow-point bullet?	A bullet with a hollow end that "mushrooms" out upon impact with a solid object (e.g., a human)

What is larger: a 22-caliber bullet or a 44-caliber bullet?

A 44-caliber bullet; caliber is basically a rough estimate of the bullet size in inches (i.e., a 44-caliber bullet is roughly 0.44 inch in diameter)

What is a shotgun?

A large-bore long firearm that shoots multiple pellets per shot (up to 50)

What is larger: a 410-gauge shotgun or a 12-gauge shotgun?

A 12-gauge shotgun barrel is much larger than a 410-gauge shotgun. (Gauge is determined by the number of lead balls the same diameter as the barrel that it takes to reach 1 pound; it takes 12 lead balls with the diameter of the 12-gauge and 41 balls for the 410-gauge to reach 1 pound)

Which pellets are larger: Number 8 shot or Number 2 shot?

Number 2 shot is larger (again, the larger number is smaller).

What is the appropriate treatment of each of the following injuries:
    Popliteal vein–penetrating injury?

Repair; do not ligate

    Suprarenal vena caval injury?

Repair; do not ligate

    Infrarenal vena caval injury?

Repair if possible; otherwise, ligate

    Internal jugular vein injury?

Lateral venography, if possible; otherwise, ligate

    Transection of the femoral vein?

Repair if possible; otherwise, ligate

    Transection of a single artery of the lower leg (calf)?

Ligate

What is bullet yaw?

The deviation of the bullet from its longitudinal projection

What is bullet tumble?

Head-over-heel somersaults

What is the formula for kinetic energy?

$\frac{1}{2}MV^2$ (thus, increasing velocity greatly increases the kinetic energy of the bullet)

What material must be sought in all shotgun wounds?

The plastic wadding—a small plastic "cup" that holds the pellets; the wadding is not sterile and may also be cardboard

What clues might indicate a close-proximity gunshot wound?

Gunpowder "tattoos" of the skin surrounding the entrance site

Can the entrance and exit wounds be reliably determined?

Exit wounds are generally larger than entrance wounds. The entrance wound can be reliably determined only by evidence of gunpowder tattoos.

What is cavitation?

When a high-powered bullet enters the body, it transfers its kinetic energy to the surrounding tissues, which are then violently thrown out from the bullet's path in a radial direction, forming a cavity and thus **injuring tissues not in the actual path of the bullet.**

What determines the amount of cavitation?

1. Kinetic energy of the bullet
2. Surface area of the bullet

What are the basic principles of patient care for abdominal gunshot wounds?

A,B,Cs
Nasogastric tube
Foley catheter
Chest and abdominal x-rays (if the patient is stable)
Cefoxitin/tetanus
Surgery

What are the basic principles of patient care for chest gunshot wounds?

A,B,Cs
Nasogastric tube
Foley catheter
Chest tube
Chest x-ray
Cefoxitin (for lower chest wounds)
Ancef (for mid/high chest wounds)

Which prophylactic antibiotics are used to treat penetrating abdominal trauma?

Wide spectrum, including anaerobes:
1. Cefoxitin **or**
2. Cefotetan **or**
3. Ampicillin-sulbactam

What type of incision is used for abdominal trauma?

Long midline abdominal incision

Why should a leg be prepped in the field in a trauma patient?

For access to a saphenous vein for vascular procedure

What action should be taken if serious bleeding is evident upon opening of the peritoneal cavity?

Pack off all four quadrants with laparotomy pads

In the patient with a single gunshot wound, what other injury should always be considered?

Another gunshot wound (totally undress the patient/log roll, and so forth)

What is the appropriate treatment of a 38-year-old woman with a gunshot wound through the rectum?

Lithotomy position:
1. Proximal diverting colostomy
2. Presacral drainage
3. Closure of the rectal defect if it communicates with the peritoneal cavity
4. Although controversial, rectal washout lavage is sometimes performed

What percentage of patients with penetrating trauma to the pancreas will have an elevated serum amylase?

Only approximately 15%

What is the appropriate treatment of each of the following wounds:

    Pancreatic contusion from a gunshot wound cavitation injury?

Hemostasis and wide external closed drainage

    Distal pancreatic duct transection from a gunshot wound?

Distal pancreatectomy

    Proximal pancreatic duct injury?

1. Distal pancreatectomy **or**
2. Roux-en-Y pancreaticojejunostomy (especially if distal resection would leave less than 15% pancreatic remnant)

Massive combined irreparable duodenal and pancreatic head injury?

Trauma Whipple

Small laceration from a gunshot wound to the small bowel?

Close in two layers in a **transverse** fashion (better short than narrow).

What are the indications for resection and anastomosis after small bowel–penetrating injury?

1. Loss of more than 50% of circumference
2. Closure that results in stenosis greater than one-third of normal lumen
3. Multiple perforations in a single segment

What is the appropriate treatment of two small-bowel perforations that are side by side?

Make into one perforation and close transversely.

Which type of retroperitoneal hematoma from a gunshot wound should not be explored?

Stable retrohepatic hematoma
Stable renal hematoma with preoperative imaging that reveals adequate function

What is the appropriate treatment of pelvic hematoma from penetrating trauma?

Open it up after proximal (aorta/vena cava) and distal (iliac vessels) control **in contrast to blunt trauma.**

What is the appropriate treatment of the following wounds:

Suprarenal vena caval injury?

Repair; do not ligate

Infrarenal vena caval injury?

Repair if at all possible; otherwise, it can be ligated

Can the portal vein be ligated?

Repair if at all possible; otherwise, it can be ligated if the injury is isolated, but with a mortality of at least 50%.

What major operative and postoperative complications can follow ligation of the portal vein?

1. **Massive** fluid sequestration in the splanchnic vascular bed; large amount of crystalloid
2. Bowel necrosis

Can the common or proper hepatic artery be ligated?

Yes, especially proximal to the gastroduodenal branch, because this artery then provides collateral flow from the superior mesenteric artery via the pancreaticoduodenal arcades

Can the right or left hepatic artery be ligated?

Yes, especially if the portal vein is intact, because the portal vein delivers approximately 50% of the liver O_2

Can a lobar bile duct be ligated?

Yes, and without jaundice in the vast majority of patients

Define lower chest wound.

Below the nipple and scapular tip and above the costal margin

What is a safe treatment of lower chest wounds?

Abdominal exploration, because of frequent diaphragm injury

What is the role of laparoscopy in penetrating abdominal surgery?

Evolving; it can be used to evaluate peritoneal penetration in tangential abdominal gunshot wounds

What percentage of solitary lung parenchymal injuries are treated solely by a chest tube?

More than 85%

What are the options for treatment of severe retrohepatic venous hemorrhage?

Atriocaval shunt
Pringle maneuver

What is the atriocaval shunt?

Usually a modified chest tube that is placed into the right atrium and descends in the IVC past a retrohepatic vena caval injury; allows treatment of retrohepatic venous injury, control of blood loss, and venous return to the heart (associated with significant mortality)

PENETRATING NECK TRAUMA

What is a superficial penetrating neck wound versus an injury that must be further investigated?

An injury that does not traverse the platysma is superficial, and one that does cross the platysma must be investigated.

What structure separates the anterior from the posterior neck triangle?

The posterior border of the sternocleidomastoid muscle

Name the neck zones associated with the following attributes:

  Highest mortality with penetrating trauma

Zone I

  Lowest mortality with penetrating trauma

Zone II

  Most common zone associated with penetrating trauma

Zone II (largest zone)

When do you place the nasogastric tube in a patient with penetrating neck trauma?

Right before induction in the OR, **not** in the ER, because the patient's bucking may dislodge a carotid artery clot

How should neck bleeding be controlled?

Pressure

Should penetrating neck wounds be probed in the ER?

No; probing may dislodge the clot

Which x-rays are indicated for a patient with a penetrating neck wound?

1. Cervical spine
2. CXR (to rule out injury/ pneumothorax caused by downward projectory/fragments)

How should a patient with a penetrating neck injury be prepped?

Neck, chest, shoulder, and contralateral leg for saphenous vein, if needed for vascular treatment

In which patients is surgical intervention needed emergently?	Shock Exsanguinating bleed Expanding hematoma Loss of airway
What is the appropriate treatment of a stable patient with signs and/or symptoms of arterial/ airway/esophagus injury?	Surgery, with or without preoperative A-gram
Which zones will receive a preoperative A-gram in a stable symptomatic patient?	Zones I and III, to define the anatomy/ injury to gain distal and proximal control
Define the signs and symptoms of the following injuries with penetrating neck trauma: 　　**Esophageal neck injury**	Odynophagia Dysphagia Subcutaneous crepitus Hematemesis
Vascular neck injury	Expanding/stable hematoma Bleeding Shock Loss of pulse Focal neurologic deficit
Laryngeal/tracheal injury	Subcutaneous air/crepitus Change in voice Hemoptysis Dyspnea
What controversy is associated with penetrating neck injuries?	The management of the **asymptomatic/ no sign of injury, stable** patient with penetrating neck trauma
What are the options for the asymptomatic, stable patient with no sign of injury?	Mandatory surgery Selective approach

Define the following terms:

Mandatory exploration — Exploratory surgery for every patient with penetrating neck trauma

Selective approach — Diagnostic work-up and operation only if significant injury is found

What is the appropriate diagnostic work-up for penetrating neck injury? — A-gram, laryngoscopy/bronchoscopy, esophagoscopy/esophagram

What injury is the most difficult to test for diagnostically? — Esophageal injury

What is the single best test for identifying esophageal injury? — **Rigid** esophagoscopy

What is the best combined diagnostic test to identify esophageal injury? — Rigid esophagoscopy **and** esophagram

CAROTID ARTERY INJURY SURGERY/ANATOMY

Which vein is located in front of the carotid artery at approximately the level of the bifurcation? — The facial vein

Which nerve crosses in front of the carotid artery at approximately 2 cm above the bifurcation? — The hypoglossal nerve (CN XII)

Which nerve runs in between the carotid artery and the jugular vein? — The vagus nerve (CN X)

Which nerve runs in front of the carotid artery at the level of the angle of the mandible? — The facial nerve (CN VII)

What clinical findings are associated with a damaged hypoglossal nerve? — The tongue deviates to the side of the injury (wheelbarrow phenomenon).

What maneuvers are used to gain additional exposure of the distal carotid artery in a Zone III injury?

Transection of the digastric muscle
Releasing of the sternocleidomastoid muscle from the mastoid
Division of the occipital artery
Anterior subluxation of the mandible

What are the indications for systemic heparinization during traumatic carotid artery repair?

Complex repair without obvious contraindication (e.g., subdural hematoma)
Shunt
(Heparin is usually not used for simple repair)

What is the appropriate treatment of an avulsed recurrent laryngeal nerve?

Implantation of the nerve into the cricoarytenoid muscle, if possible

What intraoperative techniques are used to test for esophageal injury?

Intraoperative endoscope
Methylene blue intraluminally
Filling of the wound with saline and having anesthesia bag the patient and check for bubbles

What is the appropriate treatment of an esophageal injury in the first 24 to 48 hours?

Diversion (spit fistula)
Drainage

What are the indications for A-gram, even after a decision has been made to explore the neck following a penetrating neck injury?

Zone III injury
Zone I injury
Shotgun injury (multiple pellets)
Injury from a projectile weapon that traversed the neck with possible bilateral carotid injury

What is the correlation between base deficit and fluid resuscitation?

The greater the initial base deficit (from ABG) is in the ER in the trauma patient, the greater the fluid requirement. An increasing base deficit is often caused by ongoing hemorrhage.

Are higher base deficits in trauma patients associated with more blood transfusions?

Yes

Define hypertonic saline.

7.5% NaCl saline IV solution
(remember, normal saline is 0.9% NaCl)

To maximize IV fluid infusion using large-bore IV catheters, what else must be used?

Large-bore IV **tubing**

What is the idea behind "supranormal values" for severe trauma?

The **controversial** idea of supranormal values for severe trauma is that above-normal values of CI, oxygen delivery, and oxygen consumption in the patient with shock are beneficial in the patient with inadequate tissue perfusion (i.e., "more is better").

Should ER thoracotomy be performed on the blunt-trauma patient arriving without vital signs?

No

What determines peritoneal penetration from an abdominal stab wound more accurately: probing or local exploration?

Local exploration is more accurate than probing.

What procedure must be performed with a common or proper hepatic artery ligation for trauma?

Cholecystectomy

After penetrating trauma to the abdomen, is there any benefit to administering perioperative antibiotics for more than 24 hours?

No; as long as the antibiotics have anaerobic as well as aerobic coverage, 24 hours is satisfactory

What are the risk factors for infection after penetrating abdominal trauma?

Blood transfusions
Shock
Left colon injury
Multiple organ injury

What injuries are associated with seat-belt use?

Small-bowel perforations
L-spine fracture

Are two-point (lap belt) or three-point (shoulder belt) seat-belt restraints more often associated with L-spine fractures?	Two-point seat belts are associated with more L-spine fractures than three-point restraints.
In the patient with penetrating wounds to both the stomach and the diaphragm, what should be done besides closing the holes?	Irrigation of the pleural cavity via the diaphragm hole or via a chest tube, because empyema is often a problem after this combination of injuries
Are sternal fractures in patients who were wearing shoulder seat belts associated with either heart or aortic injury?	No

TRAUMA INJURY SCALES

LIVER INJURY SCALE

What is the number of grades?	Six, but only five are valid, because Grade 6 is total liver avulsion (think: the six-letter word livers, with the "**s**" standing for sarcastic, because almost no one survives a liver avulsion)
By which two types of injuries is each grade defined?	1. Liver hematoma 2. Liver laceration
Define Grade I liver injury in association with the following conditions:	
Hematoma	Subcapsular blood less than 10% of the surface area of the liver (and nonexpanding)
Laceration	Less than 1 cm in depth, capsular tear (and nonbleeding)
Name a memory aid for Grade 1.	The number 1; Grade 1; 1 cm depth of laceration and hematoma less than 10%

Define Grade 2 liver injury in association with the following conditions:

Hematoma

Subcapsular—Less than 50% of the surface area (and more than 10%, because less than 10% is a Grade 1)

Intraparenchymal—Less than 2 cm in diameter (both nonexpanding)

Laceration

Less than 3 cm in depth and less than 10 cm in length

Name a memory aid for Grade 2 intraparenchymal hematoma size.

Grade **2** = **Less than 2** cm Intraparenchymal hematoma

Define Grade 3 liver injury in association with the following conditions:

Hematoma

Subcapsular—more than 50% of the surface area (nonexpanding); **expanding hematoma; or ruptured with active bleeding**

Intraparenchymal—more than 3 cm in diameter

Laceration

Greater than 3 cm in depth

Name a memory aid for Grade 3 laceration.

Grade **3** = **more than 3 cm in diameter**

What is the first grade to have active bleeding?

Grade 3 (expanding subcapsular hematoma or subcapsular hematoma rupture with active bleeding)

Define Grade 4 liver injury under the following conditions:

Hematoma

Ruptured central **intraparenchymal** hematoma

Laceration

Massive parenchymal destruction of less than 75% of the hepatic lobe (but more than 25%)

**Define Grade 5 liver
injury under the following
conditions:**
Laceration

Massive parenchymal destruction of
more than 75% of the hepatic lobe

Vascular injury

Retrohepatic venous injury (i.e., IVC,
major hepatic vein injury)

**Define Grade 6 liver
injury under the following
conditions:**
Vascular injury

Total hepatic avulsion (six = sarcastic
survival)

POWER REVIEW OF LIVER INJURY GRADES

**Define the grade of the
following injuries:**

Liver avulsion	6
Laceration 1 cm deep	1
Expanding 25% subcapsular hematoma	3
Nonexpanding 11% subcapsular hematoma	2
Intraparenchymal hematoma 3.4 cm in diameter	3
Central ruptured hematoma	4
Thirty-six percent parenchymal lobe destruction	4
Nonexpanding 10% subcapsular hematoma	1
Ninety percent parenchymal lobe destruction	5

Laceration 2.4 cm deep and 8 cm long	2
Retrohepatic IVC injury	5
Laceration 3.5 cm deep	3

SPLEEN INJURY SEVERITY SCALE BY GRADES (AAST)

By what two types of injury is each grade defined?

1. Hematoma
2. Laceration
(Same as liver injuries)

Define Grade 1 spleen injury in association with the following conditions:
   Hematoma

Subcapsular, less than 10% surface area, and nonexpanding
(just like liver Grade 1)

   Laceration

Less than 1 cm deep with capsular tear, but nonbleeding
(just like liver Grade 1)

Define Grade 2 spleen injury in association with the following conditions:
   Hematoma

Less than 50% surface area subcapsular, less than 5 cm intraparenchymal hematoma (both nonexpanding)

   Laceration

Capsular tear with **active bleeding,** 1 to 3 cm in depth, but must **not involve a trabecular vessel**

Define Grade 3 spleen injury in association with the following conditions:
   Hematoma

More than 50% subcapsular hematoma or expanding subcapsular hematoma; ruptured subcapsular hematoma with active bleeding; contained hematoma more than 5 cm; or contained expanding subcapsular hematoma

   Laceration

More than 3 cm deep parenchymal laceration

**Define Grade 4 spleen
injury in association with
the following conditions:**
  Hematoma   Ruptured intraparenchymal hematoma
                                  with active bleed

  Laceration   Wound involving segmental or hilar
                                  vessels with major devascularization
                                  (> 25%)

**Define Grade 5 spleen
injury in association with
the following conditions:**
  Laceration   Shattered spleen (massive)

  Vascular injury   Hilar injury that completely
                                  devascularizes the spleen

KIDNEY INJURY SCALE

**Define the following
kidney injury grades:**
  Grade 1   Kidney contusion

  Grade 2   Minor laceration

  Grade 3   Major laceration

  Grade 4   Shattered kidney

  Grade 5   Major vascular injury

**Define the retroperitoneal
trauma zones:**
  Zone 1   Central and medial aspects of the
                                  retroperitoneum

  Zone 2   Flanks

Zone 3   Pelvis

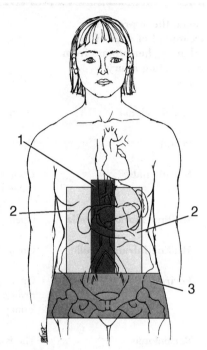

In blunt trauma, should a pelvic hematoma be opened?	No
In penetrating trauma, should a pelvic hematoma be opened?	Yes
In penetrating trauma, should a perirenal hematoma be opened?	Yes, unless a preoperative CT/IVP reveals an intact kidney
In blunt trauma, should a retroperitoneal pericolonic hematoma be opened?	Yes (unless contiguous with a pelvic hematoma)

POWER REVIEW OF RETROPERITONEAL HEMATOMAS

Name the appropriate treatment of each of the following hematomas from penetrating injury:	
Pelvic	Open
Paraduodenal	Open
Portal	Open
Retrohepatic	Do not open in stable patients with stable hematomas
Midline supramesocolic	Open
Midline inframesocolic	Open
Perirenal	Open, unless preoperative CT/IVP reveals functioning/minor injury to kidney
Pericolonic	The issue is controversial, but lumbar or muscle vessels can rebleed

What action should be taken with the following retroperitoneal hematomas from blunt trauma:	
Pelvic?	Do not open if the pelvis is fractured
Retrohepatic?	Do not open if the patient and the hematoma are stable
Portal?	Open
Pericolonic?	Open
Paraduodenal?	Open
Midline supramesocolonic?	Open
Midline inframesocolonic?	Open

Perirenal hematoma?	Do not open if CT, IVP, or U/S reveals "reasonably" intact kidney.
What is the major complication of a negative laparotomy for blunt trauma?	Small-bowel obstruction (incidence is approximately 5%)

GU TRAUMA

URETHRAL TRAUMA

Name the regions of the male urethra.	Anterior (bulbous, penile) Posterior (membranous, prostatic)
What is the most common cause of urethral trauma?	Blunt trauma
What percentage of patients with urethral injuries have pelvic fractures?	Ninety-five percent (usually involve rami or symphysis)
What percentage of patients with pelvic fractures have urethral injuries?	Approximately 10%
What is the single most important sign of possible injury?	Blood at the urethral meatus
Can it be absent?	Yes
What are the other signs/ symptoms of possible urethral trauma?	Pelvic fracture, blood at the meatus, inability to void, displaced "high-riding" prostate
What test should be done prior to attempting catheterization?	RUG—retrograde
What method is used?	Inject 15 to 20 cc water-soluble contrast retrograde into the urethra using a catheter-tip syringe; x-ray

Name the types of posterior urethral injuries.	**Type 1**—stretch injury (no rupture) **Type 2**—prostatomembranous disruption, intact GU diaphragm **Type 3**—prostatomembranous-, GU diaphragm-, and proximal bulbar–urethral disruptions
What is the appropriate treatment?	Early realignment (nonsutured over catheter) versus delayed repair (suprapubic tube), although the issue is controversial
What are the causes of anterior urethral trauma?	Straddle injuries, penetrating trauma, instrumentation
Which fascial planes limit blood and urine extravasation?	Buck's, then Colles' fascia

BLADDER TRAUMA

What are the types of rupture?	Intraperitoneal, extraperitoneal, and combined
Which is most common in adults?	Extraperitoneal
Which is most common in children?	Intraperitoneal
What are the causes?	Blunt and penetrating trauma, iatrogenic causes
What percentage of blunt trauma ruptures have associated pelvic fractures?	Ninety-seven percent
What percentage of pelvic fractures have associated bladder ruptures?	Ten percent to sixteen percent
What are the associated signs and symptoms?	Gross hematuria, low urine output, abdominal pain
What tests should be performed?	Cystography is the gold standard; CT alone is inadequate; RUG

How is this test performed?	1. Scout film 2. Instill approximately 400 cc water-soluble contrast by gravity (adjust volume for age) 3. X-ray 4. Drain out/postvoid x-ray
What are the associated intraperitoneal radiologic findings?	Contrast outlines bowel loops and paracolic gutters above the acetabular line.
What are the associated extraperitoneal radiologic findings?	"Starburst" areas below the acetabular line
What is the appropriate treatment?	**Intraperitoneal**—open surgical repair, multilayer closure, suprapubic tube **Extraperitoneal**—conservative (Foley catheter for 10–14 days), or repair if the patient is undergoing exploratory laparotomy

RENAL TRAUMA

What are the classifications?	Blunt or penetrating **Minor**—contusions, small lacerations, or hematomas **Major**—deep lacerations, vascular injuries
What is the most important sign?	Hematuria (greater than 5 rbcs/hpf; present in more than 90% of cases)
Does the degree of hematuria correlate with the severity of the injury?	No; vascular injuries may have no hematuria
What are the signs of possible renal trauma?	Contusions, seat-belt marks, lower rib fractures, transverse process fractures
What are the most important indicators of possible major injury?	Hypotension (SBP < 90) Gross hematuria
Which pediatric patients need imaging?	Those with any degree of hematuria (gross or microscopic)

Which radiologic study stages renal trauma most accurately?	CT
In patients undergoing immediate laparotomy, what study should be performed for suspected renal trauma?	"One-shot" IVP: 2 ml/kg (max 150 ml) and ER KUB film (can be performed in the OR)
What information does this study obtain?	The presence of a functional contralateral kidney
What are the absolute indications for operative management?	Hemodynamic instability from renal bleeding; expanding or pulsatile retroperitoneal hematoma at laparotomy
What are the keys to operative exploration?	Midline, transabdominal approach; early bilateral vascular control

URETERAL TRAUMA

What is the incidence?	Rare in blunt trauma; may occur in gunshot wounds or stabs
What is the best study for suspected injury?	IVP
What factors influence repair?	Site, extent of necrotic tissue, time delay to diagnosis, associated injuries (may necessitate nephrectomy)
Children may have ureteral injury secondary to what mechanism?	Hyperextension, secondary to flexibility of spine

GENITAL TRAUMA

What is fractured in penile fractures?	Erectile bodies
What are the associated signs and symptoms?	Deformity, swelling, ecchymosis, palpability of the defect
What is the appropriate treatment?	Operative repair, hematoma evacuation, and closure of tunica and Buck's fascia

With what type of skin grafts are degloving penile skin injuries repaired?	Split thickness (allow for erectile function)
What is the appropriate management of penile amputation?	Clean with saline, place in sterile saline solution on ice, perform microvascular reanastomosis
What layer is violated in testicular laceration or rupture?	Tunica albuginea
What study can evaluate the testicle in a swollen, traumatized scrotum?	U/S can often identify whether or not the tunica is ruptured.
What are the principles of repair?	Meticulous debridement of nonviable tissue, irrigation, repair of the tunica albuginea

DUODENAL INJURIES

What is the incidence?	Uncommon; present in 3% to 5% of exploratory laparotomies for trauma
What is the etiology?	Penetrating trauma—85% Blunt trauma—15%
What are the mechanisms causing blunt injuries?	Crushing impact with the vertebral column (often caused by a steering wheel) and deceleration injuries at points of duodenal attachment, the ligament of Treitz, and the ampulla of Vater
What is the associated mortality?	15% to 30%, most commonly from early hemorrhagic shock
What is the major cause of morbidity?	Fistula formation
How is the diagnosis made?	With difficulty, because of the retroperitoneal location of duodenum and because diagnosis is often delayed. Requires a high index of suspicion when significant upper abdominal impact is sustained.

CT with IV and oral contrast is the best all-around test to confirm the diagnosis.

What other studies may aid in making the diagnosis?

Plain films of the abdomen and upright CXR may reveal free intraperitoneal air, retroperitoneal air, or air in the biliary tree.

DPL may reveal blood, bile, or bowel contents, but a negative DPL does not rule out injury.

Upper GI study with water-soluble contrast is the most sensitive test, but is obviously difficult to perform in a trauma setting.

Computed tomography

Serum amylase may be elevated, but is of little value because it is not very specific.

What is the appropriate treatment of duodenal injuries?

Laparotomy, exploration, and intraoperative management of injuries identified

What are some findings at the time of laparotomy that mandate formal exploration of the duodenum?

Retroperitoneal hematoma in the right upper quadrant, (**i.e., Kocher maneuver**), crepitus or bile staining along the lateral border of the duodenum, petechiae or fat necrosis in the retroperitoneum

What is the appropriate treatment of intramural hematomas?

May be treated conservatively if perforation is excluded (i.e., nasogastric tube decompression, IV fluids, and TPN)

What are some intraoperative management options?

Primary repair after debridement, with or without tube decompression of the duodenum

Repair with diversion of gastric contents by either Roux-en-Y reconstruction or pyloric exclusion

Duodenal diverticulization

Pancreaticoduodenectomy for **severe** combined injuries

What issues are involved in the postoperative care of these patients?

Restoration of volume status

Nasogastric tube decompression (until bowel function returns, usually 5–7 days)

Frequent tending of the nasogastric tube sump, to maintain optimum decompression

Management of lateral duodenostomy tubes or retrograde jejunostomy tubes placed intra-operatively involves maintaining adequate decompression of the duodenum. They are usually removed once bowel function returns and enteral feedings are tolerated.

Resultant fistula tracts should close spontaneously over time, and failure to close should prompt consideration of distal obstruction.

Drains around the duodenum should be left in place again until enteral feedings are tolerated.

Increased output with feedings may indicate development of a leak or fistula.

What is the treatment of a fistula should it develop?

1. Bowel rest and decompression
2. TPN and IV fluids
3. H₂ blockers
4. Somatostatin analogues, to decrease GI secretions
5. Control of fistula (i.e., maintainance of adequate drainage)
6. Protection of skin
7. Radiologic evaluation of fistula (i.e., CT to rule out abscess formation and fistulogram to define fistula tract)
8. Continue treatment for at least 4 to 6 weeks prior to considering operative intervention.

BOWEL INJURIES

What is the mechanism of most bowel injuries?

Penetrating trauma (> 90%)

What is the most common organ injured in penetrating trauma?

Small bowel

Where do most blunt injuries to the small bowel occur?

Perforation of the jejunum at the ligament of Treitz, the distal ileum, or areas of previous adhesions

If traumatic perforation of the GI tract is discovered at the time of laparotomy, how long should antibiotic therapy be continued?

Twenty-four to forty-eight hours (longer coverage has not been shown to decrease the incidence of abscess, peritonitis, or wound infections)

What is the source of blood supply to the right colon?

Superior mesenteric artery

What is the source of blood supply to the left colon?

Inferior mesenteric artery (and collaterals)

Should right-sided colon injuries be treated differently than left-sided injuries?

The issue is controversial, but it appears that similar management is indicated (i.e., colostomy for high-risk patients; primary anastomosis otherwise)

Should penetrating extraperitoneal rectal injuries be repaired?

Generally not, because the rectum is relatively inaccessible. Fecal diversion and presacral drainage continue to be the standard of care. Note, however, that repair of the rectum is indicated if the injury is easily accessible or if rectal injury is intraperitoneal.

29

Burns

David D. Graham, MD

What is the first priority in treating a burn patient?

ABCs—ensure adequate airway, breathing, and circulation

What is the initial burn treatment employed, often at the scene?

Reverse the heat source (e.g., extinguish burning clothes)

Name some other important aspects of the initial management of a burn.

Obtain adequate history and physical examination. Identify the burn agent and whether the injury occurred in a closed or open space. Pertinent past medical history should include allergies, tetanus status, and current medications. Evaluate the extent of the burn. Place a Foley catheter for monitoring urine output as an indicator of adequate resuscitation. Administer IV analgesia. Obtain blood for CBC, renal profile, ABG, and carboxyhemoglobin, if inhalation injury is suspected. Lavage all burned areas to remove foreign material.

When is an escharotomy performed?

Early for circumferential burns to the extremities and chest, to prevent circulatory and respiratory compromise

When is early endotracheal intubation necessary?

Inhalation injury, deep facial burns, supraglottic obstruction, severe facial fractures, and closed head injury with unconsciousness

When is admission to the hospital indicated?

Full-thickness burns of more than 2% total body surface area (TBSA)
Partial-thickness burns of more than 15% in adults or 10% in children
Involvement of the face, hands, feet, or perineum
Electrical, chemical, or inhalation injuries

High-risk patients: age 65 or older, or 3
    years or younger; pre-existing medical
    problems
Multitrauma
Suspicion of abuse or neglect

**What is a first-degree
burn?**

It is a burn wound involving the
epidermis only. Typically, first-degree
burns are painful, erythematous, and
have no blisters. There is no systemic
response, and they usually heal by
peeling within 3 to 4 days.

**What is a second-degree
burn?**

A burn wound into, but not completely
through, the dermis; this "partial-
thickness" burn is divided into
superficial and deep types

**What is a superficial
partial-thickness burn?**

A burn wound into the papillary dermis
that is typically painful, pink in color,
blanches with pressure, and has intact
hair follicles (do not pluck easily); these
burns usually heal within 3 weeks and
do not leave a scar

**What is a deep partial-
thickness burn?**

A burn wound into the reticular dermis
that is typically multicolored (mottled
pink to white), has decreased pain
sensation, does blanch to pressure, and
has damaged hair follicles (pluck easily);
these burns usually take longer than 3
weeks to heal primarily and scar by
texture, pigmentation, or both

**What is a third-degree
burn?**

It is a burn wound involving the full
thickness of the dermis. All dermal
appendages are destroyed. These
wounds are typically multicolored,
hypesthetic, dry, leathery, and inelastic.
They require grafts for healing, unless
they are small.

**What is a fourth-degree
burn?**

A burn wound involving the underlying
adipose, fascia, muscle, or bone

How is the extent of a burn estimated?

Rule of nines—9% head and neck; 9% each upper extremity; 18% each lower extremity and each hemithorax; 1% perineal region.

How is fluid resuscitation generally instituted?

Via large-bore IV access; CVP and pulmonary catheter monitoring are reserved for patients with significant cardiac or pulmonary dysfunction

How much fluid should be given?

Many institutions use the Parkland formula, which calls for lactated Ringer's solution to be given for the first 24 hours after the injury at 4 ml/kg multiplied by the percentage of burn. Half of the total should be given over the first 8 hours, followed by the second half over the next 16 hours. Regular assessment of the adequacy of resuscitation should be done, and rate of fluid administration adjusted accordingly.

What parameters should be followed in order to assure adequate resuscitation?

Urine output of at least 0.5 to 1 cc/kg/hr in adults; 1 to 2 cc/kg/hr in children
Pulse less than 120 bpm; normal blood pressure; normal pH
Normal mental status
Warm, well-perfused extremities

What causes inhalation injury?

Usually exposure to carbon monoxide, chemical irritants, and toxic gases (rarely caused by thermal injury)

When should an inhalation injury be suspected?

If the burn occurred in a closed space (house fire), or with the presence of facial burns, singed nasal hairs, bronchorrhea, carbonaceous sputum, wheezing and rales, tachypnea, progressive hoarseness, and difficulty clearing secretions

What may result from inhalation injuries?

The upper airway may become obstructed secondary to edema within the ensuing 48 hours; the lower airway may develop pulmonary edema and chemical tracheobronchitis secondary to noxious gases

What is the appropriate treatment of inhalation injury?

Assisted ventilation, oxygen supplementation, and bronchoalveolar lavage to remove debris; steroids are contraindicated

How is carbon monoxide poisoning diagnosed?

Signs and symptoms of hypoxia; serum carboxyhemoglobin level greater than 10% (nonsmoker) or 20% (smoker)

What is the appropriate treatment of carbon monoxide poisoning?

100% oxygen

Typically, which topical agents are used to treat burn wounds?

Mafenide acetate cream, silver sulfadiazine, bacitracin, silver nitrate

What side effect must be looked for when using mafenide acetate cream?

Because it is a carbonic anhydrase inhibitor, mafenide acetate cream absorption may cause a hyperchloremic metabolic acidosis (think: **m**afenide = **m**etabolic acidosis). It has a broad spectrum, excluding most fungi, penetrates eschar well, but is **painful** on application.

In what type of patient is silver sulfadiazine contraindicated?

Those with glucose-6-phosphate dehydrogenase deficiency

What is the major side effect of silver nitrate?

Electrolyte wasting (salt, calcium, potassium; think of silver nitrate as two electrolytes and, thus, electrolyte wasting is the side effect)

How are first-degree burns treated?

Typically, only minor care is required, such as application of bacitracin to the injured area. Symptomatic pain control may also be necessary. Healing is complete and without scar formation.

How are superficial second-degree burns treated?

Wounds are initially cleaned with an antiseptic soap to remove foreign material and dead skin. Blisters are generally unroofed, although this is a point of controversy, and a topical antibiotic is applied prior to dressing the wounds.

How are deep second-degree and third-degree (full-thickness) burns treated?	These burn wounds are treated initially just as superficial second-degree wounds, with cleansing and application of topical agents. This treatment is followed by early excision of eschar and grafting within the first week of hospitalization.
What is the conservative approach to burn-wound excision?	Waiting until the burn wound forms an eschar sparation
What is early burn-wound excision?	Removal of burn wound and coverage early after admission (usually performed within 72 hours)
Which approach to burn wounds is used most often by treatment centers: early excision or conservative?	Early excision has now replaced the conservative approach, because data have revealed a lower mortality rate associated with early excision, especially in young burn victims.
What are the advantages of early excision and grafting?	Allows for early mobilization and rehabilitation, improved joint function, and short hospitalization
What is an autograft?	A skin graft from the same individual
What is an allograft?	A skin graft from an individual of the same species (cadaver)
What is a homograft?	Same as an allograft
What is a xenograft?	A skin graft from a different species (porcine)
What are the indications for homograft usage?	Must be used (if available) if there is an insufficient amount of autologous skin available, such as with large surface area burns; allow for **temporary** wound coverage prior to autologous skin grafting
What are mesh grafts used for?	These autografts may be used instead of homografts when there is insufficient autologous skin. The cosmetic result is not optimal, and this treatment is therefore typically used on the back, flanks, or other less-visible areas. The graft is meshed to allow greater coverage.

What is the most common cause of combined burns and major trauma?

Automobile accidents

Which bacteria are silver sulfadiazine ineffective against?

Gram-positive and *Pseudomonas*

What are the signs of burn-wound infection?

1. Peripheral wound edema
2. Conversion of second-degree burn to a third-degree burn
3. Ecthyma gangrenosum
4. Hemorrhage of underlying tissue
5. Green fat
6. Black skin around the wound
7. Rapid eschar separation
8. Focal areas on a burn wound that turn black, brown, or purple-red, or show generalized discoloration

What is the most common viral infection of burn wounds?

Herpes (type I)

What tissue organism counts correlate with the absence of burn-wound invasive infection?

Less than 10^6 organisms per gram of burn-wound tissue correlate with the absence of invasive infection.

If tissue counts reveal more than 10^6 organisms per gram of burn tissue, what percent will have an invasive burn-wound infection?

Only about 50%; histology of tissue with invasion of organisms into **living** tissue is necessary to diagnose an invasive infection

What is the appropriate treatment of thrombophlebitis in burn patients?

Complete excision of the vein/pus (change IV sites every 3 days to help prevent this complication)

Which IV fluid is administered to burn patients on the second postoperative day?

Albumin 5% at 0.5 cc, multiplied by body surface area (BSA), multiplied by weight in kg, infused in 4 to 8 hours

30

Ostomies

Mark J. Pidala, MD

What is an ostomy?

An intestinal diversion that brings out a portion of the GI tract through the abdominal wall

Name the types of ostomies.

Colostomy or ileostomy
Temporary or permanent
End or loop
Continent or incontinent

What is another name for continent ileostomy?

Kock pouch

What is the average daily ileostomy output?

500 to 800 cc

What is the usual sodium concentration in ileostomy effluent?

~115 mEq/L

What advantages are offered by an extraperitoneal colostomy?

Lower incidence of pericolostomy hernia, prolapse, and recession

Which type of ostomy closure is associated with lower morbidity: loop ileostomy or loop colostomy?

Loop ileostomy

In the immediate postoperative period, what IV fluids should be used to replace ileostomy output?

Normal saline or lactated Ringer's with 40 KCl/L at equal volumes (cc for cc)

Patients with ileostomies in general have what type of overall body fluid abnormality?

Mild dehydration with a chronic state of sodium and water depletion

Which type of stomas are candidates for the irrigation method of bowel control?

Descending colon and sigmoid colostomies

What is the average sodium excretion per day from ileostomy?

~60 mEq

Under what circumstances is an ostomy indicated?

Permanent diversion of the GI tract after complete distal resection (i.e., abdominoperineal resection [APR])
Protection of distal anastomosis
Decompression
Temporary diversion when it is not safe to reanastomose the GI tract (i.e., emergent Hartmann for diverticulitis)

What are the most common situations requiring ileostomy?

Total proctocolectomy with end ileostomy for inflammatory bowel disease
Loop ileostomy to protect colorectal anastomosis
Temporary diversion of the fecal stream from the distal inflammatory process

What are the most common situations requiring colostomy?

APR
Hartmann procedure for colon perforation/diverticulitis
Radiation proctitis
Protection of distal anastomosis

Name two indications for cecostomy.

Colonic decompression (i.e., Ogilvie's)
Cecal volvulus

What are the most common indications for permanent end colostomy?

Rectal cancer treated by APR
Severe anorectal Crohn disease
Anorectal agenesis in infants
Severe anorectal trauma
Incontinence

What procedure is the most common indication for an end ileostomy?

Total proctocolectomy

What are the indications for repair of parastomal hernias?

Repair/relocate for pain, obstruction, inability to fit appliance adequately, cosmetic reasons (note: not all hernias require repair)

What does the eversion technique of Brook ileostomy help prevent?

Serositis, leading to obstruction and high-output ileostomy diarrhea with associated dehydration/electrolyte abnormalities; protects skin

What does placing the ostomy through the rectus muscle help to prevent?

Parastomal hernia
Prolapse

In general, ostomies should be placed through the anterior abdominal wall within a triangle composed of what landmarks?

Umbilicus, pubis, and anterior superior iliac spine

Upon completion of an end ileostomy, how far beyond the skin should the "bud" protrude?

2 to 3 cm

Through which muscle should proper ileostomy formation always place the ostomy?

Rectus abdominis muscle

In general, a stoma in a very obese patient with numerous skinfolds should be placed in what section of the abdomen: upper or lower?

Upper abdomen, above the panniculus

What length of ileum should be brought out above skin to fashion an end ileostomy?

4 to 6 cm

When creating a stoma, how many "average"-size fingers should be able to be admitted through fascia and skin?

Two

What simple bedside technique is used to assess the viability of a stoma?	Insert a glass test tube into the ostomy and use a flashlight to assess the mucosa down to the rectus fascia. Puncture with a needle to assess for bleeding. Examine with an endoscope.
What is the average incidence of small-bowel obstruction following loop ileostomies?	Ten percent
Is the incidence of small-bowel obstruction with loop ileostomies higher or lower than for loop colostomies?	Higher
Is parastomal hernia more common in ileostomy or colostomy?	Colostomy
What is the most common dermatologic problem associated with stomas?	Chemical irritation from effluent
What is the most common organism associated with peristomal skin infection?	*Candida albicans*
What is the recommended treatment for ischemia of an ileostomy superficial to rectus fascia?	Observation
Name the most common colostomy complications.	Ischemia Retraction Stenosis Prolapse Peristomal hernia
What is diversion colitis?	Inflammation of the distally diverted portion of the colon
What is the cause of diversion colitis?	It is thought to be secondary to a lack of trophic factors to mucosa, particularly short-chain fatty acids.

What is the appropriate treatment of diversion colitis?	Reversal of the colostomy is curative (if feasible).
What are the possible complications of ileostomy?	Retraction Prolapse Hernia Fistula Profuse ileostomy diarrhea causing fluid/ electrolyte abnormality Ulceration Stenosis Bleeding
What is the best surgical option for parastomal hernia?	Relocation of the stoma
What sodium and potassium abnormalities do patients with profuse ileostomy diarrhea usually have?	Hyponatremia and hypokalemia
What is the most common cause of colostomy stenosis?	Ischemia
How is pericolostomy hernia surgically managed?	Local repair, with or without mesh Relocation, if possible (most successful)
What is the most common cause of pericolostomy abscess?	Perforation caused by an irrigating device
What is the most common technical error in stoma construction leading to peristomal hernia?	Stoma brought out laterally to the rectus
What is the most common complication following closure of a colostomy?	Wound infection
What is the most frequent cause of ileostomy fistulas?	Crohn disease

What is the most common cause of venous obstruction in colostomy?

Tight fascial opening
Tension on mucocutaneous junction from inadequate proximal colon mobilization

What is the most common cause of arterial insufficiency in colostomy?

Excessive clearance of mesentery from the bowel

What is the appropriate treatment of mild colostomy strictures?

Dilatation

What mortality rate is associated with Hartmann closure?

Up to 5%

How can the depth of ischemia/necrosis be assessed in an ileostomy?

By inserting a small test tube into the stoma and illuminating with a flashlight to assess mucosa down to and below the fascia

Why do patients with ileostomies have increased incidence of gallstones?

Ileal disease or resection interrupts the enterohepatic circulation by decreasing the availability of bile acids and favoring precipitations of cholesterol stones.

Which limb is usually involved in prolapse of a loop colostomy?

Distal

High ileostomy output can result in which type of acid–base disorder?

Metabolic acidosis, secondary to excessive bicarbonate loss from ileostomy

What is the most common type of urinary stone in ileostomy patients?

Uric acid stones (60%)

31

Stomach and Duodenum

Naveen Reddy, BA
Lorne H. Blackbourne, MD

UPPER GI BLEEDING

What are the associated symptoms?	Hematemesis, melena, syncope, shock symptoms, fatigue, coffee-ground emesis, hematochezia, epigastric discomfort
Why does hematochezia occur?	Because blood is a cathartic
What are the associated signs?	Hypotension, positive hemoccult
What are the risk factors?	NSAIDs, liver disease, alcohol, smoking, burn/trauma, peptic ulcer disease/ esophageal varices, sepsis, vomiting, steroids, splenic vein thrombosis, or previous bleed
Name the causes and the percentage of occurrence for each.	Peptic ulcer disease (45%); duodenal ulcers (25%); gastric ulcers (20%); acute gastritis (20%); esophageal varices (20%); Mallory-Weiss tear (10%); other (< 5%)
Which diagnostic tests are indicated?	History, NGT aspiration, abdominal x-ray, EGD (endoscopy)
Which laboratory tests are indicated?	CBC, liver function test (LFT), Chem 7, PT/PTT, amylase, bilirubin, type and cross
Why are BUN levels elevated?	Because of absorption of blood by the GI tract

What is the appropriate initial treatment?	1. IV fluids (16 gauge or larger peripheral IV × 2) 2. Foley catheter (monitor fluid status) 3. NG suction (to determine rate and amount of blood) 4. Water lavage (use warm H_2O to dissolve clots) 5. Endoscopy (to determine the etiology/location of bleed and possible treatment)
What are the indications for surgical intervention in UGI bleeding?	Profuse bleeding with hypotension; recurrent bleeding

PEPTIC ULCER DISEASE

What is it?	Gastric and duodenal ulcers
What is the incidence in the United States?	Ten percent of all Americans will have peptic ulcer disease in their lifetime.
What are the consequences?	Hemorrhage, obstruction, perforation, and pain
Which type of bacteria is associated with peptic ulcer disease?	*Helicobacter pylori*

DUODENAL ULCERS

What is the mean age of occurrence?	Peaks at 45 to 60 years
What is the incidence compared with that of gastric ulcers, and in men as opposed to women?	Higher than that of gastric ulcers; two times as frequent in men than women
What is the most common location?	The majority are within 2 cm of the pylorus in the duodenal bulb on the posterior duodenal wall.
What is the most common cause?	Increased basal gastric acid secretion

What are the risk factors?

Smoking, NSAIDs, *H. pylori* infection, uremia, Zollinger-Ellison syndrome

What are the associated symptoms?

Epigastric pain, which occurs several hours after a meal and is relieved by food, milk, or antacids
Back pain (may indicate pancreatic involvement)
Nausea and vomiting
Anorexia

What percentage of patients with a duodenal ulcer are asymptomatic?

Up to a third!

What are the associated signs?

Tenderness in the epigastrium, guaiac-positive stool, melena, hematochezia

What are the differential diagnoses?

Acute abdomen, pancreatitis, cholecystitis, Zollinger-Ellison, gastritis, MI, gastric ulcer

Which diagnostic tests are indicated?

History and physical examination are necessary. EGD is the preferred modality, because of increased sensitivity and specificity compared with barium contrast UGI series. Endoscopy allows visualization, biopsy, and possible treatment. Lesions are erosive, edges are sharply demarcated, submucosa is exposed, ulcer base may be smooth or have adherent exudate, if acute. UGI series shows retention of contrast in the ulcer.

What preventive measures can be taken?

Avoid aspirin/NSAIDS, nicotine, alcohol, reserpine, caffeine/xanthines (e.g., chocolate)

What is the appropriate treatment?

H₂ receptor antagonists
Antacids (intensive treatment will heal 78% of ulcers in 4 weeks by buffering gastric pH and promoting healing)
Sucralfate (an acid medium that becomes viscous and adheres to mucosa, provides a protective barrier, coats ulcer)
Omeprazole (an H–K ion pump inhibitor)
H. pylori treatment

When is surgery indicated?	**Failed medical treatment** (intractability) **Massive bleeding** **Perforation** **Obstruction (gastric outlet)**—acutely occurs as a result of edema and inflammation in the pyloric channel, suggested by recurrent vomiting, dehydration, and hypochloremic alkalosis. Resolves with supportive measures (i.e., IV fluids, NG suction, H_2 blockers) in 72 hrs. Chronic obstruction occurs with repeated episodes of ulceration and healing, eventually leading to pyloric stenosis.
What is the saline load test?	A test for gastric obstruction: Saline (750 cc) is instilled via an NGT into the stomach; fluid is aspirated 30 minutes later. If the residual is greater than 400 cc, obstruction is present.
What is the goal of surgery?	Decrease gastric acid secretion and correct any anatomic abnormalities.
What types of surgical procedures are most widely used for duodenal ulcer?	Truncal vagotomy and drainage, truncal vagotomy and antrectomy, and proximal gastric vagotomy
What is vagotomy?	Truncal vagotomy involves resection of 1 to 2 cm of each vagal trunk at the diaphragmatic hiatus. Denervation results in decreased acid secretion and impaired gastric emptying. Basal acid secretion is decreased by 80%.
If truncal vagotomy is performed, what else must be done?	Drainage procedure (pyloroplasty, antrectomy, or gastrojejunostomy)—vagal fibers provide relaxation of the pylorus; if cut, the pylorus will not open
What are vagotomy and pyloroplasty?	Vagotomy compensates for decreased gastric emptying. Heineke-Mikulicz pyloroplasty is performed by making a longitudinal incision of the pyloric sphincter extending 2 cm into the antrum and duodenum, and the incision

is closed transversely, thus creating a larger pyloric lumen. **Finney** pyloroplasty combines gastroduodenostomy with pyloric transection. **Jaboulay** pyloroplasty employs a side-to-side gastroduodenostomy for cases in which the pylorus cannot be completely transected.

What are vagotomy and antrectomy?

Removal of the antrum in addition to vagotomy to effect a further decrease in acid secretion; reconstruction as a Billroth I-gastroduodenostomy or a Billroth II-gastrojejunostomy with an afferent limb (associated with higher mortality)

What is a proximal gastric vagotomy?

Preserves vagal fibers to the pylorus, as well as hepatic and celiac divisions of the vagal nerve
Transect only fibers to the fundus and skeletonize 5 to 7 cm of the distal esophagus.
No drainage procedure is needed.
Has a low rate of dumping syndrome
Also known as high selective vagotomy and parietal cell vagotomy (PGV)

What is the procedure of choice in individuals who have failed medical treatment for a duodenal ulcer?

Proximal gastric vagotomy (PGV)

Does PGV affect gastric motility?

Only slightly

Does PGV inhibit gastric bicarbonate production?

No

Is PGV the operation of choice for prepyloric ulcers?

No (associated with a higher recurrence rate)

Which ulcer operation has the highest ulcer recurrence rate and the lowest dumping rate?

Proximal gastric vagotomy

Which ulcer operation has the lowest recurrence rate and the highest dumping rate?

Vagotomy and antrectomy

What are the most common postgastrectomy syndromes?

Dumping and alkaline reflux gastritis
Stomal stenosis, afferent loop syndrome, and delayed gastric emptying

What is dumping?

It is a syndrome characterized by GI and vasomotor symptoms including nausea, epigastric discomfort, borborygmi, palpitations, dizziness, and syncope occurring immediately following a meal (early dumping). Late dumping occurs 1 to 3 hours after a meal and includes reactive hypoglycemia. This syndrome is apparently caused by rapid gastric emptying of foods high in carbohydrate content into the proximal small bowel after vagotomy and pyloric alteration. Most cases resolve with time; few cases have been ameliorated with somatostatin. Severe dumping should be surgically treated with conversion from Billroth I or II to a Roux-en-Y gastrojejunostomy.

What is alkaline reflux gastritis?

It is a triad consisting of:
1. Postprandial epigastric pain associated with nausea and vomiting
2. Evidence of reflux of bile into the stomach
3. Histologic evidence of gastritis. Diagnosis is confirmed via endoscopy (reflux can be quantitated using Tc HIDA radionuclide scans). The only proven treatment is diversion of intestinal contents from the gastric mucosa using Roux-en-Y gastrojejunostomy, with the afferent limb divided and then reanastomosed 60 cm downstream from original

gastrojejunostomy to prevent reflux of intestinal contents.

What medication is used to treat bile reflux?

Carafate binds the ulcer crater and **binds bile.**

PERFORATED PEPTIC ULCER

What are the associated symptoms?

Acute onset of severe epigastric, upper-abdominal, or lower-quadrant pain, or diffuse pain, as in acute abdomen; radiation to the right subscapular area is common

What causes pain in the lower quadrants?

The passage of perforated fluid along colic gutters

What are the associated signs?

Tympanic sound over the liver (air), peritoneal signs, intensely tender/rigid abdomen, and decreased bowel sounds

What are the signs of posterior erosion?

Bleeding from the gastroduodenal artery (and acute pancreatitis)

What are the signs of anterior erosion?

Free air (more common with anterior than posterior perforation)

What is the differential diagnosis?

Acute pancreatitis, acute cholecystitis, perforated acute appendicitis, colonic diverticulitis, MI, any perforated viscus

Which diagnostic tests are indicated?

X-ray (to check for free air under the diaphragm or in the lesser sac in upright CXR, or air over the liver in left lateral decubitus AXR)
Peritoneal lavage (in the obtunded patient)
Exploratory laparotomy

What are the associated laboratory findings?

Leukocytosis, high amylase in peritoneal fluid/serum (secondary to absorption into blood from the peritoneum)

What is the appropriate initial treatment?

NGT (to decrease contamination of the peritoneal cavity)
Antibiotics and IV fluids
Surgery

When should a definitive ulcer operation be performed?

It is indicated if there is history or anatomic evidence of chronic disease, no preoperative shock or life-threatening coexisting illness, and perforation has been present less than 48 hours. If these criteria are not met, Graham patching and peritoneal debridement is preferred, with definitive surgery at a later date when the patient has recovered.

What mortality rate is associated with perforation?

Ten percent

What factors contribute to increased mortality?

Advanced age, female gender, gastric perforation, blood loss

Why may a duodenal rupture be painless?

Fluid can be sterile with a nonirritating pH of 7.0.

What nonoperative treatment can be administered?

(Controversial) NGT, H_2 blockers, nothing by mouth, IV fluids, antibiotics

What late complications can occur after ulcer surgery?

Recurrent ulcer (marginal ulcer at anastomotic site is common), dumping syndrome, vitamin deficiency, afferent loop syndrome, postvagotomy diarrhea

GASTRIC ULCERS

What is the mean age?

Peaks at 40 to 70 years (rarely develops before 40)

What is the most common location?

Ninety-five percent are on a lesser curvature and sixty percent of these ulcers are at or above the incisura angularis.

Type I—along a lesser curvature
associated with large volumes of
secretion

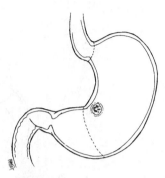

Type II—in the body of the stomach in
combination with a duodenal ulcer
(think: Type II = 2 ulcers)

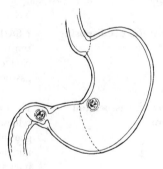

Type III—prepyloric ulcer (think: Type
III = **pre**pyloric)

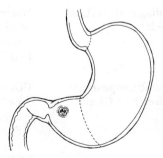

Type IV—next to the GE junction

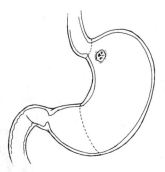

What causes gastric ulcers?	Decreased cytoprotection (decreased mucus and bicarbonate production)
How is acid production affected?	Levels are normal or low.
What are the predisposing factors?	NSAIDs, smoking, alcohol, steroids, sepsis, CNS tumors, intraarterial chemotherapy, shock, burns, trauma, gastric stasis, *H. pylori* infection
What are the associated symptoms?	Recurrent cycles of quiescence and relapse are characterized by dull, gnawing, burning pain localized to the midline or left upper quadrant. Pain recurs within 30 minutes of eating. Also, nausea and vomiting, anorexia, and weight loss are common.
Which diagnostic tests are indicated?	History and physical examination EGD with multiple biopsies (97% sensitivity) UGI barium studies (90% sensitivity)
Describe the appearance of an ulcer on UGI and EGD.	**UGI**—radiolucent line 1 mm in width, partially or completely traversing the orifice of an ulcer or mucosal folds that radiate to the edge of the ulcer crater. **EGD**—smooth and flat ulcer base; raised and erythematous ulcer margin; symmetrical mucosal folds

Describe the common appearance of malignancy on UGI or EGD.

UGI—tumor in the vicinity of ulcer or mass with central ulceration, nodular or irregularly shaped ulcer base
EGD—exophytic mass, disrupted mucosal folds, necrotic ulcer crater, bleeding from the edge of the crater, or heaped-up margins

Which types of gastric ulcers should be biopsied?

All gastric ulcers should be biopsied to rule out gastric cancer. If an ulcer does not heal in 6 weeks after medical treatment, the biopsy should be repeated.

What is the appropriate medical treatment?

Same as that of duodenal ulcers; treat *H. pylori* with triple regimen (e.g., bismuth, metronidazole, and tetracycline)

What are the indications for surgery?

1. Hemorrhage
2. Perforation
3. Obstruction
4. Intractability (i.e., failure of ulcer to heal after 12 weeks of medical treatment, recurrence after 2 initial courses of treatment, or inability to exclude malignancy)

What are the most common operations for each of the following types of ulcers:
Type I?

Distal gastrectomy with Billroth I (3% recurrence rate) (15% recurrence)

Type II?

Antrectomy with truncal vagotomy (because acid secretion is elevated, as evidenced by the duodenal ulcer), truncal vagotomy and pyloroplasty, or truncal vagotomy and drainage

Type III?

Antrectomy and vagotomy with incorporation of the ulcer in the specimen

Type IV?

Excision of the ulcer or distal gastrectomy with vertical extension of the resection specimen to include the ulcer

Is it necessary to perform a vagotomy with a type I ulcer in a patient with no history of duodenal ulcers?	No
What is a Dieulafoy ulcer?	A gastric vascular malformation in which a small (2–4 mm) mucosal defect bleeds from a submucosal large artery, resulting in painless hematemesis
What is the appropriate treatment of a Dieulafoy ulcer?	Endoscopic coagulation or surgical resection

STRESS ULCER/GASTRITIS

What are the causes?	Major physical trauma, shock, sepsis, hemorrhage, respiratory failure, severe burns, renal failure
What is it?	Multiple superficial, nonulcerating erosions that begin in the proximal stomach and progress distally
What is Cushing ulcer?	PUD/gastritis associated with CNS trauma or tumor
What is Curling ulcer?	PUD/gastritis associated with major burn injury
What is a marginal ulcer?	An ulcer at an anastomosis
What are the associated signs?	Painless UGI bleeding, lowered hematocrit, hemoccult (+)
How is the diagnosis confirmed?	Via EGD—multiple, shallow areas of erythema with adherent clot appear within 24 hours and late lesions resemble healing mucosa around a gastric ulcer

GASTRIC CANCER

What is the incidence?	Rare in the United States (higher in Japan)

What are the risk factors?

Diet (e.g., smoked meats, high nitrites, low fruits and vegetables, alcohol, smoking)

What is the mean age of discovery?

Greater than 60 years

What is the male to female ratio?

2:1

Which premalignant lesion is associated with gastric cancer?

Adenomatous polyps—The risk for development of malignancy is related to size, number, and histology. Atypia and mitotic figures are more prominent. Over time, dysplasia and cancer in situ may develop. A 10% to 20% risk of developing cancer is observed. Excision is recommended for sessile lesions larger than 2 cm or proven invasive cancer.

Is atrophic gastritis associated with gastric cancer?

There is an increased incidence of gastric cancer in patients with chronic gastritis and pernicious anemia. If the disease is active more than 5 years, the corresponding risk of developing gastric cancer is doubled.

What are the associated symptoms?

Postprandial epigastric pain that is constant, nonradiating, and unrelieved by feeding; anorexia, nausea and vomiting, weight loss, dysphagia, melena, hematemesis

What are the associated signs?

Anemia, melena, positive hemoccult, epigastric mass, hepatomegaly, coffee-ground emesis, Blumer's shelf, Virchow node, enlarged ovaries (Krukenberg tumor), Irish's node

Which diagnostic tests are indicated?

EGD—most definitive method, biopsy all gastric ulcers at operation and endoscopy
UGI series with double contrast has a diagnostic yield of 90%. Findings include ulceration, gastric mass, loss of mucosal detail, or distorted gastric silhouette.

What is the histology?

The majority are adenocarcinoma.

What is the morphology?

Ulcerative (25%)—ulcerate through all layers

Polypoid (25%)

Superficial spreading (10%)—early cancer; only through mucosa and submucosa; best prognosis

Linitis plastica (10%)—"leather bottle" caused by early spread through all layers; stomach is impliable

Advanced cancer—extends beyond the stomach

What is the appropriate treatment?

Surgical resection is the only cure, but most patients present with advanced disease that is not amenable to resection. Objectives are to provide a cure for localized tumor or to provide effective palliation for advanced disease. Requires resection with wide margins (6 cm); usually, total or subtotal gastrectomy with lymph node dissection is required for local or regional disease. Chemotherapy is used only for disseminated disease, but has no impact on patient survival if used alone. Palliation can be achieved with either surgery or radiation.

When should a splenectomy be performed?

If splenic nodes or spleen hilum is involved

Define the stages and give the prognosis for each stage:

Stage I—to mucosa; 66% 5-year survival rate

Stage II—to muscularis propria; 33% 5-year survival rate

Stage III—with lymph nodes but without distant metastases; 10% 5-year survival rate

Stage IV—with lymph nodes and distant metastases or contiguous spread; 0% 5-year survival rate

Name the stages by TNM:
Stage I

T1 (mucosa), No, Mo

Stage II	T2 (to serosa but not through) No, Mo T3 (through serosa, with or without adjacent tissue involvement)
Stage III	T1-3, N1-3 (any lymph nodes), Mo
Stage IV	M1 distant metastases or unresectable
What percentage of patients have metastases at the time of diagnosis?	75%
Define the following lymph node dissections:	
R1	Perigastric nodes
R2	Celiac and periduodenal nodes
R3	Celiac, aortic, and esophageal nodes
What are the most common locations of cancer in the stomach?	**Antrum**—40% (mainly lesser curve, as seen with gastric ulcers) **Body and fundus**—30%

GASTRIC LYMPHOMA

At what age is the highest incidence noted?	Peaks at 60 to 70 years
What is the most common GI site?	Stomach (> 50% of GI lymphomas arise in this location; most common organ involved in extranodal non-Hodgkin lymphoma)
What are the associated symptoms?	Epigastric pain, anorexia, nausea and vomiting, weight loss
How is the diagnosis confirmed?	Endoscopy is the method of choice; biopsy with brushings provide diagnosis in more than 90% of cases
What else should be done if biopsy for lymphoma is positive?	Evaluation for systemic involvement is necessary and includes CT of the chest and abdomen, bone marrow biopsy, and biopsy of enlarged peripheral lymph nodes.

Define the following stages:

Stage I	Confined to the stomach
Stage II	Spread to the perigastric nodes
Stage III	Nodes other than perigastric
Stage IV	Spread to other abdominal organs

What is the appropriate treatment?

Surgical resection (total gastrectomy), followed by radiation to improve regional and local control; chemotherapy is required for systemic disease

Are microscopic positive margins a concern with gastric lymphomas undergoing postoperative chemotherapy and x-ray therapy?

No, they are not a marker for local recurrence

What is the prognosis?

Highly dependent upon stage at diagnosis; early stage disease has a 5-year survival rate of 95%, whereas late-stage disseminated disease has a 5-year survival rate of 15%

GASTRIC SARCOMA

What is the incidence?

Mean age is 60 to 70 years old; incidence is the same in men and women

What is the histology?

Most are leiomyosarcomas.

What are the associated symptoms?

Similar to those of adenocarcinoma; masses usually attain a large size before causing symptoms

Describe the appearance.

Grossly, they are firm, gray-white masses that occasionally contain a pseudocapsule.

What determines the behavior of these tumors?

The number of mitoses per hpf, with 5 to 10 mitotic figures/hpf demonstrating increased propensity for metastases

What is the most common route of metastasis?	Hematogenous (90%)
What is the appropriate treatment?	Surgical resection of the tumor and involved structures; negative margins must be ensured
What is the prognosis?	**Low-grade**—81% 5-year survival rate **High-grade**—32% 5-year survival rate

GASTRIC CARCINOID

What is a leading risk factor?	Pernicious anemia
What diagnostic test confirms the diagnosis?	EGD with biopsy
What are the associated findings?	Yellow or pink submucosal gastric nodules
What is the appropriate treatment?	Resection for cure

MALLORY-WEISS SYNDROME

What is it?	Severe UGI hemorrhage that occurs after retching or vomiting; longitudinal tear results through the mucosa and submucosa of stomach near the GE junction; approximately 75% are in the stomach
What causes the tear?	Increased gastric pressure, often aggravated by a hiatal hernia
What are the most common risk factors?	Alcohol (50% of patients), retching, and hiatal hernia (50% of patients)
What are the associated symptoms?	Epigastric pain, thoracic substernal pain
What are the associated signs?	Post-retching hematemesis

What is the classic order of events?	First, food and gastric contents are vomited, followed by **forceful retching,** and then bloody vomitus.
How is the diagnosis confirmed?	History and physical examination EGD (permits diagnosis and treatment)
What is the appropriate treatment?	Therapy initially involves volume resuscitation, followed by room temperature water lavage and gastric decompression. In 90% of patients bleeding stops; rebleeding is rare. Continued bleeding can be managed with electrocautery, selective vasopressin infusion, or arterial embolization. **Balloon compression** of the GE junction is **contraindicated** because it will propagate the tear. Refractory bleeds may be treated surgically by oversewing the laceration through an anterior longitudinal gastrostomy in the middle third of the stomach.

BOERHAAVE SYNDROME

What is it?	Postemetic esophageal rupture through all layers; usually does not bleed profusely
What is the most common location?	The posterolateral aspect of the esophagus on the left, 3 to 5 cm above the GE junction
What causes rupture?	Increased intraluminal pressure, usually triggered by violent retching and vomiting
What are the associated symptoms?	Pain postemesis that may radiate to the back Dysphagia
What are the associated signs?	Left pneumothorax, Hamman's sign, left pleural effusion, subcutaneous/ mediastinal emphysema, fever, tachypnea, tachycardia, signs of infection by 24 hours, neck crepitus

What is Hamman's sign?	"Mediastinal crunch" produced by the heart beating against air-filled tissues

MORBID OBESITY

What is the definition?	Body weight 100 lbs. over ideal
What is the incidence in the United States?	**Men**—5% **Women**—7.2%
What are the associated medical problems?	CAD, hypertension, type II diabetes mellitus, sleep apnea, obesity hypoventilation, hypercoagulability, necrotizing panniculitis, degenerative joint disease, cholecystitis, chronic venous stasis ulcers, stress overflow incontinence, GE reflux, sex hormone imbalances, an increased risk of uterine and breast malignancies
What factors determine surgical eligibility?	Body mass index (BMI; weight in kg/M^2) over 40 or BMI over 35 with comorbid conditions (e.g., CAD, diabetes mellitus, hypertension, degenerative joint disease)
What is a jejunoileal bypass?	Surgery initially used for morbid obesity that bypasses the ileum with an end-to-end anastamosis between the proximal jejunum and distal ileum (no longer performed today)
What complications are associated with this procedure?	Cirrhosis (from protein calorie malnutrition), bacterial ovegrowth with resultant vitamin K deficiency, interstitial nephritis, iron deficiency anemia, bypass enteritis; also, hypocalcemia, resultant severe osteoporosis, and a rheumatoid-like arthritis can develop; this operation is no longer performed because of the large number of complications
What is gastroplasty?	A procedure in which the stomach is stapled, creating a small pouch that permits the passage of food into the pylorus

What is the disadvantage of horizontal gastroplasty?

Requires ligation and division of the short gastric vessels between the stomach and spleen, with resultant risk of devascularization of the gastric pouch or spleen; associated with a higher rate of failure

What does the abbreviation VBGP stand for?

Vertical Banded Gastroplasty—two rows of staples are placed vertically in the muscular part of the stomach to create a small gastric pouch. Mesh is then wrapped around the stoma on a lesser curvature between upper and lower pouches and sutured to itself. This procedure is associated with a lower rate of failure compared with horizontal gastroplasty.

Which patients can "beat" the vertical-banded gastroplasty?

Sweets eaters!

What is gastric bypass?

A procedure in which three staple lines are placed to create a blind gastric pouch that is drained via a loop of bowel in a gastrojejunostomy or a Roux-en-Y limb

How does the gastric bypass work?

Small pouch is created; triggers dumping syndrome if too much food is eaten

What are the advantages of bypass?

Better weight reduction (60% vs. 40% after 3 years)
Half to two-thirds of excess weight is lost in 1 to 1.5 years.

What are the disadvantages of bypass?

Higher incidence of stomal ulcer, stomal stenosis, B_{12} deficiency, iron-deficiency anemia

What is the most common cause of bypass surgery failure?

Excessive, constant snacking on high calorie foods (10% to 15% of patients)

What are the potential complications of surgery?

Postoperative gastric leak
Peritonitis
Gastric necrosis
Marginal ulcer
Hernia

What is the appropriate postoperative management?	The patient receives nothing by mouth for 4 days and begins receiving clear liquids on the fifth postoperative day, if a UGI series demonstrates no leak.
What is the most common cause of leak?	Ischemic necrosis caused by stapling procedures
What sign indicates obstruction in the afferent limb or the jejunojejunostomy of a Roux-en-Y?	Frequent hiccoughs with a large air bubble noted in the stomach on AXR
What are the signs of a gastric leak?	Increasing pain, especially in the back or left shoulder, as well as fever, leukocytosis, tachypnea, and tachycardia
How is a leak diagnosed?	UGI series using water-soluble contrast (Gastrografin)

SMALL BOWEL AND APPENDIX

ILEUS

What is the definition?	Paralytic ileus is a functional obstruction of the small bowel that occurs in most patients following abdominal surgery and is caused by a combination of neural, humoral, and metabolic factors. It also occurs with inflammatory processes in the abdomen, such as pancreatitis and peritonitis, retroperitoneal hemorrhage, spine injury, electrolytes, medication
What are the associated signs?	Lack of bowel sounds and inability to pass flatus or stool
What are the other common causes of ileus?	Opiates, hypokalemia, hyponatremia
What is the order of return of motility following abdominal surgery?	1. Small intestine 2. Stomach 3. Colon
What is one theory regarding physiologic mechanism?	Sympathetic hyperactivity, which slows GI propulsion and constricts sphincters

How is the diagnosis confirmed?	History and physical examination Abdominal plain film demonstrating air throughout the GI tract with or without air–fluid levels
What is the appropriate treatment?	Conservative: Nothing by mouth, NGT, IV fluids until patient passes flatus, electrolyte replacement, as needed

SMALL BOWEL OBSTRUCTION

What is it?	Mechanical obstruction of the bowel lumen, resulting in stimulated activity proximal to and inhibited activity distal to obstruction; results in accumulation of fluid and gas proximally with distension
What are the physiologic changes that occur with obstruction?	Distension results in decreased absorption (lumen to blood) and increased secretion (blood to lumen), thereby leading to further distension, as well as fluid and electrolyte abnormalities (third-spacing). Bacterial proliferation occurs because of stasis, but this has no role in the clinical picture of simple mechanical obstruction, because neither bacteria nor their toxins cross the normal intestinal lumen acutely.
What gas accumulates proximally?	Nitrogen from **swallowed air** (cannot be absorbed by the bowel)
At what pressure does net secretion occur in the small bowel?	When intraluminal pressure exceeds 20 cm H_2O
Why do patients vomit?	As fluid accumulates proximally, it refluxes into the stomach, causing irritation and resulting emesis.
What is the most common translocating bacterium in small-bowel obstruction?	*E. coli*

What causes small-bowel obstruction?

Mechanical (obstruction of the lumen)—polypoid tumors, intussusception, gallstone ileus, impacted feces, meconium, bezoar
Intrinsic—congenital, neoplastic, or inflammatory (Crohn) lesions of the bowel; iatrogenic strictures
Extrinsic—postoperative adhesions, inflammation, hernias, neoplastic masses, abscesses, volvulus

What disease does small-bowel obstruction commonly mimic?

Paralytic ileus

How are small-bowel obstructions commonly categorized?

They are either partial or complete. Depending on the cause, partial ones are often managed conservatively (i.e., without surgery) because the risk of ischemic necrosis is much lower than with complete obstruction. Complete obstruction requires operative intervention.

What is the difference between a simple and a strangulating obstruction?

A simple mechanical obstruction is one that disrupts the bowel lumen. Strangulation obstruction is a closed-loop blockage with vascular compromise of the involved intestinal segment.

What is the most common cause of small-bowel obstruction in adults?

Postoperative adhesions

What is the most common cause of large-bowel obstruction in adults?

Colon cancer

What is the most common pediatric cause?

Hernias

What is the incidence of adhesions?

Sixty-seven percent, following laparotomy

What percentage of patients undergoing a laparotomy will subsequently develop small-bowel obstruction caused by adhesions?

Approximately 5%

What is the clinical presentation?

Crampy, paroxysmal abdominal pain (colic); vomiting obstipation; abdominal distension; borborygmi (high-pitched bowel sounds) separated by relatively quiet periods; tachycardia and hypotension in relation to the degree of hypovolemia resulting from third-spacing of fluids into the bowel lumen

What is the radiographic presentation?

Distended bowel proximal to the obstruction, air–fluid levels, foreign bodies, minimal or complete lack of gas in the colon/rectum, "stair stepping," "string of pearls"

Which radiologic test differentiates partial from complete small-bowel obstruction?

Enteroclysis (contrast study from above), but contrast studies do not differentiate between simple and strangulation obstruction

What are the signs of a strangulated bowel?

Fever, peritoneal signs, shock, acidosis (increased lactic acid), severe/continuous pain, hematemesis, abdominal free air, gas in the bowel wall or portal vein, peritoneal signs

What are the lumenal contents of a strangulated bowel?

Bacteria, toxins, necrotic tissue, and blood

What is the appropriate management?

Initially, IV fluids, electrolyte and acid–base correction, NG decompression; patient must show objective improvement within 4–6 hrs

If obstruction does not resolve, timing of surgery depends on:

1. The duration of the obstruction (i.e., severity of fluid, electrolyte, and acid–base abnormalities); complete versus partial
2. The need to improve vital organ function prior to surgery
3. The risk of strangulation

What are the clinical parameters that will lower the threshold to operate on a small-bowel obstruction?

1. Increasing WBC
2. Fever
3. Tachycardia
4. Abdominal pain/tenderness (peritoneal signs mandate exploration)

GALLSTONE ILEUS

What is it? Mechanical intestinal obstruction that results from gallstones eroding through the biliary system via fistulization into the intestine (usually the duodenum)

What is the mean age? Peaks at 60 to 70 years (most commonly a cause of obstruction in the elderly)

What is the usual size of a stone? At least 2.5 cm in diameter lodged, usually in the terminal ileum (the narrowest portion of the small bowel)

Describe the common presentation. Intermittent symptoms of small-bowel obstruction as stones lodge at various levels of the small intestine, followed by repeated impact and disimpact

What are the associated radiologic findings? Pneumobilia (air in the biliary tree) Intestinal obstruction; visualized stone

What is the appropriate treatment? Initially, management is the same as for other causes of small-bowel obstruction, as well as definitive treatment by removal of the stone. The entire small intestine must be examined to rule out other stones in the small bowel, with or without cholecystectomy and fistula closure.

What is the most common cause of recurrence? Missed stones during the first operation

What is the operative mortality rate of definitive repair of biliary/intestinal disease (fistula)? Five to ten percent, because patients are frail and elderly

ANTICOAGULANT-INDUCED OBSTRUCTION

What is it? Patients taking warfarin may develop an intramural hematoma of the small bowel.

What is the most frequent site? Proximal jejunum

What are the associated signs/laboratory findings?	Elevated PT, ecchymoses, hematuria
What are the associated radiologic findings?	Affected segment appears narrow and rigid; "picket fence" appearance of mucosa
What is the appropriate treatment?	Discontinuance of the anticoagulant Vitamin K NG suction/IV fluids

MECKEL'S DIVERTICULUM

What is it?	Remnant of the omphalomesenteric duct/vitelline duct that connects the yolk sac with the primitive midgut in the embryo
What is the usual location?	Within 2 feet of the ileocecal valve on the antimesenteric border of the bowel
What is the major differential diagnosis?	Appendicitis
Is it a true diverticulum?	Yes; all layers of the intestine are found in the wall
What is the incidence?	Present in approximately 2% of the population at autopsy, but most cases are asymptomatic
What is the gender ratio?	Three times more common in men than in women
What is the average age of the onset of symptoms?	Most frequently in the first 2 years of life, but can occur at any age
What are the potential complications?	**Intestinal hemorrhage (painless)**—50%; accounts for half of all lower GI bleeding in patients under 2 years old; bleeding is caused by ectopic gastric mucosa–secreting acid, leading to ulcers and bleeding **Intestinal obstruction**—25%; most common complication in adults; includes herniation, volvulus, intussusception, and Littré's hernia **Inflammation (with or without perforation)**—20%

What is the "rule of 2's"?	Two percent of patients are symptomatic. Located about 2 feet from ileocecal valve Found in 2% of the population
What is a Meckel's scan?	A scan for ectopic gastric mucosa in a Meckel's diverticulum that uses technetium pertechnetate IV, which is taken up preferentially by gastric mucosa

SMALL-BOWEL TUMORS

What are the differential diagnoses of benign tumors of the small intestine?	Leiomyoma, lipoma, lymphangioma, fibroma, adenoma, hemangioma
What is the most common benign tumor of the small intestine?	Leiomyoma (followed by lipoma and adenoma)
What are the differential diagnoses of malignant tumors of the small intestine?	Adenocarcinoma, carcinoid tumor, lymphoma
What is the most common malignant small-bowel tumor?	Adenocarcinoma
What is the incidence of neoplasms?	Less than 2% of all maligancies arise in the small bowel.
What factors are important in preventing malignancies in the small bowel?	Fast transit time, thus limiting contact of carcinogens with mucosa Alkaline pH and decreased bacterial contamination High activity of benzopyrene hydroxylase, which detoxifies carcinogens Rapid turnover of mucosal cells Secretory IgA
What is the usual presentation?	Insidious onset, weight loss, anorexia, malabsorption with steatorrhea, dull aching pain, symptoms of obstruction, occult or massive bleeding

| How is the diagnosis confirmed? | UGI series with enteroclysis
EGD for duodenal lesions |

ADENOCARCINOMA OF THE SMALL BOWEL

What is the incidence?	Most common small-bowel neoplasm; accounts for 30% to 50% of all small-bowel cancers
What is the mean age?	Peaks at 60 to 70 years (parallels colonic adenocarcinoma)
What is the most common location?	Occurs most frequently in the duodenum, especially in the periampullary region, which accounts for two-thirds of all small-bowel adenocarcinomas; occurs least frequently in the ileum
What are the signs of duodenal/ampullary adenocarcinoma?	Extrahepatic biliary obstruction
What is the usual presentation?	**Duodenal/Periampullary—** Obstructive jaundice **Jejunoileal—**slow, progressive obstruction
What is the appropriate treatment?	Surgical resection with removal of draining lymph nodes Radical pancreaticoduodenectomy (Whipple resection) for duodenal lesions; segmental resections for small proximal and distal duodenal lesions Segmental resection and mesenteric lymphadenectomy for jejunoileal lesions
What is the prognosis?	Usually poor because patients present with advanced disease **With lymph node metastases—**5-year survival rate of 15% **Without lymph node metastases—**5-year survival rate of 50% to 70%

| How does the prognosis of periampullary neoplasm compare with that of pancreatic cancer? | More frequently resectable for cure than pancreatic cancer; 5-year survival rate is 40%, compared with a rate of less than 10% for pancreatic cancer |

LYMPHOMA OF THE SMALL BOWEL

What is the incidence?	Accounts for 10% to 15% of all small-bowel malignancies Primary involvement of the small bowel is the second most common site after the stomach.
What is the mean age of occurrence?	Peaks at 50 to 60 years
What is the associated cell type?	Virtually all primary small-bowel lymphomas are non-Hodgkin B-cell lymphomas
What is the most common location in the small bowel?	Ileum
What is the usual presentation?	Fatigue, malaise, weight loss, abdominal pain, obstruction (Fever and night sweats are rare and usually indicate secondary small-bowel involvement by diffuse lymphoma.) Malabsorption is also common from diffuse mucosal involvement, guaiac-positive stool.
How is the diagnosis made?	UGI series with enteroclysis (demonstrates submucosal nodules, ulcerations, or diffuse mucosal thickening) CT (demonstrates bulky nodes and bowel wall thickening)
What are the associated medical conditions?	Celiac disease, Crohn disease, AIDS, SLE, Wegener disease, X-linked agammaglobulinemia

What is the staging?

Follows Ann Arbor classification
Stage I—confined to the small bowel
Stage II—with regional lymph nodes
Stage III—with nonresectable lymph
  nodes beyond regional nodes
Stage IV—metastases to other organs in
  and beyond the abdomen

**What is the appropriate
treatment?**

Surgery, for diagnosis, staging, relief of
  obstruction, and resection/debulking
Intraoperative staging involves liver
  biopsy and sampling of lymph nodes
  outside of the field of resection.
Surgical treatment mandates resection of
  the involved bowel with wide, en bloc
  lymphadenectomy.
Widespread or diffuse involvement is
  best managed with debulking.

What is the prognosis?

Stage I or II—80% 5-year survival rate

ENTERIC INFECTIONS

**What type of diarrhea is
associated with enteric
infections?**

Stool mass greater than 250 g/day

**Through what mechanisms
do these infections act?**

Osmotic
Secretory (i.e., cholera)
Inflammatory (i.e., *Shigella*)

**Which diagnostic tests are
indicated?**

Stool smear, Wright's stain for WBCs,
hemoccult testing, stool culture,
examination for ova and parasites

**What are the sites of
intestinal involvement?**

Small intestine (cholera, *E. coli, Giardia,*
viruses)
Ileum and colon (*Salmonella, Yersinia,
Campylobacter*)
Colon (*Shigella, E. coli* [invasive,
hemorrhagic], *Amoeba, Giardia*)

**What is the most common
cause after drinking from
a mountain stream?**

Giardia

What causes food poisoning?	Preformed toxins elaborated by *Staphylococcus aureus, Clostridium perfringens,* or *Bacillus cereus*
What part of the history differentiates gastroenteritis?	Vomiting is followed by pain and diarrhea.

MALABSORPTION SYNDROMES

What are the causes?	Postgastrectomy, postvagotomy, pancreatic insufficiency, enzyme deficiency, cholestasis, blind-loop syndrome, short bowel syndrome
What are the symptoms?	Weight loss, diarrhea, steatorrhea, tetany, osteomalacia, pathologic fractures, bleeding, neuropathies
How is the diagnosis confirmed?	Appearance of stool (bulky, malodorous, and floats) Sudan stain for fecal fat D-xylose test to measure the absorptive capacity of the jejunum Schilling test to evaluate for B_{12} absorption
Which vitamins and minerals are often deficient?	Fat-soluble vitamins: A, D, E, and K Calcium Vitamin B_{12}

BLIND-LOOP SYNDROME

What is it?	It is a bacterial overgrowth in the small intestine. The organisms that tend to overgrow are not the normal flora of the small bowel. Rather, they are more representative of colonic flora (such as gram-negative bacteria [*E. coli*]). There is often overgrowth of strictly anaerobic bacteria, such as *Clostridium* and *Bacteroides.*
What are the causes?	Anything that disrupts the normal flow of intestinal contents (i.e., causes stasis), such as strictures of the intestine, Crohn disease, postvagotomy, scleroderma, small-bowel diverticula, decreased gastric acid secretion, and incompetent ileocecal valve

What are the associated signs/symptoms?	Diarrhea, steatorrhea, malnutrition, abdominal pain, hypocalcemia, B_{12} deficiency, and resultant megaloblastic anemia
What is the pathogenesis of B_{12} deficiency?	1. Bacterial utilization of B_{12} 2. Bacterial toxins inhibit the absorption of B_{12} across the small-bowel mucosa.
Which diagnostic tests are indicated?	**Schilling test**—demonstrates an intrinsic factor–resistant B_{12} malabsorption **Hydrogen breath test**—lactose is swallowed and expiration of hydrogen is monitored; with bacterial overgrowth, there is an increased H_2 production earlier than normal
What is the appropriate treatment?	Surgical correction of the underlying disorder, if feasible; otherwise, antibiotics to inhibit bacterial overgrowth
What are the other causes of B_{12} deficiency?	Gastrectomy (decreased secretion of intrinsic factor) and excision of terminal ileum (site of B_{12} absorption)

AFFERENT LOOP SYNDROME

What is it?	Partial or total obstruction/kink of the afferent limb following a Billroth II, with accumulation of bile and pancreatic secretions in the afferent limb
What are the associated signs/symptoms?	Postprandial right upper quadrant pain, bilious vomiting, anemia, steatorrhea; pain often resolves suddenly after decompression of the afferent limb; vomiting often relieves symptoms
When does it usually occur?	Approximately 66% present in the first postoperative week; otherwise, it can occur anytime
How is the diagnosis confirmed?	UGI series (afferent loop will not fill with contrast because of the obstruction) EGD

What is the appropriate treatment?	Balloon dilatation, surgical reanastomosis (e.g., Roux-en-Y)

APPENDICITIS

What is it?	Obstruction of the appendiceal lumen producing a closed loop with resultant inflammation that can lead to necrosis and perforation
What are the causes?	**Fecalith (appendolith)**—35% **Lymphoid hyperplasia**—60%
What is the pathophysiology?	Following obstruction, mucus continues to be secreted into the lumen. Stasis leads to bacterial proliferation and secretion of toxins that enable organisms to penetrate the wall of the appendix and establish inflammation. Increased intraluminal pressure leads to impeded arterial/venous flow and, ultimately, necrosis and gangrene.
What is the usual presentation?	Onset of (referred) periumbilical pain, followed by anorexia, nausea, and vomiting (Note: Unlike gastroenteritis, **pain precedes vomiting.** Pain later migrates to the right lower quadrant, where it becomes more intense and localized because of local peritoneal irritation. Pain and tenderness are maximal corresponding to the anatomic location of the appendix, and thus vary from patient to patient. (If the patient is hungry and can eat, seriously question the diagnosis of appendicitis.)
What is McBurney's point?	A point located one third of the way on a line drawn from the anterosuperior iliac spine to the umbilicus; represents location of maximal tenderness in appendicitis
How is the diagnosis made?	History and physical examination (a clinical diagnosis)

What are the associated signs/symptoms?

Signs of peritoneal irritation may be present (guarding, rebound tenderness, muscle spasm, rigidity, obturator/psoas/ Rovsing sign, low-grade fever rising to high-grade if perforation occurs)

What are the differential diagnoses?

Intussusception, volvulus, Meckel's diverticulum, Crohn disease, ovarian/ testicular torsion, ovarian tumor/cyst, epididymitis, perforated ulcer, pancreatitis, pelvic inflammatory disease, ruptured ectopic pregnancy, mesenteric lymphadenitis, mittelschmerz, acute gastroenteritis

Which laboratory tests are indicated?

WBC (> 10,000/mm^3 in > 90% of cases; elderly patients often have normal WBC count)
UA (mild hematuria and pyuria are common in appendicitis with pelvic inflammation)

Which radiographic studies are indicated?

Often none; most adult patients receive:
CXR, to rule out right middle lobe (RML) or right lower lobe (RLL) pneumonia
Abdominal plain films (usually nonspecific, but calcified fecalith is present in approximately 5% of cases)

What is the appropriate treatment?

Without perforation—prompt appendectomy with preoperative cefoxitin to avoid perforation; ABX continued for 24 hours postoperative
With perforation—triple ABX, fluid resuscitation, and immediate appendectomy; all pus should be drained and cultures obtained; postoperative ABX is continued for 5 to 7 days; wound is left open in most cases of perforation after closing the fascia (heals by secondary intention or delayed primary), with or without drain

What are the steps in laparoscopic appendectomy?

1. Appendix is held up for retraction.
2. Mesoappendix and appendiceal artery are stapled with a vascular load gastrointestinal anastomosis (GIA) or electrocoagulated.

3. Appendix is transected with staples from GI-load GIA or endo loops.

What is done if a normal appendix is found?

Additional exploration to eliminate other possible causes (i.e., Meckel's diverticulum, Crohn disease, intussusception, gynecologic causes), then appendectomy

What percentage of patients have a normal appendix at laparotomy?

Approximately 10% to 20%

What is the risk of perforation?

Approximately 25% after 24 hours from the onset of symptoms
Approximately 50% by 36 hours
Approximately 75% by 48 hours

What are the signs of a perforated appendix?

Increasing abdominal pain, diffuse pain, increased muscle spasm, tachycardia; temperature rises from 39° to 40° C; patient appears "toxic"

What is the most common general surgical abdominal emergency in pregnancy?

Appendicitis (approximately 1/1750); because of enlarged uterus, **the appendix may be in the right upper quadrant**

What are the potential complications of appendicitis/ appendectomy?

Abscess, free perforation, hepatic abscess, wound infection, appendiceal stump abscess, wound/inguinal hernia, minor bleeding, portal pyelothrombophlebitis (very rare)

APPENDICEAL TUMORS

What is the most common appendiceal tumor?

Carcinoid tumor (accounts for 90% of all primary appendiceal cancer)

What are the differential diagnoses of appendiceal tumors?

Carcinoid tumor, adenocarcinoma, malignant mucoid adenocarcinoma

What is the usual presentation?

Similar to that of acute appendicitis

When is a right hemicolectomy indicated versus appendectomy for appendiceal carcinoid?

If the tumor is more than 2 cm, right hemicolectomy is indicated. If no signs of serosal involvement are present and the tumor is less than 2 cm, appendectomy is indicated.

32

Postgastrectomy Syndromes

Lorne H. Blackbourne, MD
Paul Shin, BA

What is a postgastrectomy syndrome?	A syndrome of morbidity following gastric surgery
Name the types of postgastrectomy syndromes.	1. Alkaline reflux gastritis 2. Dumping syndrome 3. Afferent loop syndrome 4. Efferent loop syndrome 5. Postvagotomy diarrhea 6. Roux stasis syndrome 7. Chronic gastric atony 8. Small gastric remnant syndrome

AFFERENT LOOP SYNDROME

What is it?	**Obstruction** of the afferent loop of a Billroth II (afferent loop is the proximal duodenum/jejunum loop draining bile toward the gastrojejunostomy)
What is the efferent loop?	The distal loop draining away from the stomach (think: **e**fferent = **e**gress)
What is the incidence?	Less than 1%
What are the causes?	Kinking, intussusception, adhesions, volvulus, hernias of the afferent loop
What are the associated risks?	**Long afferent loop** Antecolic anastomosis Anastomosis to a lesser curvature of the stomach
What are the signs/symptoms of acute onset?	Abdominal pain, epigastric mass, **nonbilious** (usually in the first week), vomiting, nausea, fever

What are the signs/ symptoms of chronic disease?	Abdominal pain relieved by **pure bile emesis** (from decompression of the obstructed afferent loop)
What are the possible complications?	Duodenal stump blowout Pancreatitis
What mortality rate is associated with acute onset?	Approximately a third! (**surgical emergency**)
How is the diagnosis of acute disease confirmed?	Fluid-filled epigastric mass on ultrasound or CT
How is the diagnosis of chronic disease confirmed?	EGD (to rule out alkaline reflux gastritis)
What is the appropriate treatment?	Convert Billroth II to a Roux-en-Y of the afferent loop 40 to 50 cm from the gastrojejunostomy on the efferent limb

EFFERENT LOOP SYNDROME

What is the efferent loop syndrome?	Obstruction of the efferent loop or at the anastomosis of the gastric remnant to the efferent loop
What causes it?	Adhesions, volvulus, hernia, omental wrap with fibrosis of the omentum, tight mesocolon tunnel, anastomotic stricture
How is the diagnosis confirmed?	Upper GI barium series, EGD
What is the appropriate treatment?	Surgical correction of the obstruction Balloon dilatation of anastomosis

POSTVAGOTOMY DIARRHEA

What is it?	Diarrhea after a truncal vagotomy
What causes it?	It is thought that after truncal vagotomy, there is a rapid transport of unconjugated bile salts to the colon, resulting in osmotic inhibition of water absorption in the colon resulting in diarrhea.

What is the incidence?	Approximately one third of patients will have diarrhea after a truncal vagotomy, but only about 1% will have severe diarrhea.
What are the associated signs/symptoms?	Diarrhea
What is the appropriate medical treatment?	Cholestyramine
What is the appropriate surgical treatment?	Reversed interposition jejunal segment

DUMPING SYNDROME

What is it?	Delivery of **hyperosmotic** chyme to the small intestine (normally the stomach will decrease the osmolality of the chyme prior to its emptying); **late** dumping is thought to be caused by hypoglycemia
With what conditions is it associated?	Any procedure that bypasses the pylorus or compromises its function (i.e., gastroenterostomies or pyloroplasty), thus "dumping" of chyme into the small intestine
What are the associated signs/symptoms?	Postprandial diaphoresis, tachycardia, abdominal pain/distention, emesis, increased flatus, dizziness, weakness, weight loss, mental status changes
What is the appropriate medical treatment?	Small, multiple, low fat/ carbohydrate meals that are high in protein content Avoidance **of liquids** with meals to slow gastric emptying Lying down after eating **Octreotide** **Ingestion of carbohydrates to raise blood glucose (for late dumping syndrome)**
What percentage of patients with dumping syndrome resolve with medical treatment?	Approximately 75% in less than a year

What is the appropriate surgical treatment?	If medical therapy fails (for a trial period of usually a year), then a Roux-en-Y should be performed with possible reversed jejunal interposition loop.

ROUX STASIS SYNDROME

What is it?	Stasis of chyme in the gastric remnant
What causes it?	Loss of normal gastric motility (loss of migration of the normal pacemaker motor waves)
What are the associated signs/symptoms?	Abdominal pain, nonbilious vomiting, nausea postprandially
How is the diagnosis confirmed?	Endoscopy (to rule out outlet obstruction/ulcer) Emptying study
What is the appropriate medical treatment?	Cisapride
What is the appropriate surgical treatment?	Shorten Roux limb to 40 cm and completion of gastrectomy.

ALKALINE REFLUX GASTRITIS

What is it?	Reflux of bile into the stomach after a Billroth I, Billroth II, or pyloroplasty (Note: alkaline refers to the alkaline nature of bile in contrast to the more common gastritis caused by gastric acidic environment.)
What are the associated signs/symptoms?	Epigastric burning, abdominal pain, nausea, weight loss, anemia, bilious vomiting
How do the symptoms compare with those of afferent loop syndrome?	With reflux gastritis, the bilious vomiting does not relieve the symptoms as it does in chronic afferent loop syndrome.
What is the major risk factor for alkaline reflux gastritis?	Billroth II

How is the diagnosis confirmed?	EGD—gastritis/bile Biliary scan (pooling in stomach remnant)
What is the appropriate medical treatment?	H_2 blockers, cholestyramine, metoclopramide
What is the appropriate surgical treatment?	Conversion to Roux-en-Y

CHRONIC GASTRIC ATONY

What is it?	Delayed gastric remnant emptying following vagotomy
What are the associated risk factors?	Diabetes, smoking, alcohol, Roux-en-Y
What are the associated signs/symptoms?	Epigastric pain, nausea, pain, early satiety, weight loss, anemia, postprandial exacerbation
How is the diagnosis confirmed?	EGD (to rule out ulcer/obstruction) Gastric emptying study
What is the appropriate medical treatment?	Small meals, cessation of smoking and/or alcohol, metoclopramide/cisapride
What is the appropriate surgical treatment?	Near total gastrectomy with Roux-en-Y (Roux-en-Y without gastric resection is disastrous)

SMALL GASTRIC REMNANT SYNDROME

What is it?	Loss of gastric reservoir and vagal-mediated receptive gastric relaxation in patients with greater than 80% gastric resection and vagotomy
What are the associated signs/symptoms?	Early satiety, epigastric pain, weight loss, anemia, malnutrition
How is the diagnosis confirmed?	EGD (to rule out obstruction, ulcer, bezoar, cancer)
What is the appropriate medical treatment?	Small meals, liquid supplements

What is the appropriate surgical treatment?	Jejunal pouch reconstruction

MISCELLANEOUS

What nutritional problems can follow gastrectomy?	B_{12} deficiency by loss of intrinsic factor, folate deficiency, iron deficiency, calcium deficiency, weight loss caused by poor food intake, bacterial overgrowth, steatorrhea because of loss of pancreatic enzymes (loss of vagal stimulation)
What is the incidence of cancer following a partial gastrectomy?	Probably a slight increase in the incidence of gastric cancer following partial gastrectomy, usually after 20 years
What is the incidence of cholelithiasis after truncal vagotomy?	Increased incidence, most likely because of decreased emptying of the gallbladder and decreased opening of the sphincter of Oddi; higher incidence after truncal vagotomy **and** total gastrectomy

33

Carcinoid Tumors and Carcinoid Syndrome

Matthew Edwards, MD

What are carcinoid tumors?

Neuroendocrine neoplasms arising from primitive ectodermal stem cells in the gut (Kulchitsky cells), which are differentiated along the enterochromaffin line. These tumors can secrete a variety of humoral substances.

What are the secretory products?

Classically, serotonin (5-HT) and bradykinin; also, substance P, 5-HTP, ACTH, histamine, dopamine, prostaglandins, neuromedin A, motilin, tachykinins, and kallikrein

Are they common?

No; incidence is approximately 25 per 1,000,000, but they constitute roughly one third of all primary small-bowel neoplasms

What is the carcinoid syndrome?

A group of symptoms that can occur in patients with carcinoid tumors and includes flushing (95%), diarrhea (80%), valvular heart disease (40%), and wheezing (20%)

What percentage of patients with carcinoid tumors manifest the carcinoid syndrome?

Only 5% to 10%

What causes carcinoid syndrome to occur in some patients but not in others?

Carcinoid syndrome occurs when the secretory products gain access to the systemic circulation. Classically, this happens in the setting of hepatic metastases, which allow the humoral products to avoid the "hepatic filter" and drain systemically into the hepatic veins. Other routes include primary tumors such as ovarian, bronchial, and

409

retroperitoneal carcinoids, which drain systemically and not into the portal vein.

What are the common primary sites?

Appendix, small intestine, rectum, and bronchus

Where do most small-bowel primaries occur?

Ileum—90%
Jejunum—7%
Duodenum—2%

What are the most common metastatic sites for primary small-bowel carcinoids?

1. Regional lymph nodes
2. Liver
3. Lung

Other than the appendix, what is the most common site for a primary carcinoid tumor?

Ileum

PATHOLOGY/HISTOLOGY

Does site of origin matter?

Absolutely; carcinoid tumors are usually classified according to primitive foregut, midgut, or hindgut origin

What is the typical course of foregut tumors?

Foregut carcinoids are argentaffin-negative and commonly secrete 5-HT, histamine, and peptide hormones (e.g., ACTH). These tumors tend to metastasize to bone.

What is the typical course of midgut tumors?

Midgut carcinoids are argentaffin-positive and tend to secrete 5-HT and tachykinins. Midgut tumors are the classic carcinoids that metastasize to the liver and cause carcinoid syndrome (especially small bowel).

What are tachykinins?

Tachykinins are a family of vasoactive peptide hormones with very short half-lives.

What is the typical course of hindgut tumors?

Hindgut carcinoids are argentaffin negative and tend to be nonsecretory. Hindgut tumors (e.g., rectal) tend to metastasize to bone and are frequently asymptomatic.

What factors determine the risk of metastases?

Size—tumors less than 1 cm have a risk of 2%; 1- to 2-cm tumors have a 50% risk; tumors greater than 2 cm have 90% metastatic risk

Location—in general, the more distal the primary tumor, the higher the metastatic risk (except for the appendix)

What percentage of patients with carcinoid tumors have elevated serotonin levels?

Approximately 60%

What percentage of patients with serotonin overproduction are symptomatic?

Approximately 66%

Which primary tumor sites are most frequently associated with serotonin overproduction?

Ileum, cecum, jejunum

What are the effects of serotonin on the GI tract?

Serotonin increases small-bowel tone, motility, fluid secretion, and blood flow. It also increases exocrine pancreas secretion and decreases gastric acidity and bile flow.

Are elevated serotonin levels responsible for the carcinoid syndrome?

Not entirely—excessive serotonin levels seem to be involved in diarrhea and valvular disease; however, the other classic symptoms seem to be due to a number of other vasoactive/endocrine products

What are the associated valvular lesions?

Most commonly tricuspid, regurgitation, and pulmonic stenosis (note: **right-sided valvular lesions**)

What causes the valvular lesions?

Subendocardial fibrosis, thought to be secondary to elevated serotonin levels

Why are the valvular lesions predominantly right sided?

The lungs (like the liver) act as a filter to deactivate the bulk of the humorally active substances and thus protect the left side of the heart.

Do desmoplastic (fibrotic) changes occur at other sites as well?	Yes; the most common sites are the gut wall, mesenteric vessels, and the retroperitoneum. Other sites that may become fibrotic include the penile fascia and joints.
Can these fibrotic changes cause trouble?	Absolutely—the intense mesenteric and gut-wall fibrosis is the most common cause of bowel obstruction in carcinoid tumor patients; moreover, the mesenteric vascular fibrosis can lead to intestinal ischemia in some patients
Which humoral product causes flushing?	Bradykinin is thought to be the most likely culprit.

CLINICAL MANIFESTATIONS

How do patients with carcinoid tumors present?	Appendix—asymptomatic or appendicitis, small-bowel obstruction, diarrhea, weight loss, carcinoid syndrome, bronchus— incidental CXR finding, bronchial obstruction, pneumonia
Is GI bleeding common with carcinoid tumors?	No; carcinoids are submucosal in location and do not commonly bleed. Bleeding is seen with rectal carcinoids.
Are there any risk factors for developing a carcinoid tumor?	There are no clearly defined risk factors; however, animal studies suggest that elevated gastrin levels may be contributory. Also, there is an increased incidence among patients with pernicious anemia, other atrophic gastritides, and Zollinger-Ellison syndrome.
Is there a familial risk?	No, there is no evidence of increased risk
What disease is associated with carcinoid tumors of the ampulla of Vater?	Neurofibromatosis
In MEN-I patients, what are the most frequent locations of carcinoid tumors?	**Men**—thymus **Women**—lung

Which primary site(s) are most commonly associated with carcinoid syndrome?	Two-thirds of all cases occur with ileal primaries.

DIAGNOSIS

What is the classic lab test to diagnose carcinoid syndrome?	Twenty-four hour urinary 5-hydroxyindoleacetic acid (5-HIAA) level; level of greater than 10 mg/24 hr is 75% sensitive and 100% specific
Other than carcinoids, what can cause elevations in 5-HIAA?	Celiac disease, malabsorption, acetaminophen, phenothiazines, guaifenesin, bananas, pineapple, kiwi, walnuts, and pecans
Why is 5-HIAA elevated in the urine of patients with carcinoid syndrome?	It is the major product of serotonin breakdown by monoamine oxidase and aldehyde dehydrogenase.
Are other tests useful?	Yes; the serum serotonin, platelet serotonin, urine serotonin, serum 5-HT, urinary 5-HT, and urinary 5-HTP levels can also be measured to increase sensitivity in cases of high clinical suspicion with normal urine 5-HIAA levels
What radiologic studies are useful?	Bronchus-CXR, CT small-bowel CT, small-bowel follow-through, enteroclysis, arteriogram, I-131 MIBG and radio-labeled somatostatin scintigraphy, colon barium enema, endoscopy
What characteristic barium study findings are associated with GI carcinoids?	Filling defects, rigidity, and kinking of bowel loops
What are the characteristic arteriogram findings?	Retraction and narrowing of mesenteric vessels and poor venous pooling
Are there other potential localization tests?	Yes, selective venous sampling for serotonin and its metabolites

Is pentagastrin useful in diagnosing carcinoid tumors?	Yes; it can be used to induce GI symptoms and flushing and to elevate serotonin levels to increase sensitivity of detection of midgut tumors metastatic to the liver
What are the best tests for evaluating for liver metastasis?	Angiography (most sensitive), CT, and MRI (T2 images)

TREATMENT

What is the appropriate surgical treatment of appendiceal carcinoids?	Localized tumor less than 2 cm—appendectomy Also, appendectomy alone if the tumor is greater than 2 cm in elderly or high operative-risk patients because of the slow growing nature of the tumor Right hemicolectomy if the tumor is greater than 2 cm or if there is vascular, cecal, or mesoappendiceal involvement
Where are appendiceal carcinoids located?	**Tip**—70% **Body**—20% **Base**—10%
What is the incidence of carcinoids in appendectomy specimens?	10 to 15 per 1000 appendectomies
What are the most common tumors of the vermiform appendix?	Carcinoid
What is the 5-year survival rate for appendiceal carcinoids?	99%
How common are metastases from appendiceal carcinoids?	Very rare and if they do occur, they are almost always limited to the regional lymph nodes
What is the appropriate surgical treatment of small-bowel carcinoids?	Wide en bloc resection, including as much nodal drainage as possible. It is imperative to look for other small-bowel carcinoids (high incidence of multifocality), second malignancies, and isolated liver or nodal metastases that can be resected.

Describe the typical appearance of a small-bowel carcinoid tumor.

A small, smooth, firm submucosal nodule surrounded by intense gut-wall fibrosis and mesenteric retraction and fibrosis

What is the incidence of multifocal primary small-bowel carcinoids?

Approximately 30%

What percentage of small-bowel carcinoids are metastatic at diagnosis?

Approximately 50%

What is the most important prognostic factor?

Presence of liver metastases at initial operation
Resectable abdominal disease (including resectable nodal disease) has a 15-year median survival.
Unresectable abdominal disease (without liver metastases) has a median survival of 5 years.
Presence of liver metastases reduces median survival to 3 years.

What is the 5-year survival rate for small-bowel carcinoids?

Approximately 50%

What is the most common metachronous primary GI malignancy?

Colon adenocarcinoma

What is the median survival for patients with carcinoid syndrome?

Three years

What are the treatment options for carcinoid syndrome in the presence of liver metastases?

Octreotide
α-interferon
Hepatic artery embolization
IFN + embolization
Liver resection
Cytotoxic chemotherapy

How does octreotide work?

It is a synthetic somatostatin analog that is thought to inhibit the release of humoral products by the carcinoid.

What are the side effects of octreotide?	Steatorrhea Cholelithiasis secondary to biliary stasis
How effective is octreotide?	Response rate of 60% to 80%, with excellent relief of diarrhea and flushing; however, tachyphylaxis occurs with time in most patients because of receptor downregulation with a median response time of 9 months
How effective is α-IFN?	Response rate of 50% to 80% with symptom alleviation; tachyphylaxis also occurs with α-IFN, most likely because of the development of antibodies
What are the side effects of α-IFN?	Flu-like symptoms
In what cases should hepatic resection be attempted?	Only in low-risk patients in whom safe extirpation of more than 90% of a metastatic tumor mass can be safely performed
Can hepatic resection ever be considered curative?	Yes, if all of the primary abdominal disease and all metastatic disease is resected
Why is cholecystectomy indicated at the time of initial operation for carcinoid tumors?	To prevent potential gallbladder ischemia, if future hepatic artery embolization is necessary
What is the blood supply for most carcinoid liver metastases?	Hepatic artery (**not the portal vein)**
What is the rationale for hepatic artery embolization?	The liver has dual blood supplies and, thus, two oxygen sources. The hepatic artery branches supplying the tumor can be interrupted without causing excessive damage to the normal liver.
What are the potential side effects of embolization in carcinoid patients?	Increased release of humoral substances from the tumor Infection of necrotic liver

What precautions must be taken prior to any tumor embolization, manipulation, or anesthesia induction?	Octreotide blockade, to prevent excessive humoral product release from the tumor
What is the 5-year survival rate for colorectal carcinoids?	80% to 90%
What is the proper surgical therapy for bronchial carcinoid?	For typical carcinoids, local excision is adequate. If carcinoid is atypical, the lesion should be treated as a bronchogenic carcinoma.
What is carcinoid crisis?	Severe cramping, abdominal pain, and diarrhea, with or without cardiac disturbances (hypotension and/or tachycardia) and wheezing Crisis is caused by extremely high humoral product levels (especially serotonin, which in high levels can cause mesenteric vasoconstriction). GI symptoms are caused by ischemia, not by mechanical obstruction.
Why should catecholamines be avoided in the treatment of carcinoid bronchospasm?	There is evidence that humoral product release by enterochromaffin cells may be controlled by adrenoreceptors, and thus catechols/agonists **may actually worsen the bronchoconstriction.**
What is the appropriate therapy for carcinoid crisis?	Octreotide; fluids can be administered to alleviate hypotension acutely; aprotinin should be administered for bronchospasm, if present
What is aprotinin?	An inhibitor of kallikrein
Can carcinoid tumors cause paraneoplastic syndromes?	Yes; carcinoids are a common cause of ectopic cortisol secretion (Cushing syndrome); acromegaly and hypercalcemia have also been reported
What nutritional deficiency occasionally occurs secondary to carcinoid tumors?	Pellagra, because of excessive tryptophan consumption in making excess serotonin (tryptophan is a niacin precursor)

When is cytotoxic chemotherapy indicated?

In anaplastic variants of carcinoid, etoposide, and cisplatin yield response rates of 67%; this therapy is not useful in other variants.

34

Colon, Rectum, and Anus

Jeffrey T. Cope, MD

SURGICAL ANATOMY AND PHYSIOLOGY

What is the length of the normal adult colon?	1.3 to 1.5 meters
Where is the rectosigmoid junction consistently located?	15 to 18 cm from the anal verge
What are three gross anatomic differences between the colon and the small intestine?	1. The outer longitudinal muscle layer of the small intestine becomes three longitudinal bands in the colon, the taeniae coli 2. Haustra do not completely encircle the colon, whereas the plicae circulares (valvulae conniventes) span the entire circumference of the small intestine 3. The colon has extensions of peritoneal fat, the appendices epiploicae
True or false: the colon is a completely intraperitoneal organ?	False; the right and left colon are retroperitoneal
True or false: the rectum is a completely extraperitoneal organ?	False; the proximal rectum is invested by peritoneum
What is the site of the widest colonic diameter?	Cecum (7–9 cm)
Why is this fact significant?	By the law of LaPlace, the cecum is the most likely site of colonic perforation in the setting of distal obstruction/distention. T=PR, in which T = colonic wall

419

tension, P = intraluminal pressure, and
r = radius

Greatest risk of perforation: r > 14 cm

What is the marginal artery of Drummond?

A continuous arterial chain linking the arcades of the entire colon

What is the arc of Riolan?

Proximal collateral in the colonic mesentery that links the SMA and the IMA

Why is an end ileostomy preferable to a cecostomy?

The smaller diameter makes it easier to care for and fit with an appliance.

Should a sigmoid colostomy be brought through the rectus or oblique muscles?

Rectus muscle (lower incidence of peristomal hernias)

Which procedure has the higher morbidity, takedown of an end colostomy or a loop colostomy?

End colostomy

Which ion is preferentially absorbed from the normal colonic lumen?

Na$^+$

By what dominant mechanism is it absorbed?

cAMP-mediated active transport

Which ions are preferentially secreted by the normal colonic epithelium?

K$^+$, HCO$_3^-$

Where in the GI tract does the majority of H$_2$O absorption take place?

Ascending colon

By what mechanism?

Passive diffusion, which is linked to active Na$^+$ transport

What is the effect of bile acids on colonic epithelium?

They produce secretory diarrhea by inducing Na$^+$ and H$_2$O secretion.

What is the main nutrient to the colon?

Short-chain fatty acids

Where is the anorectal junction?

Puborectalis muscle (4–4.5 cm from anal verge)

What does the inner circular muscle layer of the rectal wall become in the anus?

Internal anal sphincter

What is the major stimulus for its relaxation?

Rectal distention

Which pelvic floor muscle is continuous with the external anal sphincter?

Levator ani

What are the major stimuli for relaxation of the external anal sphincter?

Defecation straining, micturition, massive rectal distention

What structures are located at the dentate line?

Anal valves, anal columns of Morgagni, anal ducts and crypts

Epithelium at the dentate line?

Transition zone between columnar and squamous

BENIGN COLORECTAL TUMORS AND POLYPS

What is the most frequent clinical manifestation of colonic polyps?

Occult gastrointestinal bleeding

Compare and contrast tubular and villous adenomatous polyps.

Table 34–1

	Tubular	Villous
Incidence	Common (60% to 80%)	Less common (10%)
Size	Small (<2 cm)	Large (usually >2 cm)
Attachment	Pedunculated	Sessile
Malignant potential	Lower	Higher
Distribution	Even	Left-sided predominance

What is the treatment of choice for a rectal carcinoid less than 2 cm in diameter?	Transanal excision
What is the most common type of colonic polyp?	Hyperplastic
Are they premalignant?	No
What is the etiology of inflammatory polyps (pseudopolyps)?	Colonic mucosal injury from various causes (inflammatory bowel disease, bacterial infections, amebic dysentery, schistosomiasis)

COLORECTAL CANCER

EPIDEMIOLOGIC FACTORS

Where does colorectal cancer rank among annual causes of cancer mortality?	Second (behind lung cancer)
What are the associated risk factors?	Advanced age, dietary factors (high animal fat, low grain fiber), genetic factors, polyposis syndromes, adenomatous polyps, ulcerative colitis, Crohn disease with colorectal involvement, previous history of colorectal cancer, family history
What specific factors increase the risk of colorectal cancer from ulcerative colitis?	Younger age at onset, extensive colonic involvement, duration with active disease (approximately 20% at 20 years)
What features of adenomatous polyps predict an increased risk of colorectal cancer?	Increased size and number, greater degree of dysplasia, increased villous histology
What factors may be protective?	Grain fiber, fruits, vegetables, vitamin D, calcium, aspirin, other NSAIDs

SCREENING AND DIAGNOSIS

What are the most common signs/symptoms of right-sided colon cancer?

Microcytic anemia, melena, constitutional symptoms (weight loss, lassitude), vague abdominal discomfort

What are the most common signs/symptoms of left-sided colon cancer?

Change in bowel habits (constipation, diarrhea, or both in an alternating fashion), decrease in stool diameter, colonic obstruction

What is the most common primary site of colorectal cancer in the U.S.?

Sigmoid (although incidence of right-sided lesions is increasing)

What is the range of the following diagnostic instruments:
Colonoscope?

Entire colon and distal small bowel

Flexible sigmoidoscope?

Distal 60 cm

Rigid proctoscope?

Distal 25 cm

Which is more accurate for assessing the distance of a rectal tumor from the anus: rigid or flexible sigmoidoscopy?

Rigid (especially important when trying to determine whether a rectal cancer is resectable by a low anterior resection or requires an abdominoperineal resection)

What is the value of the Valsalva maneuver when performing a digital rectal exam?

A high rectal tumor may descend within reach of the examiner's finger

Which is more accurate for detecting colonic lesions less than 1 cm in size: colonoscopy or air-contrast barium enema?

Colonoscopy (although these two modalities are comparable for lesions > 1 cm)

What is the current role of transrectal ultrasonography in rectal cancer?

To determine the depth of rectal-wall invasion by small tumors and lymph node involvement

What are the current American Cancer Society recommendations for screening a low-risk, asymptomatic individual?

Flexible sigmoidoscopy at age 50 and every 3 to 5 years thereafter

Annual digital rectal exam and fecal occult blood test beginning at age 40

What are the current American Cancer Society recommendations for screening an individual with a first-degree relative with colorectal cancer?

Colonoscopy (or flexible sigmoidoscopy combined with air-contrast barium enema to study remainder of colon) at age 35 to 40 and every 2 to 3 years thereafter

Other recommendations described in the preceding question

What are the biologic markers of colon cancer?

Carcinoembryonic antigen (CEA), CA 19–9, CA 50, CA 195, TAG-72, sialic acid, tissue polypeptide antigen, tumor-cell DNA ploidy

What is the best initial imaging modality to rule out local recurrence?

CT scan (most local recurrences are **extraluminal**); MRI may be better for rectal recurrences; colonoscopy

What is the best initial imaging modality to rule out liver metastases?

Ultrasound (or CT)

What is the main benefit of postoperative surveillance colonoscopy?

To identify **early** metachronous primaries or premalignant polyps (BE is not the preferred study because of the small size of these lesions)

What are the indications for imaging modalities after resection of colorectal cancer?

Presence of symptoms, rising CEA, abnormal follow-up colonoscopy or BE

Currently, what are the two most useful and reliable uses of CEA measurements in colorectal cancer?

1. To identify incomplete tumor resection (failure of CEA levels to decrease within 6 weeks after surgery)
2. To identify early, subclinical recurrences (first sign of recurrence in 25% to 50% of all patients, but tumor is a **local** recurrence alone in only 25% of cases)

What other conditions can cause CEA elevation?	Smoking; lung, breast, pancreatic, or gastric cancer; renal failure; liver failure; pancreatitis; inflammatory bowel disease
What is the risk of a second synchronous colonic primary?	Approximately 3% (it is therefore imperative that the **entire** colon be visualized and palpated intraoperatively)
What are the most common sites of metastases?	Liver ($\frac{1}{3}$ of all patients with colorectal cancer develop hepatic metastases), bone, lungs, brain
Which liver function test is most frequently elevated in the presence of liver metastases?	Alkaline phosphatase (many patients have normal LFTs!)
What is the proper workup prior to hepatic resection for metastasis?	Chest and abdominal CT (bone scan and head CT for specific symptoms only)

STAGING AND PROGNOSIS

Which histologic subtype has the worst prognosis?	Mucoid adenocarcinoma
What is a "signet ring" tumor?	A tumor characterized by accumulation of mucoid material within colonic epithelial cells, giving them a signet ring appearance (poor prognosis)
What is the five-year survival rate following hepatic resection for solitary liver metastasis with 1 cm margins?	Approximately 25%

SURGICAL RESECTION

What percentage of patients are potentially curable by surgical resection at the time of diagnosis?	Approximately 80%

What is the best and safest mechanical preparation for the following conditions:

Unobstructed colon?

One gallon of oral polyethylene-electrolyte lavage solution the day prior to surgery; oral antibiotics

Partially obstructed colon?

Liquid diet, oral cathartics, and electrolyte enemas for 3 days prior to surgery

Totally obstructed colon?

No mechanical preparation

Classically, what is the recommended length of a margin of normal bowel for resection of colorectal cancer?

At least 5 cm (but many surgeons now state that 2 cm is adequate, especially for low-lying rectal lesions in which sphincter preservation is an issue)

What determines the proximal margin of resection for colonic tumors?

The level of vascular ligation

Identify the location in the colon in which tumors are treated by the following procedures:

Right hemicolectomy

Cecum, ascending colon (ligation of ileocolic and right colic vessels).

Extended right hemicolectomy

Hepatic flexure (ileocolic, right colic, middle colic vessels)

Transverse colectomy

Transverse colon (middle colic vessels)

Left hemicolectomy

Splenic flexure, descending colon (inferior mesenteric vessels at their origins)

Sigmoid colectomy

Sigmoid colon (sigmoidal vessels)

What is the appropriate surgical treatment of a colorectal tumor adherent to adjacent organs?

En bloc resection

What is the proper initial surgical therapy for perforated colon cancer?

Resection and proximal colostomy

What is the recommended concomitant procedure for a postmenopausal woman undergoing resection for colorectal cancer?

Bilateral oophorectomy (7% of patients have occult ovarian metastases)

How far from the anal verge must a rectal tumor be located to facilitate low anterior resection?

Usually, at least 8 cm

What are the conservative local treatment options for rectal cancer?

1. Transanal excision
2. Radiation therapy only
3. Electrocautery fulguration

Which type of patient is an ideal candidate for conservative therapy?

Elderly, high-risk patient with small (stage 0 or 1), mobile, well-differentiated, distal (0–5 cm) rectal tumor

What is the proximal margin of an abdominoperineal resection (APR) and a low anterior resection (LAR)?

Mid-sigmoid colon

What is the distal margin of an APR?

Anal canal below levators

What is the distal margin of a LAR?

Rectum just above levators

Which procedure should come first: colostomy maturation or abdominal closure?

Abdominal closure (decreased risk of infection)

What percentage of patients are candidates for hepatic resection?

Approximately 10% to 20%

What is the procedure of choice for small metastases?

Wedge resection

What is the procedure of choice for large (> 4 cm) or multiple metastases in the same lobe?	Hepatic lobectomy
From which circulation do hepatic metastases obtain their blood supply?	Hepatic arterial

ADJUVANT AND NEOADJUVANT THERAPY

Which chemotherapeutic agents are considered standard for stage III colon cancer?	5-fluorouracil (5-FU) and levamisole
Which chemotherapeutic agents are considered standard for stage IV colon cancer?	5-FU and leucovorin
Why is radiotherapy (RT) not standard adjuvant therapy for colon cancer?	Because of frequent complications of radiation enteritis and renal injury
What is the standard adjuvant therapy for stage II and III rectal cancer?	5-FU and postoperative RT
Why is RT an important adjunct to surgery for local control of rectal cancer?	Because it is difficult to achieve wide margins in the pelvis; the field is usually away from the small bowel
What is the current role of neoadjuvant therapy for rectal cancer?	Preoperative RT for fixed and/or advanced rectal tumors (to potentially convert an unresectable lesion to a resectable lesion)

HEREDITARY POLYPOSIS AND NONPOLYPOSIS COLORECTAL CANCER SYNDROMES

What percentage of cases of colorectal cancer are hereditary?	**Hereditary polyposis syndromes**—1% **Hereditary nonpolyposis syndromes**—5% to 10%
What percentage of cases of colorectal cancer are sporadic?	Greater than 90%

List the more common hereditary polyposis syndromes.	**Adenomatous polyps**—familial adenomatous polyposis, Gardner syndrome, Turcot syndrome **Hamartomatous polyps**—Peutz-Jeghers syndrome, juvenile polyposis
Which is the most common?	Familial adenomatous polyposis (FAP)
What is the incidence of FAP?	1/5000 to 1/7500
What is the mode of inheritance?	Autosomal dominant
Is it associated with an increased risk of colon cancer?	Yes
What is the average age at onset of polyps?	Twenty-five years
What is the average age at onset of colon cancer?	Forty to forty-five years
What are the most common presenting signs/symptoms?	Abdominal pain, bleeding per rectum
What are the associated colonic features?	Hundreds to thousands of small (< 1 cm) adenomatous polyps throughout the colon (heaviest density in the left colon)
What is the procedure of choice after the diagnosis is established?	Total abdominal colectomy with mucosal proctectomy, ileoanal pull-through anastomosis with creation of reservoir pouch
Are there any other options?	Subtotal colectomy with ileorectal anastomosis for patients with very few rectal polyps End ileostomy with total abdominal colectomy Close follow-up is **imperative.**
What is the incidence of Gardner syndrome?	1/8000 to 1/12000 (thought to be simply a different phenotypic expression of FAP)

Is it associated with an increased risk of colon cancer?	Yes
What are the colonic features?	Identical to those of FAP
What are the associated extracolonic features?	Osteomas (skull, mandible, long bones), fibromas, desmoid tumors, dental abnormalities, UGI polyps, extracolonic neoplasms (thyroid, adrenal, biliary system, liver), lipomas, congenital hypertrophy of the retinal pigment epithelium
What are the features of Turcot syndrome?	Adenomatous colonic polyps and malignant brain tumors
Is it associated with an increased risk of colon cancer?	Yes
What is the genetic defect of FAP, Gardner syndrome, Turcot syndrome, and many sporadic cases of colon cancer?	Mutation or deletion of the APC gene on chromosome 5 (a tumor-suppressor gene)
What is the mode of inheritance of Peutz-Jeghers syndrome?	Autosomal dominant
What are the intestinal manifestations?	Hamartomatous polyps throughout the GI tract (heaviest density in the small intestine)
What are the extraintestinal manifestations?	Melanin deposits in buccal mucosa, lips, nose, palms of hands, and soles of feet
What are the presenting signs/symptoms?	GI bleeding, intestinal obstruction, intussusception, mucocutaneous hyperpigmentation
What is the mode of inheritance of juvenile polyposis?	Autosomal dominant

| What are the intestinal manifestations? | Three variants: hamartomas confined to the stomach, colon, or dispersed throughout the GI tract |

| What is the mode of inheritance of hereditary nonpolyposis colorectal cancer (HNPCC) syndromes? | Autosomal dominant |

| What are the other names for HNPCC syndromes? | Lynch syndromes or family cancer syndromes |

| What distinguishes type I from type II HNPCC syndrome? | Colonic cancers only in type I, extracolonic cancers as well in type II |

| What other types of cancer characterize type II HNPCC syndrome? | Ovary, endometrium, ureter, renal pelvis, stomach, pancreas, biliary tree, bone marrow, skin, larynx |

Contrast the features of the polyps of FAP with those of HNPCC syndromes.

Table 34–2

	FAP	HNPCC
Location	Concentrated in the left colon	Predilection for right colon
Size	Small	Even smaller
Number	Hundreds or thousands	Up to 100

| What is the genetic defect associated with HNPCC syndromes? | Mutations in several genes involved in DNA repair (hMSH2, hMLH1, hPMS1, hPMS2), leading to DNA instability, abnormal cell growth, and, ultimately, tumor genesis |

ULCERATIVE COLITIS

| What is the distribution of disease in ulcerative colitis (UC)? | Tends to start distally (distal colonic/rectal involvement in 90% of cases) and proceeds in a continuous pattern to involve the proximal colon |

What percentage of patients have "backwash ileitis"?

Approximately 10%

What are the histopathologic characteristics?

Diffuse, nonspecific, nongranulomatous inflammation of mucosa and submucosa with formation of inflammatory polyps, crypt abscesses, and ulcers

What are the associated BE findings in ulcerative colitis?

Loss of haustral markings
Rigid "stovepipe" appearance
Foreshortening of the colon
Wall irregularities (pseudopolyps, ulcers)

What is the most common presenting symptom?

Bloody diarrhea

What are the extraintestinal manifestations?

Arthritis
Ocular disorders (conjunctivitis, iritis, choroiditis)
Dermatologic disorders (erythema nodosum, pyoderma gangrenosum)
Hepatobiliary disorders (sclerosing cholangitis, pericholangitis, nonspecific hepatitis)

What percentage of patients with sclerosing cholangitis have UC?

Approximately 50%

When does the risk of colon cancer increase?

After 10 years with UC (approximately 20% risk at 20 years); related to both the extent and duration of the disease

Is it more or less aggressive than sporadic colon cancer?

Less

What is the primary therapy for acute UC exacerbations?

Corticosteroids

What are the indications for surgery?

Persistent massive bleeding per rectum
Toxic megacolon with perforation or imminent perforation
Fulminant acute exacerbation unresponsive to IV steroids
Stricture (25% malignant, risk of obstruction)

Suspicion of or documented colon
cancer
Failure to thrive in children with
ulcerative colitis
Chronic, unrelenting disease with
substantial lifestyle limitations (overall
most common indication for surgery)
Prophylaxis for colon cancer

What are the radiographic signs of toxic megacolon?

Massively dilated colon (most commonly
transverse) with bowel-wall thickening
and irregularity

What is the appropriate initial therapy for toxic megacolon?

Fluid resuscitation and brief (24–48
hour) trial of IV steroids to "cool down"
acute disease and thus convert operation
to elective procedure

What is the emergency operative procedure of choice?

Total abdominal colectomy with Brooke
ileostomy (preservation of rectum and
sphincters for later continence-restoring
reconstruction)

What is considered the classic "gold standard" elective operative procedure for chronic UC?

Total proctocolectomy with permanent
Brooke ileostomy

What is the preferred continence-sparing elective procedure?

Total abdominal colectomy, mucosal
proctectomy, and endorectal ileoanal
pull-through anastomosis (with creation
of J, S, or W reservoir pouch)

What are the advantages of this procedure?

Preserves fecal continence
Eliminates all involved mucosa
Eliminates need for abdominal stoma
(permanent)
Preserves sacral autonomic nerves, thus
protecting sexual and bladder function
in these patients (many of which are
young)

What are the disadvantages?

Frequent stools (~6 bowel movements
per day)
Potential fecal soiling of undergarments
Pouchitis
Pouch ischemia
Misdiagnosis of UC in a patient with
Crohn disease with ileal involvement
and late pouch failure

Why is a temporary diverting ileostomy often performed in conjunction with the above procedure?

To protect the anastomosis

Why is stomal maturation of an ileostomy or a colostomy important?

To prevent the development of an inflammatory response by the serosa, which may result in stomal stenosis

What is pouchitis?

A syndrome of indeterminate etiology after construction of a reservoir pouch, characterized by malaise, low-grade fever, increased stool frequency (often watery), and crampy abdominal/pelvic pain, with stasis and inflammation of the ileal pouch

What is the incidence?

Approximately 30% to 50% of patients with ileal pouch

What is the appropriate treatment?

Oral metronidazole

What is the most common major complication after surgery for UC?

Sepsis (bowel surgery in chronically immunosuppressed patient)

DIVERTICULAR DISEASE AND LOWER GASTROINTESTINAL HEMORRHAGE

DIVERTICULOSIS/LOWER GASTROINTESTINAL BLEEDING

Compare "true" and "false" diverticula.

Table 34–3

	True	False
Mucosal involvement	All layers	Mucosa only
Transmission	Congenital	Acquired
Location	Cecum	Sigmoid
Incidence	Uncommon	Common
Age at onset	Younger	Older

What is the incidence of diverticula in the general population?

Approximately 35% to 50%

Where are most diverticula found?	Sigmoid (90% to 95% of patients with diverticula have sigmoid involvement)
Where are most bleeding diverticula found?	Right colon in 50% to 70% of cases
What fraction of initial cases stop bleeding spontaneously?	Approximately 75% (but a third rebleed)
What percentage of patients with diverticula develop diverticular hemorrhage?	Approximately 15%
What is angiodysplasia?	Vascular ectasias in the colonic mucosa that develop with aging, also called arteriovenous malformations (AVMs)
What is the etiology?	Progressive dilatation of venules as a result of obstruction to draining veins or chronically increased intraluminal pressure
What are the associated cardiac abnormalities?	Aortic stenosis (although this association has recently been questioned)
Where are most AVMs located?	Right colon (antimesenteric border)
Where are most bleeding AVMs located?	Right colon
What is the preferred treatment of bleeding AVMs?	Colonoscopic coagulation (very difficult to localize by laparotomy)
What are the most common causes of acute massive LGI bleeding?	Diverticulosis (30% to 50%), angiodysplasia (25%, but increasing in frequency)
What are the other causes?	**Hemorrhoids,** anal fissures, polyps, ulcerative colitis, Crohn disease, Meckel's diverticula, ischemic colitis, aortoenteric fistula, infectious colitis, radiation colitis

Define LGI bleeding.

Bleeding arising distal to the ligament of Treitz

What is the most common sign of LGI bleeding?

Hematochezia (although 10% to 20% of patients with brisk **upper** GI bleeding will present with hematochezia)

What does melena normally indicate?

Bleeding proximal to the ligament of Treitz, as a result of bacterial and acid degradation of hemoglobin (although a slow colonic bleeder can also cause melena)

What distinguishes melena from clotted LGI blood?

Melena does not turn toilet water red

What fraction rebleed after spontaneous cessation?

A third

What is the appropriate management of an actively bleeding patient who remains hemodynamically stable?

Diagnostic attempts to identify the bleeding site

How would an algorithm for workup of massive LGI bleeding be illustrated?

Resuscitation (IV fluids, blood/blood products, O_2)
↓
NG lavage → (+) → EGD
↓
(−)
↓
Anoscopy/sigmoidoscopy (still must perform colonoscopy if bleeding hemorrhoids or fissure found)
↓
Colonoscopy → (+) → treat
(after rapid prep)
↓
(−) (spontaneous cessation of bleeding in 3/4)
↓
Observe
↓
Bleeding recurs (1/3)
↓
Tagged RBC scan → (−) → Observe
↓
(+)
↓
Mesenteric arteriography

What are the treatment options for acute LGI hemorrhage?	Colonoscopy (bipolar, heater probe, laser) Arteriography (vasopressin, embolization) Surgery
In what fraction of cases is the site of LGI bleeding never identified?	A third
What is the only absolute contraindication to colonoscopy in a workup of acute LGI hemorrhage?	Shock
How brisk must the bleeding be for arteriography to define the site?	Greater than 0.5 ml/min
How brisk must the bleeding be for a tagged RBC scan to define the site?	Greater than 0.1 ml/min (but not very specific in identifying the exact site of hemorrhage)
What is the role of a barium enema in the workup of acute LGI hemorrhage?	None! It can obscure attempts at visualization with arteriography or colonoscopy, and increased intraluminal pressure can disrupt any clot that might have formed.
What are the indications for surgery for LGI hemorrhage?	Persistent hemodynamic instability (in spite of colonoscopic or angiographic therapy) Transfusion of greater than 6 units in 24 hours Second bleeding episode after initial spontaneous cessation
If the site of LGI bleeding is identified preoperatively, what is the operation of choice?	Segmental colonic resection and primary reanastomosis (effective in 90%, most often is a right hemicolectomy)

DIVERTICULITIS

What percentage of patients with diverticula develop diverticulitis?	Approximately 10% to 25%

Where does diverticulitis arise?

Sigmoid in greater than 90% of patients; right colon in 5% of patients

What is the pathogenesis?

Chronic erosion of discrete sites in the colonic wall by increased intraluminal pressure and inspissated food particles, resulting in inflammation and focal necrosis/perforation

What are the signs/ symptoms of mild, uncomplicated diverticulitis?

Left lower quadrant abdominal pain and tenderness of several days' duration, low-grade fever, mild leukocytosis, abdominal distention, mild peritoneal signs, anorexia, nausea, vomiting, history of constipation

What are the causes of right lower quadrant tenderness in diverticulitis?

Right-sided diverticulitis (5%), redundant loop of sigmoid colon in the right lower quadrant containing inflamed diverticula

What complications are associated with diverticulitis?

Intestinal obstruction (colon or small bowel), perforation, abscess formation, fistulization

What percentage of patients develop complications?

25%

What is the most common complication?

Abscess formation

What are the most common types of diverticular abscesses?

Peridiverticular, retroperitoneal, pelvic, mesenteric

What are the most common types of diverticular fistulas?

Colovesical (less common in women), colocutaneous, colovaginal, coloenteric

What are the best modalities for diagnosis of colovesical fistula?

Cystoscopy, BE, CT scan

What are the signs/
symptoms of complicated
diverticulitis?

Tender lower abdominal mass (abscess),
moderate leukocytosis (WBC > 15,000),
high-grade fever (> 39°C), widespread
peritoneal signs (free perforation),
bacteriuria, pneumaturia, fecaluria, or
pyuria (colovesical fistula), abdominal
distention (obstruction)

What is the most common
cause of colonic
obstruction?

Left-sided colon cancer (sigmoid
diverticulitis is second)

True or false: free air
beneath the diaphragm on
an upright abdominal X-
ray is a common finding in
perforated diverticulitis?

False

Why are BE and
colonoscopy not
recommended in the
setting of acute
diverticulitis?

Because increased intraluminal pressure
could cause diverticular perforation

What is the radiographic
procedure of choice for
diagnosis of complicated
diverticulitis?

CT scan (may identify pericolic
inflammation, colonic-wall edema,
abscesses, fistulas, air in the bladder, or
ureteral obstruction)

What is the radiographic
procedure of choice for
diagnosis of uncomplicated
diverticulitis?

Elective BE or colonoscopy after
inflammation subsides (and after ruling
out other diagnoses requiring emergent
surgical intervention, such as
appendicitis or perforated ulcer)

What is the appropriate
treatment of mild,
uncomplicated
diverticulitis?

Clear liquid diet for several days as an
    outpatient
Oral antibiotics (metronidazole, bactrim)
Inpatient IV antibiotics and complete
    bowel rest if no improvement occurs
    on outpatient management

What are the indications
for surgical intervention?

Complicated diverticulitis (obstruction,
    free perforation, fistulization)
Recurrent bouts of acute diverticulitis
Clinical deterioration or no improvement
    with nonoperative therapy
Inability to exclude colon cancer (e.g.,
    stricture with negative colonoscopic

biopsy)
Right-sided diverticulitis (to eliminate
confusion in diagnosis of appendicitis)

What is the surgical procedure of choice under elective conditions (prepared bowel)?

Segmental resection and primary anastomosis

What is the surgical procedure of choice under emergent conditions for complications or fulminant course (unprepared bowel)?

Hartmann procedure (sigmoid resection with end-colostomy and oversewing of rectal pouch)

COLONIC VOLVULUS

What are the most common sites of colonic volvulus?

Sigmoid (75%), cecum (25%), transverse (very rare)

What are the anatomic features predisposing patients to volvulus?

Large, redundant segment of colon with a narrow mesenteric base (acquired in sigmoid, congenital in most cases of cecal volvulus)

What are the most common causes of sigmoid volvulus?

Chronic constipation (with associated laxative and enema abuse)
Neuropsychiatric disorders (sedentary state, psychotropic drugs decrease bowel motility)
Adhesions (serve as lead points)
Pregnancy (most common cause of intestinal obstruction during pregnancy)

What are the radiographic signs of sigmoid volvulus?

"Bent inner tube" or "omega loop" signs (represent the convexity of a dilated sigmoid loop pointing toward the right upper quadrant)
"Bird's beak" sign (represents the area of tapered colon at the site of obstruction, most commonly in the left lower quadrant)

What is the preferred initial treatment of sigmoid volvulus?	Attempted reduction via colonoscopy or rigid proctoscopy
What is the initial success rate?	Approximately 75%
What is the recurrence rate after reduction alone?	Approximately 50%
What is the appropriate treatment if initial endoscopic reduction is unsuccessful?	Operative reduction Elective sigmoid resection and primary anastomosis (after bowel is amenable to mechanical preparation)
What is the appropriate treatment if bowel necrosis is present at endoscopy or surgery?	Sigmoid resection
What are the radiographic signs of cecal volvulus?	"Bird's beak" in the right colon, convexity of dilated cecal loop points toward left upper quadrant
What is the preferred initial treatment?	If the bowel is viable—detorsion and cecopexy or right hemicolectomy (nonoperative reduction is rarely successful) If the bowel is gangrenous—right hemicolectomy with ileotransverse colostomy

BENIGN ANORECTAL DISEASE

RECTAL PROLAPSE

What physiologic abnormality is associated with complete rectal prolapse (procidentia)?	Idiopathic laxity of the anal sphincters
What is the cause of sphincter laxity?	Chronic stretching and resultant neuropathy of the internal pudendal nerve

What is the potential complication of untreated sphincter laxity and procidentia?	Fecal incontinence
Is procidentia more common in men or women?	Women

HEMORRHOIDAL DISEASE

What are the three anatomic components of hemorrhoids?	Prolapsed redundant anorectal mucosa Submucosal venous engorgement Protuberances at the anal margin (skin tags)
From what normal anatomic structures do hemorrhoids arise?	Cushions of vascular tissue in the submucosa underlying the squamocolumnar transition zone of the anal canal (2 on the right, 1 on the left)
From which venous plexus do internal hemorrhoids arise?	The main hemorrhoidal plexus in the submucosa of the upper anal canal (with overlying secretory columnar epithelium)
From which venous plexus do external hemorrhoids arise?	External anal plexus in the submucosa of the anal margin (with overlying squamous epithelium)
What are the common physiologic disturbances in patients with hemorrhoids?	Chronic constipation Increased internal anal sphincter pressure
What are the consequences of these disturbances?	Excessive straining at defecation, descent of pelvic floor, weakening of sphincters, extrusion of anal mucosa outside the anal margin, and stasis in the hemorrhoidal veins
What are the main complications of hemorrhoids?	Acute thrombosis and hemorrhage (important: rectal bleeding should never be attributed solely to hemorrhoids until colon cancer has been ruled out)
Why do hemorrhoids bleed?	Defecation trauma to the mucosa exposes the underlying engorged veins

What is the preferred treatment of painful acute thrombosis?	Incision and evacuation of the clot under local anesthesia
What is the preferred treatment of mildly symptomatic hemorrhoids?	Fiber laxatives and stool softeners (to avoid straining), sitz baths
What are the treatment options for moderately symptomatic hemorrhoids (frequent bleeding, reducible prolapse)?	Rubber band ligation Sclerotherapy Infrared coagulation Cryotherapy Cautery Laser therapy Surgery
What is the common goal of these therapies?	To produce submucosal fibrosis and subsequent obliteration of distended hemorrhoids
What is the appropriate therapy for severe symptoms?	Hemorrhoidectomy (5% to 10% of patients)
What are the indications for hemorrhoidectomy?	Recurrent episodes of thrombosis Substantial external component Large, prolapsed hemorrhoids with overlying squamous metaplasia Unresponsiveness to nonoperative therapy (such as dietary changes, banding, injection therapy)

ANORECTAL SUPPURATIVE DISEASE

What is the most common cause of anorectal suppuration?	Infection of anal glands in the intersphincteric space as a result of obstruction of anal ducts
What are the other causes?	Crohn disease, tuberculosis, lymphogranuloma venereum, malignancy, trauma/foreign body
What is the most common acute sequel?	Abscess
What is the most common chronic sequel?	Fistula

How do the various types of anorectal abscesses and fistulas form?

Spread of suppuration from the intersphincteric space

What are the different types of anorectal abscesses?

Intersphincteric—between the internal and external sphincters
Perianal—subcutaneous tissues of the anal margin (distal to sphincters)
Supralevator—between the sphincters, superior to the levators
Ischiorectal—ischiorectal fossa (lateral to external sphincter)
Horseshoe—circumferential in the ischiorectal fossa (most commonly), intersphincteric space, or supralevator space

What are the signs/ symptoms of anorectal abscess?

Perianal pain and tenderness, especially with defecation
Perianal swelling, skin induration, and erythema
Exquisitely tender, fluctuant mass on examination of perineum or digital rectal exam
Fever of unknown origin or unexplained sepsis (especially in immunocompromised patients or those with high-lying abscess)

How should anorectal abscesses be evaluated?

Examine perianal skin for swelling, erythema, induration, tender masses, sinuses
Perform digital rectal exam for tender, fluctuant masses
Perform anoscopy/proctoscopy for tender masses, swelling in the anal canal, internal sinus-tract opening

What should be done if the patient is too tender for a digital rectal exam?

Examine under anesthesia

What is the appropriate treatment of anorectal abscesses?

Surgical incision and drainage **immediately** after diagnosis (sepsis may develop rapidly if surgery is delayed)
Antibiotics as adjuncts to surgery, if the patient has cellulitis, diabetes mellitus, immunosuppression, heart-valve or extensive infection

How should low-lying anorectal abscesses be drained (perianal, intersphincteric, ischiorectal)?

Externally (transperineal approach)

High-lying anorectal abscesses (supralevator)?

Internally (transrectal approach)

What is the definition of a fistula?

Abnormal communication between 2 epithelial surfaces

What are the different types of anorectal fistulas?

Intersphincteric—intersphincteric spac → downward → perianal skin

Transsphincteric—intersphincteric spacer laterally across extrasphincteric sphincter → ischiorectal fossa → skin

Suprasphincteric—intersphincteric space → superolaterally → over extrasphincteric sphincter → through levator → ischiorectal fossa → skin

Extrasphincteric—rectal lumen → through levator → ischiorectal fossa → skin

What is the frequency of each type?

Intersphincteric—70%
Transsphincteric—25%
Suprasphincteric—less than 5%
Extrasphincteric—less than 1%

What are the signs/symptoms of anorectal fistulas?

Recurrent or persistent purulent or bloody drainage from a sinus in the perineum; often there is a history of an anorectal abscess that drained spontaneously or was drained surgically

What is Goodsall's rule?

If a transverse line is drawn across the anal verge, an external fistulous opening anterior to this line will lead directly into the rectal lumen in a straight, radial pattern; however, an external opening posterior to this line will lead in a curved pattern to the posterior midline of the rectal lumen.

What is the appropriate treatment of anorectal fistulas?	Incision and drainage of underlying abscess If fistula persists, re-examine under anesthesia **Low-lying fistula (does not involve external sphincter)**—primary fistulotomy **High-lying fistula (involves external sphincter)**—staged fistulotomy with Seton suture (high risk of incontinence if primary fistulotomy is performed)

ANAL FISSURES

Where are most primary anal fissures located?	Posterior midline of the anal canal (linearly through squamous mucosa)
What is the most common etiology of primary fissures?	Constipation and passage of a hard stool
Where are most secondary anal fissures located?	Location varies, often anterior or lateral
What is the etiology of secondary anal fissures?	Crohn disease, AIDS, GC, chlamydia, syphilis, pruritus ani, prior anal surgery, direct trauma, tuberculosis
What fraction of patients with Crohn disease have anal disease of all types?	Three-fourths
What are the physiologic consequences of anal fissures?	Spasm of internal anal sphincter and increased resting sphincter pressure (further aggravates the fissure)
What are the signs/ symptoms of anal fissure?	Pain during defecation, rectal bleeding
How can an acute fissure be distinguished from a chronic fissure?	"Sentinel pile" (an edematous skin tag at the distal end of the fissure) is only present in **chronic** anal fissures Duration of symptoms Transverse fibers of the exposed internal anal sphincter are present at the base of a chronic fissure

What is the preferred initial treatment of acute primary anal fissures?	Conservative measures:
	  Topical anesthetics
	  Avoidance of straining, constipation, and hard stools with a laxative
	  Sitz baths

What is the appropriate treatment if these measures fail?	Anal dilation or lateral internal sphincterotomy (enlarges the anal canal, thus avoiding continued trauma from passage of the stool)
What is the most serious complication of these procedures?	Fecal incontinence
What is the proper management of suspected secondary anal fissures?	Biopsy of the fissure (to rule out anal cancer, infectious etiologies) Biopsy of rectal mucosa (to rule out Crohn disease)

ANAL CANCER

What is the histologic type of most tumors of the proximal anal canal?	Adenocarcinoma
What is the histologic type of most tumors of the distal anus?	Well-differentiated keratinizing squamous cell carcinoma (overall most common malignant tumor of the anus)
What is the lymphatic drainage of the proximal anus?	Superior hemorrhoidal chain—pelvic nodes
What is the lymphatic drainage of the dentate line?	Submucosal nodal plexus—superior hemorrhoidal chain → pelvic nodes **or** Inferior and middle hemorrhoidal chain—hypogastric and obturator nodes
What is the lymphatic drainage of the distal anal canal/anal margin?	Superficial inguinal nodes
Which has the best prognosis: squamous cell carcinoma of the anal canal or anal margin?	Anal canal

What is the preferred initial treatment of squamous cell carcinoma of the anal canal?

Radiotherapy and chemotherapy

What is the preferred initial treatment for squamous cell carcinoma of the anal margin?

Local excision

What is the most common site of primary gastrointestinal melanoma?

Anus

35

The Liver

Lorne H. Blackbourne, MD

ANATOMY

What is the weight of the average liver?	Approximately 1500 grams
What fissure does the falciform ligament enter?	Umbilical fissure
What are the borders of the caudate lobe?	IVC, umbilical fissure Transverse hilar fissure
What are the borders of the quadrate lobe?	Transverse hilar fissure Umbilical fissure Gallbladder fossa
Do the hepatic veins follow the segmental lobar anatomy of the liver?	No
Does the portal vein have valves?	No
What is the bare area?	The area that is not covered with peritoneum on the back of the liver
What is the name of the liver ligament that crowns the bare area?	Coronary ligament
What are the lateral liver ligaments called?	Triangular ligaments (right and left)
What is the obliterated umbilical vein called?	Ligamentum teres
What percentage of left hepatic arteries are replaced entirely by a branch from the left gastric artery?	Approximately 10%

What percentage of left hepatic arteries are partially replaced by a branch of the left gastric artery?	Approximately 10%
What percentage of right hepatic arteries arise from the superior mesenteric artery?	Approximately 10% (**Is there a pattern here?**)
What percentage of right hepatic arteries pass anteriorly to the common hepatic bile duct?	Approximately 25%
What percentage of right hepatic arteries pass posteriorly to the portal vein?	Approximately 10%
What is the name of macrophages located in the liver?	Kupffer cells
What are the components of a portal triad?	1. Arteriole (hepatic) 2. Portal venule 3. Bile duct

PHYSIOLOGY

What fraction of total liver blood flow comes from the portal vein?	Approximately two thirds
What fraction of total liver blood flow comes from the hepatic artery?	Approximately one third
What percentage of total cardiac output goes to the liver?	Approximately 20%
What percentage of total liver oxygen comes from the portal vein?	Approximately 50% of liver oxygen comes from the blood via the portal vein.

What are the functions of the liver?	Carbohydrate, lipid metabolism (energy) Protein synthesis Bile production Detoxification of drugs, etc. Pathogen filtering
What protein is produced in the largest amount by the liver?	Albumin
What are the vitamin K–dependent clotting factors made in the liver?	2, 7, 9, 10 (think: 2 + 7 = 9 and 10)
What are the hepatic acute-phase proteins?	Fibrinogen, haptoglobin, C-reactive protein, complement 3, ceruloplasmin, α-antitrypsin, α-antichymotrypsin, α-acid glycoprotein, amyloid A
What are the signs/ symptoms of liver disease?	Hepatomegaly, splenomegaly, icterus, pruritis (from bile salts in skin), blanching spider telangectasia, gynecomastia, testicular atrophy, caput medusae, dark urine, clay-colored stools, bradycardia, edema, ascites, fever, Fetor hepaticus (sweet musty smell), hemorrhoids, variceal bleeding, anemia, body hair loss, liver tenderness, palmar erythema

LIVER INFECTIONS

LIVER ABSCESSES

What is the etiology?	Direct spread from the gallbladder/ biliary tract Portal spread from GI infection (e.g., appendicitis, diverticulitis) Systemic source (bacteremia) Cryptogenic, malignant obstruction
What are the two most common types?	Bacterial (most common in the United States) and amoebic (most common worldwide)
Define pyogenic.	Caused by bacteria
Define cryptogenic.	Unknown; puzzling (cryptic)

What are the possible diagnoses of liver abscess?	Pyogenic (bacterial), parasitic, fungal

BACTERIAL ABSCESSES

What are the three most common gram-negative organisms associated with bacterial abscesses?	*E. coli, Klebsiella, Proteus*
How often are streptococci species isolated from liver abscesses?	Approximately one third of the time
How often are anaerobes isolated from liver abscesses?	Approximately one third of the time
When treating a liver abscess with triple therapy, is metronidazole or clindamycin preferred?	Metronidazole, because it treats *Amoeba* (it is often difficult to distinguish between bacterial and ameobic abscesses)
What are the associated signs/symptoms?	Fever, chills, leukocytosis, right upper quadrant pain, increased LFTs, sepsis
What is the appropriate treatment?	IV antibiotics with "triples"/ drainage
What is the best way to drain a liver abscess?	The preferred method is by a percutaneous route with radiographic guidance
What are the relative contraindications for percutaneous drainage?	Multiple abscesses Biliary obstruction requiring surgery Intraabdominal source for the abscess that will require surgery Echinococcal hydatid cyst Ascites

AMOEBIC ABSCESSES

What is the etiology?	***Entamoeba histolytica;*** typically reaches the liver via the portal vein from intestinal amebiasis

What are the associated risk factors?	Patients from countries south of the U.S./Mexican border; patients who have been institutionalized
What are the associated signs/symptoms?	Same as those of bacterial abscesses; most involve the R lobe of the liver
Which laboratory tests are indicated?	Indirect hemagglutination titers for entamoeba antibodies (elevated in greater than 95% of patients)
What is the approprite treatment?	IV metronidazole
What does the amebic abscess fluid look like?	Red, brown (described as anchovy paste)
How is _E. histolytica_ spread?	Fecal–oral transmission
What is the name of the forms that live in the colon?	Trophozoites
What percentage of people infected with the amebiasis will develop liver abscesses?	Approximately 5%
What are the indications for percutaneous drainage of amebic abscesses?	Abscess refractory to metronidazole Large, left liver–lobe abscess Bacterial contamination
When should large, left-lobe abscesses be drained?	When there is risk of rupture into the pericardium
What are the indications for surgical drainage?	Free rupture into the peritoneal cavity

HYDATID LIVER CYSTS

What is it?	Usually a right-lobe cyst filled with _Echinococcus_ (e.g., _Echinococcus granulosus_)
How rare are these cysts in the United States?	Only approximately 200 new cases are reported yearly!

What are the associated risks?	Travel, exposure to dogs
List the endemic countries.	Ireland, Scotland, Italy, Spain, Greece, Turkey/South America (below Mexico), New Zealand, Australia
Which farm animal is a carrier?	Sheep
Which diagnostic tests are indicated?	Indirect hemagglutination antibody test, history of travel, CT
What findings may appear on AXR?	Calcified outline of the cyst
What is the risk of surgical removal of cysts?	Rupture or leakage of the cyst contents into the abdomen; may cause a fatal **echinococcal (hydatid)** anaphylatic reaction
What is the appropriate treatment?	Surgical resection; large cysts are often drained after injection of a toxic substance into the cyst (hypertonic saline)
What are the possible parasitolytics for intraoperative injection?	Hypertonic saline (less common: formaldehyde, H_2O_2, iodine)
What is the appropriate medical adjuvant treatment?	Mebendazole or albendazole
What contraindicates intraoperative injection of a paracytolytic?	Communication of bile ducts with the cyst (i.e., cyst drains bile)
What is the appropriate treatment of cyst rupture and bile duct obstruction?	ERCP with papillotomy
What are the layers of a hydatid cyst (3)?	1. Host pericyst 2. Ectocyst (from parasite) 3. Endocyst (from parasite)

Which layers must be removed in the OR?	The endocyst and the ectocyst, because both layers may contain live parasites
What is the recurrence rate of postoperative hydatid cysts?	Approximately 20%

LIVER TUMORS

BENIGN

What are the primary benign liver tumors?	Hemangioma (most common) Hepatocellular **adenoma** (strongly associated with birth control pills and anabolic steroids) Focal nodular hyperplasia Infantile hemangioendothelioma—teratoma Angiomyolipoma Lipoma Hamartoma Mesothelioma Bile duct adenoma

Hepatocellular Adenoma

What is it?	A benign liver tumor
What is the histology?	Hepatocytes
What are the associated risk factors?	Women, birth control pills, anabolic steroids, type I or II glycogen storage disease
What are the associated signs/symptoms?	RUQ pain/mass
What are the possible complications?	Rupture with bleeding, necrosis
Which diagnostic tests are indicated?	CT, US
What is the appropriate treatment?	Discontinue birth control pills or steriods. If the tumor regresses, the patient should be observed. If the tumor does not regress, it should be resected.

Focal Nodular Hyperplasia

What is it?	A benign liver tumor similar to hepatocellular adenoma
What are the associated risk factors?	Women are at greater risk than men
Is this type of tumor associated with birth control pills?	Birth control pills are **not** associated with causing the lesion, but if oral contraceptives are discontinued, the lesion often shrinks
Which diagnostic tests are indicated?	US, CT
What pathognomonic sign appears on CT scan?	Central filling defect or "central scar" (think: **FNH** = **f**ocal **n**ecrosis)
What is the appropriate treatment?	Observation or resection, if the patient is **symptomatic**
Do focal nodular hyperplasias ever rupture?	No

Hepatic Hemangioma

What is it?	A benign vascular tumor of the liver
What is its claim to fame?	It is the most common benign liver tumor.
What are the two types of hepatic hemangioma?	1. Capillary hemangioma 2. Cavernous hemangioma
What is the significance of capillary liver hemangiomas?	Clinically insignificant

Cavernous Hemangioma

How common are cavernous hemangiomas?	Approximately 7% incidence (autopsy studies)
What percentage of cavernous hemangiomas are multiple?	Approximately 10%

What are the associated signs/symptoms?	Right upper quadrant pain/mass, shock, CHF
What are the possible complications?	Hemorrhage, congestive heart failure, coagulopathy
Which diagnostic tests are indicated?	CT with IV contrast
Should biopsy be performed?	No; there is a chance of severe hemorrhage with biopsy
What is the appropriate treatment?	Observation or resection, if the patient is symptomatic/hemorrhaging
What are the nonoperative treatment options?	Steroids Radiation

Bile Duct Adenoma

What is it?	Benign tumors less than 1 cm composed of bile ducts and fibrous material
What is the incidence?	Nearly one third of all people have these lesions!
What is the appropriate treatment?	Leave alone

MALIGNANT TUMORS

Hepatocellular Carcinoma

What is the incidence?	Most common primary malignant liver tumor (accounts for > 75% of all primary malignant tumors)
Which populations are at risk?	African and Asian
What are the associated risk factors?	Cirrhosis, hepatitis B, alcohol abuse, hemochromatosis, schistosomiasis, aflatoxin (fungi), α-1-antitrypsin deficiency

What are the associated signs/symptoms?	Dull right upper quadrant pain, hepatomegaly, abdominal mass, weight loss, paraneoplastic syndromes, weakness
What are the associated laboratory findings?	Elevated alpha-fetoprotein (AFP)
What is the most common site of metastasis?	Lungs
What is the appropriate treatment and what is the prognosis?	Surgically resectable; approximately 25% of patients live for five years
What percentage of patients who receive a liver transplant for hepatoma will have a recurrence?	Approximately 50%
What options are available for treating a solitary, small hepatoma in a patient who is not an operative candidate?	Ethanol injection under U/S guidance
Which subtype has the best prognosis?	Fibrolamellar hepatoma (young adults); not associated with AFP elevations

PORTAL HYPERTENSION

What level of portal pressure is normal?	Less than 10 mmHg
What level of portal pressure is associated with portal hypertension?	Greater than 18 mmHg
What is the most common cause of portal hypertension in the United States?	Cirrhosis
What is the most common cause of portal hypertension in the world?	Schistosomiasis

What are the classes of portal hypertension?	Presinusoidal Sinusoidal Postsinusoidal
Give examples of presinusoidal portal hypertension.	Schistosomiasis Portal vein thrombosis
Give an example of sinusoidal portal hypertension.	Cirrhosis
Give an example of postsinusoidal portal hypertension.	Budd-Chiari syndrome (most common cause of portal hypertension and upper GI bleed in children)
What percentage of patients with an acute variceal bleed will die?	Approximately 50%
What are the signs of portal hypertension?	Caput medusae Hemorrhoids Esophageal varices Ascites Splenomegaly
Name the veins involved with the retroperitoneal collateral route of portal blood flow.	Veins of Retzius
What is a major cause of isolated gastric varices?	Splenic vein thrombosis secondary to pancreatitis
What is the appropriate medical treatment of bleeding esophageal varices?	Vasopressin or somatostatin
What is a common long-term medical treatment of portal hypertension?	Propanolol
What must be administered to patients with a history of coronary heart disease who are taking vassopressin?	IV nitroglycerin

What is the first step in treating bleeding esophageal varices?	EGD and sclerotherapy
What percentage of patients with an acute variceal bleed will stop bleeding (at least temporarily) with EGD and sclerotherapy?	Approximately 90%
If these procedures fail, what steps should be taken next?	Balloon tamponade; sclerotherapy should be repeated
If rebleeding takes place after multiple sclerotherapy episodes, what steps should be taken next?	TIPS, Shunt procedure, or transplant

What is "TIPS"?

Transjugular intrahepatic portacaval shunt: a metalic shunt is placed from the hepatic vein to the right portal vein via a catheter introduced into the venous system through the internal jugular vein

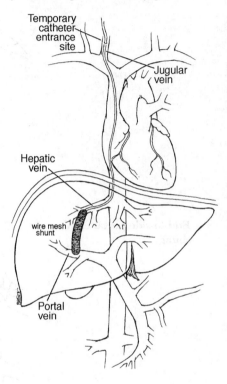

Which patients are good candidates for TIPS?

Those who will most likely undergo transplantation subsequently
Poor operative candidates

Which patients are good candidates for a shunt procedure?

Good operative candidates who are not good liver transplant candidates

Image the following
shunts:
   Mesocaval shunt "H"
   graft

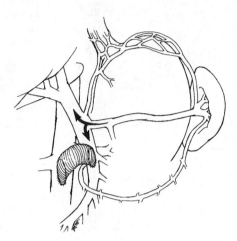

   End-to-side portal caval
   shunt

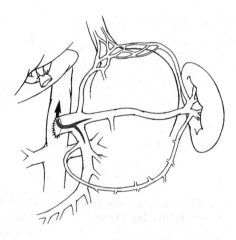

Side-to-side portocaval shunt

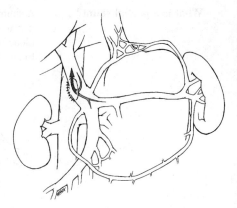

Warren distal splenorenal shunt

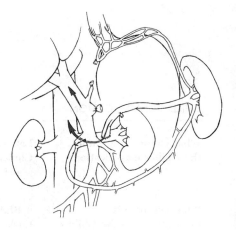

Which vein must be tied off with a distal splenorenal shunt?

The coronary vein

What is the advantage of a Warren distal splenorenal shunt?

Lower rate of encephalopathy

What are the relative contraindications for the Warren shunt?

Poorly controlled ascites (i.e., the warren shunt makes ascites), alcoholic cirrhosis

What is a partial shunt?

A shunt that does not shunt all of the portal blood (i.e., decrease variceal bleeding but allow some liver blood flow to avoid encephalopathy) as illustrated:

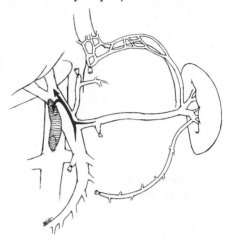

CHILD'S CLASSIFICATION

What factors determine the Child's classification?

Lab—bilirubin, albumin
Clinical—nutrition, encephalopathy, ascites

What acronym is associated with the Child's classes?

A BEAN—**A**lbumin, **B**ilirubin, **E**nchephalopathy, **A**scites, **N**utrition

Define Child's classification.

Table 35–1

	Bilirubin	Albumin	Nutrition	Encephalopathy	Ascites
A	<2	> 3.5	Excellent	None	None
B	2–3	3–3.5 controlled	Good	Minimal	Easily
C	>3	< 3 controlled	Poor	Severe	Poorly

(think: like a lettter grading system, A is better than B, B is better than C)

What is the operative mortality rate for venocaval shunt according to Child's classification:	
A?	Approximately 7%
B?	Less than 15%
C?	Approximately 33%
What is the Seqiura procedure?	Devascularization of the esophagus and splenectomy, selective vagotomy and pyloroplasty
What other tube do all patients recieving a Sengstaken-Blakemore balloon need?	Oral intubation, to protect the airway

LIVER FAILURE AND ASCITES

Why do patients with cirrhosis and portal hypertension have high aldosterone levels?	Low GFR and renal blood flow
Are sodium levels in the urine low or high?	Low
Why do patients with portal hypertension and ascites have a low GFR and decreased renal blood flow?	With portal hypertension, the splanchnic blood volume drastically increases and the intravascular volume decreases, resulting in decreased renal blood flow and decreased GFR.
What are the most common electrolyte abnormalities in patients with cirrhosis and ascites?	Hyponatremia Hypokalemia
What is the best way to prevent hyponatremia in patients with cirrhosis and ascites?	Limit H_2O intake, because total body sodium is normal or elevated.
How does spironolactone work?	It is an aldosterone antagonist agonist (sodium/H2O loss and potassium retention)

**What is a risk of
spironolactone therapy in
the patient with cirrhosis
and mild renal
dysfunction?**

Hepatorenal syndrome

MISCELLANEOUS LIVER FACTS

**What 5-year survival rate
is associated with
colorectal carcinoma
metastasis to the liver
without surgical resection?**

0% to 7%

**What 5-year survival rate
is associated with
colorectal liver metastasis
in patients who undergo
resection?**

Approximately 25% to 35% (with
negative margins)

**If a kidney from a patient
with hepatorenal
syndrome is transplanted
into a patient with normal
liver fuction, does the
kidney recover function?**

Yes

**If a patient with
hepatorenal syndrome
receives a liver transplant,
what happens to the
kidneys?**

They recover function.

**From what source do
metastatic tumors to the
liver receive their blood
supply?**

The vast majority receive their blood
from the hepatic artery

**What is the liver's
"favorite" amino acid for
gluconeogenesis (for
making glucose)?**

Alanine

**Which two serum tests are
most sensitive for liver
parenchyma damage?**

AST and ALT

What is the most sensitive and specific test for hepatocyte injury?	ALT
Which three tests are sensitive for bile duct damage or pathology?	1. Alkaline phosphatase 2. GGT **3. 5'nucleotidase**
What is the most common liver tumor?	Metastatic disease outnumbers primary tumors 20:1. The primary site is usually in the GI tract.
What is hemobilia?	Bleeding from the common bile duct
What are the signs/ symptoms of hemobilia?	Triad: 1. Right upper quadrant pain 2. Positive guaiac/upper GI bleed 3. Jaundice
What hepatic defect is associated with Dubin-Johnson syndrome?	Faulty excretion of conjugated bilirubin from the liver (think: **D**ubin = **D**epart defect)
What hepatic defect is associated with Crigler-Najjar syndrome?	Faulty conjugation of bilirubin (think: **C**rigler = **C**onjugation defect)
What hepatic defect is asssociated with Rotor syndrome?	Faulty excretion of conjugated bilirubin due to a defect in the storage of bilirubin (think: **R**otor = **R**elease defect)
Which vitamin should be administered to a patient with elevated protime and liver failure?	Vitamin K
What do the Denver and LeVeen shunts do?	Drain ascitic fluid from the peritoneal cavity to the central venous system
What dreaded complication is associated with the Denver and LeVeen shunts?	DIC (If refractory DIC occurs, the shunt must be emergently ligated!)
What type of amino acid should be limited in patients with liver failure?	The aromatic amino acids, because they are thought to be precursors of the false neurotransmitters involved with hepatic encephalopathy

Which amino acids are thought to be beneficial to patients with hepatic encephalopathy?

Branched amino acids (Leucine, Isoleucine, Valine; think: **LIV** = **LIV**er)

36

The Biliary Tract

John Pilcher, MD

BILIARY ANATOMY

What is the capacity of the gallbladder?	Approximately 50 ml
What are the valves of Heister?	The spiral folds of mucous membrane in the wall of the cystic duct
What is the function of the valves?	Unknown; it is believed that they prevent sudden distention of the cystic duct when the pressure in the gallbladder or cystic duct rises
What is Hartmann's pouch?	A sacculation of the neck of the gallbladder; common site for gallstones to lodge (also known as the infundibulum)
What are Rokitansky-Aschoff sinuses?	Branching evaginations from the lumen into the mucosa and muscularis of the gallbladder
What is their clinical significance?	They play a part in acute cholecystitis and gangrene of the gallbladder.
What causes these sinuses to form?	Increased intraluminal pressure in the gallbladder
Is the predominant blood supply to the bile ducts arterial or venous?	Arterial
Describe the anatomy of the arteries to the bile duct.	Two main vessels running axially at approximately three o'clock and nine o'clock Arise mainly from retroduodenal artery below, and right hepatic artery above Majority of the axial blood supply to the common bile duct is from below

Where does the lymphatic drainage of the gallbladder occur?	To the glands along the right side of the common bile duct, and then inferiorly to the head of the pancreas
What is the source of afferent innervation of the gallbladder?	Arises from spinal levels T5 through T11 The pain fibers travel with the splanchnic nerves, through the sympathetic ganglion, and then course with the sympathetic nerves to the target tissues.
What is the origin of sympathetic and parasympathetic nerves to the extrahepatic biliary system?	Arise from T7 through T10 spinal segments
What are the effects of vagal innervation on the gallbladder?	Excitatory (emptying), but this effect may not be clear cut
What is the effect of sympathetic stimulation on the gallbladder?	Predominantly inhibitory motor effect on the gallbladder
What is the effect of sympathetic stimulation on the sphincter of Oddi?	Excitatory

BILE METABOLISM/PHYSIOLOGY

What are the main chemical components of bile?	Water, electrolytes, bile salts, cholesterol, lecithin, bile pigments (bilirubin)
What does bile do?	Emulsifies fats
What is the volume of bile secreted per day?	Approximately 600 ml
What are the main sources of bile secretion?	Contributions from hepatocytes and from bile ductular cells: **Hepatocytes**—bile salt dependent (225 ml) plus bile salt independent (225 ml) **Bile ductular cells**—150 ml

What is the difference between bile salt–dependent and bile salt–independent flow?

Bile salt–dependent—secreted against a concentration gradient by energy-dependent active transport; water follows the osmotically active bile salts, causing a correlation between bile salt secretion and total bile flow
Bile salt–independent—deduced because of extrapolation to zero
Bile salt output leaves a component of bile salt flow, which is driven by active secretion of other osmotically active organic solutes, such as glutathione and bicarbonate.

From what substance are bile acids formed?

Cholesterol

What is the source of this substance?

Cholesterol is synthesized de novo in the liver, diet

What are the two primary bile acids?

Cholic acid and chenodeoxycholic acid

What are the two secondary bile acids?

Lithocholate and deoxycholate

What makes the secondary bile acids?

Bacterial action

What step do the primary bile acids undergo prior to secretion as bile salts?

They are conjugated in the liver with glycine or taurine.

What is a bile salt?

Conjugated bile acid at a neutral pH results in an ionic salt and thus a bile salt.

What weight of bile salt is formed daily to replace that which is lost in the feces?

0.5 gm

What is the total bile salt pool size?

2.5 gm

What is the enterohepatic circulation?

Secretion of bile salts into the gut, reabsorption, and return to the liver

In what part of the bowel are the bile salts reabsorbed?

In the **terminal ileum,** by active transport

What is the main bile pigment?

Bilirubin glucuronide

From what substance does it arise?

Eighty to eighty-five percent of bilirubin is derived from the catabolism of senescent red blood cells by the reticuloendothelial system (from heme).

Which enzymes participate in this conversion?

1. Heme oxygenase converts heme to biliverdin
2. Biliverdin reductase converts biliverdin to bilirubin

What is bilirubin conjugated to?

Glucuronic acid, by glucuronic transferase

What is the significance of urobilinogen in the urine?

Urobilinogen is produced in the terminal ileum from the breakdown of bilirubin glucuronide by bacterial action. Some of it is reabsorbed into the bloodstream. If urobilinogen is present in the urine (after being absorbed from the GI tract), then complete biliary obstruction must not be present.

What modifications does the gallbladder make to bile composition?

The composition of bile within the gallbladder is changed by absorption and/or secretion by the gallbladder mucosa:

Water and electrolytes are absorbed
Bile is acidified because of acid secretion
Mucus is secreted
Immunoglobulins are added to the gallbladder contents

What is the relative absorptive capacity of the gallbladder mucosa?

Greater than that of any other mucosal surface in the body

What are the primary stimuli for gallbladder contraction?

CCK
Vagal stimulation

What inhibits gallbladder emptying?

Somatostatin

Sympathetic stimulation (it is impossible to digest food and "flee" at the same time)

What are the effects of the female reproductive processes on gallbladder contraction?

Efficiency of gallbladder contraction is significantly reduced during the latter half of the menstrual cycle and in the last trimester of pregnancy.

What is the level of bilirubin at which clinical jaundice is usually evident?

Usually, 2.5 to 3.0 mg/dl

Classically, at what anatomic site is jaundice first clinically evident?

Under the tongue

What is the difference in jaundice associated with stone obstruction versus malignancy?

In patients with choledochal stones, jaundice often increases to moderate levels and tends to fluctuate, because stones rarely produce complete obliteration of the bile duct lumen.

In contrast, in patients with a tumor of the pancreatic head, jaundice progresses continuously until serum bilirubin levels reach approximately 20 to 25 mg/dl.

What is the approximate maximum bilirubin?

When urinary daily losses of bilirubin match bilirubin production, the intensity of jaundice stabilizes at a level of approximately 30 mg/dl.

What enzyme is found in the biliary endothelium?

Alkaline phosphatase

Are NSAIDs useful in treating cholecytitis?

NSAIDs may be particularly effective in treating the pain of acute cholecystitis; they block the prostaglandin-stimulated secretion of fluid into the gallbladder lumen, which occurs in the setting of cystic duct obstruction.

BILIARY IMAGING

What are the ultrasonographic signs of acute cholecystitis?

1. A positive sonographic Murphy's sign (pain upon pushing the ultrasound probe right over the gallbladder)

2. Thickened gallbladder wall (nl < 3 mm)
3. Pericholecystic fluid
4. Distended gallbladder
5. Gallstones (supportive data)

How often can US diagnose cholelithiasis?

More than 98% of the time

How often can US diagnose ductal dilatation?

More than 80% of the time

How often can US diagnose choledocholithiasis?

Only about one third of the time!

How often can US diagnose the cause of biliary obstruction?

Only about 50% of the time

What is distal obstruction versus proximal biliary obstruction?

Proximal bile ducts are in or near the liver and distal is near the duodenum

What are the differential diagnoses of proximal bile duct obstruction?

Cholangiocarcinoma, lymphadenopathy, metastatic tumor, gallbladder carcinoma, sclerosing cholangitis, gallstones, parasites, postsurgical stricture, liver tumor, benign bile duct tumor

What is the differential diagnosis of distal bile duct obstruction?

Gallstones, pancreatic carcinoma, pancreatitis, ampullary carcinoma, lymphadenopathy, pseudocyst, postsurgical stricture, ampulla of Vater dysfunction, lymphoma, benign bile duct tumor, parasites

What diagnostic tests are available to further evaluate dilatation of the CBD after it is diagnosed by U/S?

Percutaneous transhepatic cholangiography (PTC)
Endoscopic retrograde cholangiopancreatogapy (ERCP)

What diagnostic and therapeutic modalities are available from both of these tests?

Imaging of obstruction
Drainage of biliary system, including stents
Tissue diagnosis by brushing or biopsy

When should PTC be used versus ERCP?

Proximal obstruction—PTC; also better as intraoperative guide and as a stent across anastomosis

Possibly better as a long-term stent for palliation because of easier access to the stent for routine changes to prevent cholangitis

Distal obstruction—ERCP; allows visualization of the ampulla of Vater and papillotomy if appropriate (but also depends on local expertise)

What is the rate of cholangitis associated with PTC and ERCP?

PTC—4%
ERCP—3%

What is the rate of pancreatitis after ERCP?

Mild self-limiting pancreatitis occurs following approximately 3% of ERCPs; more severe life-threatening pancreatitis occurs after less than 0.1%.

What is the mechanism of action of iopanoic acid (used in oral cholecystogram)?

Iopanoic acid is administered orally and is readily absorbed into the bloodstream. The hepatic microsomes conjugate the iopanoic acid with glucuronic acid and it is excreted in this form into bile (this test is rarely used today).

What are the causes of failure of gallbladder opacification in oral cholecystogram?

Cystic duct obstruction (true positive)
Failure of absorption from the gut
Liver insufficiency

GALLSTONES

What is the incidence of cholelithiasis in the United States?

Approximately 10%

Which subpopulation in the United States is reputed to have a significantly higher rate of gallstone formation?

Pima Indians

What is the rate of symptoms in patients with gallstones?

Approximately 15% to 20%

How are gallstones classified?

Cholesterol stones (predominate in the United States)

Pigment stones, brown or black (predominate in Asia)

What percentage of all gallstones do the following classes comprise:
  Cholesterol?

Approximately 75%

  Black?

Approximately 20%

  Brown?

Approximately 5%

Which type of stone is most likely to be intrahepatic?

Approximately 95% of intrahepatic stones are pigment stones.

What are the steps in the formation of cholesterol gallstones?

1. Cholesterol saturation
2. Nucleation
3. Stone growth

What is Admirand's triangle?

A tricoordinate phase diagram describing the concentrations of bile salts, cholesterol, and lecithin (the main phospholipid)

What substances are implicated in the nucleation of cholesterol gallstones?

Calcium, gallbladder mucus

Which tumor is associated with gallstone formation?

Somatostatinoma

What factors predispose patients to pigment stone formation?

Hemolytic disorders
Cirrhosis
Biliary infections
Parasitic infection
Ileal resection
Long-term TPN

What is the mechanism of formation of pigment stones?

Unconjugated bilirubin precipitates to yield calcium bilirubinate and insoluble salts. Calcium bilirubinate is the main component in pigment stones.

What are the characteristics of "black" pigment stones?	Typically black and tarry Frequently associated with hemolysis or cirrhosis Almost always located in the gallbladder Almost never associated with infection
What are the characteristics of "brown" pigment stones?	Earthy, brown, friable Typically found in Asian patients Frequently associated with **infection** Primary common duct stones are almost invariably of this type
What is the mechanism of formation of "brown" pigment stones?	Stagnant bile with bacteria allows enzymatic hydrolysis of bilirubin glucuronide into free bilirubin and glucuronic acid. The free unconjugated bilirubin (insoluble) combines with calcium in the bile to produce a calcium bilirubinate matrix that is the predominant component of most pigment stones.
Which enzyme is involved in this process?	Bacterial b-glucuronidase
Which bacteria commonly produce this enzyme?	*E. coli* and *Klebsiella*
What common over-the-counter medicine decreases the rate of gallstone formation in animals?	Aspirin (inhibits gallbladder mucus secretion)
What is Mirizzi syndrome?	Impaction of a large gallstone in the cystic duct, with extrinsic obstruction of the adjacent CHD

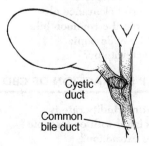

Cystic duct

Common bile duct

General Surgery

Which antibiotic is
associated with cholestatic
jaundice and gallbladder
sludge?

Ceftriaxone

CHOLECYSTECTOMY AND COMPLICATIONS

What complications are
specific to laparoscopy?

Gas embolism
Trochar injury
Respiratory and cardiac compromise

How does the mortality
rate associated with
cholecystectomy for acute
cholecystitis compare with
that of the same procedure
for uncomplicated
cholelithiasis?

Mortality rate is increased ten- to
twenty-fold in the setting of acute
cholecystitis

Is cholecystectomy
associated with colon
cancer?

Evidence in recent large studies suggests
not

CHOLEDOCHOLITHIASIS, PAPILLOTOMY/
SPHINCTEROPLASTY

What is the rate of
retained, residual, or
recurrent common bile
duct stones after
cholecystectomy?

One in twenty

What is the cause of
primary common duct
stones?

In the Western hemisphere, primary
common duct stones are usually a
consequence of biliary stasis and the
resulting colonization of the biliary tract
with enteric bacteria (e.g., *E. coli*)

What is the rate of
successful clearance of
stones in the common bile
duct by endoscopic
sphincterotomy?

Approximately 85%

ERCP EXTRACTION OF CBD STONES

What morbidity rate is
associated with endoscopic
stone extraction?

Approximately 5% to 10%

What is the associated mortality rate?	Approximately 1%
What specific complications are associated with this procedure?	GI hemorrhage Duodenal perforation Biliary sepsis Pancreatitis
What conditions prevent/ impair endoscopic stone extraction?	Prior Billroth II Stone size greater than 15 to 20 mm Large or tortuous ducts Small ducts compacted with stones

COMMON BILE DUCT EXPLORATION

What backup procedure can be used in the rare instance that a stone is impacted in the distal common duct and cannot be removed with transductal manipulation?	A transduodenal sphincterotomy
What is the correct orientation for incisions on the CBD?	Usually longitudinal (parallel to the blood supply)
Describe the ideal placement of a T-tube in biliary stone disease: the goal is to facilitate subsequent percutaneous stone extraction through tract if necessary.	Bring the stem out in a straight path to a point that is lateral and just inferior to the costal margin

GALLSTONE ILEUS

What is gallstone ileus?	Complete mechanical small bowel obstruction due to a gallstone impacted in the intestinal lumen.
How does it happen?	There is a required antecedent internal biliary fistula, which is located between the gallbladder and the proximal small intestine 95% of the time.

What is "tumbling obstruction" in gallstone ileus?	It occurs when bowel dilatation proximal to the obstructing stone releases the stone and allows it to impact further downstream.
How frequently is bowel obstruction caused by gallstone ileus?	It represents only 1% of all cases of intestinal obstruction.
In what age group is gallstone ileus a significant cause of bowel obstruction?	It accounts for 15% of simple complete obstruction in patients over the age of 70
What is the most common site of obstruction in gallstone ileus?	The terminal ileum
What are the radiographic features unique to gallstone ileus as a cause of bowel obstruction?	The diagnosis may be made by visualization of the radiopaque gallstone (approximately 15% of cases) or by air in the biliary tree (present in about 50% of cases of gallstone ileus).

BILIARY STRICTURES

What is the most common source of benign biliary strictures?	Iatrogenic (most are caused by surgeons in training)
What procedures precede postoperative benign strictures?	More than 90% result from cholecystectomies (an incidence of from 1/400 to 1/500 cases). Approximately 5% follow exploration of the biliary passages and are caused by undue handling of tissues. Partial or subtotal gastrectomy Pancreatoduodenectomy Liver resection for trauma
What are some noniatrogenic conditions causing biliary stricture?	Mirizzi syndrome Stricture or fistula in the common hepatic duct caused by inflammation associated with gall bladder calculi Radiotherapy (rare) Idiopathic

Describe the Bismuth classification of benign biliary strictures.

Grade I—stricture of CHD > 2 cm from confluence of left and right hepatic ducts
Grade II—stricture of CHD < 2 cm from confluence of left and right hepatic ducts
Grade III—stricture at confluence of left and right hepatic ducts
Grade IV—obliteration of all extrahepatic ducts by stricture

What is the success rate of biliary repair based on the Bismuth classification?

Bismuth grade I or II strictures—75% to 90% long-term success rate for repair
Bismuth grade III lesions—approximately 70% success rate
Bismuth grade IV lesions—50% of patients will have recurrent cholangitis on follow-up

Is there benefit in the use of external percutaneous transhepatic biliary drainage before surgery in cases of biliary obstruction with jaundice?

Preoperative drainage has failed to show benefit.

CHOLANGITIS

What percentage of acute cholecystitis is associated with gallstones?

Approximately 95%

What factors predispose patients to cholangitis?

Partial or complete biliary obstruction
Biliary stasis
Bacterial proliferation

What are the etiologies of cholangitis?

Common bile duct stone
Malignancy with obstruction or prostheses for drainage

Describe the bacteriologic features of normal bile.

Bile is normally sterile (but bile culture is positive in up to 16% of patients with no biliary pathology in some studies)

What is the rate of positive bile culture in patients with complete ductal obstruction, but no clinical sign of cholangitis?

Approximately 25% to 50%

What is the mechanism of biliary septicemia?

Arises from entry of organisms into systemic circulation = cholangiovenous reflux or cholangiolymphatic reflux.

What is the normal pressure in the biliary system?

7 to 14 cm H_2O

What is the biliary pressure at which cholangiovenous reflux occurs?

At duct pressure greater than 20 to 25 cm H_2O, which occurs in setting of obstruction

What condition leads to biliary hydrops ("white bile")?

Complete long-term obstruction of the cystic duct causes increased intraluminal pressure.
Biliary secretion stops when pressure is greater than 300 mm H_2O.

Which bacteria are associated with cholangitis?

E. coli (35%)
Enterococcus (16%)
Klebsiella (14%)
Proteus (12%)
Pseudomonas (9%)
Enterobacter (5%)

What is Charcot's triad?

Right upper quadrant pain, fever, jaundice

In what proportion of patients with cholangitis are these three conditions present?

Only 19%!

What is Reynold's pentad?

Abdominal pain, fever, jaundice, hypotension, delirium/mental status changes

What is the significance of its presence?

Usually indicates the more aggressive course of toxic cholangitis

What is the appropriate treatment of cholangitis?	Antibiotics Drainage Removal of infected hardware, if present
What is the recommended antibiotic therapy?	Antibiotics should cover a broad spectrum: usually a penicillin, an aminoglycoside, and an anaerobic agent.
What is the leading complication of cholangitis?	Renal failure
How does this complication affect mortality?	Three-fourths of patients who develop renal failure die.
What percentage of hepatic abscesses are caused by cholangitis?	Cholangitis accounts for about 50% of cases of hepatic abscess (highly lethal)
Are routine changes of biliary drainage catheters or endoprostheses beneficial?	The incidence of cholangitis may be reduced by the routine changing of these biliary catheters at approximately 3-month intervals.

ORIENTAL CHOLANGIOHEPATITIS

What is it?	Recurrent cholangitis, in association with recurrent formation of **primary** common duct stones
With what other disorders is it associated?	Parasitic infection: *Clonorchis sinensis, Ascaris lumbricoides, Trichuris trichiura* (Parasites may cause stasis, damage to bile ducts) Bacterial colonization with *E. coli* (produces b-glucuronidase, which causes deconjugation of bilirubin and the subsequent production of pigment stones)
What is the endemic area?	Asia
What is the appropriate therapy?	Choledochoenterostomy and antiparasitic medications

CHOLEDOCHAL CYSTS

What is the anatomic classification of choledochal cysts?

Type I—fusiform or saccular dilatation of the extrahepatic biliary tree (85% to 90%)

Type II—diverticular choledochal cyst

Type III—choledochocele, usually intraduodenal or intrapancreatic

Type IV—type I plus associated intrahepatic dilatation

Type V—segmental dilatation of the intrahepatic ducts only (Caroli's disease)

What is the usual clinical presentation of choledochal cysts?

Infantile—younger than 6 months at onset (indistinguishable from biliary atresia; usually marked by complete obstruction)

"Adult"—older than 6 months at onset, usually older than 2 years (marked by abdominal pain and jaundice; cholangitis may occur; pancreatitis is rare)

What is the risk of cancer secondary to choledochal cysts?

An estimated 10% to 15% of patients will progress to carcinoma if lesions are left in place.

Which gender/race groups are at increased risk for choledochal cysts?

Women and Asians

What causes choledochal cysts?

The majority of patients with the common form of choledochal cysts have an anomalous arrangement of the pancreaticobiliary ductal system in which the pancreatic duct enters the common duct at an abnormal angle proximal to the circular muscle of the ampulla of Vater. Reflux of pancreatic enzymes containing trypsin may flow upward into the common duct, with resulting damage to the ductal wall during intrauterine development.

What is the appropriate workup?

US; other useful tests include biliary nuclear studies, PTC, ERCP, and operative cholangiography

What is the appropriate therapy?	The current standard of management is **excision of the cyst**, with biliary drainage by Roux-en-Y hepaticojejunostomy.
What is the appropriate management of a choledochal cyst that is adherent to the portal vein?	If inflammation is severe and dissection away from the portal vein cannot be performed safely, an intramural resection can be done, leaving the outer wall of the cyst on the vein.

CAROLI'S DISEASE

What is it?	A type V choledochal cyst; congenital dilatation of the intrahepatic biliary ducts
What is the clinical presentation?	Often presents as recurrent cholangitis
Is surgical therapy recommended under any conditions?	Hepatic lobectomy is the therapy of choice if only one lobe of the liver is involved

BILE DUCT TUMORS

What are the most common sites of occurrence?	CBD ($\frac{1}{3}$ to $\frac{1}{2}$) CHD ($\frac{1}{3}$) Bifurcation ($\frac{1}{5}$) Cystic duct ($\frac{1}{20}$)
What is the survival rate?	Less than 10% five-year survival
What is a Klatskin tumor?	Adenocarcinoma at the **bifurcation** of the hepatic ducts
What is the most likely cell type of cholangiocarcinoma?	Adenocarcinoma (95%)
What conditions are strongly associated with cholangiocarcinoma?	Gallstones Sclerosing cholangitis Ulcerative colitis (not Crohn disease) Cystic abnormalities of the bile ducts Pancreatic reflux vs. bile stasis vs. stone formation vs. chronic inflammation Thorium dioxide retained in reticuloendothelial system for life; tends to cause more peripherally

located cholangiocarcinoma
Clonorchis sinensis (liver fluke)

What are the most common presenting symptoms?

Jaundice (90%); also pruritus, abdominal pain, weight loss
Cholangitis is uncommon, but arises frequently as a complication of manipulation.

What are the mainstays in workup and staging?

PTC or ERCP, depending on the level of the tumor and local expertise; also, occasional dynamic CT or angiography

When is it necessary to diagnosis tissue prior to an operation or resection?

Definitive diagnosis of malignancy is not required prior to resection, because such can be difficult or impossible to obtain. Incisional biopsies should be avoided in the OR because of the risk of spread of the tumor. Biliary drainage is necessary, regardless of the cause of biliary obstruction.

What is the operability rate?

Approximately 75% of patients are considered operable by preoperative staging.

What is the resectability rate?

Of patients who go to the OR with hopes of curative resection, approximately 40% get complete resection of gross disease.

What is the survival rate of those resected "for cure"?

Approximately 10%

What is the most common cause of death?

Cholangitis is the usual route of exit.

Is there any benefit to preoperative decompression prior to surgery?

Preoperative decompression of the biliary tree in cases of obstruction does **not** improve survival.

How effective is x-ray therapy or chemotherapy?

Cholangiocarcinoma is resistant to x-ray therapy; the only chemotherapeutic agent with a history of response is 5-FU.

What is the success rate of liver transplantation in the therapy of cholangiocarcinoma?	Less than 10% of patients who undergo liver transplantation for cholangiocarcinoma have disease-free survival up to 2 years.
What is the best technique for palliative drainage in unresectable cholangiocarcinoma?	Palliative drainage is achieved essentially equivalently by surgery (fewer returns for cholangitis or catheter maintenance) or endoprosthesis (out of the hospital sooner, fewer total hospital days).
What is "peripheral" cholangiocarcinoma?	Cholangiocarcinoma that occurs in the intrahepatic biliary system, near the periphery of the liver
What is the appropriate treatment?	Hepatic resection
What survival rate is associated with therapy?	Approximately 50% at 3 years

PERIAMPULLARY TUMORS

What is the definition?	Malignant tumors arising adjacent to or from the ampulla of Vater
What are the possible sites of origin?	Anatomically they may originate from: Distal pancreatic duct (40% to 60%) Ampulla itself (20% to 40%) Distal bile duct (10%) Duodenum (10%)
What are the most common cell types?	Adenocarcinoma is the most common cell type, but the cancer may arise from any cell type in the region.
Why are these grouped, despite these variations in anatomy and histology?	Because they have the same mode of presentation (jaundice) and the same operation (pancreatoduodenectomy) is performed for curative intent
How do periampullary tumors usually present?	Jaundice is the most common sign, occurring in 80% to 90% of patients; 75% of patients lose weight
What is the tumor marker for periampullary tumors?	CA 19–9 is the tumor marker with the best sensitivity and specificity (both close to 90%)

What is the operative mortality rate of pancreatoduodenectomy, past and present?	The operative mortality has decreased from 25% in older reports to 1% to 2% in most current series.
What is the survival rate after pancreatoduodenectomy performed "for cure"?	Five-year survival rate is dependent on cell type: Pancreatic (15% to 20%) Distal bile duct (40%) Duodenal (40%) Ampullary (50% to 70%)

GALLBLADDER TUMORS

What is the incidence of gallbladder cancer in comparison with cancer of the common bile duct?	Gallbladder cancer is about four times as common.
What is the rate of incidental presentation of gallbladder cancer?	Approximately 1% of all biliary tract operations
What proportion of all gallbladder cancer is discovered incidentally?	Approximately 20% to 30%
What are the symptoms of gallbladder cancer?	Pain, nausea/vomiting, weight loss, jaundice
How effective is US in diagnosing gallbladder cancer?	Approximately 75% of gallbladder cancers can be diagnosed by US, but approximately 50% of ultrasound diagnoses of gallbladder cancer are false positives.
What is the most common cell type?	Adenocarcinomas (85%), with the remainder composed of undifferentiated or squamous carcinoma
What percentage of patients with gallbladder cancer also have gallstones?	Approximately 75% of patients with gallbladder cancer have gallstones, although the cause and effect are not clear.

What is the rate of resectability at presentation?	The majority of patients present with advanced disease characterized by extensive local invasion and a low (25%) resectability rate.
What are the most frequent routes of spread?	Lymphatic (to nodes along the right side of common bile duct) and vascular (venous drainage is into segment IV of the liver); in addition to direct invasion, liver involvement by gallbladder carcinoma may occur by means of short veins that drain the gallbladder into the gallbladder bed or into the venous plexus around the common duct
What is the prognosis?	**Overall**—2% to 5% five-year survival rate **Asymptomatic tumors diagnosed by cholecystectomy**—approximately 15%–50% **Patients who undergo resection for a symptomatic tumor**—approximately 3% **Patients with unresectable disease**—3 to 6 months
What is the margin of resection?	Controversial; anatomic and pathologic facts support the wide excision of the gallbladder bed and lymph node dissection for the treatment of gallbladder cancer
What is the appropriate management of porcelain gallbladder?	Resection upon identification, because 25% to 75% of patients develop malignancy

HEMOBILIA

What are the causes?	Trauma, other disease, accidental tumors, blunt or penetrating trauma, operative/interventional aneurysms, gallstones, and inflammation
What is the appropriate workup?	Arteriography, which is often therapeutic by means of embolization

PRIMARY BILIARY CIRRHOSIS

What is the etiology/
histology?

An autoimmune disease causing
granulomatous destruction of the
medium-sized intrahepatic bile ducts

What is the final common
pathway?

The final event is an attack by cytotoxic
T cells on biliary epithelium. Suppressor
T cells are reduced in number and
function.

What is the usual
presentation/clinical
course?

Ductal destruction leads to cholestasis,
with later cirrhosis, portal hypertension,
and liver failure.

What are the associated
signs/symptoms?

Fatigue and pruritis (usually occur
    early)
Jaundice (usually occurs later; does not
    always correlate with the pruritis)
Xanthelasmas and xanthomas (appear
    as signs of chronic liver disease
    manifest)
**Evidence of an associated
    extrahepatic autoimmune disorder**,
    such as Sjögren syndrome or
    rheumatoid arthritis (incidence of up
    to 80%)

Is the disease more
common in men or
women?

Women account for 90% of cases, with
peak incidence between 40 and 50 years
of age.

What is the difference in
clinical course between
genders?

The clinical course is similar in men and
women.

What laboratory findings
are associated with the
disease?

Consistent with cholestasis;
antimitochondrial antibody is present in
95% of cases

Is medical therapy
effective?

No; a variety of immunosuppressive
drugs and penicillamine have proved
unsuccessful

What is the appropriate
surgical therapy?

Liver transplant; primary biliary cirrhosis
(PBC) is the most frequent indication
for transplantation in the cholestatic
group of patients

What is the risk of disease recurrence after transplantation?	Antimitochondrial antibodies persist after liver transplantation.

PRIMARY SCLEROSING CHOLANGITIS

What is it?	An inflammatory/ischemic disease of the bile ducts of unknown etiology
Is the disease more common in men or women?	It usually occurs in young men.
What other diseases is it associated with?	Inflammatory bowel disease, predominantly ulcerative colitis (70% of patients with primary sclerosing cholangitis have ulcerative colitis)
What are the most common initial symptoms of primary sclerosing cholangitis?	Jaundice, pruritis, and fatigue
What are the early physical findings?	Hepatomegaly and splenomegaly are common findings on initial physical examination.
What laboratory findings are associated with the disease?	Patients have a cholestatic biochemical profile. Serum markers of autoimmune disease, such as antimitochondrial or antinuclear antibodies, are usually absent.
What histologic characteristics are present?	Periductal fibrosis, pericholangitis, focal proliferation and obliteration of the bile ducts, copper deposition, and cholestasis
What are the effects on the liver and ducts?	Progressive bile duct obliteration leads to jaundice and recurrent cholangitis. If untreated, it will progress to cirrhosis with portal hypertension and/or hepatic failure.
What are the differential diagnoses?	Other processes that cause sclerosis of the bile ducts: AIDS (with viral or fungal superinfection) Intraarterial chemotherapy for colon metastases

Fistulization of hydatid cysts into the biliary tree with leakage of a scolecoidal agent (e.g., formaldehyde, hypertonic saline)

(Liver transplantation with hepatic artery thrombosis causes the same clinical, chemical, and radiologic picture)

What are the most important factors in the diagnosis?

Characteristic cholangiographic: diffuse, multifocal stricturing of the intrahepatic and/or extrahepatic ducts gives a "beaded" appearance

Is medical therapy effective?

No; copper chelation has been attempted because of the markedly elevated copper in the liver, and immune therapy has been attempted because of association with and similarity to autoimmune/inflammatory diseases. None of these methods has shown a symptomatic or survival benefit.

What is the appropriate surgical therapy?

Other than liver transplantation, surgery does not affect survival, but it can address biliary obstruction in focal extrahepatic disease as a temporizing measure.

Is colectomy useful in treating patients with ulcerative colitis?

The timing of colectomy does not alter the symptoms, progression, or course of the disease; most patients die of liver failure, variceal bleeding, or sepsis. Colectomy should therefore be performed only for symptoms related to colitis or cancer prevention.

Is the disease associated with an increased cancer risk?

Slight predisposition to cholangiocarcinoma

37

Pancreas

Thomas G. Gleason, MD
Lorne H. Blackbourne, MD

PANCREATIC EMBRYOLOGY

Within which pancreatic bud does the common bile duct form?	The ventral pancreatic bud
Which pancreatic bud migrates to fuse with the other bud?	The ventral bud migrates posteriorly to the left to fuse with the dorsal bud.
What does the ventral pancreatic bud form in the adult pancreas?	The uncinate process and the inferior aspect of the pancreatic head
What does the dorsal pancreatic bud form?	The superior aspect of the pancreatic head, the body and the tail of the pancreas
From which pancreatic bud does the small accessory pancreatic duct of Santorini form?	From the dorsal bud; the main duct of Wirsung forms from the entire ventral pancreatic duct, which fuses with the distal pancreatic duct of the dorsal bud
What abnormality arises if the ventral pancreatic bud migrates posteriorly and anteriorly to fuse with the dorsal pancreatic bud?	Annular Pancreas

ANATOMY

Name the parts of the pancreas.	Head (uncinate process), neck, body, and tail
On what structure does the pancreatic head rest?	The inferior vena cava (IVC), renal vessels

On what structure does the uncinate process (a prolongation of the pancreatic head) rest?	The aorta
What lies behind the pancreatic neck?	The superior mesenteric vessels
How is blood supplied to the head of the pancreas from the celiac axis?	The gastroduodenal artery branches into the **superior** posterior and anterior pancreaticoduodenal arteries.
How is blood supplied to the pancreatic head from the SMA?	The SMA branches into the **inferior** posterior and anterior branches of the pancreaticoduodenal arteries.
Which arteries supply the body and tail of the pancreas?	The dorsal pancreatic artery from the splenic artery branches and joins a branch from the SMA to form the inferior pancreatic artery. Multiple branches from the splenic artery, along with the inferior pancreatic artery, supply the tail.
Into which veins do the pancreatic veins drain?	The splenic vein and into the portal vein
Which nodal groups drain the pancreas?	From the head, nodes in the pancreaticoduodenal groove drain into subpyloric, portal, mesocolic, and aortocaval nodes. From the body and tail, retroperitoneal nodes in the splenic hilum drain into the celiac, mesocolic, mesenteric, or aortocaval nodes.

PANCREATIC PHYSIOLOGY

What do the islets of Langerhans produce?	**Insulin**—β-cells **Glucagon**—α-cells **Somatostatin**—δ-cells Pancreatic polypeptide, gastrin, and VIP
What types of cells comprise the exocrine pancreas?	Acinar, centroacinar, intercalated ductal, and ductal cells

Describe the composition of pancreatic secretions.	Clear, isotonic, pH = 8, sp. gr. = 1.007–1.035, concentration of HCO_3 = 30 - 120 mEq/L, Cl = 30–100 mEq/L, **Enzymes**—inactive forms of peptidases: trypsin, chymotrypsin, elastase, kallikrein, carboxypeptidase A and B **Other substances**—phospholipase, lipase, colipase, carboxylesterase, amylase, ribonuclease, deoxyribonuclease
What stimulates exocrine secretion?	Vagal efferents and secretin stimulate HCO_3 secretion; cholecystokinin and acetylcholine stimulate enzyme secretion.
What other GI hormone is structurally similar to cholecystokinin?	Gastrin, which may explain why it is a weak stimulator of pancreatic enzyme secretion
How are the peptidases activated?	Intraluminally by enterokinase

ACUTE PANCREATITIS

What percentage of acute pancreatitis is idiopathic?	Approximately 10%
Which commonly used medicines can cause pancreatitis?	Metronidazole, ranitidine, cimetidine, azathioprine, furosemide, acetaminophen, erythromycin, tetracycline
What are metabolic causes of pancreatitis?	Hyperlipidemia, hypercalcemia
What other surgical diseases may cause pancreatitis?	Perforating peptic ulcer Crohn disease of the duodenum
Which diagnostic GI test may cause pancreatitis?	ERCP
Which arachnid bite can cause pancreatitis?	Scorpion (found on some exotic islands, not in the United States)
Which worms cause obstructive pancreatitis?	*Ascaris, clonorchis sinensis*

Which enzyme, when activated, is thought to initiate many of the deleterious events associated with pancreatitis?	Trypsin
Which lipolytic enzyme causes pancreatic necrosis in the presence of bile?	Phospholipase A
Which enzyme is responsible for creating intrapancreatic hemorrhage?	Elastase
What causes fat necrosis in pancreatitis?	**Lipase,** especially in the presence of bile
What is the most important risk factor for severe necrotizing pancreatitis?	Obesity (more fat for the lipase)
What percentage of patients with cholelithiasis will develop gallstone pancreatitis?	Between 4% and 8%
What peritoneal tap findings are associated with severe necrotizing pancreatitis?	Dark brown, sterile, nonfoulsmelling fluid
Do NG tubes reduce the length of hospital stay or decrease pain in cases of acute pancreatitis?	No; they should be used as needed (vomiting/ileus)
Somatostatin has been shown to decrease pancreatic fistula output. Is it helpful in acute pancreatitis?	There is **no** evidence to show that it is helpful.
What is the cause of coagulopathy in pancreatitis?	Released proteases

What is the appropriate treatment?	Fresh frozen plasma as required
What is the proposed mechanism by which phopholipase A₂ causes pulmonary dysfunction during acute pancreatitis?	Digests pulmonary surfactant
What is the appropriate treatment?	Mechanical ventilation, as required
How is pancreatic necrosis diagnosed?	Abdominal CT scan: pancreatic tissue that does not enhance with IV contrast is necrotic.
What percentage of patients with necrotic pancreatic tissue eventually develop pancreatic infection?	Approximately 50%
What is the most common bacteria that infect the necrotic pancreatic tissue?	Gram-negative rods from the GI tract
What is the appropriate treatment of infected pancreatic tissue?	Surgical debridement, antibiotics
How do patients with acute pancreatitis present?	Epigastric pain and tenderness, often radiating to the back; abdominal distension; fever; tachycardia; jaundice (when associated with gallstone pancreatitis)
What are the most common causes?	Alcoholism, gallstones
When do Ranson's criteria play a role?	In the first 24 to 48 hours, they help stratify the severity and thus prognosis of the pancreatitis.

Table 37–1

Number of signs	Mortality
0–2	0%
3–4	15%
5–6	50%
7–8	100%

What tests aid in the diagnosis of acute pancreatitis?

Serum, peritoneal fluid and urinary amylase, serum lipase, WBC, T. bilirubin, liver function test, abdominal x-ray, US, CT

What is a sentinel loop?

An adynamic, dilated loop of small bowel associated with a **focal** area of inflammation initially described in relation to pancreatitis-associated ileus

When can patients with pancreatitis be fed?

Most surgeons agree that early PO feeding causes reactivation and thus is ill-advised.

Should antibiotics be used in the treatment of acute pancreatitis?

For mild, alcoholic pancreatitis they are probably not indicated unless there is documented infection; however, with necrotizing pancreatitis, studies have shown a decreased rate of both pancreatic and extrapancreatic infection with prophylactic use of antibiotics (imipenem/cilastatin).

How many patients with acute pancreatitis develop complications requiring surgery?

Approximately 10%

Does early use of mini-dose heparin prevent intravascular thrombosis during acute pancreatitis or alter the course of the pancreatitis?

Probably not

Does peritoneal lavage alter the clinical course of severe or necrotizing pancreatitis?

Controversial; a recent study showed that patients with five or more of Ranson's criteria had reduced incidence of sepsis and death with 7 days of early peritoneal lavage.

What are the indications for operative management (necrosectomy) of severe or necrotizing pancreatitis?

Unresponsiveness to aggressive ICU care beyond 3 days; sepsis; refractory shock; infected necrosis; greater than 50% pancreatic necrosis; bile duct stricture; bowel obstruction

Should sterile pancreatic necrosis be resected without other indications for surgery?	No
How should pancreatic abscesses be managed?	A well-circumscribed abscess should be drained percutaneously with radiographic guidance. Operative drainage should ensue if this procedure fails. If infected necrotic pancreas and/or septated collections are present, then operative debridement should be performed.
How should patients with severe pancreatitis be nourished?	Initially, most surgeons believe they should be supplied by TPN; however, once peristalsis returns, nasoenteric or enteric feeding tubes may offer better nutrition without worsening the pancreatitis (ideally, feeding beyond the ligament of Treitz).

GALLSTONE PANCREATITIS

What is it?	Pancreatitis and cholelithiasis, probably caused by the passage of a gallstone through the common bile duct
What are the theories that explain the causes of gallstone pancreatitis?	Bile reflux into the pancreas Reflux of duodenal succus from a loose sphincter of Oddi Stone blockage of the pancreatic duct
If surgically untreated, what percentage of patients with gallstone pancreatitis will have a recurrence within 8 weeks?	Approximately 33%
What other causes of pancreatitis must be ruled out in a patient with gallstones?	Alcohol abuse, medications, and hyperlipidemia, hypercalcemia

What is the appropriate treatment of mild gallstone pancreatitis (< 3 Ranson's criteria)?	Laparoscopic cholecystectomy and intraoperative cholangiogram on the third through the fifth hospital days, if the pancreatitis **resolves**

CHRONIC PANCREATITIS

What is the definition of chronic pancreatitis?	Recurrent bouts of acute pancreatitis with chronic pain and both exocrine and endocrine dysfunction; pathologically, irreversible parenchymal fibrosis occurs
What are the signs/symptoms of chronic pancreatitis?	Abdominal pain, diabetes, steatorrhea, pancreatic calcification
What anatomic pancreatic changes are associated with chronic pancreatitis?	Sclerosis with duct stenosis and dilatation; loss of acinar tissue
What is the most common cause of chronic pancreatitis in the United States?	Alcohol abuse (75% of cases)
What CT findings are associated with chronic pancreatitis?	Dilated pancreatic duct Calcifications Parenchymal atrophy (many patients also have pseudocysts)
What findings associated with chronic pancreatitis are evident on ERCP?	"Chain of lakes"
What is the most sensitive test for chronic pancreatitis?	ERCP
What factors indicate surgery for chronic pancreatitis?	There are probably no absolute indications other than for the complications of pancreatitis previously described; however, there are many relative indications: refractory, disabling pain, frequent recurrent acute exacerbations, possible presence of malignancy, GI or biliary obstruction, splenic vein thrombosis with portal hypertension

How are patients with chronic pancreatitis managed nonoperatively?

Treatment of pain, pancreatic exocrine replacement, and insulin therapy

What are the operative options?

Sphincteroplasty, for patients with proximal stenosis or pancreatic divisum

Retrograde drainage with distal resection and end-to-end pancreaticojejunostomy

Peustow procedure with side-to-side pancreaticojejunostomy

Distal or subtotal distal pancreatectomy for isolated distal disease (usually secondary to trauma)

Modified Whipple procedure (pylorus-preserving pancreaticoduodenectomy)

Resection of the pancreatic head with duodenal preservation and Roux-en-Y pancreaticojejunostomy

Total pancreatectomy, with or without pancreas transplantation

Splanchnicectomy or celiac ganglionectomy, for pain

PSEUDOCYSTS

What are pseudocysts?

Pancreatic juice enclosed by a false capsule of fibrous or granulation tissue that arises as a consequence of pancreatitis or trauma

What percentage of patients with acute pancreatitis form pseudocysts?

Approximately 20%

What percentage of patients with chronic pancreatitis develop pseudocysts?

Approximately one third (20%–40%)

What percentage of patients with acute pancreatitis develop persistent pseudocysts?

Only approximately 4%

What is the most common cause of pancreatic pseudocysts in children?

Trauma

What are the signs/ symptoms of pancreatic pseudocysts?

Persistant pain, persistent vomiting/ nausea, weight loss, abdominal mass, persistent amylase elevation, jaundice (bile duct obstruction), distention (bowel obstruction)

What percentage of patients with pseudocysts have persistent abdominal pain?

More than 90%

What percentage of patients with pseudocysts have an abdominal mass?

Up to 50%

What is the appropriate treatment of an infected pseudocyst (pus in the pseudocyst, also known as a pancreatic abscess)?

External drainage

On average, how long does it take for a pseudocyst less than 4 cm to resolve?

Approximately 2 to 3 months

How should pancreatic pseudocysts be managed?

Wait 6 to 12 weeks from the onset of development or resolution of acute pancreatitis. If cysts are small (< 5 cm) or asymptomatic, they can be watched with serial US or CT. If cysts are large or symptomatic, internal drainage is preferred with cystojejunostomy, cystogastrostomy, or cystoduodenostomy. External drainage should be used in cases with gross infection. In all cases, a **biopsy** of the pseudocyst wall or involved tissue should be sent to confirm that there is no malignancy.

What complications can be associated with a pseudocyst?

Hemorrhage, infection, leak, gastric outlet obstruction, bile duct obstruction

What is the appropriate treatment of an unstable patient with hemorrhage into a pseudocyst?	Surgery
What is the appropriate treatment of a stable patient with hemorrhage into a pseudocyst?	Arteriogram with possible embolization

PANCREATIC FISTULAS

How are pancreatic pleural and peritoneal effusions managed?	Initially, they are treated nonoperatively with no oral feeding, repeated evacuation percutaneously, and TPN.
What defines a high-output pancreatic fistula?	More than 200 cc/day
How should pancreaticocutaneous fistulas be managed?	Initially by nonoperative modalities with TPN, electrolyte replacement, and skin care. **Octreotide** may help reduce output. Sinogram and ERCP will help define anatomy if operative closure becomes necessary. The majority of fistulas will close spontaneously. Refractory distal duct fistulas are best managed by distal pancreatectomy, proximal duct fistulas with pancreaticojejunostomy.
What side effect is associated with somatostatin?	Gallstones and gallbladder sludge

PANCREATIC DIVISUM

How does pancreas divisum occur?	The primordial ductal systems do not fuse.

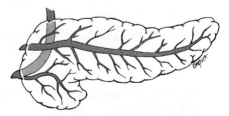

What percentage of the population has pancreatic divisum?	Approximately 6% to 10%
What percentage of patients undergoing ERCP for idiopathic pancreatitis has pancreatic divisum?	Up to 50%

PANCREATIC CARCINOMA

What is it?	A malignant tumor arising in the exocrine portion of the pancreas
What is the incidence?	In 1994, 27,000 new cases, or 9/100,000
What is the ratio of women to men?	1.0:1.3
In what ethnic group and in what city is the highest incidence of pancreatic cancer in the United States found?	Koreans in Los Angeles (16/100,000)
What are the associated risk factors?	Advanced age and smoking Diabetes mellitus (especially in women) Heavy alcohol use Exposure to the chemicals benzidine and B-naphthylamine (possibly) Partial gastrectomy (possibly)
What is the most common type?	Over 90% are adenocarcinomas; other types include cystadenocarcinoma and acinar cell carcinoma.
What is the most common location?	Two thirds arise in the head of the pancreas and one third arise in the body and tail.
What are the signs/symptoms?	Pain, weight loss, nausea, anorexia, and painless jaundice (if the tumor is in the head of the pancreas)
What are the associated tumor markers?	Ca-19–9, Ca-50

Which diagnostic test is indicated?	CT scan
Which diagnostic tests should be considered for patients with jaundice?	US ERCP, with or without brushings for cytology or biopsy CT
Why is tissue diagnosis important, even in advanced cases?	Because differential diagnoses include lymphoma, sarcoidosis, tuberculosis, choledocholithiasis, pancreatitis, etc.
What is the disadvantage of percutaneous fine needle aspiration (FNA)?	Potential needle-tract seeding ot peritoneal seeding
When should tissue diagnosis of potentially resectable tumors be performed?	In the OR (FNA)
Which patients are the best candidates for percutaneous needle biopsy of a periampullary tumor?	Nonoperative candidates
Which primary tumor location is associated with the most major vessel tumor involvement?	Head of the pancreas
What is the value of preoperative A-gram?	May determine vascular involvement, defines vascular anatomic variants
What are the most common sites of metastasis?	Liver, peritoneum (laparoscopy is helpful)
What factors contraindicate resection in pancreatic cancer?	Liver metastases Peritoneal metastases Periaortic node metastases Celiac node metastases Tumor involvement of the SMA, SMV

If lymph nodes in the planned resection specimen are positive for a tumor, is the patient's tumor unresectable?

No; the goal should be cure

How does the surgeon determine if the SMA is involved?

Kocher maneuver, **then:**
If the hand cannot identify a normal tissue plane between the pancreas and the SMA

What intraoperative maneuvers simplify visualization of the portal vein?

Cholecystectomy
Transection of the common hepatic duct

What is the appropriate treatment of distal pancreatic cancer?

Distal pancreatectomy with splenectomy

What is the appropriate treatment of cancer of the head of the pancreas?

Whipple procedure, if resectable

What is a treatment option of unresectable pancreatic cancer?

Radiation therapy and 5-fluorouracil

What is an option for postoperative adjuvant treatment?

5-fluorouracil and radiation therapy have been shown to improve survival.

Is the pylorus-preserving Whipple procedure associated with any survival disadvantage?

No

What is the current operative mortality rate associated with a Whipple procedure?

Less than 3% (1%–10%)

What is the most common postoperative complication after a Whipple procedure?

Delayed gastric emptying (33%)

What is the appropriate treatment of delayed gastric emptying?	Often responds to metoclopramide
What percentage of patients develop a postoperative pancreatic fistula?	Up to 20%
What is the appropriate treatment of a pancreatic fistula?	Controlled drainage, with or without somatostatin
What potential complications are associated with standard Whipple procedure?	Gastric delayed emptying (1/3) Pancreatic fistula (1/5) Abscess (1/10) Wound infection (1/12) Bile leak (1/20) Pancreatitis (1/20)
What is the prognosis for pancreatic cancer patients after resection?	Up to 20% are alive after 5 years
What are the most important postresection prognostic factors?	Positive lymph nodes **Need for blood transfusions** Clear margins Vascular invasion by histology

OTHER PANCREATIC TUMORS

Name the various endocrine tumors of the pancreas.	Insulinoma, glucagonoma, VIPoma, somatostatinoma, gastrinoma; also, tumors secreting pancreatic polypeptide, calcitonin, and neurotensin
Which of the pancreatic endocrine tumors is most common?	Insulinoma
How do insulinomas classically manifest?	Whipple's triad: fasting blood sugar less than 50 mg, symptoms of hypoglycemia when fasting, symptomatic relief following glucose replacement

How is insulinoma diagnosed?	Monitored 72-hour fast with blood glucose and insulin levels, insulin/glucose ratio greater than 0.4, elevated C-protein and proinsulin
Should an imaging study be performed with a presumed pancreatic endocrine tumor?	Yes, CT with contrast often helps localize the tumor
Where are insulinomas located?	Head ($\frac{1}{3}$) Body ($\frac{1}{3}$) Tail ($\frac{1}{3}$)
How should insulinomas be treated?	Resection: enucleation for small lesions, distal pancreatectomy for large lesions
What is the role of diazoxide for patients with unresectable disease?	It can attenuate hypoglycemia.
What is Zollinger-Ellison syndrome?	Peptic ulcers in unusual places, refractory hypersecretion of gastric acid, pancreatic endocrine tumor that secretes **gastrin** (gastrinoma)
Is there a hereditary factor associated with Zollinger-Ellison syndrome?	Yes, in some cases; although the majority of cases are sporadic, some cases are associated with the MEN I syndrome
How is a diagnosis of gastrinoma confirmed?	Secretin stimulation test
Where are they typically located?	The gastrinoma triangle: (1) the confluence of the cystic and common bile ducts, (2) the junction of the second and third portions of the duodenum, (3) the junction of the neck and body of the pancreas
What is their malignant potential?	Up to 60% are malignant at the time of diagnosis (in Zollinger-Ellison syndrome).
How should gastrinoma be treated?	If possible, resection with medical anti-acid production therapy (H_2 blockers or omeprazole)

How should gastrinomas be localized?	CT with contrast, intraoperative ultrasound, duodenotomy, somatostatin indium scan

What is Verner-Morrison syndrome?	WDHA syndrome:
	  Watery **D**iarrhea
	  Hypokalemia
	  Achlorhydria, associated with vasoactive intestinal peptide tumors, **VIPoma**

Where are VIPomas located?	Typically in the body and tail
Should VIPomas be resected?	Yes, although more than half of patients have metastases at diagnosis.
What action should be taken if no tumor is identified in a patient with watery diarrhea, hypokalemia, achlorhydria syndrome (WDHA)?	Occasionally, there is diffuse islet-cell hyperplasia, which can cause WDHA. In this case, subtotal pancreatectomy is an option.
What condition would a patient with diabetes and a migratory rash be likely to develop?	**Glucagonoma** is the characteristic necrolytic migratory erythema associated with this tumor. These patients may also have anemia, glossitis, and weight loss.
How is it diagnosed?	Elevated serum glucagon level
Where are these tumors usually found?	Body and tail
How should they be treated?	Resection for cure is possible in only one third of cases. Steroids, zinc, and octreotide have helped in treatment of the rash. Octreotide may also help control hyperglycemia.
What is a somatostatinoma and what is the appropriate treatment?	It is a very rare tumor, usually of the head of the pancreas, which may present with diabetes, steatorrhea, and gallstones. If possible, it should be treated by excision **with** cholecystectomy.

Are nonfunctional islet-cell tumors malignant?

Yes, in 90% of cases; however, they usually run an indolent course.

What is the most common benign neoplasm in the pancreas?

Cystadenoma

What is the most common cystic lesion of the pancreas?

Pancreatic pseudocyst

What is the appropriate management of cystic lesions of the pancreas that are incidentally found?

Tissue diagnosis must eventually be confirmed; it is impossible to distinguish malignancy radiographically. If the lesion is not associated with pancreatitis (i.e., not a pseudocyst) it should be resected.

How is pancreatic lymphoma diagnosed and treated?

Percutaneous radiographically guided needle biopsy with appropriate staging, followed by chemotherapy

38

The Breast

Paul J. Mosca, MD, PhD

ANATOMY/HISTOLOGY

What are the bony landmarks outlining the base of the normal female breast?

The second through the third rib to the sixth through the seventh rib; sternal edge to the anterior or midaxillary line

Name the two muscles that the breast directly overlies.

Two thirds of the breast are superficial to the **pectoralis major,** one third is superficial to the **serratus anterior.**

What are the three types of tissue in the breast?

1. Glandular epithelium
2. Fibrous stroma/supporting structures
3. Adipose tissue

List the tissue layers of the breast from the most superficial to the deepest.

Epidermis, dermis, superficial layer of the superficial fascia, Cooper's ligaments, glandular tissue, deep layer of superficial fascia, retromammary space, deep investing fascia, pectoralis major muscle

In what layer is the glandular tissue of the breast located?

Superficial fascia (within the "hypodermis")

When raising a skin flap, between which layers should dissection be performed?

In the bloodless plane located just subdermally; the final thickness of the flap should be approximately 4 mm at the edge and less than 6 mm at the base

What structure is responsible for the mobility of the breast, and between what layers of fascia is it located?

Retromammary bursa, formed by the deep layer of superficial fascia and deep investing fascia of the pectorales major muscle

What eponym refers to the mammary "tail"?

Axillary tail of Spence

What three primary arterial systems supply the breast?

1. Perforating branches of the internal mammary artery
2. Lateral branches of the posterior intercostal arteries
3. Branches from the axillary artery

What are the three routes of venous drainage of the breast?

1. Intercostal veins
2. Axillary vein
3. Internal mammary vein perforators

What is the name of the anastomotic venous network of the nipple?

Circulus venosus

What plexus probably mediates much of breast cancer metastasis to the skull, vertebral column, CNS, and pelvis?

Batson's vertebral plexus of veins: this network encircles the vertebrae from skull to sacrum and communicates with thoracic, abdominal, and pelvic viscera

What nerves provide sensory innervation to the breast?

Lateral and anterior cutaneous branches of intercostal nerves 2 through 6

Describe the three levels of lymph nodes and the group(s) included in each.

Level I—Lateral to the lateral border of the pectoralis minor muscle, including the external mammary, scapular, and some of the central axillary group nodes
Level II—Deep to the pectoralis minor muscle, including the remaining central axillary nodes
Level III—Subclavicular nodes **medial** to the pectoralis minor muscle

What are Rotter's nodes and where are they located?

Interpectoral nodes, located between the pectoralis major and minor muscles

Name the following nerves:

   Medial axilla, innervates the serratus anterior.

Long thoracic nerve (external respiratory nerve of Bell)

   Lateral axilla, innervates the lateral dorsi.

Thoracodorsal nerve

Lateral region of the pectoralis minor muscle, innervates the lowest third of this muscle.	Lateral pectoral nerve
Name the types of cells found in the lumen of a lactiferous duct.	Epithelial cells and myoepithelial cells
What are clusters of milk-forming glands, or acini, together with their ductules, called?	Lobules
How many lactiferous duct orifices are there on the nipple?	Approximately 15 to 20
At what stage of the menstrual cycle do breasts tend to be engorged and painful, and what additional clinical significance does this have?	Late luteal (i. e., premenstrual) phase; breasts may be rather nodular, possibly causing concern for malignancy
When collecting secretions via the nipple from a typical nonlactating breast, what components might be found?	Exfoliated ductal epithelial cells, as well as other cell types Substances such as α-lactalbumin immunoglobulins, lactose, cholesterol, steroids, and fatty acids
What exogenous substances might be found?	Ethanol, caffeine, nicotine, barbiturates, pesticides, technetium, etc.

PHYSIOLOGY

Which cells produce LH and FSH?	Basophilic cells of the anterior pituitary
Which cells produce prolactin (PRL)?	Acidophilic cells of the anterior pituitary
What hormone stimulates secretion of LH and FSH, and what is its anatomic origin?	Gonadotropic-releasing hormone (GnRH), from the hypothalamus

What is the primary regulatory hormone for GnRH, LH, and FSH release?	Positive and negative feedback by estrogen (E) and progesterone (P)

PRL SECRETION

What hormone primarily controls the secretion of prolactin?	Dopamine
What two other hormones also affect PRL levels?	Estrogen and TSH can promote secretion.
What is the role of each of the following hormones in mammary development:	
Estrogen?	Starts **ductal development,** up-regulates epithelial E and P receptors
Progesterone?	Involved in epithelial cell differentiation and **lobule development**
Prolactin?	Involved in the development of **mammary epithelial** and adipose tissue; up-regulates E receptors; synergizes with E in ductal development and with P in lobular development
What changes in the hypothalamic–pituitary axis are important for the onset of menarche?	Increased sensitivity to positive feedback of E; decreased sensitivity to negative feedback of E and P; increased GnRH; increased LH and FSH; increased E and P

PERIPARTUM FORMATION OF MILK

What role does prolactin have in this process?	Promotes differentiation of lactogenic cells and synthesis of milk
What other hormones are needed for these effects?	Insulin, growth hormone, epidermal growth factor, and cortisol
Would normal pubertal breast development occur in the absence of pituitary function, as long as estrogen is supplied?	No, probably because of a lack of ACTH and TSH

MILK "LET DOWN"

How does oxytocin affect this process?	Causes **contraction** of perialveolar myoepithelial cells
What is the anatomic origin of oxytocin?	Posterior pituitary
What stimuli cause release of oxytocin?	Stimulation of sensory nerve endings in nipple-areolar complex (e.g., suckling); anything that elicits the thought of nursing; vaginal stimulation
What are the two general classes of galactorrhea?	Those associated with hyperprolactinemia and those with normal prolactin levels
What is the most common setting for galactorrhea?	Idiopathic with nl PRL, especially persistent in postpartum lactation because of increased sensitivity of the breast to PRL

BENIGN BREAST CONDITIONS

What is the frequency of developing a palpable mammary cyst?	Approximately one woman in fifteen
Approximately what percentage of these cysts are multiple or recurrent?	Approximately 50%
What is the age range in which breast cysts are most common?	Between 35 and 55 (with regression after menopause)
Is the formation of carcinoma within breast cysts a common occurrence?	No; approximately 0.1% of cysts (1 in 1000 cysts)
Does the occurrence of cysts increase the risk of breast cancer in the case of small/microscopic cysts?	No

Does the occurrence of cysts increase the risk of breast cancer in the case of large cysts?	Controversial
What two organisms are most frequently isolated from nipple discharge in the inflamed breast?	*S. aureus* and *Streptococcus*
Which of these organisms tends to be particularly invasive, suppurative, and multilocular?	*S. aureus*
Describe three treatments of a breast abscess that might be used in succession if necessary.	Antibiotics; incision and drainage; excision of diseased ducts
What location is typical for a breast abscess?	Subareolar
Why might needle aspiration be ineffective for treatment of a breast abscess?	Breast abscesses are frequently loculated.
What are the signs and symptoms of mastitis?	Typically, there is tenderness and hyperemia, pus sometimes can be expressed from the nipple, and the patient may be febrile.
In what setting does mastitis usually occur and what organism is responsible?	During lactation/breast-feeding; typically caused by *S. aureus*.
What is the appropriate treatment of mastitis?	Discontinuation of breast-feeding; also, ice, heat and a breast pump have been used; antibiotics should be prescribed if infection persists
Why is careful follow-up for mastitis extremely important?	Because inflammatory carcinoma is a differential diagnosis

What important information should be obtained regarding the nature of a nipple discharge?

Uni- or bilateral?
Milky?
Coming from one or more than one duct?
Bloody or blood-streaked?

What type of discharge suggests an underlying malignancy?

Unilateral, bloody (or heme-positive) discharge coming from one duct

What is the likelihood that such a discharge indicates an underlying carcinoma (in the absence of a palpable mass)?

Cancer is found in only about 5% of cases.

What is the most common etiology of a spontaneous bloody nipple discharge?

Intraductal **papilloma**

Is breast pain frequently a symptom of breast cancer?

No, although it is a common complaint

ADOLESCENT PHYSIOLOGIC GYNECOMASTIA

What percentage of pubertal boys experience physiologic gynecomastia?

Approximately 66%

How long does regression take?

Approximately 1 to 2 years

NEONATAL GYNECOMASTIA

Is gynecomastia normal in the neonate?

Yes

What is the cause?

Maternal and placental estrogens

How long does resolution of neonatal gynecomastia require?

A few weeks

ADULT GYNECOMASTIA

Roughly what percentage of men experience gynecomastia at some point in their lives?

Approximately 50% to 66%

What is the likely etiology of this senescent gynecomastia?	It is probably caused by a relative increase in estrogen, as well as an increase in adipose tissue
Define gynecomastia in nonobese male patients at least 12 years old.	Condition in which at least 2 cm of glandular tissue can be pinched (> in density than adipose tissue of axillary folds)
Into what four groups are pathologic causes of gynecomastia classified?	1. Decreased testosterone (production/action) 2. Increased estrogen (production/action) 3. Drug-induced (e.g., cimetidine, spironolactone, marijuana, etc.) 4. Idiopathic
What is the first critical judgment that should be made in the workup of a man with a breast mass or breast enlargement?	If there is reason on physical examination to suspect cancer
What is the only setting of gynecomastia that clearly has been shown to increase a man's risk of breast cancer?	Klinefelter syndrome (47, XXY)
What percentage of American women will eventually be diagnosed with breast cancer in their lifetimes?	Approximately 10%
What percentage of American women will die of breast cancer?	Approximately 4%
What are the odds of a 30-year-old woman developing breast cancer over her next decade of life?	Less than 1 in 200
What are the odds at age 40?	Approximately 1 in 60

What are the odds at age 50?	Approximately 1 in 40
In what age range is breast cancer the leading cause of death in women?	Between 40 and 55 years
What percentage of all breast cancers occur in men?	Approximately 1%
What percentage of all cancers in men does breast cancer comprise?	Approximately 0.2%
In what areas of the world is the incidence of breast cancer lower than that of the United States?	In economically poor areas and the Far East, presumably because of dietary and other environmental factors
How does the incidence in Japan compare with that of the United States?	It is approximately 20% of the incidence in the United States.
In the following regions, is the incidence of breast cancer increasing or decreasing?	
The United States	Increasing
Regions of lower incidence	Increasing
What is at least partly responsible for the rapid rate of increase in the incidence of breast cancer during the 1980s?	Screening mammography
What is relative risk?	Ratio of [risk of disease in the presence of some characteristic] to [risk in the absence of the characteristic]
What relative risk of breast cancer is associated with the following factors:	
Family history of a mother with breast cancer less than 60 years old?	2

Family history of two first-degree relatives (i. e., mother or sister) with breast cancer?	5
Age of menarche less than 15 versus 16 years old?	1.3
Nulliparous versus age at first childbirth less than 20 years old?	2
Menopause past 55 years versus 45 to 54 years?	1.5
Atypical hyperplasia versus never biopsied?	4

Is a strong genetic predisposition to breast and ovarian cancer linked to a specific chromosomal locus?

It appears that there may be such a "breast-ovarian cancer gene" on 17q (BRCA1).

What percentage of breast biopsies without cancer show atypical hyperplasia?

Approximately 5% to 10%

What is the lifetime risk of breast cancer for a woman who tells you her sister had the disease in both breasts prior to age 50?

Greater than 50%

By approximately how much does screening probably reduce overall mortality?

25%

What age group clearly benefits from screening?

Between 50 and 69 years (40–49 year old patients possibly benefit too, but the issue is controversial and under study)

What age group tends to be least compliant with undergoing screening mammography?

Patients over 50

What screening guidelines are generally recommended for the early detection of breast cancer?

Physical examinations annually past 35 years of age

Baseline mammogram between 35 and 40 years, mammograms every 1 to 2 years after 40 and then annually over the age of 50 (although note that guidelines for mammographic screening of those < 50 are the subject of current controversy)

MAMMOGRAMS

What type of mass is likely to be missed, and in what kind of breast?

Large, noncalcified lesions in radiographically dense breasts (common in pre-menopausal women)

What percentage of palpable masses are missed by mammography?

Approximately 5% to 15%

For the mammographic diagnosis of breast cancer, what is the:
   Sensitivity?

Greater than 90%

   Specificity?

Greater than 90%

   Positive predictive value?

between 10% and 40%

How many more cancers are likely to be detected if mammograms are "double-read" (read by two different radiologists)?

Approximately 15%

What percentage of breast cancers are detected by mammograms as a mass and/or cluster of calcifications?

Approximately 80%

Practically speaking, how big must a breast mass be to be detected mammographically?

5 mm (theoretically, as small as 2 mm)

Do breast cancers tend to be more or less radiodense than normal breast tissue?

Cancer is usually more radiodense

How often does a radiolucent lesion turn out to be cancer?

Rarely

What mammographic quality of a lesion is most highly suggestive of breast cancer?

An irregular or spicular margin

How frequently will a mass with a sharp margin be cancer?

Approximately 5% of cases

What percentage of breast cancers have mammographically detected calcifications?

As many as 50%

Roughly what percentage of clustered microcalcifications in the absence of a mass will ultimately prove to be cancer?

Up to 33%

From the 1989 to 1990 Mayo Clinic study, what were the radiographic findings that yielded cancer in more than 20% of cases of nonpalpable lesions (there were 7)?

1. Calcification, malignancies (~90%)
2. Irregular mass with calcification (~70%)
3. Structural distortion with calcification (~60%)
4. Structural distortion without calcification (~50%)
5. Irregular mass without calcification (~40%)
6. Asymmetry with calcification (~30%)
7. Calcification, "indeterminate" (~20%)

The mammographic report for a patient indicates that cancer cannot be excluded and biopsy is suggested. What should be done?

Most experts would advise biopsy, to be safe; other factors that might raise suspicion are:
Increasing size of mass
Indistinct margins
More than 5 microcalcifications/cm²
Recurrence of cyst after aspiration
Structural distortion

Any microcalcification in irradiated breast

What is presently touted as a cost-effective alternative to open surgical biopsy of a breast lesion?

Percutaneous large-core biopsy

BREAST CANCER STAGING

What does an "x" indicate?

Parameter cannot be assessed

What does an "O" indicate?

No evidence for that feature

What does Tis represent?

Carcinoma in situ or Paget disease of nipple with no other tumor

What are the key divisions in diameter that separate T1 through 3?

T1—less than 2 cm
T2—2 to 5 cm
T3—more than 5 cm

Define T4.

Invading chest wall and/or skin (any size) or inflammatory carcinoma

Define N1 through N3.

N1—ipsilateral; positive axillary nodes
N2—same as N1, but matted or fixed
N3—ipsilateral; positive internal mammary nodes

Define M1.

Distant metastases or **positive supraclavicular nodes.**

STAGES 0 THROUGH IV

What is stage IV?

M1 plus anything else

What is stage 0?

<Tis/N0

What is stage I?

T1/N0

What is stage IIIB?

The worst T (T4) with any N, or the worst N (N3) with any T (**think:** 3B = worst N or T). Now you can forget about T4 and N3!

What primarily separates stages II and III?	Once you've gotten up to **N2 or T3N1,** you are in stage III
What is the difference between IIA and IIB?	**IIA**—sum of T and N is less than or equal to 2 **IIB**—sum of T and N is 3 (**think:** IIB = 3) (Remember, no N2s in this stage)
What is stage IIIA?	N2 with any T, but add **T3N1**
Why is staging important?	It provides a framework for developing and choosing the optimal treatment of breast cancer patients, as well as for estimating prognosis.
Which staging factor most reliably predicts long-term survival?	Number of **pathologically** positive nodes (physical examination is not reliable prognostically)
What is the approximate 5-year survival rate for each of the following numbers of pathologically positive axillary nodes: **None?**	80%
1 to 3?	60%
More than 3?	30%
What is the most common distant site to which breast cancer metastasizes?	Bone metastases are present in approximately 50% of cases
What are some other common sites to which breast cancer metastasizes?	Lung (20%), pleura (15%), soft tissues (10%), and liver (10%)
What constitutes a reasonable approach to clinical staging?	Good history and physical examination Bilateral mammography Laboratory tests, including liver enzymes CXR Other radiologic tests, such as CT and bone scan, if indicated

NODAL METASTASES

What is the general sequence in which levels I through III become positive?

I - II - III

Which level is an ominous sign if positive?

III

What does the term invasive neoplasm mean?

The tumor cells penetrate the basement membrane, unlike the case of **noninvasive** biological characteristics of breast neoplasms.

What is the difference between the terms ductal carcinoma in situ (DCIS), intraductal carcinoma, and infiltrating ductal carcinoma.

DCIS and intraductal carcinoma are **identical.** Unlike these neoplasms, infiltrating ductal carcinoma is invasive.

How might DCIS be detected and what are the histopathologic features that allow for the detection of these lesions.

The avascular central region may undergo necrosis and **calcification,** which may be detected by **mammography.**
If **many ducts** are involved, a mass may be **palpable.**

What is lobular carcinoma in situ (LCIS)?

Noninvasive carcinoma that originates from the breast acini, as opposed to ducts

How is LCIS generally discovered and why?

It is found incidentally in specimens obtained during biopsy for other reasons, because it does not calcify and is never palpable.

What two pathologic types of breast cancer most frequently are found to be the predominant cell type in breast neoplasms (and roughly what percentage of all breast cancer do they comprise)?

1. **Infiltrating ductal carcinoma**— Approximately 80%
2. **Lobular carcinoma**—Approximately 10%

How do the 5- and 10-year survival rates for the various morphologic types of invasive cancers compare?	For both scirrhous and lobular cancer, only about 50% of patients live beyond 5 years and only 33% live beyond 10 years. For the other types, approximately 60% to 80% live beyond 5 years and 50% to 60% live beyond 10 years.
What staging factor seems to inversely correlate well with these survival statistics?	The percentage of patients with positive nodes correlates inversely with survival.
A patient has a palpable mass in her breast. Answer the following questions: **What action should be taken?**	Core biopsy, FNA, or open biopsy
What should be done if FNA biopsy is negative for malignancy?	Open biopsy (usually excisional), because the sensitivity of FNA is inadequate to rule out cancer
What should be done if the FNA is positive for malignancy?	A definitive operation for malignancy should be performed.
What if cystic fluid is obtained?	If bloody, open biopsy; if nonbloody, follow closely with exams, mammography, etc.
What if a dominant mass remains after aspiration of the cyst?	It must be treated as any other mass and biopsied, etc.
What if the cyst returns after drainage?	Repeat cyst aspiration. If it recurs, excision of the cyst should be performed.

BIOPSY INCISIONS

How should the incision for excisional biopsy of a subareolar mass be performed to produce an optimal cosmetic result?	Concentrically with respect to the areola (i. e., along Langer's line)

Should the incision for a peripheral lesion still be placed in a circumareolar location?

No; this location may expose more breast tissue to the tracking of tumor cells.

What is a radical mastectomy (RM)?

Resection of the breast/overlying skin and pectorales major and minor muscles and dissection of axillary node groups I through III

In what decade did the number of RMs performed decrease dramatically and the number of modified RMs (MRMs) sky-rocket?

The 1970s

In what rare cases might an RM still be performed today?

T2 through T4 lesions with gross invasion of the skin or pectoralis major muscle

Tumors close to the clavicle in patients who are not candidates for radiation therapy

Define the following terms and provide the standard indication (none is generally used in the case of metastatic disease):
Extended radical mastectomy

RM with removal of internal mammary vessels, nodes, underlying chest-wall soft tissue, and bony structures (e. g., sternocostal ends of ribs 2–4 or 2–5 plus ipsilateral edge of the sternum, associated intercostal muscles); used for patients at risk of internal mammary lymphatic involvement (central or medial lesions that are T3 or T4 or have axillary node involvement)

MRM

This procedure is similar to RM, except that the pectoralis major muscle is spared. The breast, nipple–areolar complex, and axillary nodes are removed en bloc. Generally, the pectoralis major muscle and level III nodes are also spared (Auchincloss method), although the pectoralis major fascia is removed. The pectoralis major muscle and level III nodes may be sacrificed, as well

	(Patey method). MRM is used for T1 or T2 tumors that are not fixed to the pectoralis major muscle.
Total (simple) mastectomy	Mastectomy, as in RM and MRM, but the pectoralis major muscle is not removed and axillary node dissection is not performed
Quadrantectomy	Removal of essentially the whole quadrant, along with skin and muscular fascia
Wide local excision (i. e., **lumpectomy, segmentectomy, tylectomy, tumorectomy**)	Removal of the tumor (only) with grossly (or by frozen section) tumor-free margins (typically at least 1 cm); used for stages I or II, provided breast size is adequate
How long should (closed) suction catheter drains be left in place?	Generally, until drainage is reduced to 30 to 40 ml/day
Define the following types of recurrence:	
Local	Regrowth of malignancy in ipsilateral– lateral breast, skin, chest wall, underlying muscles, and other associated soft tissues
Regional	Regrowth of malignancy in regional nodes (i. e., internal mammary, axillary, supraclavicular, and/or Rotter's)
Answer the following questions according to the National Surgical Adjuvant Breast and Bowel Project protocol B-04 (NSABP B-04), initiated in 1971:	
What were the three limbs of the (clinically) node negative group, and what were the differences in 10-year survival and recurrence rates?	RM versus total (simple) mastectomy with immediate axillary irradiation versus total mastectomy with delayed axillary dissection (only if eventually found to be enlarged) No difference in 10-year survival rate noted. The only difference noted was a 15% ten-year local recurrence rate for

delayed axillary dissection versus less than 10% for other types of dissection.

What were the two limbs of the node-positive group and what were the differences in 10-year survival and recurrence rates?

RM versus total mastectomy with axillary irradiation; no differences noted

After several randomized, prospective trials including NSABP B-06, what can be concluded about the differences in survival rates after MRM versus lumpectomy plus irradiation, versus lumpectomy alone?

There are no differences in survival rates. Lumpectomy alone, however, yields a higher local recurrence rate than the other two treatments.

What do these studies suggest about the biological characteristics of breast cancer that renders it a fatal disease for some patients, and what therapeutic approach must be used to address this problem?

What kills patients is **metastatic disease** that has developed, regardless of local treatment; thus, adjuvant systemic treatment is necessary in selected patients.

What are the surgical options generally offered to patients with stage I or II disease?

MRM or lumpectomy/radiation; all patients receive axillary dissection for staging

DCIS

What surgical options are generally offered to patients with DCIS?

Spectrum: segmentectomy, with or without irradiation for smallest tumors to simple mastectomy

What is the risk of eventual recurrence after simple mastectomy for DCIS, and what percentage of these tumors are invasive?

Approximately 3% recurrence, half of which are invasive

If untreated, what percentage of patients with DCIS would develop invasive cancer during the 20 years after diagnosis?	Between 30% and 50%, generally in the ipsilateral breast (i. e., it is thought to be a precursory lesion)

LCIS

What is it?	Lobular carcinoma in situ
What is the risk of invasive cancer after a patient is diagnosed with LCIS and what is the percentage risk in each breast?	Overall incidence of 30%, including approximately 15% in both ipsilateral and contralateral breasts
How valuable is local excision of LCIS?	Not valuable at all; the risk of cancer includes all breast tissue in **both** breasts
What are the management options for a patient with LCIS?	Close follow-up; bilateral total mastectomy is also an option, as well, especially in light of modern breast reconstruction technique, particularly in very young patients with a **strong** family history

RADIOTHERAPY

How long after surgery for breast cancer is radiotherapy initiated?	Between 2 and 3 weeks
What is adjuvant treatment?	Treatment given after surgery to enhance the likelihood of long-term survival
What is endocrine treatment?	Any treatment aimed at abolishing tumor cells by abrogating the trophic effect of sex hormones on breast cancer cells
What are the three types of endocrine treatment?	1. Ablative (e. g., oophorectomy) 2. Competitive (e. g., tamoxifen) 3. Inhibitory (e. g., LHRH analogues)

What is the "flare" reaction associated with endocrine treatment?

Approximately 5% to 10% of patients have increased symptoms associated with metastasis, such as pain, swelling, or erythema. Hypercalcemia associated with bone metastases may also occur. Flare may start within days to approximately one month after treatment is begun. Treatment should be continued, unless dangerous hypercalcemia occurs.

Overall, approximately what fraction of patients respond to endocrine therapy versus chemotherapy?

Endocrine therapy—one third
Chemotherapy—two thirds

What factors render a patient more likely to respond to endocrine therapy?

Tumor with E and/or P receptors
Disease-free survival at least 2 years
Metastasis only to bone, soft tissue
Postmenopausal or late premenopausal status
Prior response

What is the primary goal of treatment for metastatic breast cancer?

Palliation, although some studies have shown a modest (6 month) increase in median survival with chemotherapy

How should patients with metastatic disease be treated?

Chemotherapy (e. g., CMF, CAF, or experimental treatment)
Radiotherapy for selected metastasis (e. g., brain, bone), especially if the patient is symptomatic
Surgical reduction/fixation of pathologic fracture or impending fracture

Which patients with metastatic breast cancer should receive adjuvant chemotherapy?

Based on **risk of recurrence**; accepted indicators of increased risk are:
Positive axillary nodes
Large tumor size
High pathologic grade
E and P receptor negativity
Unfavorable histopathologic subtype

What group of patients with metastatic breast cancer should receive adjuvant chemotherapy regardless of the other prognostic factors?

Premenopausal patients with **positive** nodes

For what group of patients is tamoxifen the standard treatment?

Postmenopausal patients with positive nodes and positive receptors

What are the common side effects of tamoxifen?

Nausea, hot flashes, transient leukopenia, or thrombocytopenia

What has been learned about the effect of adjuvant therapy on survival in node breast cancer from: NSABP-13, NSABP-14, and the Early Breast Cancer Trialists' Collaborative (meta-analysis) Study?

Either chemotherapy or endocrine therapy (i. e., tamoxifen or oophorectomy) appears to increase disease-free and overall survival by 5% to 10% at 5 to 10 years in node-negative breast cancer patients.

Why shouldn't all women with breast cancer, regardless of how early, receive some form of adjuvant therapy?

The chemotherapeutic agents presently in use are too toxic to expose a large percentage of low-risk breast cancer patients to the risks of chemotherapy; thus, prognostic factors are important. For tamoxifen, the benefits may outweigh the long-term risks, but it is too early to be certain.

What agents comprise the chemotherapy combination CMF?

Cyclophosphamide
Methotrexate
5-Fluorouracil

What agents comprise the chemotherapy combination CAF?

Same as CMF, but adriamycin is used in place of methotrexate

What may be an advantage of CAF over CMF?

Adriamycin (doxorubicin) is associated with a better response rate in metastatic disease; half of studies show a 3- to 6-month increase in survival compared with CMF.

List the major side effects of the following chemotherapeutic drugs:
    Cyclophosphamide

Alopecia, GI toxicity (e. g., nausea and vomiting), **hemorrhagic cystitis**

    Methotrexate

Myelosuppression, GI toxicity (e. g., mucosal ulceration)

5-fluorouracil	GI toxicity (e. g., anorexia, nausea/vomiting/diarrhea, stomatitis, mucosal ulceration), myelosuppression; if given as a bolus injection, alopecia
Adriamycin	Myelosuppression, GI toxicity, alopecia, **cardiotoxicity** (acute, reversible, and chronic from as little as a 250 mg/m^2 cumulative dose)
What new mitotic spindle poison may be a promising new chemotherapeutic agent for breast cancer?	Taxol
What means of treating myelosuppression resulting from high-dose chemotherapeutic regimens is (still) currently being investigated?	Autologous bone marrow transplantation (ABMT) and G-CSF (neither have met with great success yet)

INFLAMMATORY BREAST CANCER (IBC)

On what three findings is the diagnosis of IBC generally based?	1. Erythema/warmth 2. Peau d'orange and skin ridging 3. Rapid onset (< 3 mos.), with or without pathologic findings
What is the median survival rate of patients with IBC?	Approximately 1.5 years
Currently, what appears to be the optimal treatment for IBC?	Combination therapy, including doxorubicin-containing chemotherapy with a subsequent "toilet" mastectomy and radiotherapy

ESTROGEN RECEPTOR (ER) AND PROGESTERONE RECEPTOR (PR) LEVELS EXPRESSED IN BREAST CANCERS

Is ER/PR positivity generally more common for breast cancers in pre- or postmenopausal women?	Postmenopausal women

Roughly what percentage of breast cancers are positive for both ERs and PRs?	About half (45% in premenopausal women, 65% in postmenopausal women)
Roughly what percentage of breast cancers are negative for both ERs and PRs?	Approximately 10% (15% in premenopausal women, 5% in postmenopausal women)
Give the approximate response rate to endocrine therapy in patients with the following ER and PR status:	
ER+ PR+	80%
ER+ PR–	35%
ER– PR+	45%
ER– PR–	10%

HER-2/NEU (C-ERB B2)

In what fraction of breast cancers is it amplified (and overexpressed)?	One third
To what receptor is it homologous?	The epidermal growth factor (EGF) receptor
What is its purported prognostic significance in breast cancer?	Overexpression correlates with **decreased** disease-free survival.

CATHEPSIN D

What is it?	Lysosomal protease secreted by estrogen-stimulated breast tumor cells
What process is it thought to facilitate in the natural history of breast cancer?	Metastasis
What is its purported prognostic significance?	Higher levels correlate with **decreased** disease-free and overall survival.

What oncogene is amplified (in genec-copy #) in 20% to 30% of breast cancers?

Myc

Why is this fact important?

Portends a poor prognosis.

TUMOR SUPPRESSOR GENES/PROTEINS

What tumor suppressor is (at least functionally) missing in about half of breast cancers?

p53

What does it normally do?

Prevents DNA replication if DNA damage is detected

Why is this function important?

It helps prevent widespread mutations/ rearrangements of genomes and, hence, transformation to malignancy.

What process that probably accounts for the high frequency of homozygous mutations in tumor-suppressor genes has served as a clue in the search for other such genes?

Loss of heterozygosity (LOH), as can occur by the "chance" gain of an extra mutated gene during nondisjunction and subsequent "chance" loss of the only normal (wild-type) copy left

What are five procedures for breast reconstruction?

1. Breast prosthesis
2. Expandable prosthesis
3. Lateral dorsi myocutaneous flap
4. Transverse rectus abdominis musculocutaneous (TRAM) flap
5. Gluteal musculocutaneous free flap

39

Endocrine

A Lucktong, MD
Brian Ferris, MD

THYROID

ANATOMY

Name the three arteries supplying the thyroid.

Superior thyroid artery
Inferior thyroid artery
Thyroid IMA–aortic arch (12% of the population)

Which veins provide drainage?

Superior, middle, and inferior thyroid veins

To what nodes does lymphatic drainage from the thyroid go?

Anterior and posterior triangle, tracheo-esophageal groove, antero- or paratracheal nodes of mediastinum

Which important nerves are located in this region?

Recurrent laryngeal nerve, superior laryngeal nerve (vagus nerve in carotid sheath)

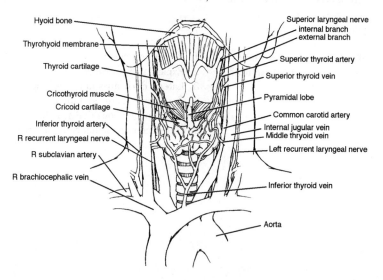

Hyoid bone
Thyrohyoid membrane
Thyroid cartilage
Cricothyroid muscle
Cricoid cartilage
Inferior thyroid artery
R recurrent laryngeal nerve
R subclavian artery
R brachiocephalic vein

Superior laryngeal nerve
  internal branch
  external branch
Superior thyroid artery
Superior thyroid vein
Pyramidal lobe
Common carotid artery
Internal jugular vein
Middle thyroid vein
Left recurrent laryngeal nerve
Inferior thyroid vein
Aorta

What is a nonrecurrent laryngeal nerve?

Variant in which the laryngeal nerve passes from the vagus directly into the larynx at the level of inferior horn of thyroid cartilage

How common are nonrecurrent laryngeal nerves?

1/200 cases

On what side is a nonrecurrent laryngeal nerve likely to be found?

Almost always on the **right** (can be seen with an aberrant right subclavian artery)

How common is the presence of the pyramidal lobe?

Common (75% of the population)

What is the ligament of Berry?

Posterior superior suspensory ligament of the thyroid directly adjacent to the cricoid cartilage on the posterior surface of the thyroid

What is the function of the superior laryngeal nerve?

Motor to the cricothyroid and sensory to the supraglottic pharynx

What structure is closely associated with the superior thyroid nerve?

Superior thyroid artery

To avoid damaging the superior laryngeal nerve, where should the superior thyroid artery be ligated?

The point at which the superior thyroid artery enters the thyroid gland

Describe the relationship of the posterior recurrent laryngeal nerve to the inferior thyroid artery.

Variable; nerve is inferior to the thyroid artery between the branches of the artery (7%); the nerve is superficial to the artery (20%)

Where is aberrant thyroid found?

Anywhere along the embryologic path of descent
Along the midline from the base of the tongue down into the mediastinum

What is the incidence of lingual thyroid?

1/3000

What is the usual presentation?

Dysphagia or problems speaking because of goiter enlargement

What is the appropriate management?	Suppression of TSH with thyroid replacement is often effective (glottic thyroid is usually **hypo**functional). Surgical removal, if the condition is obstructive and medical treatment is ineffective
What is a thyroglossal duct cyst?	Cystic remnant of the thyroid's embryologic downward migration
What are the most common presenting signs/ symptoms?	Solid or cystic, midline mass Can present at any age, but is most common in children May present with inflammation from infection
What is the appropriate management?	Radical excision including the hyoid bone and proximal duct extending to the base of the tongue (Sistrunk procedure)

PHYSIOLOGY

Outline the basic steps in thyroid and release.	1. Iodine uptake by synthesis in the GI tract and conversion to I^-; I^- concentrated by thyroid
	2. Peroxidases couple I^- to tyrosine residues on thyroglobulin, forming mono- and di-iodotyrosine, (MIT) and (DIT)

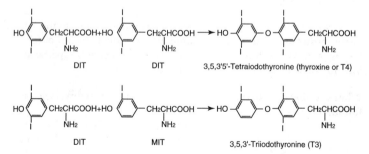

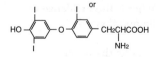

3,3'5'-Triiodothyronine (reverse T3)

3. Coupling of MIT and DIT forms T_3; DIT and DIT form T_4 (still attached to thyroglobulin)
4. Upon secretion, lysosomal enzymes cleave T_3 and T_4 from thyroglobulin.

What is Wolff-Chaikoff-White block?

The phenomenon in which iodine binding by thyroid and production of T_3 and T_4 are **inhibited** as plasma iodine levels **accumulate** beyond a critical level (~25 mic/100 ml)

Clinically, why is this relevant?

Iodine is the most effective means to rapidly decrease thyroid hormone levels (Lugol's solution, Na ipodate).

What is Lugol's solution?

Potassium iodide

What is the physiologic response to thyroid hormone?

Increase metabolic rate
Augment action of catecholamines

Which has more activity, T_3 or T_4?

T_3

Where is the majority of T_3 produced?

From **peripheral** conversion of T_4 to T_3 in the liver, heart, and kidney

Where is T_4 produced?

Thyroid gland (only source)

What do the parafollicular cells of the thyroid secrete?

Calcitonin, in response to increased serum Ca^{2+}

What does calcitonin do?

Inhibits osteoclast activity

What do osteoclasts do?

Resorb bone

What do osteoblasts do?

Form bone

What is reverse T_3 (rT_3)?

More inactive form of T_3 produced by the same enzyme that converts T_4 to T_3

When is rT_3 elevated?

Severe illness (e.g., sick euthyroid states)

What is a sick euthyroid state?

Change in thyroid hormone regulation resulting from severe illness, trauma, or stress

What is the appropriate treatment of sick euthyroid?

None indicated

THYROID FUNCTION TESTS

What does serum T_4 measure?

Total serum T_4

What does FT_4 measure?

Circulating, unbound T_4

In what situations is FT_4 useful?

It is the test of choice for following thyroid after treatment of hyperthyroidism.

What does resin T_3 uptake measure?

Relative levels of **thyroid-binding globulin** (TBG)

What does an elevated RT_3U indicate?

Hyperthyroid or decreased TBG

What does a decreased RT_3U indicate?

Hypothyroid or increased TBG

What are the differential diagnoses for increased ^{123}I uptake by the thyroid?

Graves disease, toxic nodular goiter, early Hashimoto nephrotic syndrome, pregnancy, iodine-deficient diet

What are the differential diagnoses for decreased ^{123}I uptake?

Subacute thyroiditis, thyroid gland damage (from surgery, radiation, thyroiditis), circulating iodine contrast dyes, ectopic thyroid, hypopituitarism, severe Graves disease

What test is the single most sensitive and specific indicator of thyroid function?

TSH

Name some causes of elevated TSH hypothyroidism.

1. **Severe illness** (17% of hospitalized adults have abnormal TSH on admission); in these cases, TSH levels are usually above 0.05 micro U/ml
2. Psychiatric illness, especially mania; elevated in 14% of patients with acute psychiatric admissions
3. **Dopamine** treatment; a short course of thyroxine may be required during treatment
4. **Acute glucocorticoid treatment** (normalizes with chronic use)
5. Delay in normalization of TSH following thyroid replacement dose adjustment; a minimum of 8 weeks must be allowed for TSH to accurately reflect new levels
6. **Pregnancy** and HCG-secreting trophoblastic tumors
7. Hypothalamic or pituitary tumors (very rare)

HYPERTHYROIDISM

What are the most common causes of hyperthyroidism (in descending order)?

1. **Graves disease**
2. Thyroiditis
3. Toxic multinodular goiter
4. Toxic thyroid adenoma
5. Exogenous hyperthyroid (includes iatrogenic, iodine-induced, and factitious causes)
6. Excess TSH (HCG-and TSH-secreting tumors)
7. Ectopic thyroid hormone production (struma ovarii, metastatic thyroid cancer)

Who is most likely to develop the disease?

Graves disease is more common in young women (7 to 1 women:men ratio)

What are the signs/ symptoms of hyperthyroidism?

Tachycardia (100%), goiter, nervousness, skin changes (warm, thin, and moist), tremor, increased sweating, **heat intolerance, palpitations**, fatigue, weight loss, dyspnea, eye signs, weakness, increased appetite, leg swelling, increased bowel frequency

What are the associated laboratory findings?	**Decreased TSH, elevated T_3 or T_4,** abnormal T_3-suppression and TRH-stimulation tests
What is apathetic hyperthyroidism?	Hyperthyroidism without adrenergic and hyperkinetic symptoms; commonly seen in elderly patients who may present with only cardiac failure or arrhythmias
What extrathyroidal manifestations are associated with Graves disease?	Exophthalmos, pretibial myxedema, periodic hypocalcemic paralysis, vitiligo
What are the treatment options for hyperthyroidism?	Antithyroid medication (PTU and methimazole) Radioiodine therapy Surgery
How do PTU and methimazole work?	Inhibit organification of I^- and coupling of iodotyrosines
In what way are their actions different?	PTU: Inhibition of T_4 to T_3 conversion in periphery
What is the incidence of side effects from PTU/ methimazole?	Less than 10%
What is the most potentially dangerous side effect of PTU/ methimazole?	Agranulocytosis (0.2%), marked by fever, diarrhea, or sore throat
What type of patient should receive radioiodine treatment?	Patients over 40 Patients who have poor surgical risk Patients who are unresponsive to drug therapy
In whom is this treatment contraindicated?	Pregnant women and children
Is radioiodine therapy associated with subsequent malignancies?	No significant association has been identified with leukemia, thyroid cancer, or congenital anomalies.

Is radioiodine therapy associated with benign lesions?	Yes; the incidence of benign thyroid tumors is **increased** following radioiodine therapy
What is the incidence of subsequent hypothyroidism following radioiodine therapy?	Approximately 70% of patients develop hypothyroidism within 10 years of treatment
How long is a patient at risk after therapy?	Risk persists **indefinitely** and rises approximately 3% each year
What are the indications for subtotal thyroidectomy for hyperthyroidism?	**Large goiter** or multinodular goiter with low radioiodine uptake **Nodule suspicious** for malignancy Treatment of **children** Treatment of **pregnant** patients or women who wish to become pregnant within 1 year **Noncompliance** with medical management
What is the appropriate preoperative preparation before thyroidectomy in patients with hyperthyroidism?	1. **PTU or methimazole** until the patient is euthyroid (usually 6–8 weeks) 2. β-blocker started concurrently with previously listed therapy to maintain a heart rate at 70 to 80 beats per minute 3. **Lugol's solution** or KI for 10 to 15 days in conjunction with antithyroid drugs to decrease friability and vascularity (begin only after the patient is euthyroid; otherwise, iodine may serve as a substrate for increased thyroid hormone production. Administer up until the day of surgery, then discontinue.)
What medicinal changes are recommended after thyroidectomy?	Discontinue PTU **Taper** β-blocker over 1 week to avoid rebound tachycardia

THYROIDITIS

ACUTE THYROIDITIS

What is it?	Inflammation of the thyroid gland, usually caused by bacterial infection (most uncommon form of thyroiditis)

What is the etiology?	**Suppurative infection,** usually arising from contiguous structures of thyroid; may be caused by hematogenous seeding local trauma (rare)
What is the most common cause of recurrent cases?	Piriform sinus fistula
Is the condition associated with hyperthyroidism?	No; usually TFTs are normal
What are the associated signs/symptoms?	Sudden-onset, diffuse, painful enlargement of thyroid with **fever, chills, and dysphagia**
What is the most common infection prior to acute thyroiditis?	Almost always follows upper respiratory infection in children and adolescents
What are the associated diagnostic findings?	Normal TFTs, normal radioiodine uptake Ultrasound may show abscess
What are the most common causative organisms?	*Streptococcus, Staphylococcus, Pneumococcus*
What is the appropriate treatment?	Surgical drainage and antibiotics Fistulectomy, if indicated Recovery usually occurs within 48 to 72 hours

SUBACUTE THYROIDITIS

What is another name for this disorder?	**De Quervain** thyroiditis
What is the etiology?	Viral
Who is most likely to develop this condition?	Adults 30 to 50 years of age; women are five times more likely than men
What are the associated signs/symptoms?	Diffuse enlargement, sore throat
Hyperthyroid or hypothyroid?	**Both**–transient hyperthyroid, followed by euthyroid, then hypothyroid

What are the associated laboratory findings?	Elevated ESR and serum γ-globulin; normal or elevated thyroid hormones; low radioiodine uptake
What is the appropriate treatment?	Self limiting within 2 to 6 months NSAIDS, β-blockade (antithyroid drugs are not effective in treating the hyperthyroid phase)

CHRONIC THYROIDITIS

What is another name for this disorder?	Hashimoto thyroiditis
What is the incidence?	Common (1.5/1000) Most common cause of goitrous hypothyroidism in adults
Who is most likely to develop this condition?	Women are ten times more likely than men; peak age occurs at 30 to 50 years
What is the etiology?	Autoimmune
What are the associated signs/symptoms?	Painless, diffusely enlarged gland, sometimes with nodularity; hypothyroidism
What are the associated diagnostic findings?	Increased serum antimicrosomal and thyroglobulin **antibody**; T_3 and T_4 may be within normal limits; decreased radioiodine uptake
What is the appropriate treatment?	Long-term thyroid hormone replacement

FIBROUS THYROIDITIS

What is another name for this disorder?	Reidel thyroiditis
What is the incidence?	Very rare
What is the pathophysiology?	Thyroid replaced by fibrous tissue; unknown etiology

What are the associated signs/symptoms?	**Stony** hard gland, with or without **invasion** into adjacent structures; pressure symptoms, hypothyroidism (differential diagnosis is malignancy)
What is the appropriate treatment?	Surgery, if pressure symptoms require relief Subtotal thyroidectomy may be required, although surgery may be difficult because of extensive fibrosis

POWER REVIEW: THYROIDITIS

What is another name for subacute thyroiditis?	De Quervain's thyroiditis
What is another name for chronic thyroiditis?	Hashimoto
What is another name for fibrous thyroiditis?	Reidel
What is the cause of acute thyroiditis?	Bacterial
What is the cause of subacute thyroiditis?	Viral
What is the cause of chronic thyroiditis?	Autoimmune
What is the cause of fibrous thyroiditis?	Unknown
Which type of thyroiditis is painless?	Hashimoto, often de Quervain
Which thyroiditis is associated with hyperthyroidism?	Subacute (de Quervain)
Which thyroiditis is associated with hypothyroidism?	Chronic (Hashimoto)
What are the major differences between acute and subacute thyroiditis?	Acute = Bacterial Subacute = Viral (Think: alphabetically A, B, and S, V)

THYROID GOITER AND NODULES

What is the etiology of goiter?

1. Environmental—iodine deficiency, drugs (e.g., lithium, amiodarone)
2. Immunologic
3. Genetic
4. Viral
5. Neoplastic

What are the associated signs/symptoms?

Usually a mass is noted, but otherwise the condition is asymptomatic; patients may have dysphagia, dyspnea, and/or impaired venous return

What is the appropriate management?

Usually thyroid replacement

What are the indications for surgery?

Large goiter with **airway compromise** (once obstructive symptoms occur, response to medical management is unlikely)
Cosmetic problems
Substernal goiter (rarely regresses with medical treatment)

What incision is commonly used for substernal goiter?

Cervical, in most cases

What is the most common cause of thyroid enlargement?

Multinodular goiter (present in 10% of the population; most patients are asymptomatic)

What are the differential diagnoses of thyroid nodule?

Adenoma ($\sim\frac{1}{3}$)
Carcinoma ($\sim\frac{1}{10}$)
Cyst
Multinodular goiter ($\sim\frac{1}{2}$)
Inflammatory thyroid disease
Developmental abnormalities

What is the etiology of multinodular goiter?

Adenomatous hyperplasia secondary to chronic TSH stimulation during hypothyroid states

What are the associated laboratory findings?

TFTs are usually within normal limits
Radioiodine uptake is variable in nodules

What is the appropriate treatment?	T$_4$ replacement or observation If large or obstructive symptoms are present, thyroid replacement and possibly surgery are indicated, especially if malignancy is a possible concern
What is the incidence of cancer in detectable nodules?	Approximately 5% to 15%

WORKUP OF THYROID NODULE

What does initial workup involve?	History and physical examination, thyroid panel, calcitonin (if medullary cancer is suspected), fine needle aspiration (FNA)
How accurate is FNA?	Approximately 70% to 97% (**varies** with the experience of the surgeon and cytopathologist)
What is the false-positive rate associated with FNA?	Approximately 6%
What is the false-negative rate associated with FNA?	Approximately 5%
What percentage of FNAs are positive?	Approximately 10%
What percentage of FNAs are negative?	Approximately 70%
What proportion of FNAs are indeterminate?	Approximately 20%
Of the indeterminate lesions, what percentage turn out to be malignant?	Approximately 20%
Is a radionuclide scan necessary as an initial test?	Usually **not**; does not reliably distinguish between malignant and benign nodules
When is a radionuclide scan most useful?	In patients with indeterminate cytology on FNA

How is radionuclide scanning useful?	Patients with indeterminate cytology and **hyper**functional nodules almost always have benign lesions
When is ultrasound useful?	Localizing nodules for biopsy Determining if nodules are solid, cystic, or mixed in composition (90% accuracy) Follow-up: distinguishes between nodular growth and intranodular bleeding (Many surgeons always perform ultrasound before FNA.)
When is surgery indicated?	Malignant lesions Indeterminate, hypofunctional lesions Local symptoms Neck disfigurement
What is the exception?	In patients with nodules from childhood radiation exposure, thyroxine after removal of the nodule decreases the recurrence rate $4\frac{1}{2}$ times
What is the appropriate nonsurgical treatment of benign nodules?	Observation and/or thyroxine treatment
How long should a patient be treated with thyroxine for a benign nodule?	For a 6-month trial; if nodule size decreases, treatment should be continued
What is the major risk of long-term thyroxine replacement?	Osteoporosis, especially in postmenopausal women
What is an indication for surgery in patients treated with thyroxine?	**Nodular growth** is a strong indication for surgery (associated with a high incidence of malignancy)

THYROID CARCINOMA

What are the risk factors for cancer in patients with a thyroid mass?	Male gender Extremes of **age** Rapid growth Local **invasion** (i.e., fixation, hoarseness) Exposure to external **radiation** (as little as 6.5 rads) **Hypofunctional** nodule

	Family history of papillary or medullary thyroid cancer Familial polyposis
Which diagnostic tests are indicated?	TSH (to rule out hyperthyroidism) Calcitonin (if medullary cancer is suspected) Needle aspiration Ultrasound (radionuclide scanning)
What are the differential diagnoses?	Lymphoma, sarcoma, metastases from kidney, breast, and lung cancer (all rare)
Name the type and relative incidence of all thyroid cancers?	Papillary (85%) Follicular (10%) Medullary (4%) Anaplastic (1%)
What are the treatment options?	Resection, with or without adjuvant therapy (e.g.,TSH suppression, postoperative radioiodine [I^{131}], and external beam radiation)

ADJUVANT THERAPY

POSTOPERATIVE RADIOIODINE, I^{131}

Which thyroid cancers concentrate I^{131} and often respond to this treatment?	Papillary and follicular carcinomas

EXTERNAL BEAM RADIATION (CONTROVERSIAL)

What are the relative indications?	Locally invasive follicular cancer Medullary cancer with nodal disease

THYROID SUPPRESSION TREATMENT (E.G., THYROXINE)

What type of tumor does this therapy benefit?	Well-differentiated carcinoma (recurrence and survival rates are improved with postoperative thyroxine)
What is the optimal dosage?	Controversial If tumor is completely removed, TSH should be suppressed to **low** normal levels If metastatic or invasive tumor is present, TSH levels should be suppressed to subnormal

PAPILLARY CARCINOMA

What type of patient is most likely to develop this disease?	Young adults and children Women over men Strongly associated with radiation in childhood **Occult,** up to 35% of autopsy and surgical specimens; generally not clinically significant
What is the route of metastasis?	Lymphatic
How often is this type of tumor multifocal?	Approximately 75% of cases
Is survival influenced by the presence of regional nodal metastasis?	No
Is survival influenced by distant metastasis?	Yes
What is the most common site of distant metastasis?	Lung
What is the prognosis?	**Twenty-year survival rate—90%** **Three-year survival rate with distant metastases—50% to 60%**
What factors indicate poor prognosis?	Extrathyroid extension Poorly differentiated histology Prolonged duration prior to treatment
What is the characteristic histology?	**Psammoma** bodies
What is a psammoma body?	Lamellar mineral deposits around a single necrotic cell
What is the appropriate treatment of papillary cancer?	Total thyroidectomy versus subtotal thyroidectomy (controversial); Postoperative I^{131}
When is total thyroidectomy absolutely indicated?	Extrathyroidal disease **Bilateral** disease

In the absence of extrathyroidal disease or obvious bilobar tumor, does total thyroidectomy result in survival benefit over subtotal thyroidectomy?	**No**, although it is associated with a lower incidence of recurrence
How much higher is the recurrence rate in subtotal versus total thyroidectomy?	Two times

FOLLICULAR ADENOCARCINOMA

Who gets it?	It peaks in the fifth and sixth decade; women are at greater risk than men.
What distinguishes follicular carcinoma from follicular adenoma?	Capsular or vascular invasion
Is FNA adequate for diagnosis?	**No**; intact architecture must be seen to detect the presence of an invasive tumor
What are the possible routes of metastasis?	Hematogenous (> 90%) Lymphatic involvement (< 10%)
What are the most common sites of metastasis?	Bone, brain, lung, and liver
What is the prognosis?	The 5-year survival rate is **60% to 90%**; studies are poorly controlled for the extent of the disease Influenced by **stage** and degree of peritumor **invasion** (locally invasive tumors are most aggressive) With moderate local invasion, the 5-year survival rate is 34% Skeletal metastasis can appear 10 to 20 years after resection of the primary tumor.
What is the usual treatment?	**Total** thyroidectomy is almost always indicated. Postoperative **radioiodine,** as previously described, reduces recurrence rate and is effective in treating metastasis.

Why is total thyroidectomy strongly recommended?	Survival is correlated with local recurrence.

HÜRTHLE CELL TUMOR

What is it?	A variant of follicular neoplasm
What are the treatment considerations?	**Controversial** Total thyroidectomy with node sampling and neck dissection, if malignant Hürthle cell tumor is found Lobectomy with close follow-up for benign-appearing lesions

MEDULLARY CARCINOMA

Where do these tumors originate?	C-cells (parafollicular) Neuroendocrine tissue
What is the serum tumor marker?	Calcitonin
What percentage of cases are sporadic?	Approximately 80% (fifth and sixth decade)
What percentage of cases are associated with MEN II?	Approximately 10% to 15% (second and third decade)
What percentage of sporadic cases are found to be familial?	Approximately 20%
What evidence is suggestive of MEN?	Usually is the first manifestation of MEN IIa and IIb Age at presentation is usually 20 to 40 years, versus 50 to 60 years for spontaneous cases Disease is multifocal
What screening is necessary for families in which MEN is suspected?	**Calcitonin** (basal or after provocative agent, i.e., pentagastrin); increases surgical curability by early detection
What are the characteristic symptoms?	Diarrhea (30%) caused by calcitonin, flushing, or Cushing syndrome(2%–4%)

What is the route of metastasis?	Lymphatic
Which nodes are the first to receive metastasis from medullary tumor?	Caudal pretracheal and paratracheal nodes, then cephalad to upper cervical nodes
What percentage of patients have positive nodal disease at the time of surgery?	Between 50% and 75%
What is the prognosis without nodal disease?	Five-year survival rate of 85%
What is the prognosis with nodal disease?	Five-year survival rate of 50%

What are the special treatment considerations?

1. **Total thyroidectomy** because of a high incidence of multifocal tumors
2. **Central neck dissection** at the time of resection; high incidence of nodal involvement
3. **External beam** radiation is sometimes considered (**controversial**)

What action should be taken if central neck dissection reveals more disease?	Full neck dissection
What is the characteristic histology?	Amyloid

ANAPLASTIC CARCINOMA

What type of patient is most likely to develop this disease?	Elderly patients(seventh or eighth decade) More common in areas of endemic goiter and in individuals with long-standing nodular goiter
What are the associated signs/symptoms?	Rapidly growing, sometimes painful mass; often present with cervical adenopathy

What are the treatment options?	Surgery, if possible for cure (usually it is too late at the time of presentation) Palliative combined chemotherapy/ external beam radiation Avoid tracheostomy (tumor often invades the tracheostomy site)
What is the prognosis?	Dismal (0% survival after 1 year)

POWER REVIEW: THYROID CANCER

Which type metastasizes hematogenously?	Follicular cancer
Which type secretes calcitonin?	Medullary
What is the most common type?	Papillary (85%)
What is the least common type?	Anaplastic (1%)
Which type has the best prognosis?	Papillary
Which type has the worst prognosis?	Anaplastic
Which type is associated with MEN II?	Medullary
Which types concentrate radioiodine?	Papillary and follicular
What is the characteristic histology of papillary cancer?	Psammoma bodies
What is the characteristic histology of medullary cancer?	Amyloid

SURGICAL COMPLICATIONS

POSTOPERATIVE HEMORRHAGE

What preventative steps should be taken?	Bloodless intraoperative field Reassess hemostasis following Valsalva maneuver prior to closure Closed-suction drain for the first 24 hours postoperative
What is the appropriate management of postoperative hematoma?	If the patient is in severe respiratory distress, open the wound at the bedside; otherwise, re-explore in the OR; if small, monitor and observe.

RECURRENT LARYNGEAL NERVE INJURY

What action should be taken preoperatively?	Assess nerve function and document any abnormalities
What is the risk of damage to the recurrent laryngeal nerve during thyroidectomy?	Less than 5%
What preventative steps should be taken?	Identify the nerve and its intraoperative course
What are the points at which risk of injury to the recurrent laryngeal nerve is greatest?	Dissection around the ligament of Berry Ligation of the inferior thyroid artery Dissection around the thoracic inlet
How can recurrent laryngeal nerve injury be diagnosed?	Postoperative laryngoscopy
What findings are associated with unilateral injury?	Cord on the affected side is in the paramedian position
What findings are associated with bilateral injury?	Both cords are in the midline position (airway compromise with stridor)

In cases of temporary paralysis, when should function be expected to return?	Within 6 to 8 weeks
If the nerve is obviously injured intraoperatively, should repair be attempted?	**Controversial;** repair is associated with less cord atrophy, but more cord adductor spasm because of random reinnervation

SUPERIOR LARYNGEAL NERVE INJURY

What are the associated signs/symptoms?	**Weak voice** with loss of projection, often unnoticed but potentially disastrous for singers and orators On examination, cord on affected side appears **flaccid**, with asymmetrical glottic aperture (Many surgeons evaluate cords preoperatively)
What preventative steps should be taken?	Ligation of the superior thyroid artery close to point of entrance into the thyroid gland

POSTOPERATIVE HYPOPARATHYROIDISM

What are the associated risk factors?	**Magnitude** of surgery (i.e., risk of total thyroidectomy is greater than that of isthmectomy) **Previous** thyroid surgery Surgery for large thyroid cancer with **lymphadenectomy**
What is the incidence?	Between 0.6% and 17% (depending on the experience of the surgeon)
What is the most common cause?	Devascularization of the parathyroid gland
What is the major source of blood supply to the parathyroids?	Inferior thyroid artery (80%)
How can postoperative hypoparathyroidism be prevented?	Avoid ligating the inferior thyroid artery at the main trunk. Ligate branches close to the thyroid gland.

THYROID STORM

What is thyroid storm?	Uncontrolled production and release of thyroid hormone **(medical emergency)**
What are the associated signs/symptoms?	Similar to those of hyperthyroidism but more accentuated; **fever,** cardiac failure, neuromuscular excitation, **delirium, jaundice**
What type of patients typically develop thyroid storm?	Undiagnosed or inadequately treated hyperthyroid patients who are undergoing major stress (e.g., surgery, medical illness, trauma)
What is the appropriate management?	1. ICU and fluids 2. β-blockers (short-acting) 3. PTU 4. Iodine (oral KI or IV NaI) 5. Antipyretics and/or cooling blanket (**not** aspirin, which displaces hormone from TBG) 6. Corticosteroids (**controversial**) 7. Treatment of underlying cause (e.g., infection, drugs, surgery, trauma)
Which drug is the only agent that prevents release of preformed stores of thyroid hormone?	Iodide
What other types of patients must be treated similarly?	Those with suspected or partially treated hyperthyroidism who require emergent nonthyroid surgery (risk of thyroid storm and cardiac arrhythmias)

ADRENALS

ANATOMY

What is the normal weight?	Approximately 4 g
What is the source of arterial supply?	**Variable**; usually from the inferior phrenic renal arteries and branches directly off of the aorta

Venous drainage

What is the venous course on the right side?	Anterior gland to the posterolateral **IVC**
What is the venous course on the left side?	Lower pole of the gland to the left **renal vein**
What embryologic tissue gives rise to the adrenal cortex?	Mesoderm
What are the three histologic layers of the adrenal cortex?	1. Zona **g**lomerulosa (think "salt") 2. Zona **f**asciculata (think "sugar") 3. Zona **r**eticularis (think "sex") (Think: GFR = salt, sugar, sex)
What is produced in the zona glomerulosa?	Mineralocorticoids (e.g., aldosterone) = "salt"
What is produced in the zona fasciculata?	Glucocorticoids = "sugar"
What is produced in the zona reticularis?	Androgens and estrogens = "sex"
What embryonic tissue gives rise to the adrenal medulla?	Neural crest
What is produced in the adrenal medulla?	Catecholamines
What are the most common sites for ectopic adrenal medullary tissue?	Sympathetic paraganglia along the aorta Mediastinum
What is the organ of Zuckerkandl?	Sympathetic paraganglia near the aortic bifurcation; common location for extra-adrenal pheochromocytoma.
What are the most common sites for extra-adrenal cortical tissue?	Ovary, testes, and kidney

GLUCOCORTICOIDS

Where are they produced?	Zona fasciculata

How are they regulated?	Adrenocorticotropic hormone (**ACTH**), from pituitary cortotropin-releasing factor

MINERALOCORTICOIDS

Where are they produced?	Zona glomerulosa
How do they act?	Increase renal **K⁺ and H⁺ secretion** Increase renal **Na⁺ reabsorption** Increase fluid volume Increase blood pressure
How are they regulated?	**Renin-angiotensin** system Release is also stimulated by high levels of ACTH
Where is renin produced?	Juxtaglomerular (JG) apparatus of the kidney
What is it produced in response to?	Decreased blood volume or osmolarity, manifested by: 1. Decreased renal perfusion pressure 2. Increased sympathetic stimulation 3. Decreased Na delivery to JG cells
What does renin do?	Cleaves angiotensinogen into angiotensin I
Where is angiotensin I converted into angiotensin II?	The lung
What does angiotensin II do?	1. Increases aldosterone secretion 2. Increases ADH secretion and stimulates thirst 3. Increases peripheral vasoconstriction

HYPERALDOSTERONISM

What are the possible etiologies?	Renovascular disease Adrenal **adenoma** Adrenal **hyperplasia** ACTH hypersecretion Adrenal carcinoma Ovarian tumor with ectopic aldosterone secretion

What is the classic diagnostic triad for hyperaldosteronism?

Hypertension, hypokalemia, low plasma renin

What are the other signs/ symptoms of hyperaldosteronism?

Weakness, cramps, polydipsia, polyuria
Marked hypokalemia (< 3.0 mEq/L) on K-wasting diuretics
Occasional carpopedal spasms and paresthesias caused by hypokalemic alkalosis

What is primary hyperaldosteronism?

Low renin hyperaldosteronism

What is secondary hyperaldosteronism?

Hyperaldosteronism secondary to high renin states (i.e., renovascular disease)

What percentage of hypertension is caused by primary hyperaldosteronism?

Approximately 1%

What proportion of untreated patients with both hypertension and hypokalemia have primary hyperaldosteronism?

Up to 40%

What tests are appropriate for initial evaluation of suspected primary hyperaldosteronism?

Serum K$^+$, urine K$^+$, plasma renin activity (PRA), plasma aldosterone concentration (PAC), captopril-suppression test

What is the most common cause of hypokalemia in hypertensive patients?

Diuretics

What proportion of patients with primary hyperaldosteronism have K$^+$ greater than 3.6 mEq/ L?

Up to 40%

What is the single best test for identifying primary hyperaldosteronism?

Twenty-four hour **urinary aldosterone** excretion following salt loading (> 14.0 micrograms/24 h); sensitivity 98%, specificity 96%

Which drugs can interfere with accurate renin and aldosterone values?

Spironolactone, ACE inhibitors, other diuretics, estrogens, prostaglandin synthase inhibitors, cyproheptadine, vasodilators, Ca$^+$ channel blockers

What are the two causes of hyperaldosteronism?

Adrenal **adenoma** (60%)
Primary adrenal **hyperplasia** (40%)

Why is primary hyperaldosteronism caused by hyperplasia less amenable to surgery?

Adrenal hyperplasia is usually **bilateral** (at least microscopically) making unilateral adrenalectomy ineffective.
Bilateral adrenalectomy has **high morbidity** of adrenal insufficiency, which is often more difficult to treat than hyperaldosteronism.

Once the diagnosis of primary hyperaldosteronism has been made, how can adenoma be differentiated from hyperplasia?

Imaging studies—Adenoma usually presents as a discrete unilateral adrenal mass, whereas in hyperplasia, adrenals may look normal or show bilateral nodularity
Posture study—Adenoma is less responsive to changes in angiotensin II levels, hyperplasia very sensitive to changes in angiotensin II levels that occur on standing
18-OHB levels—Adenoma generally has 18-OHB levels greater than 100 ng/dl
Dexamethasone suppression—Adenoma, unlike hyperplasia, is sensitive to ACTH; suppression of ACTH with dexamethasone, in a patient with adenoma, will return aldosterone levels to normal
Response to spironolactone—HTN caused by adenoma tends to respond better to spironolactone

What is 18-OHB?

18-hydroxycorticosterone, a precursor of aldosterone

What tests are used to localize the tumor?

CT and MRI
Dexamethasone suppression and NP-59 scintigraphy
Adrenal venous sampling, if other studies are nondiagnostic

What is the diagnostic accuracy of CT?	Approximately 70%
What size is the smallest detectable tumor?	Usually > 7 mm
What is NP-59?	6-β[^{131}I]iodomethyl-19-norcholesterol, an aldosterone precursor
What is the disadvantage of NP-59 scintigraphy?	Less useful with small adenomas; sensitivity is dependent on tumor size
What is the appropriate preoperative preparation?	1. Correction of hypokalemia 2. Spironolactone or amiloride, to control hypertension 3. Na$^+$-restricted diet, supplemented by K$^+$
How does spironolactone work?	Competitive **aldosterone antagonist** to the renal tubules; inhibits aldosterone-stimulated Na$^+$ reuptake and K$^+$ secretion
How does amiloride work?	Inhibits renal tubular ion transport, resulting in decreased Na$^+$ reuptake and K$^+$ secretion
What operation is performed for primary hyperaldosteronism caused by adrenal adenoma?	Unilateral adrenalectomy via posterior or lateral extraperitoneal approach is best. Because of accurate localization tests, bilateral exploration via midline approach is rare.
What are the associated postoperative complications?	Hyperkalemia, postural hypotension, weight loss, transient hypoaldosteronism; persistent hypertension is usually self-resolving within several weeks
Why do patients develop hypoaldosteronism postoperatively?	Because of long-term suppression of **normal** adrenal
What is the appropriate treatment of postoperative hypoaldosteronism?	1. **Preoperative spironolactone** helps to allow reactivation of the renin–angiotensin system by blocking aldosterone feedback 2. **Fludrocortisone** (aldosterone agonist); recovery usually occurs within 1 month

General Surgery

PHEOCHROMOCYTOMA

Where are catecholamines produced?	In the adrenal medulla
What normally controls catecholamine synthesis and release?	Sympathetic innervation
What are the four adrenergic receptor subtypes?	α-1, α-2, β-1, and β-2
What does α-1 receptor mediate?	**Vasoconstriction**, pupillary dilation, intestinal relaxation, and uterine contraction
What does α-2 receptor mediate?	Vasoconstriction, feedback inhibition of NE release from sympathetic neurons; inhibits renin release and insulin release
What does β-1 receptor mediate?	Increases force and rate of **cardiac** muscle contraction Increases lipolysis Increases amylase production
What does β-2 receptor mediate?	**Relaxes smooth muscle** Increases **glycogenolysis** Increases **insulin** and glucagon secretion Increases **renin** secretion
What is pheochromocytoma?	Tumor of chromaffin tissue secreting dopamine, epinephrine, or norepinephrine; most often located in the adrenal **medulla**
What percentage of hypertensive patients have pheochromocytoma?	1/1000
What type of patient is most likely to develop the disease?	Peak incidence is in the fourth to fifth decade Approximately 80% to 90% are **sporadic** Can be associated with **familial** syndromes

Which familial syndromes are associated with pheochromocytoma?

Isolated familial pheochromocytoma
MEN IIa
MEN IIb
Von Recklinghausen neurofibromatosis

Do patients with pheochromocytoma have nonepisodic hypertension?

Yes; half of patients may have sustained hypertension only as a manifestation of pheochromocytoma

THE RULE OF 10%

What proportion of pheochromocytomas are bilateral?

Approximately 10%

What proportion of pheochromocytomas are malignant?

Approximately 10%

What proportion of pheochromocytomas are extra-adrenal?

Approximately 10%

What proportion of pheochromocytomas are multiple?

Approximately 10%

What proportion of pheochromocytomas occur in children?

Approximately 10%

Where are extra-adrenal pheochromocytomas most commonly found?

Most occur intra-abdominally; only approximately 2% are found in the thorax and neck

What is the incidence of extra-adrenal tumor in children?

Approximately 30%

What is the incidence of extra-adrenal tumor in familial cases of pheochromocytoma?

Greater than 50%

What is the incidence of malignancy in extra-adrenal tumors?

Approximately 40%

What comprises the classic triad?

Hypertension, associated with **palpitation** and **diaphoresis**

What are the other signs/symptoms?

Anxiety, chest or abdominal pain, tremor, pallor, fatigue, weight loss, headache

Absence of flushing (so rarely associated with this condition that if present, pheochromocytoma is not likely to be the cause)

In what other situations should diagnosis of pheochromocytoma be considered?

Malignant hypertension
Hypertension occurring during **induction, surgery, parturition,** or thyrotropin–releasing-hormone testing
Hypertension in response to certain **drugs** (TCAs, antihypertensives)

What are the possible sequelae of untreated disease?

Complications of hypertension (e.g., cardiomyopathy, CVA, MI)
Decreased blood volume
Ventricular dysrhythmias: cardiac compromise or sudden death

What are the appropriate tests to screen for suspected pheochromocytoma?

Plasma and urine catecholamines
Urine metanephrines and VMA

Which test is the most reliable screening tool for pheochromocytoma?

Twenty-four hour urine metanephrine; should be confirmed with urine catecholamines

Which tests are used to localize the tumor?

CT and MRI
MIBG radionuclide study

What is the best study for localizing adrenal pheochromocytomas?

Abdominal CT(> 90% accuracy)

In what cases is MRI useful?

Patients who are pregnant or have extra-adrenal tumors

If unable to localize with CT, what test is best for finding extra-adrenal pheochromocytomas?

Radionuclide study with MBIG

What is phenylethanolamine-N-methyltransferase (PNMT)?

The enzyme responsible for converting norepinephrine to epinephrine

Why is this enzyme important?

Extra-adrenal pheochromocytomas **do not** have this enzyme; therefore, they **cannot** produce epinephrine, thus making it possible to distinguish between adrenal and nonadrenal tumors.

What suggests malignancy on serology and urine studies?

The presence of multiple **vasoactive peptides** (e.g., VIP, somatostatin)

What treatment options are available?

Surgical resection, with preoperative **α**- and **β-blockers** and anxiolytics
For unresectable tumors, adrenergic block with external beam rads, therapeutic embolization; chemotherapy has not been demonstrated to be effective so far (under study)

What is the appropriate preoperative preparation?

Principles include:
α-adrenergic block
β-blockade
Volume replacement

What are the advantages of preoperative treatment?

Controls HTN and morbidity related to HTN preoperatively
Limits severe fluctuations in intraoperative blood pressure
Preoperative vasodilation allows intravascular volume reexpansion and decreases hypotension following removal of the tumor

In what type of patient is α-block indicated?

Those at high risk because of severe hypertension

When is preoperative β-blockade recommended?

Controversial; some surgeons prefer routine use, others prefer selective use because of potential side effects

In what cases is preoperative β-block clearly indicated?

Significant tachycardia
History of arrhythmias
Persistent PVCs
Tumors secreting mainly epinephrine

Which should be given first, α- or β-blockers?	α-blockers
Why?	If given first, β-blockade may result in **hypertensive crisis** because of unopposed α-adrenergic (vasoconstrictive) action.
What is the preferred choice for α-block?	Phenoxybenzamine (long duration); partial block is achieved in most patients
How does phenoxybenzamine work?	Noncompetitive α-antagonist (α-1 > α-2)
When should α-block be started?	Between 10 and 14 preoperative days
When should β-block be started?	Between 3 and 7 preoperative days
What approach?	If the tumor is well localized to the adrenal gland, lateral or posterior approach may be used Otherwise, **midline** anterior (**thoracoabdominal** incision, rarely)
When would a midline approach be more appropriate?	Large tumor Recurrent pheochromocytoma Bilateral disease Extra-adrenal tumor
What are the possible intraoperative complications?	**Hypertensive** crisis Ventricular **dysrhythmia** during manipulation Profound **hypotension** following removal of the gland (All conditions are less severe with appropriate preoperative preparation)
What are the possible postoperative complications?	Persistent hypertension Hypotension Hypoglycemia Bronchospasm

What is the possible etiology of postoperative hypertension?	Incomplete removal of pheochromocytomas Renal damage from chronic hypertension Renal artery injury
What causes postoperative hypotension?	Relative lack of circulating catecholamines; decreased vascular tone with hypovolemia
What is the treatment of choice for postoperative hypotension?	Fluid expansion
Why does hypoglycemia occur?	Decreased circulating catecholamines; increased insulin release
Why does postoperative bronchospasm occur?	Decreased β-2 activation after removal of pheochromocytoma
What is the recurrence rate after resection?	Approximately 5% to 10% (monitor catecholamine levels annually for the first 5 years)

HYPERADRENOCORTICALISM

What is Cushing syndrome?	A condition caused by an excess of adrenocortical hormones from **all** causes
What is Cushing disease?	Cushing syndrome caused by **pituitary** hypersecretion of ACTH
What is the main cause of Cushing syndrome?	1. **Autonomous** adrenal tumor (20%) 2. **Pituitary** adenoma (60%) 3. **Ectopic** ACTH production (10%) 4. **Iatrogenic** Cushing 5. Adrenocortical cancer (rare)
Which type of patient is most likely to develop Cushing syndrome?	Middle-aged adults Women (ratio of women:men = 3:1) occurrence in children, if not iatrogenic, suggests adrenocortical malignancy
What are the associated signs/symptoms?	Truncal obesity, hirsutism, acne, moon facies, buffalo hump, prominent purple striae, fatigue, weakness, abnormal menses, hypertension, hyperglycemia

What skin finding suggests pituitary etiology?

Increased skin **pigmentation** (caused by increased secretion of melanocyte-stimulating hormone)

What commonly used test screens for suspected Cushing syndrome?

Overnight low-dose dexamethasone-suppression test

How does this test work?

Normally, 1 mg of dexamethasone will suppress ACTH secretion by **feedback inhibition.** This dose will **not** suppress autonomous adrenals or hypersecretion of cortisol owing to the presence of excess ACTH.

What is dexamethasone?

A highly potent, synthetic glucocorticoid

What is the purpose of a 24-hour urine free cortisol test?

Confirms Cushing syndrome in patients who fail to suppress cortisol production following dexamethasone administration

Once a diagnosis of Cushing syndrome is made, what is the next step in determining the cause?

Measure **plasma ACTH** levels

What does high ACTH indicate?

Pituitary or **ectopic** ACTH tumor (likely etiology for Cushing syndrome)

What are the most common sites of ectopic ACTH secretion?

Bronchial carcinoid
Thymic carcinoid
Adenocarcinoma or small-cell carcinoma of the lung

What does low ACTH indicate?

Hypersecretion from primary adrenal source is the likely etiology

What is the purpose of a high-dose dexamethasone-suppression test?

Distinguishes between pituitary and ectopic sources of ACTH secretion

What does this test demonstrate in patients with pituitary source?

Less than 50% **suppression** of 24-hour urinary cortisol levels

What response to high-dose dexamethasone suppression is seen in patients with ectopic source for ACTH?	No response to high-dose dexamethasone suppression
Which studies localize adrenal cortisol-secreting tumors?	CT, MRI, NP-59 (iodocholesterol scanning)
Biochemically, what findings would be suggestive of adrenocortical malignancy?	Increased production of mineralocorticoids or androgens (vast majority of benign tumors produce glucocorticoids only)
What is the appropriate treatment of Cushing disease?	**Excision** of pituitary adenoma via transsphenoidal approach
What is Nelson syndrome?	Late **complication** of bilateral adrenalectomy for Cushing disease involving marked **pituitary expansion** and compressive sequelae
What proportion of Cushing syndrome is caused by adrenal adenoma?	Between 10% and 20%
What is the appropriate treatment of Cushing syndrome caused by adrenal adenoma?	Medical management may be effective for a prolonged time in adrenal adenoma. Adrenalectomy for adenoma is usually curative, although patients may remain hypertensive and obese.
What drugs are used in medical treatment?	Metyrapone, ketoconazole, aminoglutethimide, and mitotane
How does mitotane work?	Reversible **adrenolytic**; selective for zona fasciculata and reticularis; causes atrophy and necrosis to glands; blocks 11–β-hydroxylation
How does ketoconazole work?	Inhibits steroid formation at multiple sites

How does aminoglutethimide work?	Inhibits conversion of cholesterol to pregnenolone
What special risks are associated with adrenalectomy in Cushing patients?	Increased risk of postoperative complications related to **chronically elevated circulating steroids** (e.g., poor wound healing, infection, thromboembolism hemorrhage, peptic ulcers)
When do patients require replacement corticosteroids following adrenalectomy?	Immediately
Why?	Because the hypothalamic–pituitary axis is impaired from chronically elevated glucocorticoid levels; contralateral adrenal gland cannot produce adequate amounts of corticosteroids
What is the appropriate management of corticosteroid replacement for patients undergoing unilateral adrenalectomy?	One to two 100-mg doses of hydrocortisone preoperatively Postoperative hydrocortisone 100 mg every 4 to 6 hours for the first 48 hours Taper as tolerated to oral maintenance dose Mineralocorticoid replacement is usually not necessary after adrenalectomy for Cushing syndrome. If mineralocorticoid deficiency is evident, add fluorohydrocortisone daily
How long does the pituitary–hypothalamic axis take to recover after unilateral adrenalectomy for Cushing syndrome?	Approximately 6 to 12 months; patients require long-term replacement

ADRENOCORTICAL INSUFFICIENCY

What eponym refers to this disorder?	Addison disease
What is the most common cause?	**Iatrogenic** suppression of ACTH secretion by exogenous steroids

What other causes are possible?	Autoimmune disease Histoplasmosis Bilateral adrenal hemorrhage Bilateral adrenal TB Adrenal fungal infection
What is Waterhouse-Friderichsen syndrome?	Acute **hemorrhagic** adrenal **necrosis** caused by bacteremia, usually *Meningococcus*
What is an Addisonian crisis?	Acute adrenocortical insufficiency (medical emergency)
What type of patient is most likely to develop this condition?	Patients with chronic insufficiency who are subjected to stress (e.g., surgery)
Describe the pathophysiology.	In response to stress, inadequate mineralocorticoids and glucocorticoids result in an inability to retain Na^+, secrete K^+, and maintain adequate intravascular volume. Hypovolemia and electrolyte imbalance are exacerbated by vomiting.
What are the associated signs/symptoms of adrenocortical insufficiency?	Weakness, fatigue, weight loss, nausea, vomiting, hypotension, abdominal pain, fever, diarrhea; progresses rapidly to lethargy, weakness, and cardiovascular collapse
What are the associated laboratory findings?	**Hypo**glycemia, **hypo**natremia, **hyper**kalemia, **acidosis, elevated** BUN, **decreased** chloride, depressed plasma cortisol
What is the appropriate initial treatment?	1 L NS plus 200 mg hydrocortisone over 30 minutes Followed by NS plus 100 mg hydrocortisone/L, with glucose, replace electrolytes Identification and treatment of underlying causes (e.g., infection, trauma)

What preventative measures should be taken in cases of patients with known adrenal insufficiency undergoing surgery?	Stress-dose steroids: 100 mg cortisol IM or IV on the day of surgery and then every 8 hours Taper as tolerated postoperatively to maintenance dose

POWER REVIEW

What is another name for hyperaldosteronism?	Conn disease
What is another name for hyperadrenocorticalism?	Cushing syndrome
What is another name for adrenocortical insufficiency?	Addison disease
What is the rule of 10% for pheochromocytoma?	10% bilateral 10% malignant 10% extra-adrenal 10% multiple 10% in children
What are the appropriate screening tests for the following disorders: **Primary hyperaldosteronism?**	24-hour urinary aldosterone excretion (post salt loading)
Pheochromocytoma?	24-hour urinary metanephrine, vanillylmandelic acid (VMA), epinephrine, norepinephrine
Cushing syndrome?	Dexamethasone suppression test
What is the preoperative preparation for patients with primary hyperaldosteronism?	Correct hypokalemia Spironolactone or amiloride to control hypertension Na$^+$-restricted diet, supplemented by K$^+$
What is the preoperative treatment for patients with pheochromocytoma?	α-blockade β-blockade

ANATOMY OF THE THYROID AND PARATHYROID GLANDS

When does the thyroid gland develop?	Between the fourth and seventh weeks in utero
What is the embryonic origin of the thyroid gland?	The area between the **first** and **second** pharyngeal pouches (it is an endodermal diverticulum of the ventral pharyngeal surface)
What remnant is present in adults?	The foramen cecum (the apex of the sulcus terminalis on the dorsum of the tongue)
What is the embryonic origin of the parathyroid gland?	The third and fourth pharyngeal pouches (it is an endodermal proliferation of the dorsal tip of each pouch)
Which pouch develops into the inferior and superior parathyroids?	**Third pouch**—inferior glands **Fourth pouch**—superior glands
What also develops in the third pharyngeal pouch?	Thymus
What also develops in the fourth pharyngeal pouch?	The parafollicular or **"C" cells** from the ultimobranchial bodies
Into what do the ultimobranchial bodies develop?	**Lateral** lobes of thyroid
Where do the inferior parathyroids migrate to?	To the border of the lower thyroid (third pharyngeal pouch)
What is the anatomic relationship of the inferior parathyroids to the superior parathyroids and thyroid?	The inferior glands are more ventral than the superior glands and are usually located near the inferior pole of the thyroid.
Where do the superior parathyroids migrate to?	The area where the inferior thyroid artery enters the gland **or** where the artery intersects the recurrent laryngeal nerve

What is the anatomic relationship of the superior parathyroids to the thyroid?

They are found on the posterior surface of the upper thyroid lobes.

Are glands embedded in thyroid tissue?

Rarely

Which glands, superior or inferior, are found in more variable locations?

Inferior parathyroids

Give the size, weight, and color of the parathyroid gland.

Size—5 mm to 6 mm by 3 mm by 1 mm to 2 mm
Weight—35 g to 40 g
Color—yellow–brown (distinct from normal adipose tissue)

What size parathyroid suggests hyperplasia or adenoma?

Dimensions greater than 6 mm by 3 mm by 2 mm

What percentage of people have three parathyroid glands?

Approximately 10%

What percentage of people have five parathyroid glands?

Approximately 5%

What percentage of parathyroids are found in the mediastinum?

Approximately 1%

What anatomic feature can help identify a mediastinal parathyroid?

A vascular pedicle from the neck to the mediastinal gland

Which anomalies in thyroid anatomy are important to the surgeon?

Pyramidal lobe
Lingual thyroid
Thyroglossal duct cysts
Isolated neck or mediastinal tissue (**rare**)

From what structure does the pyramidal lobe derive?

The distal thyroglossal duct

What is important about it?	It may be missed at thyroid resection
What causes a lingual thyroid?	Failure of migration
What is important about it?	It may cause a mass effect at the base of the tongue and it may be the patient's only thyroid tissue
What is the source of thyroid vascular supply?	Superior and inferior thyroid arteries and, occasionally, the thyroid IMA artery
What percentage of patients have a thyroid IMA artery?	Approximately 2%
What is the origin of the superior thyroid artery?	The first branch of the external carotid
What is the origin of the inferior thyroid artery?	Thyrocervical trunk
What is the origin of the thyroid IMA artery?	Aortic arch or innominate artery
What is the source of parathyroid vascular supply?	Usually branches from the **inferior thyroid artery**; occasionally supplied from superior thyroid and esophageal arteries
Into which vein does the superior thyroid vein drain?	The internal jugular vein
Into which vein does the middle thyroid vein drain?	Internal jugular vein
Into which vein does the inferior thyroid vein drain?	Innominate vein or internal jugular vein (note: two arteries and three veins)
What are the important associated nerves and what are the results of damage to them?	**Recurrent laryngeal nerve** (damage causes vocal cord paralysis and hoarse voice) **External superior laryngeal nerve** (innervates cricothyroid muscle; damage causes a weak voice)

What are the anatomic relationships of the recurrent laryngeal nerve?

Variable relationship to the inferior thyroid artery, often deep; tracts medially to the thyroid lobe, crosses the cricoid cartilage, and passes under the cricothyroid muscle

How common is a nonrecurrent laryngeal nerve and on what side is it usually found?

Rare; usually found on the **right** side

HYPERPARATHYROIDISM

Define primary hyperparathyroidism.

An **adenoma** or **multigland hyperplasia** of unknown etiology that secretes excess PTH

What is the frequency of adenomas in primary hyperparathyroidism?

Approximately 80%

What is the frequency of double adenomas?

Approximately 2%

Define secondary hyperparathyroidism.

Hyperplasia, often secondary to renal failure or:
Carcinoma with bone metastasis
Multiple myeloma
Osteogenesis imperfecta
Paget disease
Pituitary basophilism

Define tertiary hyperparathyroidism.

Continued abnormal hypersecretion of PTH following resolution of etiology causing secondary hyperparathyroidism

In what kind of patient is tertiary hyperparathyroidism most common?

Renal transplant patients

How are most patients currently diagnosed with hyperparathyroidism?

Slightly elevated calcium levels are evident on routine lab studies.

What is the incidence of hypercalcemia in the general population?

Between 0.1% and 0.5%

What is the most likely diagnosis for this type of patient?	Hyperparathyroidism
What is the incidence of hypercalcemia in hospitalized patients?	Approximately 5%
What is likely diagnosis for this type of patient?	**Cancer** (calcium tends to be higher in these patients)
What types of cancer are most common?	Breast and lung cancer Multiple myeloma and lymphoma Adenocarcinoma of the ovary or kidney
Do these types of cancer all result in bony metastases?	No; some, such as adenoma of the ovary or kidney, may secrete a PTH-related peptide, causing hypercalcemia
What are the differential diagnoses of hypercalcemia?	Malignancy Sarcoidosis Vitamin D and A excess Hyperthyroidism Thiazides Lithium Addison disease Immobilization Familial hypocalciuric hypercalcemia Milk–alkali syndrome **Lab error**
What is the incidence of hyperparathyroidism?	1/1000 patients overall Ratio of women:men = 3:1 1/500 in women over 40 years old (most common in postmenopausal women)
What is the possible etiology?	Low-dose radiation of primary disease Chronic furosemide use MEN Genetic anomaly (change in gland set-point or renal anomaly)
What are the common symptoms of hypercalcemia?	Fatigue Arthralgia Myalgia Bone pain **Constipation**

What are the symptoms by system?	**Bone**—osteitis fibrosa cystica **Renal**—stones **GI**—ulcers, pancreatitis, cholelithiasis, constipation **CV**—hypertension, shortened QT, decreased heart rate, heart block **Neuromuscular**—weakness, fatigue, atrophy **Psychiatric**—depression
What are the classic symptoms?	Painful **bones** Renal **stones** Abdominal **groans** Depression, psychiatric **"moans"**
What laboratory findings suggest disease?	High total serum calcium and two elevated PTH readings High alkaline phosphatase (without liver disease, this finding suggests sig. bone disease) Low phosphorus (high in renal failure) Elevated serum chloride/phosphate ratio greater than 30
What is the significance of the calcium–phosphate product?	If the product is greater than **40**, there is a chance of salt precipitation in tissues.
What is the normal calcium level?	Between 9 and 10.3 mg/dl
How much calcium is ionized?	Approximately 50%
What is the normal PTH level?	Approximately 20 meq/ml or less
What PTH levels are associated with hyperparathyroidism?	Approximately 60 meq/ml or more
How is PTH analyzed?	Radioimmunoassay Midmolecular weight PTH Double antibody–IRMAS (Tests now have more sensitivity and are less affected by renal failure)

What are the principal regulators of calcium metabolism?	PTH, vitamin D, and calcitonin (not considered essential)
How does PTH work?	Increases bone resorption of calcium and phos Increases renal resorption of calcium Increases renal secretion of phos Stimulates vitamin D formation
What stimulates PTH secretion?	Decreasing calcium
How does vitamin D work?	Increases intestinal calcium and phos absorption
How does calcitonin work?	Inhibits bone resorption and probably increases urinary excretion of calcium
Where is calcium absorbed?	Duodenum and proximal jejunum
What is the appropriate medical management of hyperparathyroidism?	IV fluids (most patients will be dehydrated) Furosemide (only after IV fluids) D/C thiazides or vitamin D (dietary intake should also be limited) In difficult to control cases: 　Bisphosphonates 　Estrogen/progesterone (in the postmenopausal patient) 　Mithramycin 　Steroids 　Gallium 　Dialysis 　Chloroquine (for sarcoid)
How does mithramycin work?	Inactivates osteoclasts, inhibits RNA synthesis
What clinical symptoms indicate failure of medical management?	Skeletal fractures Extraosseous calcification Intractable pruritus Nephrolithiasis

What percentage of patients with hyperparathyroidism require surgery?

Between 10% and 25%

What disease can mimic hyperparathyroidism?

Familial hypocalciuric hypercalcemia (surgery should not be performed)

How is this condition diagnosed?

Urinary calcium less than 200 mg/day

What is hypercalcemic crisis?

Sudden increase in PTH leading to Ca^{2+} in the 16 to 20 mg/dl range

What causes hypercalcemic crisis?

Usually, surgery to treat another condition

What are the symptoms of hypercalcemic crisis?

Polyuria, dehydration (leading to increased calcium), muscle weakness, nausea, vomiting, lethargy, coma

What is the appropriate treatment of hypercalcemic crises?

Fluids
Furosemide (if hydrated)
Calcitonin

What are the indications for surgery in secondary hyperparathyroidism?

Failure of medical therapy

What parathyroid imaging techniques are available?

Ultrasound
CT
MRI
Thallium^{231}–Technetium^{99} scan
Angiography or venous sampling (second line)
Sestamibi scan

What situation always warrants preoperative localization?

Reoperations

Should localization be performed on first operations?

The issue is **controversial;** localization is not thought to increase the success of surgery if care is taken for adequate exposure and visualization of the glands by an experienced surgeon.

What is the most common surgical option for treatment of hyperplasia?

Total parathyroidectomy with autotransplantation into forearm

What is the appropriate treatment of secondary hyperparathyroidism?

Parathyroidectomy with autotransplantation

What are the indications for parathyroid autotransplantation?

Primary parathyroid hyperplasia
Secondary hyperparathyroidism
Persistent or recurrent hyperparathyroidism
Often used with radical head and neck surgery, including total thyroidectomy

What are the advantages of autotransplantation?

Easy revision, if hyperparathyroidism persists or recurs

What are the disadvantages of autotransplantation?

If hypercalcemia remains or recurs, it is often difficult to determine if it is from the graft or from remaining tissue in the neck or ectopic site.

What are the disadvantages of total parathyroidectomy?

Risk of osteomalacia
Requires calcium and vitamin D

Define persistent hyperparathyroidism.

Patients remain hypercalcemic in the immediate post-operative period.

Define recurrent hyperparathyroidism.

Patients become hypercalcemic after at least 3 months of being normocalcemic.

What is the appropriate treatment of parathyroid adenoma?

Resection of adenoma and biopsy of normal glands

What is the purpose of biopsy?

To rule out hyperplasia

When removing a single adenoma, is bilateral exposure necessary?

The issue is controversial, but bilateral exposure is considered necessary to help rule out hyperplasia, which may be asymmetric

What is the appropriate treatment of parathyroid cancer?

En bloc resection

What is the risk of recurrent laryngeal nerve injury at first operation?	Approximately 5%

PARATHYROID CARCINOMA

What is the incidence?	Less than 1% of patients with primary hyperparathyroidism **(very rare)**
What is the ratio of men:women with this disease?	Approximately 1:1, versus 1:3 for benign disease
What is the average age at onset?	The fourth decade (usually younger than that of benign disease patients)
What are the associated signs/symptoms?	Symptoms marked by severity **Palpable neck mass** Recurrent laryngeal nerve injury Node invasion Local invasion or metastatic disease
What signs/symptoms are usually present at diagnosis?	Hypercalcemia and PTH **increased more than in benign disease** Osteomalacia (approximately 50% of patients, versus 10% of patients with benign disease) Malaise **Polydypsia/uria** Loss of appetite Muscle weakness Pancreatitis Constipation
What intraoperative evidence suggests cancer?	Hard multilobular consistency Adherent/invading adjacent tissue Cervical node involvement
Is local recurrence after surgery for hyperparathyroidism always indicative of cancer?	No; seeding of benign cells may occur
What histologic findings are associated with parathyroid cancer?	Increased mitotic frequency (may not be present in cancerous tissue and may be present in benign tissue) Capsule or blood vessel invasion Low fat content in gland

What other findings suggest cancer?	Hand x-ray showing subperiosteal resorption greater than 25% Increased hCG (or of a subunit)
Describe the appearance of tissue at surgery.	**Dense, fibrous,** and **adherent to or invading** the surrounding tissue
What is the appropriate treatment?	En bloc resection with possible node resection
What precautions must be taken by the surgeon?	To prevent seeding, the gland capsule must not be entered.
When should a node dissection be performed?	Only if cervical nodes appear involved (uncommon)
Does mithramycin help?	It only aids in controlling hypercalcemia, but does not affect cancer cells.
How common are metastases or nodes?	Approximately one third of cases or less
Where are metastases most commonly found?	Lungs
What follow-up studies should be performed?	Serum calcium and PTH
What is the rate of recurrence?	Approximately 50%, but second operations may eliminate disease
What is the survival rate?	The 5-year survival rate is approximately 50%; in most of these cases, patients die from the effects of hypercalcemia due to metastatic disease or local recurrence.

NEUROENDOCRINE GI TUMORS

What are the cells of origin?	APUD cells (amine precursor, uptake, and decarboxylation); tumor = APUDoma
What is the etiology?	Sporadic Familial (MEN I) Approximately 5% of insulinomas are associated with MEN Approximately 30% of gastrinomas are associated with MEN

What is the overall incidence?	Less than 10 cases per million per year
What is the average age at diagnosis?	Fourth decade
What is the most common source of symptoms?	Usually caused by a single secreted hormone; a mass effect is rare
Are multiple hormones secreted from a single tumor?	Rarely
What is the appropriate treatment?	Surgical removal
How does octreotide work?	This somatostatin analogue inhibits hormone release.
What is the major complication of octreotide?	Gallstones, in 25% to 30% of cases
What is the best way of preventing complications?	Cholecystectomy at the time of surgery for those undergoing chronic octreotide treatment

GLUCAGONOMA

From which islet cells do these tumors arise?	α-cells
What percentage of all islet cell tumors do they comprise?	Approximately 1%
What is the clinical triad for diagnosing glucagonoma?	1. Necrolytic migratory dermatitis 2. Diabetes mellitus 3. Weight loss
What laboratory test confirms the diagnosis?	Elevated plasma glucagon greater than 150 pg/ml (many patients will be > 1000 pg/ml)
What is the rate of malignancy?	Two-thirds of cases

What is the most common location?	Pancreas
Which test is used for localization?	CT
What is the appropriate treatment?	Surgical; removal of the tumor should include a rim of normal tissue (e.g., a distal pancreatectomy, if location is in the tail of the pancreas)
What other treatments may be beneficial?	Chemotherapy or octreotide
What is the appropriate treatment for metastases?	Surgical removal, if possible
What are the most common metastatic sites?	Liver and nodes
What is the prognosis?	Only one third of patients are cured; recurrence is common. Aggressive therapy may be indicated because the tumor is slow growing. Overall, the 5-year survival rate is 50%.

INSULINOMA

What percentage of islet cell tumors do they comprise?	Approximately 25%; almost all are small, single adenomas
From what islet cell do these tumors arise?	β-cells
What classic triad is associated with insulinoma?	**Whipple's triad:** Hypoglycemic symptoms with fasting Blood glucose 50 or less Reversal of symptoms with glucose treatment
How is the diagnosis made?	Elevated insulin with low glucose during prolonged fast (up to 72 hours, or when symptoms develop)

How can insulinoma be distinguished from factitious hyperinsulinemia?	**Insulinoma**—C-peptide:insulin = 1:1 **Factitious disease**—C-peptide:insulin less than 1:1
What is the normal insulin:glucose ratio?	Less than or equal to 0.25; useful for detecting abnormal insulin secretion in the setting of normal insulin levels
What is the rate of malignancy?	Approximately 10%
How is malignancy determined?	Only by evidence of local invasion or metastases to the nodes or liver
What tests provide localization prior to surgery?	CT and MRI (poor tests) Endoscopic ultrasound Angiography Venous sampling Octreotide indium scan
What is the appropriate treatment?	Surgery, ranging from enucleation to subtotal pancreatectomy, depending on location
What is the appropriate medical treatment?	Possibly diazoxide, octreotide, or 5-FU/streptozotocin
What is the prognosis?	Up to 95% cure rate

GASTRINOMAS

What is another name for gastrinomas?	Zollinger-Ellison syndrome
What percentage of all islet cell tumors do they comprise?	Approximately 10%
How is the diagnosis made?	Fasting gastrin **Secretin stimulation test**
What is the secretin stimulation test?	Gastrin increases, instead of decreases, after stimulation with secretin.
What levels are considered positive?	Gastrin levels greater than 200 pg/ml

What is the normal gastrin concentration?	Less than 100 pg/ml
Is a normal fasting gastrin level sufficient to rule out gastrinoma?	No; up to 50% of gastrinomas will have normal fasting levels
What are the differential diagnoses of increased gastrin?	Hypo/achlorhydria Gastric outlet obstruction Antral hyperplasia Postvagotomy status Chronic renal failure Post small bowel resection **(Secretin stimulation test should be performed)**
What are the most common locations?	One third are in the pancreas Two thirds are outside of the pancreas (usually the duodenum, but also in the stomach and jejunum)
What is the gastrinoma triangle?	An anatomic area where most tumors are found; apices are: 1. Cystic duct and common bile duct junction 2. Junction of the second and third parts of the duodenum 3. Junction of the neck and body of the pancreas
What is the rate of malignancy?	Approximately two thirds
How is malignancy determined?	Only by evidence of metastases or local invasion; histology is not helpful
What is the usual number of primary tumors?	Single tumor in sporadic cases; multiple primaries occur with MEN I
What percentage of patients with gastrinomas have MEN syndrome?	Approximately 25%
What percentage of MEN I patients have gastrinomas?	Approximately 50%

Is metastasis common?	Yes, frequently to the nodes and liver (later metastasis occurs only if the tumor is located in pancreas)
Is preoperative localization indicated?	Yes (these tumors are usually small)
Which diagnostic tests provide localization?	CT, MRI Intra-operative ultrasound Octreotide-I^{123} scan, CCK-enhanced MRI (experimental, changes in pancreas tissue density)
What is an octreotide-I^{123} scan?	"Hot" octreotide binds to somatostatin receptors and is visualized by γ-scintiscan
What surgical procedures are used?	Resection; possibly enucleation of the mass if it is located in the head of the pancreas Excision of suspicious nodes Vagotomy and/or gastrectomy, if the tumor is not removed and medical therapy fails Duodenotomy and palpation (for high prevalence of duodenal gastrinomas) Whipple procedure (rare)
Is aggressive surgical treatment recommended for metastatic disease?	Yes (tumors grow slowly); prolongs survival from gastrinomas (e.g., debulking, liver resection)
What is the prognosis?	Ten-year survival rate of approximately 90%, if the tumor is resectable Five-year survival rate of 40%, if the tumor is unresectable
Before performing an adrenalectomy for any adrenal mass, what evaluation must be performed?	Pheochromocytoma must be ruled out

NONFUNCTIONING ISLET CELL TUMOR

What is it?	An islet cell tumor that does not cause a syndrome related to excess hormone secretion

What percentage of all islet tumors do they comprise?	Up to 30% (second to insulinomas among APUDomas)
What is the average age at onset?	Sixth decade (as opposed to fourth decade for other islet cell tumors)
What are the associated histologic findings?	Islet cell type staining for neuronal specific enolase or chromograffin
What are the associated signs/symptoms?	Vague epigastric or back pain, usually from mass effect, or possibly jaundice
What is the rate of malignancy?	Almost 100%
What is the usual size of tumors?	Large (approximately 10 cm)
Are metastases common?	Yes, to the liver, nodes, peritoneum, bones, and lung
How is the diagnosis made?	History, normal serum hormone levels, and histologic findings
What tests provide localization?	Ultrasound, CT, MRI
What is the most common location?	Pancreas
What is the appropriate treatment?	Surgical resection, depending on location (e.g., subtotal or total resection of the pancreas)
What is the appropriate nonsurgical treatment?	Possibly 5-FU and streptozotocin
What is the prognosis?	Variable, but 10-year survival rate may be as high as 50%

VIPomas

What does VIP stand for?	Vasoactive intestinal polypeptide
What is a VIPoma?	A tumor arising from VIP-secreting cells of the GI tract

What are the other names for this condition?	Verner-Morrison syndrome
	WDHA syndrome:
	  Watery diarrhea
	  Hypokalemia
	  Hypochlorhydria (achlorhydria)
	  Acidosis

What percentage of all islet cell tumors does it comprise?	Less than 2% (rare)
What are the associated signs/symptoms?	Severe secretory diarrhea, leading to dehydration, hypokalemia, and acidosis, achlorhydria
What are the associated laboratory findings?	Usually VIP will be increased Electrolyte abnormalities, especially hypokalemia and acidosis
What other hormones may be elevated?	Pancreatic polypeptide Neurotensin Prostaglandin (PGE_2)
What tests provide localization?	Ultrasound, CT (often tumor is 3 cm or larger) Angiography (second line)
Where is it usually found?	Pancreas (approximately 90% of cases)
What is the rate of malignancy?	Approximately 50%
What is the appropriate treatment?	Enucleation or surgical resection, depending on location

SOMATOSTATINOMAS

From what cells do these tumors arise?	δ-islet cells
What percentage of all islet cell tumors do they comprise?	Less than 1%
Where are they usually found?	**In the pancreas—50%** **Outside of the pancreas** (e.g., duodenum or ampulla of Vater)—50%

Is metastasis common?	Yes, usually to the liver and nodes
What is the usual number and size of primary tumors?	Single and large (approximately 5 cm)
Is there a relationship between somatostatinomas and MEN I syndrome?	Yes; approximately 50% of patients with somatostatinomas have MEN I
What are the associated clinical symptoms?	Usually none, but there is an associated inhibitory syndrome triad: Mild diabetes mellitus Cholelithiasis Diarrhea
How is the diagnosis made?	Markedly elevated somatostatin level
What is the normal somatostatin level?	Less than 100 pg/ml
Is localization necessary prior to surgery?	Yes; CT, ultrasound, or angiography is sufficient, because this type of tumor is often large
What is the appropriate treatment?	Resection
What is the appropriate management of unresectable disease?	Debulking
What is the appropriate medical therapy?	Possibly streptozotocin and 5-FU
Is cure possible?	Yes, for localized disease Prognosis is poor for advanced disease (15% 5-year survival rate)

MULTIPLE ENDOCRINE NEOPLASIA

What is it?	Endocrine tumors in two or more glands and occasional neuronal, muscular, or connective tissue disease

What is the etiology?	Autosomal-dominant gene anomaly with high penetrance
	    Chromosome 11 for MEN I
	    Chromosome 10 for MEN II

What are the general types of tumors?	Hyperplasia Adenoma Carcinoma (often multicentric or bilateral)
Do the tumors occur simultaneously?	No; tumors can be temporally independent

MEN I

What is the incidence of each of the tumor types in this syndrome?	Pituitary tumors (15%–90%) Parathyroid hyperplasia (95%) Pancreatic islet cell tumors (30%–80%)
What is another name for MEN I?	Wermer syndrome
How do MEN I patients most commonly present?	Approximately 95% of patients first present with **hyperparathyroidism** 70% to 80% are asymptomatic
What percentage of primary hyperparathyroidism patients have MEN I?	Up to 10%
What is the most common type of pancreatic tumor in MEN I?	Gastrinoma (Zollinger-Ellison syndrome), often multiple tumors
How common are multiple gastrinomas?	Approximately 50% of MEN I patients
What percentage of MEN I pancreatic tumors are gastrinomas?	Approximately 50%
What is the rate of malignancy?	Approximately 50%
What is the second most common pancreatic tumor in MEN I?	Insulinoma

What percentage of MEN I pancreatic tumors are insulinomas?	Approximately 33%
Can insulinomas and gastrinomas be found in the same patient?	Yes
What other types of pancreatic tumors are found in MEN I?	Glucagonoma (rare) VIPoma (rare)
What are the most common pituitary tumors in MEN I (in order of decreasing frequency)?	Prolactinoma (**most common**; think: **p**rolactinoma = **p**opular) GHoma Inactive tumor ACTHoma
What are the symptoms of prolactinoma?	Galactorrhea, amenorrhea, infertility
What other tumors rarely occur with MEN I?	Adrenocortical Carcinoid Lipomatous Ovarian
Which condition should be corrected first in MEN I, gastrinoma or hyperparathyroidism?	Hyperparathyroidism (which can worsen ulcer disease)
What is the appropriate therapy of MEN I hyperparathyroidism?	Total parathyroidectomy with autotransplantation (40% of patients will have recurrent hyperparathyroidism after 10 years)
What therapy is indicated for multiple tumors in the pancreas?	Enucleation of palpable tumors in the head of the pancreas and resection of the body and tail, if tumors are found in this location.
What surgical therapy is indicated for insulinoma?	Enucleation of solitary tumor or partial pancreatectomy
What is the appropriate treatment if surgery fails?	Possibly diazoxide, octreotide, or streptozotocin/5-FU

What therapy is recommended for pituitary tumors in MEN I?	Transsphenoidal surgery
What medical therapy is recommended for prolactinomas?	Bromocriptine
What does bromocriptine do?	Decreases prolactin secretion, resulting in decreased size of prolactinoma and restoration of gonadal function
What is the major source of morbidity and mortality in MEN I?	Zollinger-Ellison syndrome
Is screening for MEN I necessary?	Yes; it is indicated for the family of MEN patients
What tests should screening include?	History and physical examination, calcium, PTH, gastrin, glucose, insulin, prolactin, GH

MEN II

How many types of MEN II are there?	Three
What is another name for MEN II?	Sipple syndrome
Which type of MEN II is most common?	MEN IIa
What is MEN IIa?	Pheochromocytoma Parathyroid hyperplasia Medullary thyroid carcinoma
What is MEN IIb°?	Pheochromocytoma Medullary thyroid carcinoma Marfanoid habitus Mucosal neuromas (found on conjunctiva, eyelids, tongue, lips, GI tract) °incomplete penetrance occurs

What is the third MEN II variant?

Medullary thyroid carcinoma only (more common than MEN IIb)

How do patients with MEN II most commonly present?

Medullary thyroid carcinoma (MTC)

Describe the histology of MTC in MEN II.

Diffuse C-cell hyperplasia persisting for years prior to progression to multicentric carcinoma

What stimulation test is used for MTC?

Pentagastrin stimulation test

How does pentagastrin work in this test?

Detects increased stimulation test calcitonin secretion (> 300 pg/ml) after administration

Can this test detect MTC?

Yes; it can detect MTC prior to subclinical development of carcinoma

What is the appropriate therapy for MEN II MTC?

Total thyroidectomy

What is the incidence of pheochromocytoma in MEN IIa?

Approximately 50%, often diagnosed after MTC

What is the incidence of MEN II in patients with pheochromocytoma?

Approximately 5%

What is the malignancy rate of a pheochromocytoma in MEN II?

Approximately 1%, versus 10% malignancy in non-MEN cases

What is the most common location of pheochromocytomas in MEN II?

Usually bilateral and **almost never** extra-adrenal

What are the associated symptoms?

Similar to those of sporadic cases:
  Hypertension
  Headache
  Sweating
  Palpitations

How frequently do symptoms occur in MEN patients?	Approximately 50% of patients are asymptomatic and normotensive; symptoms tend to be milder compared with sporadic cases.
How is the diagnosis made?	Measurement of urinary catecholamines, VMAs, metanephrines
Which localization tests should be performed?	Ultrasound, CT, MRI, or I^{131}–metaiodo benzyl-guanidine (MIBG) scan
What is the appropriate therapy for MEN II pheochromocytoma?	Surgery: possibly bilateral adrenalectomy instead of unilateral removal (if the tumor is localized to one side preoperatively and closely monitored)
What is the incidence of primary hyperparathyroidism in MEN IIa?	Between 10% and 20%
What is the appropriate therapy for hyperparathyroidism in MEN IIa?	Removed at MTC thyroidectomy or total parathyroidectomy, with autotransplantation
What condition can cause morbidity with GI mucosal neuromas in MEN IIb?	Small bowel obstruction
What is the prognosis of MEN IIa?	Five-year survival rate of 85% Ten-year survival rate of 70% (Death is usually caused by MTC.)
What is the prognosis of MEN IIb?	Five-year survival rate of 80% Ten-year survival rate of 60% (Death is usually caused by MTC.)
What percentage of patients with symptoms of MEN II are incurable?	Approximately 85%
What type of screening for MEN II should be performed?	Screen suspected patients and families beginning at the earliest possible age and check yearly.

What are the appropriate screening tests?

Urine catecholamines, calcium, PTH, and **calcitonin**

Is screening helpful?

Yes; most patients can be cured early on

40

The Spleen

Oliver A. R. Binns, MD

What are the anatomic surface projections of the spleen?

It underlies the ninth, tenth, and eleventh ribs on the left. Normally, the spleen does not extend below the costal margin and is therefore not palpable unless pathology is present.

What is the largest single mass of lymphatic tissue in the body?

The spleen

By which ligament is the spleen attached to the stomach?

The gastrolienal ligament

What important structures are contained in the gastrolienal ligament?

The short gastric vessels and the left gastroepiploic vessel

Which ligament attaches the spleen to the kidney?

The lienorenal ligament

Which organ is in close proximity to the spleen?

The tail of the pancreas (i.e., it is prone to injury during splenectomy); the tail is classically said to "tickle" the spleen

What is the normal weight range of the spleen?

Between 100 and 175 grams

Does the spleen contain any muscle tissue?

Yes; both the capsule and the trabeculae contain smooth muscle, allowing a very small degree of autotransfusion to take place with hypovolemia

What is the arterial supply of the spleen and where does it arise?

The splenic artery, which is the largest branch of the **celiac trunk**

What arteries arise from the splenic artery?	The left gastroepiploic, pancreaticomagna, and the short gastric arteries
Why is the spleen prone to infarction?	Its arterial supply is via "end arteries," with little collateral supply
What is the venous drainage of the spleen and into what vessel does it empty?	The splenic vein leaves the hilum and is joined by the inferior mesenteric vein; these then join the superior mesenteric vein to form the portal vein
What is the lymphatic drainage of the spleen?	Via lymph vessels that pass along the splenic blood vessels into the pancreaticosplenic lymph nodes (along the superior and posterior surface of the pancreas)
How is the spleen innervated?	Autonomics arise from the celiac plexus and have vasomotor regulatory functions.
In what percentage of the population do accessory spleens occur?	Approximately 20%
Where do accessory spleens usually occur?	Near the hilum, tail of the pancreas, or in the gastrolienal ligament

What are the functions of the spleen?	RBC and WBC production during fetal life
	Removal of senescent or diseased RBCs
	Maturation of reticulocytes
	Production of IgM and several opsonins (i.e., properdin and tuftsin)
	Removal of the following from RBCs:
	   Howell-Jolly bodies (nuclear remnants)
	   Pappenheimer bodies (iron granules)
	   Heinz bodies (denatured Hgb)
	   Bacteria and other foreign debris (by macrophages and histiocytes; enhanced by the presence of opsonins)

What portion of the circulating platelets are usually within the spleen?	Approximately one third

What conditions are associated with rupture of the spleen?

Infectious mononucleosis
Malaria
Sepsis
Blunt upper abdominal trauma

What are the indications for splenectomy?

Divided into two major categories:
Disease treatment:
  ITP > TTP
  Primary tumors or cysts
  Rupture
  Hereditary spherocytosis
  Autoimmune anemias
Treatment of associated hypersplenism:
  Lymphoproliferative disorders
  Felty syndrome
  Sickle cell disease
  AIDS
  Splenic vein thrombosis
  Hairy-cell leukemia
  Gaucher disease
  Thalassemia major

What is the most commonly injured intra-abdominal organ in blunt trauma?

The spleen (although recent studies state that the liver is most common)

What are the late complications of splenic injury?

Delayed rupture (usually occurs approximately 2 weeks after injury, i.e., during the "latency period of Baudet"); occurrence of this condition, however, is controversial and many cases probably represent delayed diagnosis of an injury that was present earlier

What are the signs/ symptoms of acute splenic injury?

Hypotension, left upper quadrant pain, peritoneal signs, Kehr's sign (referred pain to the left shoulder)

What is Ballance's sign?

Presence of a palpable, tender, enlarged mass in the left upper quadrant from a splenic subcapsular or extracapsular hematoma

How is an acute splenic injury diagnosed?

Unstable patients—History and physical examination, followed by a diagnostic peritoneal lavage and laparotomy, if positive

Stable patients—History and physical examination, followed by a CT scan

What are the treatment options?

Increasing efforts at splenic salvage to avoid total splenectomy; options include partial splenectomy, capsular repair, and splenorrhaphy

What is the indication for nonoperative management in blunt trauma?

Patient must be hemodynamically stable and all other possible intra-abdominal injuries must be ruled out or diagnosed.

What is the incidence of concomitant injuries requiring operative intervention?

In blunt trauma—37%
In penetrating trauma—94% (i.e., treatment of penetrating splenic injuries requires laparotomy)

What are the complications of splenectomy?

Atelectasis (left lower-lobe atelectasis is the most common complication)
Left pleural effusion
Subdiaphragmatic abscess
Bleeding
Hematoma formation
Injury to the tail of pancreas
Postsplenectomy sepsis
Gastric ileus

Which vaccines should be administered prior to splenectomy, if possible?

Pneumovax
Haemophilus influenzae
Neisseria meningitidis

When is it appropriate to drain the splenic bed after splenectomy?

If injury to the pancreas has occurred (note that routine placement of JP drains is not indicated after **isolated** splenic trauma)

What effects does splenectomy have on blood composition?

Thrombocytosis and leukocytosis

What are Howell-Jolly bodies?

Nuclear remnants of RBCs, usually removed by the spleen

What is the significance of the absence of Howell-Jolly bodies present on a patient's blood smear following splenectomy?

They may signify the presence of unresected accessory splenic tissue

DISEASES OF THE SPLEEN

IMMUNE THROMBOCYTOPENIC PURPURA (ITP)

What is the etiology of ITP?	Circulating IgG exists that is directed against platelet-associated antigen, resulting in destruction of platelets by the reticuloendothelial system.
What are the associated signs/symptoms?	Persistently low platelet count, easy bruising, petechiae, mucosal bleeding, menorrhagia, increased megakaryocyte counts on bone marrow aspirate
Is ITP more frequent in men or women?	Women (particularly young women)
What is the appropriate treatment?	Prednisone Platelet transfusions may be necessary for bleeding complications Plasmapheresis
What is the indication for splenectomy in ITP?	Splenectomy is indicated in patients who are refractory to medical management
What percentage of patients eventually require splenectomy ?	Approximately 75%
What is the prognosis after splenectomy?	Approximately 80% of patients have platelet counts that return to normal by the sixth postoperative week. Another 15% improve sufficiently to no longer require steroids.
What condition may cause thrombocytopenia to recur after splenectomy for ITP?	The presence of an **accessory spleen** that was not resected during the initial splenectomy

THROMBOTIC THROMBOCYTOPENIC PURPURA (TTP)

What pentad of clinical manifestations is associated with TTP?	1. Thrombocytopenia 2. Fever 3. Neurologic changes 4. Renal failure 5. Microangiopathic hemolytic anemia

What is the etiology of TTP?	Unknown
Describe the typical patient with TTP.	A woman between 30 and 40 years of age
What are the histologic findings associated with TTP?	Capillary and arteriole occlusion by aggregates of fibrin and platelets
What is the current medical treatment of TTP?	Antiplatelet agents, fresh frozen plasma, and corticosteroids
What is the indication for splenectomy in the setting of TTP?	Failure to respond to medical treatment
What percentage of patients will respond to medical treatment?	Approximately 80%

FELTY SYNDROME

What are the clinical manifestations?	Triad of: 1. Splenomegaly 2. Rheumatoid arthritis 3. Granulocytopenia
What is the underlying cause?	Formation of antibodies against granulocytes

HEREDITARY SPHEROCYTOSIS

What is the etiology?	A genetic defect resulting in an abnormal RBC membrane, which leads to increased trapping and destruction of RBCs by the spleen
What is the associated molecular deficit?	Defect of the membrane skeletal protein **spectrin**
What are the associated signs/symptoms?	Anemia, fatigue, jaundice, **pigmented gallstones**, and splenomegaly
What is the appropriate treatment?	Splenectomy for **all** patients, cholecystectomy if indicated

SPLENIC ARTERY ANEURYSM

What is the most common etiology in women?	Medial dysplasia of the artery wall
What is the most common etiology in men?	Atherosclerosis
What is the significance of pregnancy in a patient with a splenic artery aneurysm?	High incidence of rupture; therefore, these aneurysms should be resected, especially in women of childbearing age who are acceptable operative candidates

SPLENIC VEIN THROMBOSIS

What is the most common etiology?	Pancreatitis
What are the associated signs?	Isolated gastric varices, episodes of UGI bleeding
How is the diagnosis made?	Celiac angiography or US
Is splenic vein thrombosis an indication for splenectomy?	Yes
What are the types of hypersplenism?	**Primary**—underlying disease unknown (i.e., diagnosis of exclusion) **Secondary**—caused by disease (i.e., cirrhosis or other causes of venous hypertension)
What are the diagnostic criteria for hypersplenism?	Anemia, leukopenia, thrombocytopenia, splenomegaly, **compensatory increase in bone marrow activity**, and improvement after splenectomy
What disease is the most common cause of hyposplenism?	Sickle cell anemia (also seen with Graves disease)
What is the risk of hyposplensim?	Predisposes patients to infection by encapsulated organisms and lethal sepsis

What is the most common primary tumor of the spleen?

Benign hemangioma

What is the most common primary lymphoid tumor of the spleen?

Lymphoma (note: tumors may diffusely involve the spleen and present as splenomegaly rather than as mass lesions)

What are the types of splenic cysts?

Post-traumatic
Parasitic (usually *Echinococcus*)
Primary cyst (epithelial lined)

What are the indications for excision of a "true" splenic cyst?

If the cyst is larger than 10 cm in diameter, it should be removed because the risk of rupture and subsequent hemorrhage is greatly increased.

41

Surgical Hypertension

Joseph McShannic, MD

What causes surgically correctable hypertension?

Coarctation of the aorta
Pheochromocytoma
Conn syndrome
Cushing syndrome
Renal artery stenosis
Unilateral renal parenchymal disease

What percentage of hypertensive patients has one of these conditions?

Between 5% and 10%

Who should be evaluated for one of these conditions?

Young patients with hypertension
Patients with no family history of hypertension
Patients with diastolic blood pressure greater than 110 mm Hg that cannot be controlled medically

What is the appropriate initial evaluation?

History and physical examination
Serum electrolytes
Serum BUN and creatinine

COARCTATION OF AORTA

What is this condition?

Narrowing of the aorta in the area of the ligamentum arteriosum

What is the incidence?

Accounts for 5% to 10% of all congenital cardiac lesions
2% of all hypertension
1 in 4,000 people overall

What are the two types?

Preductal
Postductal

How is each type defined?

The location of the stenosis as compared with the ligamentum arteriosum

When do the two types present?	**Preductal**—infancy, early childhood **Postductal**—adulthood
How does each type present?	**Preductal**—congestive heart failure, hypotension, oliguria, metabolic acidosis (after the PDA closes) **Postductal**—sustained diastolic hypertension in the second to third decade of life
Are the "preductors" associated with other anomalies?	Yes; usually other cardiac anomalies
With what other conditions does postductal coarctation present?	Endocarditis Aortic dissection
What are the classic physical findings?	Difference in blood pressure between arms, or between arms and legs Rib notching on CXR (secondary to collateral blood vessels) Reverse 3 sign on CXR
How is the diagnosis confirmed?	Aortogram or transesophageal echocardiogram
What conditions can occur if coarctation is left untreated?	Ruptured aorta Endocarditis Complications of hypertension
What are the treatment options?	Resection with graft interposition Subclavian patch Resection with end-to-end anastomosis
Do these treatments always correct hypertension?	No; in 30% of patients, hypertension is not corrected and they must be monitored for life

PHEOCHROMOCYTOMA

What is the incidence in patients with hypertension?	Between 0.1% and 0.2% of patients with diastolic hypertension
When does it present?	The third through the fifth decade of life

How does it present?	Between 50% and 70% of patients present with paroxysmal hypertension; 50% present with sustained diastolic hypertension.
What are the symptoms?	Headache, sweating, palpitations (all secondary to elevated catecholamines)
How is the diagnosis made?	Urine is tested for elevated catecholamine or breakdown products.
What are the breakdown products?	Metanephrine, normetanephrine, vanillylmandelic acid (VMA)
Of what is VMA a breakdown product?	Normetanephrine, metanephrine, norepinephrine, epinephrine, and 3,4-dihydroxymandelic acid
What of these findings is the most reliable?	Elevated epinephrine and norepinephrine levels (90%)
Which product is most likely to be falsely elevated?	VMA (dietary sources)
What foods can elevate the urine VMA level?	Coffee, tea, raw fruits, and some drugs, such as α-methyldopa
Can patients with essential hypertension have a borderline test result?	Yes; a clonidine-suppression test or glycogen-stimulation test should be given
What is a clonidine-suppression test?	Clonidine is administered to suppress autogenous catecholamines. The production of pheochromocytoma is **not** affected.
Who should receive this test?	Well-hydrated patients; all β-blockers need to be discontinued
What constitutes a normal test?	Serum plasma levels of norepinephrine and epinephrine fall below 500 ng 2 to 3 hours following an oral dose of 0.3 mg of clonidine.

What is a glucagon test?

Glucagon is administered to stimulate the release of catecholamines.
This test may be dangerous, and is therefore used infrequently.

How are pheochromocytomas located?

1. CT scans are effective, but may miss lesions smaller than 1.0 cm.
2. MRI scan (often able to distinguish between malignant adrenal cortical carcinoma and pheochromocytoma)
3. ^{131}I-metaiodobenzylguanidine (MIBG) scan, a norepinephrine analogue

What are the treatment options?

Surgery, if the patient is an operative candidate

What should be done before surgery?

Treat the patient with an α-blocker for 2 weeks, then add β-blocker, if the patient is tachycardic.
Hydrate the patient well before surgery.

Are these tumors malignant?

Between 10% and 20% of sporadic (non-MEN) tumors are malignant

Which tumors are at risk of being malignant?

Extra-adrenal rests
Sustained hypertension

How often are tumors extra-adrenal?

Approximately 10% of all cases

Where are they located?

Paraganglionic areas
Organ of Zuckerkandl
Bladder

Where is the organ of Zuckerkandl most frequently located?

Aortic–iliac bifurcation

With which MEN syndrome is pheochromocytoma associated?

MEN IIA and IIB
IIA—pheochromocytoma, medullary carcinoma of thyroid, parathyroid hyperplasia
IIB—pheochromocytoma, medullary carcinoma of thyroid and mucosal neuromas

How is it genetically transferred?	Autosomal dominant inheritance
How often is pheochromocytoma clinically relevant?	Approximately 50% of cases

CONN SYNDROME (PRIMARY HYPERALDOSTERONISM)

What is the incidence?	Between 0.1 and 0.4% of cases of surgical hypertension 1% of all patients with diastolic hypertension
With what symptoms do these patients present?	**Hypertension (diastolic > 100 mm Hg)**—90% **Serum K⁺ < 3.5 mEq/L** **Elevated urinary potassium** (30–40 mEq/day)
Why do patients present with low potassium?	Elevated aldosterone levels promote absorption of sodium and excretion of potassium in the renal tubule cell.
What causes Conn syndrome?	**Solitary, unilateral adrenal cortical adenoma**—80% **Bilateral adrenal cortical hyperplasia**—15% **Adrenal cortical carcinoma, ovarian neoplasms, glucocorticoid-suppressible aldosteronism**—5%
What is the best test for localizing these lesions?	CT/MRI
What is the appropriate therapy?	Surgery for solitary adenoma and carcinoma
Is any preoperative preparation recommended?	Administer potassium or spironolactone; if the patient responds, surgery has a 90% chance of success in treating hypertension.
Should bilateral idiopathic hyperplasia of the adrenal glands be treated with surgery?	No; surgery is only effective 20% to 30% of the time; medical treatment is recommended

CUSHING SYNDROME

What are the hallmarks of Cushing syndrome?

Central obesity (90%), hypertension (80%), hirsutism, plethora, buffalo hump, osteoporosis, glucose intolerance, psychiatric changes

How is the disease diagnosed?

Documentation of elevated cortisol loss of diurnal variation

What are the possible causes of Cushing syndrome?

Pituitary adenoma (Cushing disease)—60% to 70% of patients
Adrenal cortical—10% to 20% of patients
(Of the adrenal cortical causes, 80% adenomas, 20% hyperplasia)

Can the source of the exogenous ACTH be located anywhere else?

Yes; ectopic ACTH produces elevated cortisol in 15% of patients with Cushing syndrome

Where are these sources usually found?

Carcinoma of the lung—50%
Pancreatic islet-cell tumors—10%
Thymoma—10%
Bronchial adenoma—5%
Medullary carcinoma of the thyroid
Pheochromocytoma

Are any of the sources of elevated cortisol malignant?

Yes; adrenocortical carcinoma occurs in less than 5% of cases, presents third through the fifth decade, and is more common in women

What is the appropriate treatment of Cushing disease/syndrome?

Removal of the source, if possible (i.e., pituitary or adrenal resection)

Should patients have bilateral adrenalectomy for Cushing syndrome?

No; 10% to 15% of patients who have this procedure develop Nelson syndrome

What is Nelson syndrome?

A pituitary tumor caused by hypertrophy because of reduced feedback inhibition after bilateral adrenalectomy

RENOVASCULAR HYPERTENSION (RVH)

What is the incidence of RVH?

Occurs in 5% of all cases of hypertension and 15% to 25% of mild to severe hypertension (diastolic > 115 mm Hg)

Is there a race predominance?

Yes; white patients are more likely to develop the disease than African-American patients

Are men and women affected equally?

In men, the disease is most often caused by atherosclerosis; in women, it is most often caused by fibromuscular hyperplasia.

Who should be evaluated for this disease?

Patients who develop hypertension **early** in life, have a negative family history, and have an abdominal **bruit**

What is the best test to diagnose renal artery stenosis?

Aortography (gold standard)

Does aortography determine the clinical significance of lesions?

No; renal vein renin levels must be checked

What other tests should be obtained?

Captopril renal scan
Duplex scan
[Both tests are good at detecting renal artery disease, not polar vessel (segmental) disease.]

How does a captopril renal scan work?

Captopril vasodilates the efferent arteriole system of the kidney, thereby reducing the perfusion pressure of the glomerules, causing a decrease in filtration rate, which is measured by the renal scan.

What are the treatment options?

Antihypertensives, angioplasty, and operative reconstruction

Which antihypertensives should be used to treat RVH?

Calcium channel blockers, β-blockers, centrally acting drugs

Which drugs should be avoided?

ACE inhibitors

Who should receive aggressive treatment?

Patients who are poorly controlled medically

Patients with declining renal function (impending dialysis)

Young patients early in the course of the disease with a good chance of recovery

42

Lymphoma and Sarcoma

Sung W. Choi, MD
Janice Ryu, MD

LYMPHOMA

What is it?

A malignant neoplasm of lymphoid or reticular endothelial origin

What is the incidence?

53,000 cases per year

Non-Hodgkin lymphoma is five to six times more common than Hodgkin disease

Lymphoma causes 23,000 deaths per year, making it the fifth leading cause of cancer death in men and the sixth leading cause of cancer death in women.

HODGKIN DISEASE

What is it?

A **histologic** diagnosis based on the recognition of Reed-Sternberg cells surrounded by a pleomorphic infiltrate of lymphocytes, histiocytes, granulocytes, plasma cells, and fibroblasts

What are Reed-Sternberg cells?

Multinucleated giant cells whose nuclei contain large nucleoli

How do patients with Hodgkin disease usually present?

Approximately 60% of patients present with asymptomatic lymphadenopathy.

Which nodes are initially involved?

Sites of initial nodal involvement include the cervical (65%–80%), axillary (10%–15%), and inguinal (10%) regions. The mediastinum is initially involved in more than 50% of cases.

How is the disease spread?

Via lymphatics; metastasis initially occurs in a predictable pattern to contiguous lymph node groups and lymphatic organs

How is the diagnosis made?

Cervical or axillary lymph node biopsy The largest and most centrally located node should be selected for excision; those with only mediastinal involvement should have a mediastinoscopy or thoracotomy to obtain a biopsy.

What are the appropriate steps in an initial workup of a patient with possible Hodgkin disease?

Complete history and physical examination—the patient should be carefully evaluated for symptoms and lymphadenopathy

CBC with platelets and differential—look for a mild, normochromic normocytic anemia, increased neutrophils and eosinophils, and normal platelets; later, leukopenia and thrombocytopenia are common

ESR, renal and liver function tests, alkaline phosphatase, LDH, uric acid, serum copper

Biopsy, as previously described

Radiographic studies—CXR, and chest and abdominopelvic CT scans

When are lymphangiograms indicated?

If CT scans are negative, bipedal lymphograms may be helpful in the evaluation of retroperitoneal and pelvic lymph node involvement (especially in preparation for surgery or radiation therapy). Lymphangiograms are more sensitive and specific than CT scans and can detect nonenlarged nodes with structural defects (whereas CT scans simply detect enlargement).

What is a staging laparotomy?

It is a laparotomy to distinguish between low-stage and advanced disease to determine proper therapy. It involves:
1. A midline abdominal incision
2. Liver examination to rule out gross disease; sedge biopsy of the free margin of the R lobe; Trucut needle biopsies three times of both

the R and L lobes; and biopsies of
any suspicious lesions
3. Splenectomy plus biopsy of the
splenic hilar nodes; splenic vessels
should be transected medially and
clipped with a radiopaque clip
4. Biopsy of celiac, portal, mesenteric,
para-aortic, and iliac lymph nodes
with excision of any suspicious
nodes (nodes may appear
suspicious either by examination or
by CT/lymphangiogram); each
nodal site should be marked with a
radiopaque clip, except for the
mesenteric nodal site, which may
move considerably during
subsequent x-ray for radiation
therapy planning
5. Bilateral bone marrow biopsies
from the iliac crest
6. Oophoropexy (women of
childbearing age)

What is oophoropexy?

Surgical fixation of an ovary
If the patient is of childbearing age,
ovaries are marked with metallic clips
and tacked to the pelvic sidewalls. If
this procedure is anatomically
impossible, the ovaries are secured
behind the uterus for protection from
radiation.

**Prior to a staging
laparotomy, what
prophylaxis must the
patient receive?**

Because a staging laparotomy includes a
splenectomy, the patient should receive
preoperative vaccinations against:
1. *Pneumococcus*
2. *Meningococcus*
3. *Haemophilus influenzae* type B

**When is a staging
laparotomy indicated?**

Controversial:
Low clinical stage (i.e., stage I and II)
20% of stage I and 30% of stage II
patients have occult subdiaphragmatic
involvement, which would alter
therapy when found on laparotomy
Those patients who will receive
chemotherapy as a primary treatment
modality (e.g., ≥ stage III, large

mediastinal disease, and those with multiple extranodal areas of involvement) need not have laparotomy. **Improved imaging and more liberal use of chemotherapy are making staging surgeries much less common.**

What are the risks of a staging laparotomy for Hodgkin disease?

There is minimal morbidity and even less mortality (< 0.5%).
The risks include:
1. Postsplenectomy sepsis, especially by encapsulated organisms (10% in those not pretreated with pneumococcal vaccine)
2. Increased occurrence (2 times) of secondary acute nonlymphocytic leukemia (ANLL), especially in those who receive alkylating agent chemotherapy (9 times greater risk)

Define the following stages according to the Ann Arbor staging classification of Hodgkin disease:

Stage I

Single lymph node or extralymphatic region

Stage II

Two or more lymph node or extralymphatic regions **on the same side of the diaphragm**

Stage III

Involvement on **both sides** of the diaphragm

Stage IV

Diffuse and/or disseminated disease (visceral involvement)

Stage A

Asymptomatic (think: **A** = **A**symptomatic)

Stage B

Symptomatic—weight loss of more than 10% in 6 months, fever greater than 38°C, night sweats (think: **B** = **B**ad)

Stage E

Extranodal site (think: **E** = **E**xtranodal)

What are the four histopathologic types of Hodgkin disease?	1. Nodular sclerosis 2. Mixed cellularity 3. Lymphocyte predominant 4. Lymphocyte depleted
What is the most common histopathologic type?	Nodular sclerosis
Which type has the best prognosis?	Lymphocyte predominant
Which type has the worst prognosis?	Lymphocyte depleted
What treatments are used for the various stages of Hodgkin lymphoma?	**Low stage (I–IIA)—** external beam radiotherapy **High stage (IIIA or above)—** combination chemotherapy (adjuvant radiotherapy is sometimes used)
Are radiation therapy and chemotherapy ever combined in the treatment of Hodgkin disease?	Yes, for bulky mediastinal disease
What percentage of patients with Hodgkin disease are cured?	Approximately 80%

NON-HODGKIN LYMPHOMA (NHL)

What is it?	A lymphoma other than Hodgkin disease NHL has an established cellular origin (usually monoclonal B cells, but may also originate in T cells) based on the stages of lymphocyte differentiation.
How is NHL classified?	Nodular (low grade) versus diffuse (high grade); the Working Classification groups NHL according to natural history and therapeutic response
Which is worse, high grade or low grade?	High grade

How does the presentation differ compared with that of Hodgkin disease?

Patients with NHL are usually older and more debilitated, but less often have B symptoms. NHL often presents with peripheral nodal (especially epitrochlear) or extranodal disease. It may present as a retroperitoneal or mesenteric mass or as hepatomegaly and/or splenomegaly.

How does NHL spread?

Via the bloodstream, thereby involving noncontiguous areas

What are some of the more dramatic presentations of NHL?

SVC syndrome
Acute spinal cord compression syndrome
Ureteral obstruction
Meningeal involvement

How is the diagnosis made?

Biopsy

What are the most common malignancies requiring abdominal surgery in AIDS patients?

Non-Hodgkin lymphoma, Kaposi sarcoma

When is splenectomy indicated in NHL?

Symptomatic splenomegaly
Pancytopenia, secondary to hypersplenism
Recurrent splenic infarcts

Define hypersplenism.

Hyperfunctioning spleen
Documented loss of blood elements (WBCs, hematocrit, platelets)
Splenomegaly
Bone marrow

GASTRIC LYMPHOMA

What is the most common site of extranodal NHL?

The stomach

What are the signs/ symptoms of gastric lymphoma?

Abdominal pain and weight loss (80%)
B signs (40%)
Nausea, vomiting, and malaise (possibly)
Upper GI bleeding (rare)

What are the major differential diagnoses?

Gastric adenocarcinoma
Menetrier disease
Zollinger-Ellison syndrome
Hypertrophic gastritis

Which diagnostic tests are indicated?	Upper GI endoscopy with biopsy is the method of choice. Grossly, the lesions are superficial, well-demarcated, stellate ulcers that involve a large area of the stomach.
What signs appear on upper GI series?	May show a mass, ulcers, enlarged mucosal folds, and/or decreased gastric mobility
What is the appropriate treatment of disease confined to the stomach and regional nodes (stage IE/IIE)?	Surgical resection (total or subtotal gastrectomy) Postoperative adjuvant radiation therapy or chemotherapy (Note: recent studies have shown that chemoradiation therapy alone provides equal long-standing remission rates for low-stage gastric lymphoma.)

THERAPEUTIC OPTIONS FOR LYMPHOMAS

What roles do the following treatments have: Hematopoietic growth factor?	Allows higher doses of chemotherapy and shortened intervals between these doses, thereby causing a more effective response
Autologous bone marrow transplant?	This technique is being used experimentally in the treatment of refractory or recurrent lymphoma, both Hodgkin disease and NHL. It involves aspiration of BM from the posterior iliac crests while the patient is laid prone on the OR table under general anesthesia. The aspirated bone marrow is concentrated and purged. Before re-infusion, the patient receives a marrow ablative regimen consisting of high-dose cytotoxic chemotherapy, with or without total body irradiation.

SOFT TISSUE SARCOMA (STS)

What is it?	Soft tissue tumor derived from the mesoderm

How common is it?	Accounts for 1% of all malignant tumors; incidence peaks before age 15
What are the associated risk factors?	History of radiation exposure (5%) History of chemotherapy with alkylating agents Immunosuppression (e.g., Kaposi's sarcoma in patients with AIDS)
What type of tumor is associated with polyvinyl chloride and arsenic exposure?	Hepatic angiosarcoma
Where is polyvinyl chloride found?	In plastic industries
What type of tumor is associated with asbestos exposure?	Mesothelioma
What are the signs/ symptoms of STS?	Soft tissue mass; pain from compression of adjacent structures
What is the most common site of adult STS?	Extremities
How do most sarcomas metastasize?	Hematogenously (via the bloodstream)
What is the most common location and route of metastasis?	Lungs, via the hematogenous route
What is the overall incidence of lymph node metastases?	Approximately 5%
What are the most common types in adults?	1. Malignant fibrous histiocytoma 2. Liposarcoma (20%)
What are the most common types in children?	1. Rhabdomyosarcoma (50%) 2. Fibrosarcoma (20%)
What is Stewart-Treves syndrome?	An angiosarcoma that develops in an edematous extremity, classically following radical mastectomy and axillary lymph node dissection for breast cancer

How do sarcomas invade locally?

Usually along anatomic planes, such as fascia and vessels

What are the steps in diagnostic evaluation?

Extensive imaging workup:
1. X-ray of the affected part; look for soft tissue calcifications and for bony destruction or remodeling
2. Local MRI/CT (MRI allows for better soft tissue contrast and for multiplanar images)
3. Chest CT, CXR
4. Biopsy

What type of biopsy is indicated for STSs less than 3 cm?

Excisional biopsy

What type of biopsy is indicated for STSs greater than 3 cm?

Incisional biopsy

How is incision biopsy performed?

If the tumor is on an extremity, the incision should be made **parallel** to the longitudinal axis of the extremity. If it is not on an extremity, the incision should follow the direction of the underlying muscle fibers. The incision should be made over the most prominent part of the tumor, taking the most direct route possible. The major vessels and nerves should not be disturbed when approaching the tumor mass, because the biopsy tract must later be encompassed by the definitive resection.

What is an adequate incisional biopsy specimen?

A 1 x 1 x 0.5 cm specimen is usually adequate. When obtaining the specimen, areas of necrosis should be avoided.

When is a core needle biopsy (CNBX) used?

To confirm metastatic sarcoma to the lung, liver, bone, and soft tissue
To avoid open biopsy of large, deep-seated, and/or unresectable tumors in the pelvis, mediastinum, and retroperitoneum

When is an open biopsy indicated and how is it performed?	If CNBX fails for a large, deep-seated tumor When performing an open biopsy, an attempt to establish a diagnosis may be made by frozen section. If the pathology is not definite, definitive therapy is usually deferred until after a tissue diagnosis is made. Exceptions are made for easily removable tumors.
What is the most common system of staging soft tissue sarcomas?	The American Joint Committee on Cancer, based on: 1. Tumor size 2. Tumor grade 3. Presence or absence of regional or distant metastases
What is the prognosis?	**Histologic grade** of the primary lesion is the most important factor. Also, size less than 5 cm and location in a distal extremity predict a better outcome.
What is the treatment of choice for localized soft tissue sarcomas?	Surgery with wide excision; radiation therapy is added for all high-grade STSs and for all low-grade STSs greater than 5 cm
What is a pseudocapsule and what is its importance?	It is the outer layer of a sarcoma that represents compressed malignant cells. Microscopic extensions of tumor cells invade through the pseudocapsule into adjacent structures. Thus, definitive therapy must include a wide margin of resection to account for this phenomenon.
What is a limited-margin excision?	Excision of the tumor and pseudocapsule, such that the margin is very close to the tumor
What are the indications for this procedure?	Excisional biopsy
What is a wide-margin (or wide local) excision?	Excision of the tumor and negative margins of normal tissue

What are the indications for this procedure?	Low-grade sarcoma Function-sparing therapy (e.g., limb-sparing therapy, sarcoma next to major functional structures that are to be spared)
What is a compartmental resection?	Removal of an entire anatomic compartment, including tendon, bone, nerves, and vessels
What determines the resectability of a soft tissue sarcoma?	Anatomic location Vascularity Invasiveness and adherence to surrounding structures Tissue plane destruction and scar formation from previous surgery

GENERAL SURGICAL PRINCIPLES

What type of resection should be performed?	En bloc resection: tumor mass and involved tissues, biopsy track, hematoma, and surrounding normal tissue should be removed as one piece.
What type of margins should be obtained?	Surgical free margins; with any surgical resection, the surgeon must weigh the relative value of wide free margins and of preservation of function, ideally
How should fascial planes be handled?	Preserve free fascial planes whenever possible. If a major nerve or vessel is close to the tumor but not involved, the sheath should be entered proximally and distally to the tumor mass. The contents of the sheath should be freed, thus allowing the sheath to be removed en bloc with the tumor.
How should dissection be approached?	Follow the path of least resistance. Dissect easier areas first, allowing improved exposure and mobilization of harder-to-reach areas.
What is the importance of surgical clips?	The sites of highest risk or recurrence should be marked with radiopaque clips for radiation therapy.

How can wound morbidity be minimized?	Handle tissues gently. Minimize intraoperative bleeding. Avoid leaving dead space in the wound. Avoid tension when closing the wound. Use drains as needed. Apply pressure on the wound and immobilize the involved structure.
When should a flap closure be performed?	When primary closure will not cover the entire wound or will not be tension free. The flap should be composed of tissue that has not been previously irradiated.
What are the risk factors for local recurrence?	High tumor grade Less than adequate margins Limb-sparing surgery Large size

STS OF THE EXTREMITIES

What is the general principle for local excision?	Longitudinal elliptical incision should encompass the biopsy site completely.
What is the general principle for compartmental resection?	Muscle resection is usually from origin to insertion.
What is the general principle for amputation?	When indicated, amputation should be above the joint proximal to the tumor. Sarcomas have a high propensity to spread along tissue planes, and involved fascia may be contiguous with the joint.
Which is better, radical excision (amputation) or limb-sparing therapy (wide local excision plus radiation therapy)?	The survival rates are the same, but limb-sparing therapy is associated with higher rates of local recurrence.
Which types are most common?	1. Liposarcoma 2. Malignant fibrous histiocytoma
What is the recommended surgical approach, midline or flank incision?	A midline incision is favored over a flank incision because it allows better control of blood supply to retroperitoneal sarcomas. The affected side should be raised by padding beneath the patient, and a midline incision should be made from the xiphoid to below the umbilicus.

Which approach is preferred: transperitoneal or extraperitoneal?

A transperitoneal approach provides better exposure than an extraperitoneal and allows for en bloc resection.

What type of incision is recommended in cases of diaphragmatic involvement?

A modified thoracoabdominal incision is preferred, and is made by extending the midline incision obliquely into one of the lower intercostal spaces.

What type of incision is recommended for sarcomas with lateral fixation in the greater or lesser pelvis?

An abdominopelvic incision is recommended. An incision from above or below the umbilicus to the pubic symphysis is made and then extended laterally from the symphysis to the midpoint of the inguinal ligament and continued vertically over the femoral vessels.

Is radiation therapy recommended for retroperitoneal sarcomas?

Yes, for both incompletely and completely resected tumors; however, the retroperitoneal location limits dose delivery, and radiation therapy should not be used in all cases.

What is the 5-year survival rate with complete resection?

Approximately 40%

What is the 5-year survival rate with incomplete resection?

Approximately 3% (compared with other locations, retroperitoneal sarcomas have the lowest 5-year survival rates)

Why do retroperitoneal sarcomas have such a poor prognosis?

Large size—by the time of diagnosis, retroperitoneal sarcomas have grown large because they are hidden in the abdominal cavity
Difficulty of resection
Difficulty of attaining adequate radiation therapy

What is the risk of local recurrence?

Ten-year survival rate of 90%

RADIATION THERAPY

What are the complications?	Poor wound healing (preoperative radiation) Fractures Fibrosis Nerve/vascular damage Limb edema
What are the theoretical advantages of preoperative radiation?	Decreased vascular seeding/ autotransplantation of tumor cells at the time of operation Decreased tumor mass Decreased size of radiation field (versus postoperative radiation) (The volume of tissue that is to be irradiated preoperatively is planned based on clinical and radiographic data. The postoperative radiation field includes the original tumor volume plus all of the surgically manipulated tissues.)
What are the disadvantages of preoperative radiation?	Poor wound healing (compared with postoperative radiation) Poor histologic sample Delay in definitive resection
What are the advantages of postoperative radiation?	No delay in wound healing Better pathologic classification and staging No delay in removal of the tumor
What steps should be taken to prepare for postoperative radiation?	Radiopaque clips should be placed at the resection margins during surgery to guide the radiation oncologist.
Is preoperative or postoperative radiation therapy preferred for local recurrence?	In general, preoperative radiation is better for local recurrences. A twice-operated field has more anatomic distortion and therefore responds less readily to radiation therapy.

PULMONARY METASTASES

What is the appropriate treatment?	Isolated pulmonary metastases may be resected. Aggressive resection of pulmonary involvement improves survival.

What factors are associated with an improved prognosis?	Slower doubling time Unilateral disease On CT, 3 nodules or less
Is pneumonectomy indicated?	No; the procedure is associated with a higher mortality rate than single- or multiple-wedge resections

MALIGNANT FIBROUS HISTIOCYTOMA (MFH)

What is it?	A sarcoma that originates from fibroblastic cells (histiocytes)
Where does it present?	Most commonly in the deep soft tissues of the extremities and in the abdominal/retroperitoneal areas
How common is it?	It accounts for approximately 20% of all cases of adult STS. Pleomorphic MFH is the most common postradiation sarcoma.
What is the rate of local recurrence?	Approximately 25%
What are the routes of metastases?	Via blood (majority of cases), most commonly to the lung (90% of cases) Via lymphatics (rare)
What is the appropriate treatment?	Radical surgery plus adjunctive radiation therapy or chemotherapy

LIPOSARCOMA

What is it?	A sarcoma that originates from adipose cells
What is the usual presentation?	More common in men than women Often develops singularly in the thigh or retroperitoneum, but may be multicentric Rarely found in subcutaneous tissue
What is unique about this type of sarcoma?	Common adult soft tissue sarcoma (23%) Largest sarcoma (on average) Most common retroperitoneal sarcoma

Describe the various types.	Well-differentiated—does not metastasize; extensive local recurrence; 10-year survival rate between 40% and 60%; may de-differentiate Myxoid Pleomorphic/round cell—metastasizes early; poor prognosis (< 20% 5-year survival rate)
What is the appropriate treatment?	Surgery plus radiation therapy

RHABDOMYOSARCOMA (RMS)

What is it?	A sarcoma that originates from skeletal muscle cells
How common is it?	Embryonal RMS is the most common soft tissue sarcoma in infants and children
Describe the various types.	**Embryonal**—one of the "malignant small blue cell" tumors of children; occurs in the first 2 decades of life; presents in the head, neck, or GU regions **Alveolar**—seen in teenagers/young adults **Pleomorphic**—rare; seen in adults
Name the other "malignant round blue cell" tumors.	Lymphoma, Ewing sarcoma, and neuroblastoma
What is sarcoma botryoides?	An embryonal RMS consisting of grape-like masses that involve the mucosal surface or tubular viscera
What percentage of patients with RMS have lymph node metastases?	Approximately 10%
What percentage of patients with RMS have distant metastatic disease at diagnosis?	Approximately 30%

What is the appropriate treatment of localized (stage I) RMS?	Complete surgical resection plus adjuvant chemotherapy
What is the appropriate treatment of advanced (stage II or higher) RMS?	Combined modality therapy involving surgical resection, radiation therapy, and chemotherapy is indicated. It the tumor is considered initially unresectable, primary chemotherapy, or primary chemotherapy with radiation therapy may be administered, followed by surgery and adjuvant chemotherapy.
What is the 5-year survival rate for embryonal RMS?	Between 80% and 90%
What is the 5-year survival rate for alveolar RMS?	Aproximately 50%

FIBROSARCOMA

What is it?	A sarcoma originating from inter/intramuscular fibrous tissues, fascial tendons, and aponeuroses
How common is it?	Second most common sarcoma in children; less common in adults
What type of patient is at greatest risk?	Black men
What is the usual presentation?	Occurs most frequently in the deep soft tissues of the extremities
What is the 5-year survival rate?	Approximately 50%
What is the appropriate treatment?	Wide excision plus radiation therapy

DESMOID TUMORS

What are they?	Benign fibrous tumors occurring in fascial tissues; may occur in areas of previous scarring

What is the most common location?	The anterior abdominal wall
Is this type of tumor likely to metastasize?	No; desmoid tumors are nonencapsulated and spread by local invasion
What are the possible complications?	Pain, intestinal/ureteral obstruction, fistulas
What is the appropriate treatment?	Wide surgery excision; chemotherapy and radiation therapy, when surgery may cause major disability or require sacrifice of functionally important structures
What is the prognosis?	Likelihood of local recurrence is high (19%–77% with adequate margins; 90% with minimal margins)
With what syndrome are desmoid tumors associated?	Gardner syndrome (familial adenomatous polyposis)—an autosomal-dominant disease characterized by adenomatous polyps of the colon and rectum, epidermal cysts, desmoid tumors, and osteomas If untreated, patients almost always develop adenocarcinoma of the colon.

KAPOSI SARCOMA (KS)

What is it?	A vascular sarcoma involving endothelial cell proliferation with reactive lymphoreticular elements
How does it usually present?	Begins as blue to purple patches, which become plaques and nodules
Describe the various types.	**Classic**—affects patients of Mediterranean and European–Jewish ancestry **African**—affects young black men in the sub-Sahara **Iatrogenic/immunosuppressed**—affects renal transplant recipients **Epidemic**—affects HIV-positive individuals (AIDS)

How do the classic and epidemic forms differ in presentation?

The classic type affects elderly males on their lower extremities, with only occasional visceral involvement. The epidemic type has a preferential distribution in the head, neck, and truncal areas, with oral/perioral mucosal involvement in 55% of cases.

How do they differ in prognosis?

Classic KS is slowly progressive, and a 10- to 15-year survival rate is average. Epidemic KS is rarely the cause of death in HIV-positive individuals, and its treatment is palliative.

What is the appropriate treatment of localized lesions?

Local radiation therapy or intralesional vinblastine

What is the appropriate treatment of disseminated KS?

Chemotherapy plus immunotherapy

How often does GI involvement occur in epidemic KS?

Approximately 40% of cases

What are the associated signs/symptoms of GI involvement?

Abdominal pain, massive hemorrhage, perforation, malabsorption, protein-losing enteropathy, bowel obstruction, obstructive jaundice, tenesmus, ulcerative colitis–like syndrome, or dysphagia

What is the most common tumor associated with AIDS?

Kaposi sarcoma

43

Melanoma

D. David Graham, MD

From what embryologic tissue do melanocytes arise?

Neural crest cells

Where do melanocytes reside in normal skin?

In the basal layer of the epidermis

What is malignant melanoma?

A malignant neoplasm arising from melanocytes

How common is melanoma?

It is the eighth most common cancer diagnosis in the United States, accounting for 1% of all cancer deaths.

In terms of patient age, what group of patients is most affected by melanoma?

The mean age for diagnosis is 48 years; the large majority (81%) present between 25 and 65 years of age.

Describe the change in incidence of melanoma over the past several decades.

The incidence in the United States has been on the rise over the past several decades (1/1500 lifetime risk in 1935 to 1/150 in 1985). The projected **lifetime** risk in the year 2000 is between 1/75 and 1/90.

Currently, how many new cases occur annually?

Approximately 34,000

Describe the population generally at most risk for melanoma.

The majority of melanomas arise in patients with fair skin, blue eyes, freckles, and red or blond hair.

Name some of the known risk factors for melanoma.

Sun exposure, dysplastic nevus syndrome, xeroderma pigmentosum, history of non-melanoma skin cancer, high socioeconomic status, and a family history of melanoma

What chromosomal abnormalities have been associated with melanoma?

Abnormalities of chromosomes 1, 6, and 9 have been implicated.

What type of nevi are at risk of melanoma transformation?

Dysplastic nevi

What is dysplastic nevus syndrome?

It is an autosomal dominant disorder characterized by the presence of hundreds of nevi, which tend to be large, have variations in color, show indistinct borders, and usually remain macular.

What is the risk of developing melanoma with this syndrome?

The probability that a single dysplastic nevus will become a melanoma is small, but in a patient with dysplastic nevus syndrome and a family history of melanoma, the risk of developing melanoma approaches 100%.

What are the clinical characteristics of xeroderma pigmentosum?

It is clinically characterized by skin aging and a predisposition to cutaneous neoplasms.

What is the environmental factor most associated with melanoma?

Sun exposure (i.e, UV radiation)

What evidence implicates sun exposure as a risk for melanoma?

Although prospective, randomized trials of factor sun exposure in humans do not exist, epidemiologic evidence includes the following: 98% of melanomas in the United States occur in white patients; the incidence of melanoma is increased at lower latitudes; most melanoma arises on sun-exposed areas; the increase in melanoma in the United States is coincident with a greater emphasis on outdoor leisure and sun-tanning during the past several decades; and a history of severe sunburn in childhood has been associated, although weakly, with the subsequent development of melanoma.

Where do most melanomas arise from?

The majority of melanomas arise de novo, but they may arise from pre-existing nevi in 10% to 50% of cases.

What is the usual presentation?

Melanoma usually presents as a pigmented skin lesion that has recently changed. Lesions usually have irregular borders; variegated pigmentation ranging from pink to blue to black; and a raised, irregular surface.

What are some characteristics of advanced lesions?

These lesions may present with itching and bleeding, presumably signaling that the lesion has invaded into the cutaneous nerve plexus or superficial capillary bed. Such lesions may also be ulcerated.

What should one look for in examining a patient for melanoma?

ABCD—Asymmetry of pigmentation, **B**order irregularity, **C**olor variation, **D**iameter (usually > 6 mm or increasing in size)

What is an amelanotic melanoma?

Occurs when malignant transformation of the melanocyte results in loss of pigment production

Patients present with nonpigmented melanomas, which may go unnoticed and untreated for an extended period of time.

Are these melanomas more aggressive than other pigmented lesions?

Perhaps; absence of pigment may be an indication of a poorly differentiated state that may be more aggressive

What body sites are generally involved in melanoma?

Skin—90%
Unknown primary—5%
Ocular—2% to 5%
Mucous membranes (anus)—1%
Visceral sites—less than 0.1%

Describe the metastatic patterns of melanoma.

After resection of a primary lesion, the patient may experience recurrence of disease locally, regionally, or systemically.

What is local recurrence?

A tumor that is less than 5 cm from the primary site (occurs in about 16% of cases); the risk of local recurrence is a function of tumor thickness and adequacy of excision.

What is regional recurrence?

Typically, lymph node metastases, which are the most common manifestation of recurrent melanoma

What are the most common sites of distant metastases in melanoma?

The lungs and liver

Name the four major histologic types of melanomas in order from most common to least common.

Superficial spreading—70%
Nodular melanoma—15% to 30%
Lentigo maligna melanoma—less than 10%
Acral lentiginous melanoma—less than 10%

Describe the growth pattern of superficial spreading melanoma.

The most common forms of melanoma grow radially for months to years, with little or no surface elevation. They eventually enter a vertical growth phase, with a nodular component becoming evident.

Is nodular melanoma more common in men or women?

Men; it appears first as a nodule with a vertical growth phase, lacking a radial growth phase. It is usually diagnosed when thick, and carries a correspondingly less-favorable prognosis than the superficial spreading type.

From what classic lesion does lentigo maligna melanoma typically arise?

This type of melanoma is more common in the elderly and in women. It typically arises from a lentigo: a macular brown lesion that is often large in diameter and has been present for many years (**Hutchinson freckle**).

On what sites do acral lentiginous melanomas usually arise?

The lesions are histologically similar to superficial spreading and lentigo maligna melanoma, with a prolonged radial growth phase. They most commonly arise on the glabrous (nonhairbearing) skin of the palms and soles, in a subungual site, or on mucous membranes.

What is the most important screening practice for patients with melanoma?

History and physical examination; approximately 80% of management and follow-up of patient's first recurrences are to local or distant skin or to regional nodes, and are best identified by physical examination of the primary site, skin, and draining nodal basins.

In general, how can tumor-involved nodes be distinguished from reactive nodes?

Tumor-involved nodes usually are nontender, round, and hard. They can be detected at 1 to 2 cm, but can be much larger. Reactive nodes may also be palpable, but are usually oblong, tender, and rubbery. They are not usually larger than 2 cm.

In a patient with a history of a primary melanoma, what should be done in the case of palpable nodes?

A complete lymph node dissection may be performed if suspicion is high. If the nodes appear reactive, FNA may be performed on the most prominent node, or the patient's node status should be followed closely on a monthly basis until the nodes resolve or increase in size. If they change or if they are still present after 2 to 3 months, an FNA or excisional biopsy should be performed.

Is FNA reliable in the diagnosis of indeterminate palpated masses in melanoma patients?

Yes; a skilled pathologist and clinician can obtain accuracy rates for positive cytology in more than 90% of cases.

What radiologic evaluation is useful in the initial workup of a patient with melanoma?

A CXR is a useful and cost-effective screening tool to detect hematogenous metastases. Remember that one of the most common visceral sites of metastatic disease is the lung.

Are any blood tests useful as screening tests in the initial workup of a patient with melanoma?

Yes; liver function tests, particular LDH or alkaline phosphatase, are useful and cost-effective screening tests for hepatic metastases, which are the second most common visceral sites of metastatic melanoma.

Are additional studies, such as CT scans of the brain, chest, and abdomen; bone scans; MRI, or liver–spleen scans indicated as part of the initial workup of melanoma patients?

No; such tests performed simply for staging purposes are not cost effective. Distant metastases not found by history and physical examination, CXR, or LFTs are rare. Only 5% to 10% of first metastases are located outside the local site, regional nodes, lung, or liver. CT scan, MRI, bone scan, and liver–spleen scan should be reserved for patients with specific symptoms, such as bone pain, or with clinical evidence of metastatic disease.

What are the four stages of the AJCC staging system for melanoma?

I—Localized; less than 1.5 mm thick
II—Localized; greater than 1.5 mm thick
III—Nodal metastases involving only one regional nodal basin or one to four in-transit nodes
IV—Advanced regional metastases or any distant metastases

What is the principal prognostic factor associated with melanoma?

Breslow thickness

How is Breslow thickness measured?

From skin surface to the deepest point of invasion

How is thickness related to prognosis?

Thin lesions (< 0.76 mm) have the best prognosis (< 10% mortality at 10 years); intermediate lesions (0.76–4.0 mm) have an intermediate prognosis; thick lesions, (> 4.0 mm) have the worst prognosis (> 50% mortality at 10 years).

What is the Clark lesion based on?

Level of invasion into and through the layers of the skin

Describe Clark levels I through V.

I—In situ melanoma confined to the epidermis (i.e, above the basement membrane)
II—Invasion into the papillary dermis
III—Invasion through the papillary dermis, without invasion into the reticular dermis
IV—Distinct invasion into the reticular dermis

V—Invasion through all layers of the dermis and into the subcutaneous tissue

How is Clark level related to prognosis?

Lesions with a higher Clark's level are more invasive and carry a less-favorable prognosis.

What other factors affect the prognosis of patients with melanoma?

Ulceration, primary site, histologic type, age, gender, and race

How do each of these factors affect prognosis?

Ulceration—ulcerated lesions have a poor prognosis

Primary site—Extremity lesions have a better prognosis than axial lesions. Mucous membrane lesions have a poor prognosis.

Histologic pattern—Acral lentiginous is associated with a poorer prognosis than superficial spreading and nodular melanoma, which have a slightly poorer prognosis than lentigo maligna melanoma. Much of this difference, however, is explained by thickness of the lesion.

Age—In a number of studies, advanced age has been associated with independent increased risk of death owing to malignancy.

Gender—Women have a slightly increased risk of melanoma, but have an improved outcome compared with men. Part of this decreased risk is explained by the fact that women are more likely to develop lesions on an extremity than are men.

Race—White patients are more likely to develop melanoma than African-American patients, but African-American patients who develop melanoma have a markedly poorer prognosis.

Are acral melanomas (palms, soles of feet, subungual) more common in African-American patients than are other cutaneous lesions?

Yes; 17% of patients with acral melanomas are black, compared with less than 1% for other cutaneous melanomas

Which mucous membrane sites are commonly affected by melanoma?

Melanomas of the mucous membranes are roughly equally divided among the oral and nasal mucosae, anorectum, and the female genital tract.

Are such lesions common?

No; they account for approximately 1% of all melanomas

What percentage of melanomas are ocular lesions?

Between 2% and 5%

Where in the eye does ocular melanoma occur?

In the uveal tract (iris, ciliary body, and chorioid), the conjunctiva, or the retina

What is the most common site of metastasis from an ocular-tract lesion?

The liver; the uveal tract lacks lymphatic drainage

Are visceral primaries common among melanoma patients?

No; they account for less than 0.1% of all melanomas

What sites have been reported as sites of visceral primaries?

Adrenals, lung, and esophagus

What percentage of melanomas present as metastases from unknown primaries?

Approximately 5%

How do most unknown primaries present?

With lymph node metastases

What is the appropriate management of such lesions?

Cutaneous, ocular, or mucous membrane primary lesions must be ruled out. Then, metastases must be treated, usually by resection.

How can an occult primary be ruled out?

Thorough examination of the skin, including the scalp, subungual and volar surfaces of the hands and feet, anorectum (proctoscopy and anoscopy), female genital tract, perineum, oropharynx, nasopharynx, sinuses, conjunctivae, and eyes

How does the prognosis of a patient with an unknown primary compare with that of a patient with a known primary?	Prognosis is equivalent to or improved in patients with a similar extent of disease and a known primary, compared with patients with an unknown primary.
How is the diagnosis of the primary lesion typically made?	Full-thickness biopsy is advised wherever there is suspicion of melanoma in a skin lesion. A punch or incisional biopsy may be used in cases of large lesions or lesions in cosmetically relevant areas (e.g., face).
Is cautery or freezing a reasonable option for treating lesions such as primary melanoma?	No; destructive treatments prevent histologic evaluation and leave the patient at risk of developing metastatic disease without adequate staging
Once the diagnosis of melanoma has been made, how should the primary lesion be treated?	A wide local excision should be performed to reduce the risk of local recurrence.
How wide should the excision be?	Based on randomized, prospective comparisons, most investigators and clinicians believe that margins of 2 to 3 cm or less are adequate for most lesions.
What are the advantages or theoretical advantages of an elective lymph node dissection (ELND)?	May cure the disease if micrometastases are in the nodes, but not yet in distant sites May prevent the need for future surgery or palliation that comes with the development of significant nodal disease Provides prognostic information
What are the disadvantages of an ELND?	May hinder the patient's immune response to the tumor Lymphedema, complications
What surgical complications are associated with an ELND?	The most common complication is wound infection. Another notable complication is lymphedema, which is particularly frequent in the lower extremities following a groin dissection.

Is an ELND indicated in patients with thin melanomas (< 0.76 mm)?

No; these lesions have such a low risk of recurrence and mortality (up to 5% recurrence rate) that any potential benefit from ELND would be very small.

Is an ELND indicated in patients with thick melanomas (> 4.0 mm)?

No; thick melanomas metastasize so frequently to distant sites that resection of clinically negative nodes is not considered likely to alter the risk of mortality. Studies have documented that ELND for lesions thicker than 4 mm does not have an impact on patient outcome.

Is an ELND indicated in patients with melanomas of intermediate thickness (0.76–4.0 mm)?

The issue is controversial. Data from retrospective studies show no survival benefit for patients with similar lesions who undergo ELND versus those who do not. Also, a number of prospective, randomized trials have failed to show any survival benefit associated with ELND.

How is an ELND prognostically valuable?

A patient's prognosis is substantially worse if an ELND reveals tumor-involved nodes.

How is lymphoscintigraphy useful as a guide to ELND?

Technetium-99 antimony sulfur colloid is used as a means of mapping the lymphatic drainage of a primary site and, therefore, determining the nodal basins of ELND.

What is the sentinel node concept?

A novel approach to ELND that involves identifying the first node in the draining basin to which the lesion will drain (sentinel node), followed by selective node dissection, if that node contains metastases.

Is the sentinel node approach useful in the management of melanoma?

Preliminary results suggest that the false-negative rate for sentinel node biopsy is approximately 2%. Clinical trials begun recently should indicate whether or not improvement is noted.

Is chemotherapy useful in the adjuvant mode for melanoma patients?

No; its use is reserved for treatment of unresectable advanced disease

What is the most active single chemotherapeutic agent in the treatment of melanoma?

Dacarbazine (DTIC), with an overall response rate of up to 20%

What is the most successful chemotherapeutic regimen to date?

DTIC, BCNU, cisplatin, and tamoxifen

Is melanoma radiosensitive?

Melanoma is considered to be weakly radiosensitive.

What types of immunotherapy have been used in the treatment of melanoma?

Specific active immunotherapy (i.e, vaccination) is currently used experimentally in the adjuvant mode for patients at high risk of recurrence after complete excision of primary and/or regional disease. Adoptive immunotherapy with lymphokine-activated killer (LAK) cells, with or without IL-2, has shown a modest 20% response rate. Use of cytokines alone, such as IL-2, has shown results similar to those of LAK cell trials. As primary therapy for advanced disease, α- and γ-interferon have demonstrated 10% to 15% response rates. Therapy with monoclonal antibodies has also been attempted, but the results have been disappointing.

True or false: the survival rate after melanoma that occurs during pregnancy is worse than that of nonpregnant patients with melanoma?

False; recent reports have indicated that although patients who present with melanoma during pregnancy may have a predilection to develop lymph node metastases, survival of these patients is comparable to that of matched controls.

What mortality rate is associated with pulmonary metastases?

Pulmonary metastases are associated with a 70% mortality rate within 1 year and a 4% five-year survival rate.

How should isolated pulmonary metastases be managed?

A new lung nodule on the CXR of a melanoma patient may be resected by thoracotomy, biopsied by transthoracic needle aspiration, or monitored. Isolated pulmonary metastases may be resected.

Are GI metastases common in melanoma patients?

No; they are considered rare

How are GI metastases generally discovered?

Usually, they cause bleeding, intussusception, or small bowel obstruction

In the melanoma patient with blood per rectum and negative upper and lower endoscopy, which diagnostic test should be performed next?

Enteroclysis, for visualization of the small bowel

What is the appropriate therapy for patients with symptomatic metastases?

GIGI metastases are often associated with unresectable disease, but resection of intussuscepting, bleeding, or obstructing lesions may provide significant palliation.

44

Critical Care Medicine

Donald B. Schmit, MD
A Lucktong, MD

NEUROLOGIC SYSTEM

What are the components of the Glasgow Coma Scale (GCS)?

Eye opening (remember: "four eyes")
  Spontaneous—4
  To verbal command—3
  To noxious stimuli—2
  No response—1
Verbal response
  Oriented and conversant—5
  Disoriented and conversant—4
  Inappropriate words—3
  Incomprehensible sounds—2
  No response—1
  Intubated—T
Motor response (remember: "six cylinder")
  Obeys verbal commands—6
  Localizes to pain—5
  Withdrawals to pain—4
  Abnormal flexion to pain (decorticate rigidity)—3
  Extension to pain (decerebrate rigidity)—2
  No response—1

What are the three most important prognostic indicators in head injury?

1. Age
2. GCS score
3. Severity of injury on head CT

What is the exception to the previous question?

Early decompression of a subdural or epidural bleed can dramatically improve prognosis.

What is the appropriate management of increased intracranial pressure (ICP)?

Hyperventilation
Elevation of the head of the bed
Sedation
Placing the head in the midline position, reverse Trendelenburg if the spine is OK

Making sure the cervical collar is not too tight
Administration of mannitol, furosemide
Fever suppression
Barbiturate coma
Ventriculostomy, when indicated
Craniectomy, when indicated

What are the determinants of cerebral perfusion pressure (CPP)?

CPP = MAP – ICP

What are the goals in ICP monitoring?

CPP > 60 mm Hg
ICP < 20 mm Hg

What are the determinants of brain death?

(Check your hospital's protocol). Basics:
Lack of brain-stem reflexes
Lack of motor response to noxious stimuli (excluding spinal reflexes)
Lack of pupillary light reflex
Lack of vestibulo-ocular reflexes
Apnea (Pco_2 > 60 mm Hg)

What other restrictions apply?

No narcotics, sedatives, anesthetics
No muscle relaxants
Lack of severe metabolic dysfunction
Normothermia

RESPIRATORY SYSTEM

Define tidal volume (V_T).

The volume of gas exchanged in one "normal" breath

What is "normal" V_T (1) when breathing spontaneously, and (2) when mechanically ventilated?

1. Between 7 and 8 cc/kg
2. Between 10 and 15 cc/kg

Define vital capacity (VC).

The volume of maximal inspiration

Wnat is normal VC?

Between 30 and 70 cc/kg

Define functional residual capacity (FRC).

The volume remaining in the lungs following passive expiration

What is normal FRC? Between 15 and 30 cc/kg

Define minute ventilation (V_E). The volume of gas exchanged in 1 minute (V_T x respiratory rate)

What is normal V_E? Between 100 and 150 cc/kg

What are the two main modes of positive pressure ventilation?
1. Volume cycled
2. Pressure cycled

Describe continuous mandatory ventilation (CMV). A preset volume of gas is delivered at a fixed rate. This process is completely independent of patient effort, and breaths by the patient are neither supported nor allowed. **This mode is no longer used on modern ventilators.**

Describe intermittent mandatory ventilation (IMV). Similar to CMV in that it still uses a fixed volume and rate, but patient breaths in between fixed breaths are allowed (although not essential)

Describe synchronized intermittent mandatory ventilation (SIMV). Like CMV and IMV, it uses a fixed V_T and fixed rate. Like IMV, unassisted patient breaths are allowed. Spontaneous breaths and mandatory breaths are coordinated to avoid breath stacking. This method has largely replaced CMV and IMV on most modern ICU ventilators.

Describe assist control (AC) ventilation. Another volume-cycled mode of ventilation in which the patient initiates a breath, and the ventilator delivers a predefined volume of gas (the patient sets the rate). If the patient's rate of ventilation falls below a preset minimum, the ventilator automatically defaults to IMV.

Describe pressure support ventilation (PSV). In this pressure-cycled mode of ventilation, the ventilator delivers a set inspiratory pressure when the patient initiates a breath and holds this pressure constant as long as the inspiratory effort continues. The patient sets the rate, and the V_T is then determined by the inspiratory time, the amount of pressure support, and the pulmonary compliance.

Describe pressure control ventilation (PCV).

The pressure-cycled equivalent to AC ventilation; again, the patient is allowed to control the ventilatory rate, but the ventilator delivers a set inspiratory pressure (rather than volume) with each breath.

Describe mandatory minute ventilation (MMV).

PSV with a backup SIMV setting to assure adequate V_E

What is PEEP and why is it used?

Positive end expiratory pressure (PEEP) is the maintenance of a low level of circuit pressure during the expiratory phase of ventilation, typically in the 5 to 15 cm H_2O range. PEEP helps prevent alveolar and small airway collapse that might otherwise occur at the end of expiration.

What is auto-PEEP?

Physiologic gas trapping in the alveoli, producing PEEP, usually because of inadequate expiratory time (patients with COPD are particularly prone to this condition)

What is CPAP and why is it used?

Continuous positive airway pressure (CPAP) maintains a set airway pressure during all phases of respiration (not just expiration, as in PEEP). CPAP is typically used for patients breathing spontaneously to increase FRC.

What are the four major complications of mechanical ventilation?

1. Barotrauma, pneumothorax
2. Nosocomial pneumonia
3. Tracheal injury/subglottic stenosis due to chronic intubation
4. Cardiac dysfunction, typically due to decreased venous return from increased intrathoracic pressures (especially common with increased levels of PEEP [> 10 cm H_2O])

What is the incidence of pneumonia in ventilator-dependent patients?

Approximately 30%

What is the mechanism of injury in ventilator barotrauma?

Studies have demonstrated that the injury is primarily caused by alveolar overdistention, which typically occurs as a result of excessive tidal volumes, not simply high-peak airway pressures ("volutrauma").

What is controlled hypoventilation?

Also known as permissive hypercapnia, this strategy to avoid ventilator-induced lung injury uses lower V_T to maintain lower plateau airway pressures, often resulting in increased Pco_2.

What is ARDS?

Adult respiratory distress syndrome (ARDS) is a form of acute lung injury resulting in:
Impaired oxygenation (Pao_2/Fio_2 ratio > 200, regardless of PEEP)
Noncardiogenic pulmonary edema
Bilateral infiltrates on CXR (diffuse, fluffy)

What is the pathophysiology of ARDS?

Diffuse alveolar damage
Disruption of the endothelial barrier
Transudation of fluid into the pulmonary interstitium
Decreased effective lung volume
Impaired gas exchange
Increased dead-space ventilation

What common factors predispose patients to ARDS?

Aspiration, inhalation injury, sepsis, multiple trauma, massive transfusions

What is the mortality rate?

Between 40% and 50%, mostly from the predisposing illness

How is the diagnosis made?

CXR: bilateral, diffuse pulmonary infiltrates
CT: patchy areas of normal lung may be present
ABG: initial respiratory alkalosis with hypoxemia that is resistant to increased Fio_2
Increasing Pao_2/Fio_2 ratio, reflecting the increasingly poor gas exchange
Pulmonary capillary wedge pressures: may be normal despite pulmonary edema

What is the appropriate treatment?	Controversial: Mechanical ventilation Early fluid restriction and diuresis Frequent repositioning to best perfuse ventilated alveoli (decrease V/Q mismatch) Empiric antibiotics, if sepsis is suspected Treatment of underlying condition (e.g., sepsis)

CARDIOVASCULAR SYSTEM

What is the formula for cardiac output (CO)?	CO = heart rate x stroke volume
What is the formula for cardiac index (CI)?	$CI = \dfrac{(HR \times SV)}{[BSA]}$ body surface area
What is the normal range of CI?	Between 2.5 and 3.5 $L/min/M^2$
What is the formula for mean arterial pressure (MAP)?	$\dfrac{(SBP - DBP)}{3} + DBP$
What is the formula for systemic vascular resistance index (SVRI)?	SVRI = [(MAP − CVP)/CI] x 80
What is the normal range for SVRI?	2000 ± 400 dyne-sec/cm^5
In what states is SVRI elevated?	Cardiogenic shock, hypovolemic shock, hypertension, vasoconstrictor therapy
In what states is SVRI decreased?	Septic shock, neurogenic shock, thyrotoxicosis, vasodilator therapy, cirrhosis
What is the formula for the oxygen content of blood?	$CaO_2 = 1.36 \times HB \times SaO_2 + PaO_2 \times (0.003)$ (that is, the amount of oxygen bound to Hb plus the amount dissolved in plasma)
In what two ways can a Swan-Ganz (PA) catheter be used to assess CO?	1. Directly, by thermodilution 2. Indirectly, by measuring P_VO_2 (mixed venous oxygen)

What does P_vO_2 measure?	The amount of oxygen remaining in the blood as it returns from the body; assesses the adequacy of oxygen delivery in meeting the metabolic demands of the body
What is the normal P_vO_2?	Greater than 35 mm Hg is excellent Less than 25 mm Hg is extremely poor
What are the potential complications of PA catheterization?	Arrhythmias Pulmonary infarctions (usually small) Infection PA rupture
What is the most common symptom of PA rupture?	Hemoptysis (> 90%)

INOTROPIC AGENTS

DOPAMINE

What is the site of action and effect of each of the following doses:	
Low dose (1–3 μg/ kg°min)?	++Dopaminergic agonist: Renal vasodilation causes increased renal flow ("renal dose dopamine")
Intermediate dose (5–10 μg/kg°min)?	+ α, ++ β: Positive inotropy and chronotropy, as well as some vasoconstriction
High dose (> 10 μg/ kg°min)?	+++ α-agonist: Marked afterload increase because of arteriolar vasoconstriction Dopaminergic and β-adrenergic effects are still present, but usually overshadowed by α-adrenergic effects

DOBUTAMINE

What is the site of action?	+++ $β_1$-agonist
How does it act?	Increases inotropy, decreases afterload (SVR), mildly increases chronotropy, which can lead to increased myocardial oxygen demand (MVO_2)

What is the usual dosage?	Between 5 and 15 μg/kg/min (tolerance to dobutamine develops in approximately 72 hours because of downregulation and uncoupling of β-adrenergic receptors)

MILRINONE

What is the site of action?	Phosphodiesterase III inhibitor (PDE III); decreases the breakdown of cAMP and therefore increases intracellular cAMP and intracellular calcium
How does it act?	Increases inotropy, **decreases afterload** (SVR), little or no increase in chronotropy with no net increase in MVO_2
What is the usual dosage?	**Load**—50 to 75 mcg/kg over 10 minutes **Maintenance**—0.375 to 0.7 μg/kg/min

ISOPROTERENOL

What is the site of action?	+++ $β_1$ and $β_2$ agonist
How does it act?	Increases inotropy, increases chronotropy (+ vasodilation of skeletal and mesenteric vascular beds)
What is the usual dosage?	**Load**—0.002 to 0.06 mg (watch for hypotension) **Maintenance**—0.5 to 10 μg/min

EPINEPHRINE

What is the site of action?	$α_1$, $α_2$, $β_1$, $β_2$ agonist
How does it act?	Increases inotropy, increases chronotropy (little change in blood pressure because of peripheral vasodilation at low doses [0.04–0.1 μg/kg/min]; can cause a marked increase in blood pressure at high doses)
What is the usual dosage?	Begin at 0.5 to 1 μg/min and titrate up to 8 to 12 μg/min

INTRAVENOUS ANTIHYPERTENSIVE AGENTS

NITROGLYCERIN (Ntg)

What is the site of action?	+++ venodilation, + arteriolar dilation
How does it act?	Increased venous capacitance and decreased preload
What is the usual dosage?	Between 5 and 100 μg/min

SODIUM NITROPRUSSIDE (SNP)

What is the site of action?	+++ venodilation, +++ arteriolar dilation
How does it act?	Decreased preload, decreased afterload (allowing for blood pressure titration)
What is the usual dosage?	Between 0.5 and 10 μg/kg/min
What are the possible side effects?	Hypotension, hypoxia (due to intrapulmonary shunting), cyanide toxicity (with prolonged infusions, > 48 hours)

ESMOLOL

What is the site of action?	β-adrenergic antagonist with very short half-life (≈ 9 min), which necessitates intravenous infusion, but allows it to be easily titrated
In what cases is it indicated?	1. Control of ventricular response rate in patients with atrial fibrillation and rapid ventricular response, or with other supraventricular tachyarrhythmias 2. Control of blood pressure (often in conjunction with SNP) in patients with hypertensive emergency or with aortic dissection
What is the usual dosage?	Load with 500 μg/kg/min for 1 minute, followed by maintenance infusion of 50 μg/kg/min for 4 minutes If response is insufficient, repeat loading infusion for 1 minute, then increase maintenance infusion to 100 μg/kg/min for 4 minutes Loading may be repeated and maintenance infusion rate increased to 200 μg/kg/min, as needed

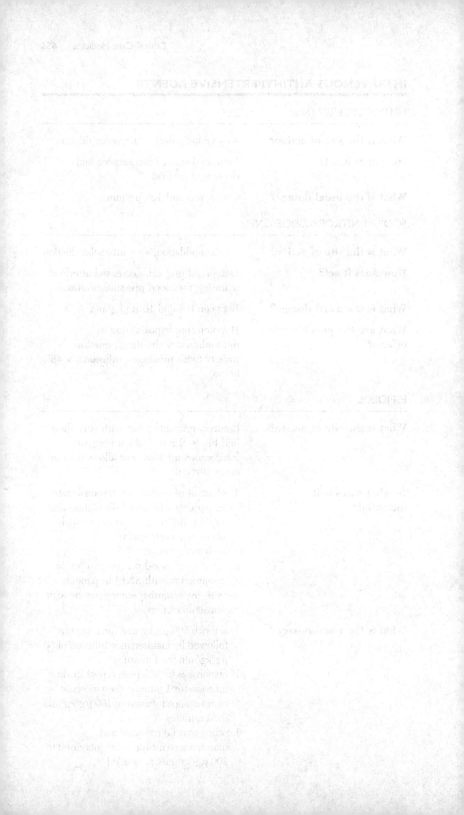

Section III

Subspecialty Surgery

45

Cardiac Surgery

Kirk J. Fleischer, MD

CONGENITAL HEART DISEASE

What is the incidence of congenital heart defects?

4 to 9 per 1000 live births

What three general physiologic disturbances are associated with congenital heart disease?

Left to right (L to R) shunts, R to L shunts, and ventricular outflow obstruction

Give examples of each type of defect.

1. L to R shunts: Ventricular septal defects (VSD), atrial septal defects (ASD), atrioventricular (AV) canal defects (i.e., "AV septal defects"), patent ductus arteriosus (PDA), truncus arteriosus, and aortopulmonary (AP) window
2. R to L shunts: Tetralogy of Fallot (TOF), tricuspid atresia, Ebstein anomaly, and pulmonary atresia
3. Ventricular outflow obstruction: Congenital aortic stenosis (AS), coarctation of the aorta, interrupted aortic arch, and congenital pulmonary stenosis (PS)

What are the three complex congenital defects (often classified as "bidirectional" shunts)?

Transposition of the great vessels, total anomalous pulmonary venous connection (TAPVC), and hypoplastic left heart syndrome. (TAPVC is sometimes classified as an L to R shunt.)

What are the three most common defects and their relative frequencies among all congenital heart defects?

1. VSD (30%–40%)
2. ASD (10%–15%)
3. PDA (10%–20%)

What defects have a relative incidence of 5% to 10%?	TOF, congenital PS, coarctation of the aorta, congenital AS, and transposition of the great vessels
What are the most common general INITIAL presentations of congenital heart lesions?	Congestive heart failure (CHF), cyanosis, and poor peripheral perfusion
Which presentation is classic for each of the classes of lesions?	CHF (acyanotic): L to R shunt, ventricular outflow obstruction Cyanosis: R to L shunt CHF and cyanosis: Complex defects. Rarely, shunts may also eventually develop into CHF, but cyanosis is the presenting sign.
How are these presentations diagnosed in the child?	CHF: Failure to thrive, tachycardia, tachypnea, hepatic enlargement (unlike adults, rales develop late) Cyanosis: Discoloration of the mucous membranes and skin
Which class of defects is characteristically associated with increased versus decreased pulmonary blood flow (PBF)?	Increased PBF: L to R shunts Decreased PBF: R to L shunts
Which shunt classically reverses if untreated, and what is the syndrome called?	L to R shunts; Eisenmenger syndrome (discussed later)
What are the basic causes of pulmonary hypertension?	1. Increased PBF 2. Obstruction of pulmonary venous drainage 3. Histopathologic changes in the pulmonary arterioles (medial hypertrophy in infants; intimal thickening and fibrosis in children and adults)
What are the common diagnostic studies for congenital heart disease, and what basic information is provided by each?	1. Chest x-ray (CXR): Gross chamber size, pulmonary vascularity and, occasionally, classic signs 2. Electrocardiogram (EKG): Chamber hypertrophy and rhythm

3. Echocardiogram with color-flow Doppler: Detailed cardiac anatomy, intracardiac flow characteristics of blood, and transvalvular gradients
4. Cardiac catheterization: Additional anatomic detail (some not visible on echocardiogram), chamber pressure, intracardiac flow characteristics of blood, transvalvular gradients, and oximetry

What is the general indication for surgery in patients with congenital heart defects?

When the morbidity and mortality rates associated with the surgical procedure are less than those of the defect or other forms of treatment

What are the other indications?

1. Worsening symptoms
2. Increasing hematocrit (Hct), suggesting worsening hypoxia
3. Echocardiographic or catheterization evidence of ventricular failure, increased shunting, increasing pulmonary vascular pressures, etc.
4. Any central nervous system (CNS) symptoms caused by emboli or significant cerebral hypoxia

Traditionally, patients with congenital heart defects undergo a palliative procedure to sustain them until they are large enough for corrective repair. What are the two basic palliative procedures and the general function of each?

1. Pulmonary artery banding: To reduce pulmonary blood flow and, thus, (a) prevent CHF and (b) reduce the risk of pulmonary vascular disease caused by reactive changes in the pulmonary vascular bed
2. Systemic to pulmonary shunt: To increase pulmonary blood flow and improve oxygenation.

As techniques and instruments improve, more defects are definitively repaired in the infant **without** an intervening palliative procedure.

What are the basic technical goals of definitive corrective surgery for congenital heart defects?

1. To separate the systemic and pulmonary circulatory systems (e.g., elimination of intracardiac shunts)
2. To relieve obstructions

Define open versus closed cardiac procedures.	Open procedures involve intracardiac lesions and require cardiopulmonary bypass (CPB). Closed procedures usually involve the great vessels (extracardiac) and do not require CPB.
What technique is often used for complex open procedures to provide a bloodless operative field?	Hypothermic circulatory arrest. The patient is cooled to 16°C to 18°C, much of the patient's blood is drained into the bypass pump, and perfusion is discontinued.
In which congenital heart defects is a PDA necessary for survival (until the primary lesion is repaired)?	1. Defects dependent on the PDA for systemic blood flow: interrupted aortic arch or severe coarctation of the aorta, hypoplastic left heart syndrome, and critical AS 2. Defects dependent on the PDA for pulmonary blood flow: Severe TOF and pulmonary atresia without VSD 3. Defects dependent on the PDA for mixing of blood: Transposition of the great vessels
How is the patency of the PDA maintained until surgery?	Prostaglandin E_1 infusion

ACYANOTIC CONGENITAL HEART DISEASE

What is the chronic ventricular response to the two classes of acyanotic lesions, and why?	L to R shunt: **Diastolic** overload resulting in ventricular **dilation** Obstructive lesion: **Systolic** overload resulting in ventricular **hypertrophy**
Compare the resultant anteroposterior CXR findings.	L to R shunts often have an enlarged cardiac silhouette; early obstructive lesions have a normal silhouette.
What are the main complications of L to R shunts?	CHF and pulmonary hypertension (± Eisenmenger syndrome)
What is the classic physical appearance of patients with L to R shunts, and why?	"Gracile habitus" (frail, thin, decreased muscular and bony development) because of decreased systemic blood flow associated with increased pulmonary flow

Which defects do patients with this habitus usually have?

VSD (most common), ASD, and PDA

CYANOTIC CONGENITAL HEART DISEASE

Compare the etiology of the central versus peripheral forms of cyanosis.

Central: Defect in oxygenation of the blood associated with an intracardiac shunt (i.e., congenital cardiac defect) **or** pulmonary lesion (e.g., pneumonia, atelectasis)

Peripheral: Vasoconstriction because of cold exposure or decreased cardiac output

What test may distinguish the causes of central cyanosis?

Hyperoxia test (100% oxygen for 15 minutes):

If PaO_2 << 150 mm Hg: Intracardiac lesion

If PaO_2 > 150 mm Hg: Pulmonary lesion

Also, pulmonary lesions tend to increase the $PaCO_2$ value, whereas the $PaCO_2$ value is usually normal in patients with an intracardiac shunt.

What are the four key factors in the development and severity of cyanosis?

Hemoglobin (Hgb) content of the blood, volume of venous blood that is shunted past the alveoli into the systemic circulation, oxygen consumption of the peripheral tissues, and aeration of the lungs

How is the Hgb content important?

The higher the Hgb content, the more hypoxic the patient must become before cyanosis is evident. The higher the Hgb content, the more intensely cyanotic the patient becomes, after reaching the stated threshold. If the Hgb level is very low, there will not be enough unsaturated Hgb to cause cyanosis.

What is the most common cyanotic congenital defect?

TOF (50% of cyanotic lesions)

Sequelae of Cyanotic Heart Disease

What are the classic sequelae of cyanotic heart disease?	Hypertrophic osteoarthropathy (clubbing), polycythemia, hypercyanotic spells, cerebrovascular accidents, brain abscesses, coagulation disorders, and endocarditis
What is hypertrophic osteoarthropathy?	Clubbing of digits (widened ends of digits because of capillary proliferation and AV malformations)
How long after the onset of cyanosis does clubbing develop?	6 to 12 months; however, clubbing is reversible with correction of the cyanotic lesion.
What is polycythemia?	Hct > 65%
Why does polycythemia develop?	Hypoxia stimulates the release of erythropoietin to increase the red cell mass (polycythemia is reversible with corrective surgery)
What are the potential complications of polycythemia?	Hyperviscosity of blood (i.e., "sludging"), with resultant tissue ischemia; hyperuricemia as a result of increased red blood cell production, with associated uric acid nephropathy and gout
What is the most common immediate cause of thrombosis in the setting of polycythemia?	Dehydration
What are hypercyanotic (or hypoxic) spells?	Abrupt increase in cyanosis associated with cerebral anoxia that may result in unconsciousness, seizure, or death
What is the usual mechanism of these spells?	Infundibular muscle spasm in the right ventricular (RV) outflow tract, resulting in a sudden reduction in blood flow to the lungs
What age-group is usually affected by these spells?	2 to 4 months

These spells are rare after what age?	5 to 6 years
These spells occur most frequently with which anomaly?	TOF ("tet" spells)
What are the mechanisms of cerebrovascular accidents in congenital heart disease?	Hypercyanotic spells, thrombosis associated with hyperviscosity, and embolic events (e.g., paradoxic emboli caused by intracardiac defect, septic emboli caused by endocarditis)
Why are brain abscesses common in patients with cyanotic heart disease?	R to L shunt permits venous blood to bypass the lungs, which are an important filter for bacteria.
What are the most common organisms in these abscesses?	Gram-positive cocci (staphylococcus and streptococcus)
Brain abscesses are most often seen with which anomaly?	TOF
Coagulation disorders have several contributing factors, but what is the most common treatment?	Phlebotomy
What is the hallmark physical finding of CHF in a child?	Hepatic enlargement
Why is CHF less common in patients with cyanotic heart defects?	There is usually only an R to L shunt, without diastolic volume overload or increased PBF

VENTRICULAR SEPTAL DEFECTS

What is the anatomic lesion?	Abnormal communication between the left and right ventricles
What are the locations ("types") of VSD?	Infundibular or canal septum (beneath the semilunar valves), membranous septum, inlet septum, and muscular septum

Which type is most common?

Membranous septum (80%–85%)

What region usually has multiple VSDs?

Muscular septum

What is a "large" VSD?

Diameter ≥ aortic orifice

What percentage of patients with VSD have additional congenital cardiac lesions?

> 50%

Give some examples of these lesions.

PDA, congenital AS, coarctation of the aorta, and complex defects (e.g., TOF, transposition of the great vessels)

What is the main physiologic problem in VSD?

L to R shunt, resulting in increased pulmonary blood flow

What primary factors determine the degree of shunting in VSDs?

Size of the VSD(s) and pulmonary vascular resistance (PVR). If the VSD is large, RV and left ventricular (LV) pressures equalize and the PVR becomes the major determinant.

What classic syndrome may develop if VSD is untreated?

Eisenmenger syndrome

Describe the murmur associated with VSD.

Harsh pansystolic murmur at the left sternal border

How does the intensity of the murmur change as the size of the VSD decreases?

Increases because of increased turbulence. Louder murmurs are often heard with smaller VSDs.

When do infants with large VSDs become symptomatic, and why?

6 weeks to 3 months. PVR must decrease from its high fetal baseline value before an L to R shunt is possible. (PVR does not reach the normal adult level until after 3 months of age.)

What diagnostic tests are performed, and what information is obtained from each?

1. Echocardiography: Size, number, and location of VSDs
2. Cardiac catheterization: PVR and pulmonary:systemic blood flow ratio (Q_p/Q_s)

What are the complications of VSD?	Large VSD: CHF and pulmonary hypertension Small VSD: Increased risk of endocarditis
Why is nonoperative management initially warranted in many cases?	Many patients (25%–50%) have spontaneous closure. The chance of closure decreases with increasing age at presentation (80% of defects noted at 1 month versus only 25% noted at 12 months).
By what age should all LARGE VSDs be repaired if spontaneous closure has not occurred?	1 year
What size VSD is well tolerated if untreated?	VSD with a diameter less than that of the aortic valve
What are the indications for surgery?	1. CHF 2. Worsening pulmonary hypertension 3. Q_p/Q_s > 2.0/1 (e.g., large L to R shunt) 4. Any canal or infundibular VSD (because of the effect on the aortic valve)
What is the primary contraindication for surgery?	Irreversible pulmonary hypertension (< 10 Wood units)
What corrective procedure is performed?	Closure of VSD + patch (prosthetic or pericardial)
What palliative procedure is performed for infants who are too small (< 3 kg) for corrective surgery or who have other medical problems?	Banding of the pulmonary artery to reduce the Q_p/Q_s. Definitive closure is performed when the child is grown. This procedure is also used for infants with "Swiss-cheese" septum or multiple VSDs.
What is the main operative complication?	Conduction defects, especially heart block, because of edema or suture injury to the conduction pathway, which travels close to the edges of the VSD. Temporary pacing wires should be placed routinely.

What is the incidence of this complication?	1% to 3%
What is the key prognostic indicator for long-term results?	Preoperative PVR. If PVR is not significantly increased, many patients have a normal life expectancy with few complications.

ATRIAL SEPTAL DEFECTS

What is the anatomic lesion?	Abnormal communication between the right and left atria
What are the types and the general location of each type in the septum?	1. Sinus venosus: high in the atrial septum 2. Ostium secundum: middle (fossa ovalis region) 3. Ostium primum: low
Which type is the most common?	Ostium secundum (80%)
What percentage of patients with ASD have additional congenital cardiac lesions?	30%
Give examples of other concurrent lesions.	VSD, congenital PS, PDA, coarctation of the aorta, TAPVC, pulmonary and tricuspid atresia
What is the main physiologic problem in ASD?	L to R shunt
Why is this problem minimal during the first few years of life?	RV hypertrophy of infancy takes time to subside. In infancy, compliance of the RV is similar to that of the LV, thus minimizing the shunt.
What are the primary factors that determine the degree of shunting in ASD?	Compliance of the ventricles, pulmonary vascular resistance, and size of the ASD. Size is less important than in VSD.

What percentage of the general population has a patent foramen ovale (PFO)?	10% to 25%
Why is PFO not considered an ASD?	It usually permits only **uni**directional (R to L) shunt because of the relation between the remnants of the septum primum and the septum secundum.

Which type of ASD is associated with:
1. **Valvular defects, and what is the combined defect called?**
2. **Lutembacher syndrome?**
3. **Right bundle branch block?**
4. **Partial anomalous venous connection?**
5. **Down syndrome?**
6. **LEFT axis deviation on EKG?**

1. Ostium primum, called a **partial AV canal defect.** (Valve defects are usually mitral valve clefts.)
2. Ostium secundum (the syndrome consists of ASD plus mitral stenosis)
3. Ostium secundum
4. Sinus venosus
5. Ostium primum
6. Ostium primum (others show right axis deviation)

At what age do UNTREATED patients with isolated ASD become symptomatic?	30 to 40 years old (usually asymptomatic until then)
At what age do UNTREATED patients with ASD show a clear increase in mortality rate?	20 years old. The survival rate (untreated) is 85% at 20 years, 40% at 40 years, and 25% at 50 years.
How does ASD present?	CHF (e.g., dyspnea)
Describe the murmur associated with ASDs.	Systolic ejection murmur at the left sternal border
What causes the murmur?	Unlike VSD, the murmur is not caused by flow across the defect, but rather by increased pulmonary blood flow (secondary to L to R shunt).
What is the other classic auscultatory finding?	Fixed, widely split S_2

What diagnostic tests are performed?	Echocardiogram (with Doppler). (Unlike VSD, cardiac catheterization is usually **not** necessary.)
When is cardiac catheterization indicated, and why?	Patients > 40 years old to rule out significant coronary artery disease **and** pulmonary hypertension
What is the primary indication for surgery for ASD?	$Q_p/Q_s > 2.0/1$
What is the primary contraindication to surgery?	Irreversible pulmonary hypertension (> 10 Wood units)
What corrective procedure is performed?	Closure of ASD by primary closure or patch (prosthetic or pericardial)
What is the main operative complication?	Injury to the conduction system

PATENT DUCTUS ARTERIOSUS

PDA is the embryologic remnant of what structure?	Sixth left aortic arch
What is the normal function of the ductus arteriosus?	Acts as an R to L shunt in the fetus to bypass the uninflated lungs (blood oxygenated at the placenta)
When does it usually close?	In the first few days of life (96% closed by 48 hours). Complete closure, through fibrosis and intimal proliferation, to form the ligamentum arteriosus takes several months.
What stimulates this initial closure?	It is theorized that increased arterial oxygen tension may constrict the muscle in the ductus.
What physiologic conditions may prevent closure of the ductus?	Hypoxia and increased levels of prostaglandins

PDA is common in what group of infants?

Premature infants, especially girls

Describe the murmur associated with PDAs.

Continuous "machinery" murmur with a late systolic peak, widely transmitted to the precordium and neck. The **diastolic** component of the murmur is absent in infancy because of elevated pulmonary vascular resistance (normal physiology); thus, it often is not continuous until 1 year of age.

What is the other classic finding on cardiovascular physical exam?

Wide pulse pressure with bounding pulse (large PDAs only)

What are the most common causes of death in adults with UNTREATED PDA?

CHF and bacterial endocarditis, especially *Streptococcus viridans*

What is the medical treatment of PDA?

Indomethacin (prostaglandin E_1 inhibitor). If unresolved in 1 week, surgery is indicated.

In which patients is medical treatment ineffective?

Full-term infants; children

What is the surgical treatment?

Ligation, clipping, or division of the PDA

What vein is divided to expose the ductus and aorta?

Left highest (supreme) intercostal vein

Care is taken to avoid injury to what nerve that courses close to the PDA?

Left recurrent laryngeal nerve

When is surgery performed?

If the PDA is large and CHF develops, surgery is performed immediately, regardless of patient age. Otherwise, surgery is performed at 1 to 2 years of age or thereafter whenever the diagnosis is made.

What is the primary contraindication to surgery, and why?	Cyanosis caused by an untreated cyanotic cardiac anomaly or severe pulmonary hypertension, both of which depend on the patency of the ductus for patient survival (one as a source of blood to the lung, the other as a means to shunt blood away from the high-pressure pulmonary bed)

TRUNCUS ARTERIOSUS

What is the anatomic lesion?	Single large vessel that straddles the ventricular septum (instead of a separate aorta and pulmonary artery), with a three- to six-leaflet truncal valve
What additional congenital cardiac lesion is always seen in these patients?	VSD, usually immediately under the truncal valve
What is the palliative surgical procedure?	Pulmonary artery banding to permit growth for infants with severe concurrent noncardiac disease (rarely used)
What is the corrective procedure?	Excision of the origin of the pulmonary artery from the main truncus and closure of the aortic defect, placement of a conduit (homograft or porcine composite graft) to establish continuity between the RV and pulmonary artery, and closure of the VSD

COMPLETE ATRIOVENTRICULAR CANAL

What is the general anatomic lesion (many variations)?	1. Low ASD (ostium primum) 2. High VSD (inlet) 3. Mitral and tricuspid valve abnormalities. (The "common AV valve" has six leaflets.)
What distinguishes a partial AV canal from a complete AV canal?	Partial AV canal lacks the VSD, so there is no intracardiac connection between the right and left sides of the heart below the AV valves.

These defects are caused by maldevelopment of what fetal cardiac tissue?	Endocardial cushion
These defects are associated with what syndrome?	Down syndrome
What is the usual presentation?	CHF in early infancy
What is the surgical treatment?	Closure of the VSD, reconstruction of the mitral and tricuspid valves by subdividing the bridging AV valve leaflets, and closure of the ASD
What factor determines the success of repair?	Amount of AV valvular tissue available for reconstruction

TETRALOGY OF FALLOT

What are the classic anatomic features?	1. Obstruction to RV outflow (infundibular or valvular pulmonic stenosis) 2. VSD 3. Overriding aorta (dextroposition of the aorta) 4. RV hypertrophy All are caused by a **single** lesion (e.g., anterosuperior malalignment of the infundibular septum), **not** four coincidental lesions.
When is this lesion also called a "double-outlet RV"?	When > 50% of the aorta arises from the RV
What is the pentalogy of Fallot?	TOF plus ASD
What is a "pink tetralogy"?	Patient with mild outflow obstruction and thus minimal R to L shunting into the aorta. (The severity of symptoms and cyanosis is directly related to the degree of RV outflow obstruction.)

What is the age of onset of the symptoms of TOF?

Approximately one-third at birth, one-third < 1 year of age, and one-third > 1 year of age

TOF is the most common cause of what complication of cyanotic heart disease?

Hypercyanotic spells ("tet" spells)

What is the classic behavior exhibited by children with TOF to relieve their symptoms, and why?

Squatting. By squatting, the patient increases systemic vascular resistance and apparently increases pulmonary circulation. The inability to increase pulmonary blood flow is the main limit for exercise tolerance in TOF.

What is the classic finding on CXR?

Boot-shaped heart shadow (concave pulmonary artery segment of the left side of the heart border because of a small pulmonary artery and a prominent upturned apex because of RV hypertrophy)

Why is an esophagogram performed?

Often detects the **right**-sided aortic arch seen in 25% of patients with TOF

What is an indication for EMERGENCY surgery in an infant, and why?

Hypercyanotic spells, which put the infant at risk for cerebral hypoxic injury and death

What is the surgical procedure for TOF?

Palliative systemic to pulmonary shunt (i.e., Blalock-Taussig subclavian artery to pulmonary artery shunt). Traditionally, a corrective procedure is performed 6 months to 2 years later to correct pulmonary outflow obstruction and closure of the VSD. Some surgeons now prefer early total correction without an intervening palliative shunt.

What is the primary contraindication to corrective surgery in infancy?

Severely hypoplastic pulmonary arteries

What coronary lesion complicates corrective surgery?

Left anterior descending artery crossing the RV outflow tract

What is the success rate of surgery?	> 95% survival; 50% have no exercise limitations!

TRICUSPID ATRESIA (TA)

What is the anatomic lesion?	Absence of communication between the right atrium (RA) and RV
What additional congenital cardiac lesions accompany TA in its classic form?	1. ASD (to permit flow into the LA) 2. RV hypoplasia Several variants involve VSD or transposition of the great vessels; the presence of VSD determines the size of the RV.
How does tricuspid atresia differ grossly from the other CYANOTIC congenital lesions?	LV hypertrophy. Others have RV hypertrophy associated with an R to L shunt.
Is tricuspid atresia associated with increased or decreased pulmonary blood flow?	Depends on whether the patient has VSD or pulmonic stenosis; 66% have decreased flow, and 33% have increased flow
What determines the severity of symptoms?	Pulmonary blood flow (e.g., if significantly reduced, cyanosis is severe)
What are the palliative surgical procedures for TA?	1. If decreased pulmonary blood flow: Systemic to pulmonary shunt 2. If increased pulmonary blood flow: Pulmonary artery banding
What is the definitive procedure?	Fontan procedure: Connection of the vena cavae (or RA) to the pulmonary artery (not usually performed until 2 to 4 years of age)
Although many centers avoid palliative procedures for other defects, why is the Fontan procedure NOT performed in infants?	Pulmonary vascular resistance in the infant is too high to permit passive flow from the RA.

EBSTEIN ANOMALY

What is the basic anatomic lesion?	Tricuspid valve is positioned abnormally low within the RV (with a large "sail" anterior leaflet and septal and posterior leaflets originating from the wall of the

RV). The RV is divided into a thin "atrialized" supravalvular portion and a normal trabeculated apical and infundibular portion. ASD is also usually present.

What are the physiologic (hemodynamic) consequences?

Tricuspid regurgitation, decreased cardiac output because of reduction in RV size, R to L shunt (through the ASD), ± RV outflow tract obstruction

What determines the severity of symptoms?

1. Size of the atrialized region (as it increases, the size of functional RV decreases)
2. Presence of RV outflow tract obstruction

What is the surgical treatment?

Tricuspid valvuloplasty, followed by reconstruction with plication of the atrialized portion of the RV, followed by ASD closure. Occasionally, tricuspid valve replacement (the procedure of choice in the past) is necessary.

PULMONARY ATRESIA

Pulmonary Atresia with Intact Ventricular Septum

What is the anatomic lesion?

RV outflow tract obstruction as a result of fusion of the pulmonary valve leaflets to form a dome-like structure

What are the common additional congenital cardiac lesions?

PFO or ASD, hypoplastic RV of variable severity, and tricuspid valve anomalies + hypoplastic pulmonary arteries

What is the primary source of pulmonary blood flow?

PDA

What is the usual presentation?

Progressive respiratory distress, cyanosis, and acidosis as the PDA closes shortly after birth

Describe the murmur associated with this lesion.

Soft, blowing pansystolic murmur at the left sternal border (because of tricuspid regurgitation)

What is the palliative surgical procedure?	Open pulmonary valvotomy to decompress the RV **plus** systemic to pulmonary shunt to augment blood flow to the lungs (i.e., modified Blalock-Taussig shunt)
What is the corrective procedure?	1. If the RV enlarges to relatively normal size, biventricular repair (closure of the PFO and ASD, ligation of the palliative shunt) 2. If the RV is too small, Fontan procedure or heart transplantation

Pulmonary Atresia with Ventricular Septal Defect

What is the primary source of pulmonary blood flow?	PDA **and** multiple aortopulmonary (AP) collaterals. The contribution of each source depends on the patient.
What is the usual presentation?	Cyanosis and CHF. These patients usually present later than those with an intact ventricular septum because the blood supply is not dependent on the PDA alone. Although CHF usually does not develop in the few patients with a ductus-dependent pulmonary blood supply, cyanosis develops earlier.
A clear understanding of what key anatomic feature is critical for successful operative intervention?	Pattern of vascularization of the lungs. The direct AP collaterals from the descending aorta, the indirect collaterals from the brachiocephalic artery, and the normal "true" bronchial arteries must be evaluated.
What is the palliative surgical procedure?	Multiple "unifocalization" procedures: Systemic to pulmonary shunts (often modified Blalock-Taussig shunt) to the "central" pulmonary trunk or largest AP collateral
What are the goals of the palliative procedure?	Provide adequate pulmonary blood flow **and** promote the growth of the pulmonary arterial tree
What is the corrective procedure?	Biventricular repair. The ASD and VSD are closed, the shunt is ligated, the RV and central pulmonary artery are connected with a conduit, a homograft if

possible. Heart–lung transplantation is a
potential option for the "inoperable"
patient.

CONGENITAL AORTIC STENOSIS

**What are the types of
congenital AS?**

1. Valvular type
2. Infravalvular or subvalvular type, with
   discrete fibrous and/or muscular
   components
3. Supravalvular type ("coarctation of
   the ascending aorta"; diffuse and
   localized types)
4. Idiopathic hypertrophic subaortic
   stenosis (IHSS)

**Which type is most
common?**

Valvular AS (80%)

**What is the anatomic
lesion in most patients
with valvular AS?**

Bicuspid aortic valve (fused
commissures)

**Which type of congenital
AS is associated with:**

**1. Increased frequency in
boys?**

1. Valvular (4:1) and subvalvular (2.5:1)

**2. LV hypertrophy on
EKG?**

2. All

**3. Poststenotic dilation on
CXR?**

3. Valvular

**4. Craniofacial anomalies,
mental retardation, and
infantile hypercalcemia?**

4. Supravalvular (if present, called
   Williams syndrome)

**5. High recurrence rate
after repair?**

5. Valvular and subvalvular

**What is the classic
presentation in the
neonate?**

Congestive heart failure and reduced or
absent peripheral pulses

**What is the classic
presentation in the older
child?**

Exertional angina, syncope, or
congestive heart failure. Most patients
are asymptomatic at rest.

**What is the primary
measure by which the
obstruction is graded?**

Transvalvular (LV–aortic) systolic
pressure gradient

What additional measure of severity is used in the valvular type?	Aortic valve area
What are the criteria for severe AS?	1. Gradient ≥ 75 mm Hg 2. Valvular area ≤ 0.5 cm^2/m^2
What are the indications for surgical treatment?	Severe stenosis or symptomatic patient
What procedure is performed for the VALVULAR type?	Commissurotomy (open technique or percutaneous balloon dilation; both techniques have similar results). Valve replacement is uncommon, but may be required later for the presenile calcification seen with the bicuspid valve.
What procedure is performed for the SUBVALVULAR type?	Resection of the fibromuscular ring and, sometimes, replacement of the aortic valve
What procedure is performed for the SUPRAVALVULAR type?	Patch graft over the stenotic region
In which group is the mortality rate particularly high (50%–100%)?	Valvular types that present in early infancy

Idiopathic Hypertrophic Subaortic Stenosis (IHSS)

What is the etiology of IHSS?	Genetically transmitted (autosomal dominant)
What is the gross lesion?	Usually asymmetric septal hypertrophy, occasionally caused by a subvalvular web
What are the symptoms?	Dyspnea, syncope, and angina
What is the most common age of patients at presentation?	30 to 40 years old; rarely symptomatic in children.
What is the classic cause of death?	Sudden death as a result of ventricular arrhythmia

What is the risk of this complication in treated versus untreated patients with IHSS?	No difference
What is the medical treatment of IHSS?	β-blockers (e.g., propranolol), which are effective for most patients
What is the rationale for the use of these drugs?	Increased contractility exacerbates stenosis by further approximating the septum and anterior mitral leaflet (the key structure responsible for the obstruction in IHSS) through Venturi forces. β-blockers are negative inotropes.
What is the indication for surgical treatment?	Refractory to medical therapy
What are the surgical options?	1. Septal myomectomy (resection of a section of the septum to form a channel of unobstructed flow from the LV) 2. Mitral valve replacement (MVR) 3. Ventricular pacing with delayed activation of the septum

COARCTATION OF THE AORTA

What is the anatomic lesion?	Narrowing of the descending aorta (± intraluminal shelf)
What is the usual location of the lesion?	Near the ductus or ligamentum arteriosum, distal to the left subclavian artery. The pathophysiology may involve extension of the fibrotic process involved in the conversion of the ductus to the ligamentum.
What are the three types?	1. Preductal (infantile) 2. Juxtaductal 3. Postductal (adult)
What is the most common type?	Postductal
What percentage of patients have a concurrent congenital cardiac lesion?	60%

Give examples of these lesions.	Bicuspid aortic valve (seen in 40%–50%); VSD (seen in 10%–15%)
What syndrome is seen in 15% to 35% of patients?	Turner syndrome (web neck, "shield" chest, gonadal streaks)
What is the presentation of coarctation of the aorta? **1. In infants?**	1. Severe CHF, diminished or absent femoral pulses, shock at the time of closure of the ductus arteriosus (caused by loss of perfusion distal to the coarctation)
2. In adults?	2. Hypertension (blood pressure of arms » blood pressure of legs), diminished or absent femoral pulses, lower extremity fatigue (although leg claudication is uncommon)
What are the most common symptoms in adults?	Usually **asymptomatic,** but headache and epistaxis are not uncommon
Describe the murmurs associated with this lesion.	Systolic murmur, radiating to the interscapular region: due to turbulence across the coarctation Continuous murmur, variable location: due to flow through the collaterals
What are the classic findings on CXR?	"Reverse 3" sign: Pre- and postcoarctation dilation seen in the region of the aortic knob Rib notching: Erosion of bone by dilated, tortuous intercostal arteries (collaterals)
What are the most common causes of death?	CHF, rupture of aortic aneurysm, rupture of intracranial aneurysm, and bacterial endocarditis
Why is the preductal type fatal in INFANCY if untreated?	Distal aorta is initially perfused by the large PDA, but as the PDA closes (normal physiology), acidosis and LV failure occur

What is the average life expectancy of patients with the postductal type, if untreated?

30 to 40 years

What is the long-term outcome of the collateral arteries, especially the intercostal arteries?

Aneurysms; eventually, rupture of the arteries may occur

What are the surgical treatment options for coarctation of the aorta?

1. Resection of the coarctation and end-to-end anastomosis
2. Subclavian artery aortoplasty (flap)
3. Patch aortoplasty
4. Bypass with a prosthetic graft

What is the procedure of choice in infants?

Subclavian artery aortoplasty (controversial)

What is the procedure of choice in the child?

Resection with end-to-end anastomosis

What is the procedure of choice in the young adult?

Bypass with a prosthetic graft (controversial)

Which procedure is now not commonly used because of the high incidence of aneurysm formation?

Patch aortoplasty. Aneurysm of the aortic wall is often seen opposite the patch.

Why is surgery hazardous in the adult?

Risk of significant (and difficult to control) hemorrhage if dilated, thin-walled intercostal collaterals are injured

What is the most feared postoperative morbidity?

Paraplegia because of spinal cord ischemia during aortic cross-clamping (approximately 1 in 200 cases)

What are two other classic complications in the immediate postoperative period?

"Paradoxic" hypertension and mesenteric necrotizing panarteritis (and GI bleeding)

Interrupted Aortic Arch

In an interrupted aortic arch, what is the anatomic lesion?

Absence of a segment of the transverse or descending aorta

What syndrome is seen in 15% to 30% of patients?	DiGeorge syndrome (i.e., no thymus or parathyroids, hypocalcemia, compromise of cellular immunity)

CONGENITAL PULMONARY STENOSIS (PS)

What is the anatomic lesion?	RV outflow obstruction because of pulmonic valvular or RV infundibular stenosis
Describe the most common type.	Fusion of the pulmonary valve leaflets to form a dome-like structure with a small orifice at the apex
What is the criterion for severe PS?	Transvalvular gradient > 75 to 80 mm Hg
What is the most common concurrent cardiac defect?	PFO (occasionally, ASD)
Describe the murmur associated with this lesion.	Loud, harsh systolic crescendo–decrescendo murmur at intercostal spaces 2 and 3
Compare the presentation of mild to moderate PS with that of severe PS.	Mild to moderate PS: Characteristic murmur discovered in **asymptomatic** patients Severe PS: Dyspnea, angina, and syncope (similar to AS); cyanosis; RV failure as a result of the **R to L shunt** (across the PFO)
What is a common cause of death in older children and young adults with untreated PS?	Sudden death (similar to AS)
What is the treatment of mild to moderate PS?	Observation
What is the treatment of severe PS?	1. Percutaneous balloon pulmonary valvuloplasty 2. Open valvulotomy–commissurotomy 3. Occasionally, infundibular resection and/or annuloplasty with a patch over the RV outflow tract

TRANSPOSITION OF THE GREAT VESSELS

What is the anatomic lesion?

Ventriculoarterial discordance (e.g., aorta originates from the RV; the pulmonary artery from the LV) with AV concordance (ventricles are connected to the appropriate atria). This condition results in parallel, rather than serial, systemic and pulmonary circulations.

What is the claim to fame of this condition?

Most common congenital defect that causes cyanosis **and** CHF in the newborn period (> 90% by day 1)

What is the classic finding on CXR?

"Egg-on-a-string" appearance (seen in 75% of cases)

What causes this appearance on CXR?

Dilated right-sided chambers: Prominent RV projecting to the left, prominent RA to the right (i.e., "egg"); superimposition of the great vessels (rather than side-by-side position), and narrow mediastinum (i.e., "string")

What is the palliative surgical procedure?

Balloon atrial septostomy. Palliative septectomy (Blalock-Hanlon procedure) is now virtually obsolete.

What are the options for corrective procedure?

1. **Atrial** switch procedure: Intra-atrial baffle to redirect venous blood toward the appropriate great vessel (i.e., Mustard procedure)
2. **Arterial** switch procedure: Switching of the aorta and pulmonary artery and reimplantation of the coronary arteries into the aorta (Jatene procedure)

What is "congenitally corrected" transposition?

In addition to the arterial transposition, ventricular inversion (ventriculoarterial concordance **and** AV discordance)

TOTAL ANOMALOUS PULMONARY VENOUS CONNECTION (TAPVC)

What is the general anatomic lesion?

No pulmonary veins directly drain into the left atrium (LA) ± pulmonary vein stenosis.

What are the three types and their relative frequencies?

1. Supracardiac: Pulmonary venous drainage into the SVC (45%–50%)
2. Intracardiac: Pulmonary venous drainage into the coronary sinus or RA (20%–30%)
3. Infracardiac: Pulmonary venous drainage into the inferior vena cava (20%)

Which type has the classic vertical vein?

Supracardiac type. The vertical vein is the left superior vena cava seen in these patients.

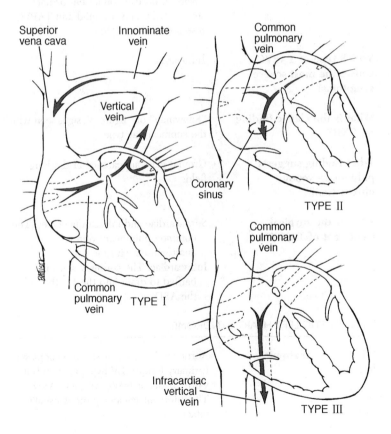

What is a partial APVC (PAPVC)?

Some, but not all, pulmonary veins empty into the LA.

What is scimitar syndrome?	PAPVC in which the pulmonary veins from the right lung join to form a single vertical vein that curves downward to join with the inferior vena cava
What additional congenital cardiac lesion is usually seen in patients with TAPVC?	ASD or PFO is essential for blood to return to the systemic circulation.
What key feature determines the severity of the presentation?	Presence and severity of pulmonary venous obstruction. If obstruction is severe, cyanosis and tachypnea are severe; if obstruction absent or not severe, symptoms are mild and TAPVC resembles a large ASD.
Which type of TAPVC causes the most severe symptoms?	Infracardiac
What is the classic finding on CXR?	"Snowman" or "figure 8" sign, seen with the supracardiac type
What finding suggests pulmonary venous obstruction?	Ground-glass appearance of the lung fields
What is the surgical treatment of TAPVC?	Supracardiac and infracardiac types: The common pulmonary vein is anastomosed with the LA. Intracardiac: The coronary sinus is baffled to drain into the LA through the ASD.

HYPOPLASTIC LEFT HEART SYNDROME

What is the anatomic lesion?	Aortic valve atresia or severe hypoplasia (primary lesion), LV hypoplasia, mitral valve atresia or hypoplasia, and ASD. The interventricular septum is usually intact.
What is the usual presentation?	Rapid development of cyanosis and CHF during the first 24 to 48 hours of life in an infant who is of normal size and **acyanotic** at birth.

What are the surgical options?	1. Complex reconstructive staged procedure: Palliative procedure followed by a modified Fontan procedure at 12 to 18 months 2. Heart transplant

VASCULAR RINGS

What is the embryonic origin of a vascular ring?	Anomalous development of the aorta and pulmonary artery from the embryonic aortic arches
What is the most common type?	Double aortic arch
What is the most prominent symptom?	Stridor as a result of compression of the trachea by vascular rings
Although a variety of anomalies and multiple operative techniques exist, what is the basic surgical procedure?	The compressive arteries are divided, and bypass performed if necessary.

ANEURYSM OF THE SINUS OF VALSALVA

What are the sinuses of Valsalva?	Outpouchings of the aortic root corresponding to leaflets (indentations where commissures meet the aortic wall)
What are the etiologies of aneurysms of these sinuses?	Congenital: Aortic wall media does not meet the aortic annulus Acquired: Endocarditis, myxomatous degeneration, syphilis, and chronic aortic dissection
What is the primary complication associated with the congenital form of the lesion?	Rupture into a cardiac chamber because these aneurysms are primarily intracardiac
What is the most common site of this complication?	Rupture into the RV in 70% and the RA in 20%

What is the average age for this complication?	30 years old
What is the usual presentation of aneurysms of Valsalva?	Asymptomatic until rupture causes CHF as a result of acute L to R shunt
What is the classic new finding on physical exam after rupture?	Continuous murmur (intercostal space 3 or 4)

EISENMENGER SYNDROME

What is Eisenmenger syndrome?	Reversal of a long-standing untreated L to R shunt (i.e., becomes an R to L shunt)
Why does it occur?	L to R shunt increases pressure in the right side of the heart. Reactive changes (e.g., medial hypertrophy, sclerosis) occur in the pulmonary arterioles, followed by pulmonary hypertension. Eventually, the shunt reverses.
What is the most common cardiac lesion associated with this syndrome, if left untreated?	VSD
What is the usual presentation?	New onset of **cyanosis** in a patient with **L to R** shunt
What is the most common cause of death?	Massive hemoptysis. Patients often die by 30 to 40 years of age.
What is the treatment?	Heart–lung transplant; thus, the condition is considered inoperable by many.

MISCELLANEOUS TOPICS

What is a common nonspecific presentation of the infant with a congenital heart defect?	Poor feeding and failure to thrive

What percentage of congenital heart defects are caused by maternal rubella?	< 2%
What defects are usually associated with rubella?	PDA (most common), ASD, and congenital PS
What is the differential diagnosis of a continuous murmur?	PDA versus other etiologies (rare). Other etiologies include AP window, ruptured aneurysm of the sinus of Valsalva, and coronary AV fistula.
What congenital defect is one of the few remaining surgical emergencies in congenital cardiac surgery because no medical treatment can palliate the defect?	TAPVC with pulmonary venous obstruction
What lesion is associated with massive hemoptysis in essentially 100% of patients by 40 years of age?	Eisenmenger syndrome
What is the most common ISOLATED congenital tricuspid valve lesion?	Ebstein anomaly
What cyanotic heart lesion has a grossly distinguishing feature on EKG?	Tricuspid atresia (left axis deviation versus right axis deviation in the rest)
A patient with congenital heart disease has headache, lethargy, and seizures. What is the most likely diagnosis?	Brain abscess
More than 50% of patients with what cyanotic defect are diagnosed by day 1 of life?	Tricuspid atresia

What is Shone syndrome?

Congenital AS, mitral stenosis (MS), and coarctation of the aorta

Which defect is associated with giant P waves on EKG?

Ebstein anomaly

Cor triatriatum (i.e., three atria) is part of the spectrum of what congenital heart defect?

TAPVC

What lesion of the reticuloendothelial system is common in congenital heart disease, and what is the classic laboratory finding in these patients?

Asplenia (no spleen). Howell-Jolly bodies are shown on blood smear.

What is the general mechanism for the development of endocarditis in congenital heart disease?

Turbulence caused by these lesions causes damage to the endocardium or aortic intima, predisposing these regions to bacterial invasion during episodes of transient bacteremia.

A patient has cyanosis for the FIRST time at 2 years of age. What is the most likely diagnosis?

TOF. Congenital cyanosis presenting for the first time at this age is almost diagnostic of TOF.

What is the most commonly diagnosed congenital heart defect in patients > 20 years old?

ASD

What rare lesion can often be diagnosed with an esophagogram?

Vascular rings (because of a characteristic pattern of posterior compression of the esophagus)

Which common lesion causes a wide pulse pressure?

PDA

Maternal lithium use increases the incidence of which lesion by 400 times?

Ebstein anomaly

Maternal thalidomide use increases the incidence of which lesion?	ASD
What lesion is associated with a characteristic shadow parallel to the right border of the heart?	PAPVC (scimitar syndrome)
What CYANOTIC heart defect is easily distinguished from the others with EKG?	Tricuspid atresia. This defect shows LV hypertrophy and left axis deviation (because of hypoplastic RV) versus other cyanotic lesions have RV hypertrophy.
What is the most common defect that is palliated with balloon atrial septostomy?	Transposition of the great vessels
Which type of pulmonary atresia (± VSD) does not respond to prostaglandin E₁ infusion, and why?	Pulmonary atresia with VSD. Most are **not** dependent on PDA for pulmonary blood flow!

ACQUIRED CORONARY ARTERY DISEASE

CORONARY ANATOMY

Identify the labeled arteries.

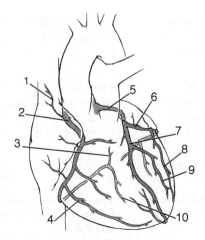

1. Sinoatrial nodal artery
2. Right coronary artery
3. AV nodal artery
4. Right marginal artery
5. Left main coronary artery
6. Circumflex artery
7. Left anterior descending (LAD) artery
8. Obtuse marginal arteries
9. Diagonal arteries
10. Posterior descending artery (PDA)

What percentage of patients with coronary artery disease (CAD) have "triple-vessel disease"?

> 50%. These patients have significant atherosclerosis in all three primary coronary arteries (right, LAD or left main, and circumflex).

Are most individuals right- or left-"dominant," and what does this designation mean?

90% are right-dominant (the PDA originates from the right coronary circulation). In left-dominant individuals, the PDA originates from the circumflex artery.

What are the multiple secondary branches off of the LAD and the circumflex artery?

LAD: Septal and diagonal arteries
Circumflex: Marginal arteries

Coronary arteries arise from what aortic region?

Sinuses of Valsalva

Which coronary artery supplies the sinus node versus the AV node?

Both are usually supplied by the right coronary artery.

Most atherosclerotic lesions are located in what general region of the coronary arteries?

Proximal one-third to one-half. This feature permits coronary artery bypass, except in the occasional patient with severe distal disease.

ISCHEMIC HEART DISEASE

What are the risk factors for atherosclerotic CAD?

Tobacco abuse, hypertension, family history, male gender, hyperlipidemia, and diabetes

Why is the heart prone to ischemia?

High myocardial oxygen extraction. Even at rest, the heart extracts 75% of blood oxygen (versus < 50% by other tissues). On exertion, extraction may approach 100%. Stenotic coronary lesions are more likely to cause a significant imbalance between oxygen supply and demand, with resultant ischemia.

What are the greatest determinants of myocardial oxygen consumption?

Heart rate, contractility, and ventricular wall tension

What are the basic sequelae of myocardial ischemia?

Reduced ventricular compliance, reduced ventricular contractility, angina, and myocardial infarction (MI)

Angina

What is stable angina?

Angina occurring with a **reproducible** level of exertion, **without** a recent change in frequency or severity, and relieved by a brief period of rest or the patient's standard dose of nitroglycerin (NTG)

How does unstable angina present?

1. Previously stable angina occurring at a lower level of exertion, with increased frequency or severity, or unrelieved by rest or NTG
2. New onset of angina in a patient with no history of angina

Which patients usually have silent myocardial ischemia?

Patients with diabetes and the elderly (autonomic neuropathy); heart transplant recipients (complete denervation of the donor heart)

What is the most common cause of sudden death in patients with CAD?

Ventricular fibrillation (not MI)

What are four EKG territories of the LV, the leads that correspond to them, and the vessel that usually supplies the region?

Lateral: EKG leads I, AVL, V5, and V6; circumflex artery
Inferior: EKG leads II, III, and AVF; right coronary artery
Anteroseptal: EKG leads V1 through V4; LAD

Posterior: Reciprocal changes in EKG
leads V1, V2; right coronary artery
The classic EKG changes of ischemia
occur in the leads that correspond to the
ischemic myocardial region.

What is the standard first-line study for the evaluation of myocardial ischemia?

Exercise stress test + thallium
radionuclide scan

What tests are performed if the patient cannot exercise?

1. Thallium scan with dipyridamole
   infusion, which mimics the reflex
   vasodilation of exercise, while the
   patient is at rest
2. Echocardiogram with dobutamine
   infusion, which mimics the increased
   catecholamine level of exercise

What is the "redistribution phenomenon" seen with the thallium scan?

Thallium (a potassium analog) is taken
up by myocardial cells. The
concentration of thallium decreases
inversely to coronary blood flow. Well-perfused areas appear more intense on
early scans, and poorly perfused areas
appear more intense on delayed scans.

What is considered a significant stenosis on coronary arteriogram?

50% reduction in diameter (i.e., 75%
reduction in cross-sectional area)
compared with adjacent normal
segments of the coronary artery

What is the most important prognostic indicator for determining operative risk?

Preoperative LV function

What studies are used to evaluate this indicator preoperatively?

Left-sided ventriculogram at the time of
coronary angiogram, echocardiogram,
and multiple-uptake gated acquisition
scanning (MUGA)

What is a normal LV ejection fraction?

> 60% to 70%

| What are the two basic physiologic goals of medical treatment of CAD? | Increase coronary blood flow and reduce myocardial oxygen consumption (MvO_2) |

What are the major drug classes used and their contribution to achieve these two goals?

Table 45–1

	↑ Blood Flow	↓ MvO_2
Nitrates	+	++
β–adrenergic blockers	. . .	++
Calcium channel blockers	+	+

What is the medical treatment of unstable angina?	Bedside monitoring, supplemental oxygen + intubation, IV nitroglycerin infusion, IV morphine, aspirin, IV heparin, ± β-blocker therapy, ± intra-aortic balloon pump (IABP)
If pain persists despite aggressive medical therapy, what steps are taken?	If the patient is an operative candidate, coronary angiogram is performed. If a correctable lesion is found, angioplasty or surgery is performed.
What acute mechanical complications of MI require surgical intervention?	1. Ventricular septal or free wall rupture 2. Mitral regurgitation as a result of papillary muscle dysfunction or rupture
What chronic complication of MI requires surgery?	LV aneurysm
What do all of these complications lead to if left untreated?	CHF and death

Percutaneous Transluminal Coronary Angioplasty (PTCA)

| What is the initial success rate for dilating a stenotic lesion? | 85% to 90% |
| What is the major disadvantage of PTCA? | **High** restenosis rate (30%–40% 6-month restenosis rate) |

CORONARY ARTERY BYPASS GRAFTING (CABG)

What is the claim to fame of this procedure?

Most commonly performed surgical procedure in the United States

Which vessels are used most often as conduits for bypass?

Internal mammary artery (IMA) and saphenous vein. Others include the gastroepiploic, inferior epigastric, and radial arteries.

Compare the 10-year patency rates of these conduits.

IMA: 85% to 95%; Saphenous vein graft (SVG): only 50%

What is the most common indication for CABG?

Unstable angina or disabling angina that is refractory to medical therapy and is not amenable to angioplasty

What are the four indications for which CABG is clearly life-lengthening (i.e., documented increased survival compared with medical therapy alone)?

1. Left main artery (or proximal LAD) disease
2. Triple-vessel disease **with decreased LV function**
3. Postinfarction angina
4. Mechanical complications of ischemic heart disease (i.e., papillary muscle rupture)

MI alone is **not** an indication for CABG. If the patient has no angina after MI, the infarction is completed, and revascularization offers no benefit to that territory. The patient must have one of the four indications for surgery.

What are the relative contraindications to CABG?

1. Diffuse distal coronary artery disease
2. Poor LV function (ejection fraction < 20%)
3. CHF refractory to medical therapy and is **not** caused by a mechanical complication of ischemic heart disease

Acute MI is not an absolute contraindication unless the patient is in cardiogenic shock.

As part of CABG, what additional procedure may be required if significant atherosclerotic disease is present at or distal to the planned anastomotic site?

Endarterectomy (A key factor in determining late patency is the rate of blood flow through the graft. Distal stenotic lesions contribute to a reduction in flow.)

What is the main risk associated with using both IMAs for CABG?

Sternal wound infection and dehiscence

Which patients are at increased risk for this complication?

Obese patients and patients with diabetes

After CABG, what percentage of patients are free of ischemia:
1. **In the early postoperative period?**
2. **At 5 years?**
3. **At 10 years?**

1. 90%
2. 75%
3. 50%

What is the most common cause of recurrence of angina < 5 years versus > 7 years after CABG?

< 5 years: Progression of atherosclerotic disease in the native coronary arteries
> 7 years: Atherosclerotic disease in the saphenous vein graft

What decreases the risk of future graft thrombosis?

Aspirin

What is the mortality rate for:
1. **Elective CABG?**
2. **Emergent CABG?**

3. **Emergent CABG in the setting of cardiogenic shock?**
4. **Elective redo CABG?**
5. **Emergent redo CABG?**
6. **Acute MI?**

1. 1% to 2%
2. 3% to 8% (often even higher in the setting of postinfarction angina)
3. > 50%

4. 7% to 8%
5. 25%
6. 10% to 25% (e.g., surgery is worth the risk to prevent or delay MI)

MECHANICAL COMPLICATIONS OF ISCHEMIC HEART DISEASE

What type of patient typically has these complications?

Patients with single-vessel disease, no history of angina, and **un**complicated MI with acute decompensation in the early post-MI period

Left Ventricular Aneurysm

What is the most common etiology of LV aneurysm?

Large transmural MI (infarcted tissue replaced by a fibrous scar that permits localized dilation of the ventricle)

What is the incidence of this complication?	5% to 15% of patients with MI
What region is most commonly involved?	Anterior–apical surface of the LV (LAD territory)
What is the most common presentation?	LV failure
How is the diagnosis made?	Dyskinesia (paradoxic outward bulge of the region during systole) seen on ventriculogram or echocardiogram. (Because of transient functional changes associated with stunned myocardium, the diagnosis of LV aneurysm **cannot** be made at the time of acute MI.)
What is the classic EKG finding?	Persistent ST elevation in the involved territory after MI (versus in pericarditis, ST elevations occur in almost all leads).
What are the usual complications?	LV failure, arrhythmias, angina and, infrequently, emboli from mural thrombus. These aneurysms rarely rupture.
What are the indications for surgery for LV aneurysm?	1. Symptomatic patient 2. Arrhythmias refractory to medical therapy 3. Aneurysm > 5 to 6 cm
What is the surgical procedure?	Aneurysmectomy **and** CABG to the ischemic territory
What is the waiting period after MI for elective repair, and why?	At least 2 months to permit the aneurysm to become well demarcated and the rim to become fibrotic (versus necrotic and difficult to suture)
What are the 5-year survival rates for treated versus untreated patients?	Treated: 75% to 80% Untreated: 20% to 30%

Acute Ventricular Septal Defect

When does acute VSD classically present?	5 to 7 days after MI

What is the classic presentation?	Acute CHF with a new, harsh pansystolic murmur and thrill at the left sternal border
What is the usual Swan-Ganz catheter finding?	"Step-up" of oxygen saturation (> 10%) between the LA (proximal port) and pulmonary artery (distal port)
What is the medical treatment?	Same treatment as acute ischemic mitral regurgitation (MR)
What is the surgical procedure for acute VSD?	Left ventriculotomy through the infarction with patch repair of the VSD and patch closure of the ventriculotomy. (Although repair was often delayed for several weeks in the past, it is now performed acutely.)
Compare the timing of surgery if cardiac output (CO) is normal versus decreased.	CO is artifactually increased in patients with VSD because the thermodilution curve is altered by the L to R shunt. CO does not affect timing.

Acute Ischemic Mitral Regurgitation

What are the mechanisms of acute ischemic MR?	Papillary muscle dysfunction or stunning (most common), annular dilation, and papillary muscle rupture (rare)
What territory is usually involved in MI associated with MR?	Posterolateral territory with injury to the posterior papillary muscle (usually circumflex coronary artery territory)
What is the classic presentation?	CHF with a new holosystolic murmur radiating to the axilla
What are the Swan-Ganz catheter findings?	Large V wave on the pulmonary capillary wedge pressure (PCWP) tracing; no "step-up" of oxygen saturation
Acute ischemic MR accounts for what percentage of early MI deaths?	1%

What is the mortality rate in UNTREATED patients with MI complicated by ischemic MR?	70% in the first 24 hours; 90% in the first 2 weeks
What key question must be answered to guide patient management?	Will the etiology of MR likely resolve with supportive medical therapy (stunning), **or** is acute surgical correction required (ruptured papillary muscle)?
What is the hemodynamic goal of medical treatment?	Afterload reduction to minimize regurgitant flow by maximizing flow from the LV. This therapy is also used to temporarily stabilize the surgical patient before repair.
What is the treatment of the normotensive patient (systolic blood pressure > 90 mm Hg)?	Sodium nitroprusside (titrated to reduce CHF while maintaining systolic blood pressure > 90 mm Hg)
What is the treatment of the hypotensive patient?	Dobutamine and IABP
What is the surgical procedure for acute ischemic MR?	MVR **and** CABG to the infarcted territory (and other territories at risk)

MISCELLANEOUS TOPICS

What is a stunned myocardium?	Transient LV dysfunction that accompanies reversible myocardial ischemia
What is a hibernating myocardium?	Chronic LV dysfunction secondary to inadequate coronary flow to perform effective contractions, but sufficient flow to maintain myocardial viability. It is reversible with coronary revascularization.
What size infarction is usually needed to cause cardiogenic shock?	40% of the LV mass, including the region of stunned myocardium (e.g., a patient in cardiogenic shock may have a 10% LV mass infarction if an additional 30% is stunned)

What is the Killip infarct classification?

Class I: No CHF
Class II: Mild to moderate CHF (+S_3, rales over < 50% of lungs)
Class III: Severe CHF (> 50%)
Class IV: Cardiogenic shock

What mortality rate is associated with each Killip class?

Class I: 6%
Class II: 17%
Class III: 38%
Class IV: 81%

What is the New York Heart Association (NYHA) classification of CHF (or angina)?

Class I: No symptoms
Class II: Symptoms with severe exertion
Class III: Symptoms with mild exertion
Class IV: Symptoms at rest

What degree of stenosis is required to stimulate the formation of coronary collaterals?

70% reduction in diameter (i.e., 90% reduction in the cross-sectional area). Thus, patients with acute occlusion of a vessel with < 70% stenosis have relatively more ischemic injury.

What appears to hasten the appearance of the mechanical complications of ischemia (e.g., occur earlier after MI)?

Thrombolytic therapy

ACQUIRED VALVULAR HEART DISEASE

AORTIC VALVE

What is the normal patent surface area of the aortic valve?

2.5 to 3.5 cm^2

What gross changes occur in the heart as a result of AS versus aortic regurgitation (AR)?

AS: LV **hypertrophy** (concentric) because of **pressure** overload
AR: LV **dilation** (and LV hypertrophy) because of **volume** overload

Compare AS with AR:
1. **Which is generally less well tolerated?**

2. **Which has a male:female ratio of 8:1?**

1. AS. Strain on the LV caused by increased intraventricular pressure is greater than that of volume overload.

2. AS

3. Which may be associated with ascending aortic dilatation?

3. Both. In AS, it may develop as a result of poststenotic turbulence. An ascending aortic aneurysm with associated dilation of the aortic annulus may cause AR.

What studies are used to diagnose and quantify the severity of AS and AR?

Echocardiogram (with Doppler) and cardiac catheterization (ventriculogram)

What variables are measured with these studies?

AS: Transvalvular pressure gradient and valvular surface area
AR: Severity of regurgitation
Valvular surface areas are calculated with the Grolin formula, using **estimates** of flow and gradients. Thus, the criteria for severity of valvular lesions are rough guidelines; the patient's symptoms are far more important!

Which patients should also have a coronary angiogram?

Any patient > 35 years old or with symptoms of MI (angina), regardless of age

What cardiac structures are at risk for injury during aortic valve replacement (AVR)?

Coronary artery ostia and the bundle of His in the membranous ventricular septum, specifically at the commissure between the right and noncoronary cusps

Which patients are at greatest risk for postoperative ventricular failure after AVR?

Patients with a low preoperative ejection fraction (< 40%)

What is the treatment of postoperative ventricular failure?

Vasodilators (for afterload reduction) and inotropic support, + IABP until the ventricle recovers or adapts

What is the target systolic blood pressure after AVR, and why?

Goal systolic blood pressure is < 120 mm Hg to reduce the risk of bleeding from the aortic suture line. (The ascending aorta is incised to gain access to the valve.)

What conduction disturbance may occur after AVR?	Heart block, usually caused by edema around the bundle of His and therefore transient. Occasionally, permanent heart block occurs because of intraoperative mechanical trauma (i.e., suture through the bundle).
What is the treatment of postoperative conduction disturbances?	Temporary pacing with pacing wires (placed intraoperatively) until the edema resolves; a permanent pacer if heart block persists
What is the 10-year mortality rate for UNtreated SYMPTOMATIC AS versus AR?	AS: ≈ 100%: AR < 40%

Valvular Aortic Stenosis (AS)

What is the claim to fame of valvular AS?	Most common isolated valvular lesion
What are the etiologies?	Calcification of congenitally bicuspid aortic valve (50%), rheumatic fever (33%), and senile (idiopathic) calcification of a normal (trileaflet) aortic valve
What are the three nonvalvular etiologies of LV outflow obstruction?	Hypertrophic cardiomyopathy (septal hypertrophy), subvalvular stenosis (focal LV outflow tract stenosis or web), and supravalvular stenosis (aortic narrowing or web)
When is valvular stenosis considered critical?	1. Transvalvular systolic pressure gradient > 50 mm Hg 2. Valvular surface area < 1.0 cm^2
How is cardiac output maintained as stenosis progresses?	Gradual LV hypertrophy to overcome increasing afterload
What is the usual age at initial presentation?	40 to 60 years of age if AS is caused by calcification of the bicuspid valve; otherwise, 60 to 80 years of age

What are the symptoms?	Angina, syncope, and exertional dyspnea as a result of CHF
What is the average life expectancy (if untreated) after the onset of each of these symptoms?	Angina: 3 to 5 years; Syncope: 2 to 3 years; Dyspnea: 1 to 2 years. Symptoms are characteristically late, and once they develop, there is rapid clinical deterioration if left untreated.
What is the usual mechanism of angina in AS?	Increased myocardial oxygen demand because of increased afterload **plus** decreased oxygen delivery because of LV hypertrophy. (Angina may also be caused by concurrent coronary artery disease.)
AS is rarely symptomatic before the valve surface area is reduced to what size?	1.0 cm^2 (about one-third of the normal area)
Why may loss of sinus rhythm cause acute decompensation in AS?	LV hypertrophy results in reduced ventricular compliance, and the synchronized atrial contraction of diastole becomes an important component of ventricular filling.
Describe the murmur associated with AS.	Crescendo–decrescendo systolic murmur in the second right intercostal space with radiation to the carotids. Intensity does **not** correlate with severity; in fact, the most severe cases often have barely audible murmurs.
What are the other classic findings of AS?	Pulsus parvus et tardus (delayed, slow carotid upstroke, with decreased amplitude); narrowed pulse pressure; paradoxic split of S_2 because of delayed closure of the aortic valve (A_2 follows P_2); decreased intensity of S_2; ejection click after S_1; LV lift or heave
What valvular lesion often masks the clinical findings of AS?	Mitral stenosis (MS)

What are the usual EKG findings?	Evidence of LV hypertrophy: S (V1 or V2) + R (V5 or V6) > 35 mm, R (V5 or V6) > 27 mm, or R (AVL) > 11 mm Evidence of LV strain: Repolarization changes (ST depression with upward convexity and T wave inversion)
What are the usual CXR findings?	Normal cardiac silhouette, except for some rounding of the apex because of LV hypertrophy, + calcifications at the level of the aortic valve, + widening of the cephalad mediastinum because of poststenotic dilatation of the aorta
When is echocardiography often inaccurate in its assessment of AS?	In the presence of concurrent MS (or AR) or low cardiac output
What is the most feared common complication of AS?	Sudden death because of ventricular fibrillation
What is the etiology of this complication?	Hypertrophy increases the risk of subendocardial ischemia and, thus, ventricular ectopy.
What are the indications for surgical treatment?	1. Symptomatic patient (angina, syncope, CHF) 2. Critical AS The surface area criteria for surgery vary from 0.5 to 1.0 cm^2, depending on the surgeon as well as the patient's overall condition. **Asymptomatic** patients are **rarely** considered for surgery.
What is the surgical procedure?	Aortic valve replacement (AVR) ± annuloplasty (incision of the annulus to accommodate placement of a larger prosthetic valve in a patient with a small aortic root)
What are the treatment options for the poor surgical candidate?	1. Percutaneous balloon valvuloplasty. Unfortunately, 50% to 75% restenose in 6 months. 2. Palliative medical therapy for CHF + angina (i.e., digitalis, diuretics, nitrates)

What is the 5-year survival rate for patients who have had AVR for AS?	80% to 90%. If ventricular function is impaired at the time of surgery, the 5-year survival rate is reduced by 15% to 25%.

Aortic Regurgitation (AR)

What are the etiologies of AR?	Myxomatous degeneration (i.e., Marfan disease), rheumatic fever, bacterial endocarditis, ascending aortic aneurysm or dissection with dilation of the aortic annulus, calcification of a congenitally bicuspid valve
What are the symptoms?	Uncomfortable palpitations as a result of arrhythmias, ectopic ventricular beats, or powerful contractions of the dilated LV against the chest wall; symptoms of left heart failure (e.g., dyspnea, orthopnea); and angina
What is the usual mechanism of angina in AR?	Increased myocardial oxygen demand caused by increased wall tension associated with LV dilation **plus** decreased oxygen delivery as a result of decreased diastolic pressure in the aortic root (the driving force for coronary perfusion) and LV hypertrophy. (Angina may also be caused by concurrent coronary artery disease.)
What is the classic presentation of ACUTE AR?	Fulminant CHF (versus adaptive changes in the LV permit gradual tolerance of chronic AR over time).
Describe the primary murmur associated with AR.	Blowing, decrescendo diastolic murmur at the left sternal border
How is this difficult-to-hear murmur accentuated?	Auscultation with the patient leaning forward while holding her breath at end-expiration
What other murmurs are associated with AR, and what is the etiology of each?	Systolic ejection murmur caused by increased flow across the aortic valve with the increased LV end-diastolic volume; MR murmur caused by "functional" MR associated with LV dilation; Austin-Flint murmur (MS

murmur, likely caused by reverberation
of the mitral leaflets as a result of AR)

**What is the classic blood
pressure finding and the
mechanism?**

Wide pulse pressure (often 80–100 mm
Hg) because of increased systolic blood
pressure associated with increased CO
and decreased diastolic blood pressure
associated with regurgitation

**How does this finding
change over the course of
the disease?**

Initially, as AR worsens, the pulse
pressure steadily widens. Paradoxically,
in late untreated AR, the pulse pressure
eventually narrows as LV diastolic
pressure increases with progressive LV
failure.

**What is the classic
character of the pulse?**

Bounding because of collapse during
diastole (Corrigan pulse); double-peaked
("bisferious" pulse); "pistol shot"
femoral pulse (excessively high femoral
compared with brachial systolic blood
pressure; Hill sign)

**What are the usual EKG
findings?**

Evidence of LV hypertrophy and strain,
as in AS

**What are the usual CXR
findings?**

Enlarged cardiac silhouette with
downward displacement of the LV apex
because of LV dilation, widening of the
cephalad mediastinum if AR is caused
by ascending aortic aneurysm

**Why is the timing of
surgical intervention more
controversial than with
AS?**

AR causes more indolent deterioration
of LV function.

**How is this problem of
timing of surgery
addressed?**

Serial CXR and EKG every 6 months.
When LV enlargement is noted, the
patient should be studied by
echocardiogram, MUGA, or
ventriculogram. If any ventricular
dysfunction is noted, surgery is
performed. As echocardiography services
become more readily available, many
cardiologists are following patients with
serial echocardiograms.

What are the indications for surgical treatment of AR?

1. Acute significant AR
2. Symptomatic patient with moderate exercise or at rest (NYHA class III or IV)
3. Asymptomatic patient with evidence of deteriorating LV function

What are the surgical options?

AVR ± tube graft for an ascending aortic aneurysm (often as a composite graft); occasionally, aortic valve repair (valve resuspension, replacement of leaflets, or simple suture closure of the cusp perforation)

What is the 5-year survival rate after AVR for AR?

75% to 80%. If ventricular function is impaired at the time of surgery, the 5-year survival rate is reduced by 15% to 25%.

MITRAL VALVE

What is the normal patent surface area of the mitral valve?

4 to 6 cm^2

Is MR or MS associated with LA enlargement?

Both are.

What are the classic signs of LA enlargement on anteroposterior CXR?

Double contour sign (round, double density noted within the cardiac silhouette), straightened left heart border, + elevated left bronchus

What is the classic EKG finding with LA enlargement?

P mitrale: broad, notched P wave in lead II

What systemic complication is associated with LA enlargement?

Systemic embolization (thrombus formation caused by stasis in the dilated low-pressure chamber)

What is the incidence of thromboembolism in MS and MR?

MS: 15% to 30%; MR: < 5%. (MS has the highest risk of thromboembolism of any valve lesion.)

What step is taken preoperatively to reduce the risk of thromboembolism?	Anticoagulation with warfarin (Coumadin)
What step is taken intraoperatively to reduce the future risk of thromboembolism?	Ligation of the left atrial appendage, which frequently harbors a thrombus
What common arrhythmia is associated with LA enlargement?	Atrial fibrillation
What is the incidence of this arrhythmia AFTER the valvular lesion is corrected?	Persists in 66% of patients because LA dilation persists
Is chronic MS or MR classically associated with LV failure?	MR
What studies are used to diagnose and quantify the severity of MS and MR?	Echocardiography (with Doppler) and cardiac catheterization (ventriculogram)
What variables are measured with these studies?	MS: Transvalvular pressure gradient and valvular surface area; MR: Severity of regurgitation (Echocardiography also provides important anatomic detail of the valve).
Which patients with mitral valve disease should also undergo coronary angiogram?	Any patient > 35 years old or with symptoms of myocardial ischemia (angina), regardless of age
What is the best indication of early LV (systolic) dysfunction (and a strong indication for surgery)?	Decrease in ejection fraction with exercise
What structures neighboring the mitral valve annulus may be injured intraoperatively?	AV node or bundle of His, circumflex coronary artery and, occasionally, the aortic valve

What diagnostic tool is used intraoperatively to evaluate mitral repairs and replacements?

Transesophageal echocardiography

Mitral Stenosis

What is the etiology of MS?

Rheumatic fever, which is noted in the patient's history only about 50% of the time because of the 20- to 30-year interval between infection and the symptoms of valvular disease

What is the criterion for critical MS?

Valve surface area < 1.0 cm^2

What is the primary physiologic effect of MS?

Pulmonary hypertension

What are the mechanisms for pulmonary hypertension due to MS?

Retrograde transmission of elevated LA pressure and increased pulmonary vascular resistance because of increased vasoreactivity of the pulmonary vascular bed associated with MS

MS may mask what other valvular lesion, and why?

AS (decreased LV end-diastolic volume results in decreased systolic murmur)

What are the symptoms of MS?

Dyspnea (most common), fatigue, orthopnea, and palpitations

Why may hemoptysis develop?

Chronic pulmonary hypertension causes dilation of the collaterals between the pulmonary and bronchial veins, forming submucosal varices in the bronchus.

Describe the murmur associated with MR.

Low-pitched ("rumble"), crescendo diastolic murmur at the apex

What feature of the murmur correlates with the severity of MS?

Duration

What are the other auscultatory findings?

Loud S_1 and opening snap after S_2 (just before the murmur)

What other cardiac lesion produces auscultatory findings similar to those of MS?	LA myxoma. Symptoms are usually more episodic and positional in nature than those of MS, and patients often have other systemic signs, including fever and weight loss.
When LV hypertrophy is seen on echocardiogram, what conclusion can be drawn?	Patient has an additional cardiovascular problem (i.e., MR, AS, systemic hypertension). MS alone does **not** cause LV hypertrophy.
What is the medical treatment of MR?	Salt restriction, diuretic therapy, digitalis, and close follow-up
What are the indications for surgery?	Multiple indications, including NYHA class III or IV, critical MS, CHF, pulmonary hypertension, atrial fibrillation, systemic emboli, endocarditis, and transvalvular gradient > 10 mm Hg
What is the first-line surgical procedure?	Open commissurotomy (sharp separation of fused leaflets)
When is this technique contraindicated?	Extensive calcification of the valve
What is the restenosis rate at 5 years?	Only 10%. Unlike in the aortic valve, mitral commissurotomy is effective in selected patients.
What procedure is usually performed if MS recurs?	MVR

Mitral Regurgitation (MR)

What are the etiologies of MR?	Rheumatic fever (40%–45%), myxomatous degeneration, severe mitral valve prolapse, senile (idiopathic) calcification of the mitral valve, infectious endocarditis, trauma, hypertrophic cardiomyopathy, and MI or ischemia (see Postoperative Myocardial Ischemia section)
What are the symptoms?	Fatigue, dyspnea, and palpitations. The symptoms are similar to those of MS, but are characteristically **insidious and late,** unless they are caused by MI.

Describe the murmur associated with MR.

Holosystolic at the apex, with radiation to the axilla

What is the characteristic finding on pulmonary artery catheter tracing?

Prominent V wave because of regurgitant systolic flow

What is the medical treatment of MR?

Salt restriction, diuretics, and digitalis. This therapy can be palliative for many years.

What are the indications for surgical treatment?

1. Acute MR (i.e., ischemic MR)
2. NYHA class III or IV status
3. Progressive increase in regurgitant fraction

What are the surgical options?

MVR or mitral valve repair, including leaflet repair, annuloplasty (reducing the size of the dilated annulus with sutures or a prosthetic ring), chorda tendineae reconstruction, or reimplantation of the ruptured papillary muscle

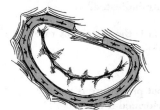

Annuloplasty

Why may LV failure develop in the early postoperative period?

LV no longer has a low-pressure vent (LA) into which it can unload blood during systole. With correction of MR, LV ejects all of its volume into the high-pressure aorta.

What is the treatment of postoperative LV failure?

Vasodilator therapy for afterload reduction; inotrope therapy + IABP

See the Mechanical Complications of Ischemic Heart Disease section for a discussion of MR caused by myocardial ischemia.

Mitral Valve Prolapse

What is mitral valve prolapse?

Bulging of the mitral leaflets into the LA during systole because of redundant MV tissue ± chorda tendineae

What is the incidence in the general population?

3% to 4%

What is the target population?

Girls and women between 15 and 30 years old. It is often seen in patients with myxomatous degenerative disorders, and it thus appears to be genetic.

What are the symptoms?

Most patients are **asymptomatic.** The most common symptoms are fatigue, nonspecific chest pain, palpitation, and dyspnea.

What is the classic auscultatory sign?

Mid to late systolic click

What percentage of these patients develop significant MR?

5% to 7%

TRICUSPID VALVE

Does tricuspid valve disease (TVD) present more frequently as tricuspid regurgitation (TR) or tricuspid stenosis (TS)?

TR (75%)

What is the most common etiology of isolated acquired TVD?

Infectious endocarditis caused by IV drug abuse. Venous return from injected veins slowly bathes the tricuspid valve before reaching the lungs, which filter many of the bacteria.

What is the most common etiology of primary acquired TVD?

Rheumatic heart disease (almost always accompanied by mitral stenosis)

What is the most common etiology of "functional" TR?

Left heart failure, which causes RV failure with associated RV dilation and concurrent dilation of the free wall segment of the tricuspid annulus (functional TR)

What is the most common etiology of TVD?

Left heart failure (functional TR)

What determines the physiologic significance of TR?

Presence of pulmonary hypertension. If pulmonary hypertension is absent or mild, TR is rarely significant.

What is the primary sequela of severe TR?

Liver congestion

What are the symptoms of TVD?

Fatigue, weakness, and extremity and abdominal swelling

Describe the murmurs associated with TR and TS.

TR: Holosystolic murmur at the left lower sternal border, with no radiation to the axilla
TS: Crescendo diastolic murmur at the left lower sternal border.
These low-intensity murmurs are difficult to distinguish from those of mitral valve disease.

What are the classic findings of RV failure on physical exam?

Hepatomegaly ± pulsatile liver, peripheral edema, ascites, prominent jugular venous pulse, and distended neck veins

What are the usual CXR findings in TVD?

Enlarged RA ± signs of LV failure in functional TR

What is the medical treatment of TVD?

Strict salt restrictions, diuretic therapy, and digitalis. In patients who undergo surgery, this preoperative medical regimen decreases hepatic congestion and significantly reduces the risk of the procedure.

What are the indications for surgery?

1. RV failure
2. RV dilation
3. Pulmonary hypertension
4. Transvalvular (tricuspid) pressure gradient > 4 mm Hg

What is the surgical procedure for functional TR?

Treatment of the primary lesion (i.e., mitral stenosis).Tricuspid valve annuloplasty or replacement (TVR) may also be necessary (controversial).

What is the surgical procedure for rheumatic TS?

TVR or open commissurotomy

What is the surgical procedure for TVD caused by infectious endocarditis?

1. Valve excision alone (TVR may not be necessary if no pulmonary hypertension is present)
2. TVR

Why is the operative mortality rate associated with TVD higher than that for other valves?

Because isolated TVD is rare, procedures are usually multivalvular (mortality rate 10%–20%)

PULMONARY VALVE

What is the most common acquired pulmonary valve lesion?

Functional pulmonary regurgitation (PR) caused by dilation of the pulmonary annulus. It usually occurs secondary to pulmonary hypertension associated with MS.

What is the classic murmur associated with pulmonary regurgitation?

Graham Steell murmur: High-pitched, diastolic, decrescendo murmur

How is this murmur distinguished from that of AR?

PR: Heard along the **left** sternal border
AR: Heard along the **right** sternal border, especially at the second intercostal space

RHEUMATIC HEART DISEASE

What is the etiology of rheumatic heart disease?

Systemic immune disease associated with antecedent hemolytic group A streptococcal pharyngitis (rheumatic fever). Patients have high antistreptolysin (ASO) titers.

What are the gross effects on the affected valve?

Leaflet fibrosis, shortening of the chorda tendineae, and commissural fusion

What are the most commonly involved valves?	Mitral valve: 85% of cases Aortic valve: 30% of cases Tricuspid and pulmonary valves: < 5% of cases

REVIEW OF ACQUIRED VALVULAR DISEASES

Which valvular lesion is associated with the following:

1. **Sudden death?**
2. **Carcinoid syndrome?**

3. **Cor bovinum?**
4. **Pulsatile liver?**
5. **Double contour sign on CXR?**
6. **Four-chamber dilation of the heart?**
7. **Angina, syncope, and CHF?**
8. **"Pistol shot" pulse?**
9. **Dyspnea, fatigue, and palpitations?**

10. **Falsely increased LV end-diastolic pressure as predicted by Swan-Ganz catheter?**
11. **Loss of x descent on central venous tracing?**
12. **Ejection click?**
13. **Opening snap?**
14. **Pulsus parvus et tardus?**
15. **Paradoxic split of S_2?**
16. **Atrial fibrillation?**

17. **Austin-Flint murmur?**
18. **Left parasternal heave?**

1. Aortic stenosis
2. Tricuspid and pulmonary valve disease (fibrosis and stenosis of valves)
3. Aortic regurgitation
4. Tricuspid regurgitation
5. Mitral stenosis and regurgitation

6. Mitral regurgitation (late)

7. Aortic stenosis

8. Aortic regurgitation
9. Mitral stenosis and regurgitation most commonly, but all valvular lesions eventually cause failure if left untreated
10. Mitral stenosis

11. Tricuspid regurgitation

12. Aortic and pulmonary stenosis
13. Mitral stenosis
14. Aortic stenosis

15. Aortic stenosis
16. Mitral stenosis and regurgitation; tricuspid regurgitation
17. Aortic regurgitation
18. Tricuspid regurgitation or pulmonary stenosis (RV hypertrophy)

PROSTHETIC VALVES

Mechanical Valves

What are the most commonly used mechanical valves?

St. Jude (low-profile, bileaflet hinged valve), Starr-Edwards (caged ball valve)

What is the primary disadvantage of these valves?

Lifelong anticoagulation (Coumadin) because of the high risk of thromboembolism. Most institutions also anticoagulate tissue valves for 3 to 8 weeks postoperatively until Dacron and suture lines endothelialize.

What are the contraindications to the use of mechanical valves (i.e., indications for tissue valves)?

Absolute: History of major bleeding
Relative: Unreliable noncompliant patient; patient > 65 years old (because of increased risk of stroke associated with anticoagulation); pregnancy (current or planned)

Tissue Valves

What is the most common type of tissue valve?

Xenograft (glutaraldehyde-fixed porcine valve)

What is the primary disadvantage of these valves?

Deterioration over time

When do 50% of the valves require replacement?

13 years

What are the contraindications to tissue valves (i.e., indications for mechanical valves)?

Rapid calcification of valve occurs in young patients (especially children, but anyone < 30 years old) and patients who are receiving renal dialysis

What three additional types of tissue valves are occasionally used?

1. Bovine pericardial valves
2. Homograft (human donor valve)
3. Autograft (autotransplant of valve)

What are the major disadvantages of homograft valves?

Limited supply and a more difficult procedure, resulting in longer cross-clamp time

What is the valve autograft procedure?

Diseased aortic valve is excised. The pulmonary valve is excised and sutured into the aortic position. A bioprosthetic valve is sutured into the pulmonary position (i.e., Ross procedure).

Complications of Valve Replacement

What are the early postoperative complications of valve replacement?

Conduction abnormalities (the AV–His bundle travels close to the valvular annuli, and multiple sutures must be placed near this region), endocarditis, systemic thromboemboli, and ventricular failure

What are the late complications of valve replacement?

Systemic thromboemboli, endocarditis, and bleeding as a result of anticoagulation

What is the most common late complication of mechanical valves?

Cerebral thromboemboli

What is the incidence of this complication?

1% to 5 % each year, even with anticoagulation. The incidence varies with the type of valve (e.g., for the St. Jude valve, only 1%–2 % per year).

Cerebral thromboemboli occur most frequently with replacement of which valve?

Mitral valve

Three-Dimensional Relation Among Cardiac Valves

On CXR, the valve that
was replaced can be
identified by its position.
In the illustrations of
anteroposterior and lateral
views of the heart on CXR,
which valves would be
placed in positions 1
through 8?

1. Tricuspid
2. Mitral
3. Aortic
4. Pulmonary
5. Pulmonary
6. Aortic
7. Tricuspid
8. Mitral

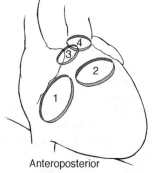

Anteroposterior

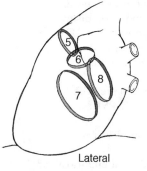

Lateral

INFECTIOUS ENDOCARDITIS (IE)

Which native valve is at greatest risk for endocarditis?	Mitral valve (accounts for 80% of cases)
What distinguishes acute from subacute native valve endocarditis (NVE)?	Acute: Rapid onset; usually caused by virulent organisms Subacute: Indolent onset; usually caused by less virulent organisms
Are normal or diseased valves the target in acute versus subacute NVE?	Acute: Normal, although some minor lesion must be present to cause the turbulence that permits the bacteria to invade the valve Subacute: Diseased (e.g., rheumatic heart disease, congenital bicuspid aortic valve)
A prosthetic valve in which position is at greatest risk for IE?	Aortic valve (accounts for 60% of cases)

Define early versus late prosthetic valve endocarditis (PVE).

Early: < 2 months after surgery;
Late: > 2 months after surgery

What is the incidence of PVE in tissue versus mechanical valves?

5% to 10% **(same for both)**

Why is aggressive therapy necessary for early PVE?

Mortality rate of 60% to 70%

What are the most common organisms responsible for IE in the following settings:
1. **Acute NVE?**

1. *Staphylococcus aureus* and group A streptococcus

2. **Subacute NVE?**
3. **Early PVE?**

2. *Streptococcus viridans,* enterococci
3. *Staphylococcus epidermidis, S. aureus,* and diphtheroids

4. **Late PVE?**

4. Enterococcus, *S. aureus,* and gram-negative bacteria

5. **Fungal endocarditis?**
6. **Right-sided endocarditis in IV drug abusers?**

5. *Candida* and *Aspergillus*
6. *S. aureus, Candida,* and gram-negative bacteria *(Pseudomonas)*

What are the most common signs of IE?

Fever and new murmur

What are the classic findings on physical exam (in decreasing order of frequency)?

Skin and conjunctival petechiae (most common), nail bed splinter hemorrhages, Osler nodes (painful nodules on the pads of the digits), Janeway lesions (painless macular lesions on the palms and soles), Roth spots (pale oval lesions on the retina with surrounding hemorrhage)

How is the diagnosis made?

1. Positive blood culture (× 3)
2. Echocardiography: Detects vegetations, regurgitation, and paravalvular leakage caused by ring abscess

What is the medical treatment?

4 to 6 weeks of IV antibiotic therapy

What is the most common indication for surgery?	CHF
What are the other indications for surgery?	Early PVE, unstable (i.e., rocking) prosthetic valve caused by PVE, positive blood culture findings after 2 weeks of IV antibiotics, fungal infections, recurrent emboli, septic shock while receiving antibiotics, and conduction defects in the heart because of ring abscess
What is the surgical procedure?	Excision of the valve and aggressive débridement of any surrounding infected necrotic myocardium, followed by valve replacement. The tricuspid valve may not require replacement if pulmonary hypertension is absent.
How long is antibiotic therapy continued after surgery?	At least 4 weeks
What is the reinfection rate of the new valve?	Only 5% to 10%

DISEASES OF THE GREAT VESSELS

THORACIC AND THORACOABDOMINAL AORTIC ANEURYSMS

What are the etiologies of thoracic and thoracoabdominal aortic aneurysms?	Atherosclerosis, myxomatous degeneration (i.e., Marfan disease), aortic dissection, and infection (i.e., syphilis)
What is the incidence of aneurysms in the various thoracic aortic regions?	Ascending aorta: > 40% Descending aorta: 35% Aortic arch: 10% (thoracoabdominal aorta: 10%)
What is the most common etiology of ascending aortic aneurysms?	Myxomatous degeneration
What is the most frequent cardiac lesion associated with ascending aortic aneurysms?	Aortic insufficiency because of dilation of the aortic valve annulus (annuloaortic ectasia). It is rarely seen in patients with an atherosclerotic etiology.

What is the gross difference in appearance between atherosclerotic and myxomatous ascending aortic aneurysms?

Atherosclerotic: Fusiform shape
Myxomatous: Pear shape

Why are aortic arch aneurysms difficult to manage?

Because they involve the aortic arch vessels, the risk of intraoperative cerebral ischemia is significant.

What is the most common etiology of descending or thoracoabdominal aortic aneurysms?

Atherosclerosis

Which etiology is classically associated with saccular aneurysms?

Syphilis

What is the most common presentation of thoracic aneurysm?

Incidental finding on CXR in an **asymptomatic** patient

What is the most common symptom of thoracic aneurysm?

Chronic dull or "boring" pain in the back or precordium

What is the classic, although less common, presentation of:
1. Ascending aortic aneurysm?

2. Descending aortic aneurysm?

1. Congestive heart failure (e.g., dyspnea) because of aortic insufficiency
2. Cough and dyspnea because of compression of the left main bronchus

What is the primary complication of aortic aneurysms if untreated?

Rupture and death

How does the rate of expansion compare with that of abdominal aortic aneurysms?

More rapid expansion as well as greater risk of rupture

What is the 5-year survival rate if untreated?

20%

What diagnostic studies are performed?

Computed tomography (CT) scan with contrast, magnetic resonance imaging (MRI), or aortogram. Some patients undergo surgery on the basis of MRI findings alone (aortogram is no longer always performed).

What are the indications for surgery for thoracic aortic aneurysms?

1. Symptomatic aneurysm
2. Asymptomatic aneurysm > 6 to 7 cm (in Marfan disease, aneurysm > 5–6 cm)
3. Rapid increase in aneurysm size. Because of the rapid rate of enlargement and the tendency to rupture, many advocate earlier surgical intervention as the morbidity and mortality rates of repair decline.

What is the usual surgical procedure?

Tube graft replacement [Dacron, homograft, or polytetrafluoroethylene (PTFE)] of the diseased segment of the aorta. Cardiopulmonary bypass (CPB) is usually required.

What procedure is often used for ascending aortic aneurysms caused by Marfan disease?

Bentall procedure: Replacement of the ascending aorta **and** aortic valve with a composite graft because of the frequency of dilation of the valve annulus.

What is the Crawford, or inclusion, technique, and where is it used most frequently?

Incorporation or implantation of a group of arteries (as an island or a cuff) into the prosthetic tube graft rather than multiple individual implantation sites. It is used primarily for arch vessels, visceral arteries, and intercostal–lumbar arteries.

What technique is necessary to minimize cerebral ischemia during the repair of aortic arch aneurysms?

Deep hypothermic circulatory arrest: Patient is cooled to 14°C to 18°C, blood is drained into a heart–lung bypass machine, and CPB (and thus, circulation of the body) is discontinued for as long as 45 to 60 minutes.

What are two alternatives to CPB in the repair of some descending and thoracoabdominal aortic aneurysms?

1. Simple cross-clamping of the aorta plus nitroprusside IV to control the resultant hypertension
2. Heparin-bonded Gott or TDMAC shunt (aortoaortic or aortofemoral)

How are most saccular aneurysms managed?

Simple excision with repair of the resultant aortic defect at the base of the aneurysm

What is the overall operative mortality rate?

< 10%

What is the most common cause of death?

Myocardial infarction

What are the postoperative complications?

Respiratory insufficiency (most common), MI, acute tubular necrosis, paraplegia, and stroke

What classic syndrome is associated with spinal ischemia?

Anterior spinal artery syndrome

Repair of which types of aortic aneurysm increases the risk of spinal ischemia?

Thoracoabdominal and descending aortic aneurysms

Why are these types at higher risk for spinal ischemia?

The primary blood supply to the anterior spinal cord is supplied by the artery of Adamkiewicz, a large intercostal or lumbar artery usually located between T8 and L4. To prevent back-bleeding into the surgical field, the intercostals and lumbars are often oversewn or ligated.

What are the signs and symptoms associated with the anterior spinal artery syndrome?

Paraplegia, incontinence (bowel or bladder), and sensory loss for pain and temperature

In addition to CPB and hypothermia, what adjunctive techniques MAY reduce the incidence of paraplegia?

1. Localization of the artery of Adamkiewicz preoperatively with selective lumbar–intercostal artery angiogram and intraoperative reimplantation of this vessel. Some centers forgo the selective angiogram and instead reimplant all patent

lumbar–intercostal arteries, often with the inclusion technique.

2. Augmentation of spinal cord blood flow with cerebrospinal fluid drainage and intrathecal papaverine (vasodilator)

What long-term medical therapy is often prescribed after aortic aneurysm surgery?

Antihypertensive agents (often β-blockers)

What is the primary reason for close long-term follow-up?

Increased risk of the development of dissection or aneurysm in any residual aorta

What is the 5-year survival rate after surgery?

50%

AORTIC DISSECTION

What are the basic histologic lesion and the resultant sequence of gross pathologic lesions?

Degeneration of the elastic fibers of the aorta media, followed by reduced intimal adherence, eventually causing intimal tears. As a result, blood dissects into the wall of the aorta, forming true and false aortic lumens. Recent evidence suggests that true "cystic medi... necrosis" accounts for only 10% of dissections.

What are the most common sites of intimal tears?

1. Proximal ascending aorta (50%)
2. Ligamentum arteriosum (35%)

Define acute versus chronic dissection.

Acute: < 2 weeks old; Chronic: > 2 weeks old

Name and describe the two classification systems.

1. **Stanford system:**
   Type A: Dissection involving the ascending aorta ± the transverse or descending aorta
   Type B: Dissection involving only the descending aorta (e.g., distal to the takeoff of the left subclavian artery)
2. **DeBakey system:**
   Type I: Dissection involving the ascending, transverse, and some or all of the descending aorta

Type II: Dissection involving only the ascending aorta

Type III: Dissection involving only the descending aorta. If restricted to the thoracic aorta, called type IIIa; if extending into the abdomen, called type IIIb.

What is the average survival rate for all patients with untreated aortic dissections?

2 weeks: 20%; 1 year: 10%. Long-term survivors have type B or type III dissections. Only 5% to 10% of patients with untreated type A or type I or II dissections survive for 2 weeks, and they rarely survive for 1 year.

The exact etiology of aortic dissection is uncertain. What is the key predisposing factor?

Hypertension (70%–90%)

What are the other predisposing factors?

Myxomatous degeneration of the aorta (i.e., Marfan disease), atherosclerosis, coarctation of the aorta, epinephrine infusion, and trauma

What is the classic initial symptom?

Abrupt onset of **severe** chest pain, often "ripping" or "tearing" in character (almost pathognomonic) ± radiation to the interscapular region of the back or the upper extremities

How is aortic dissection distinguished from MI?

Pain often **migrates** down the back as the dissection extends distally.

How helpful is an EKG, and why?

Essential. If findings are negative, MI is ruled out; if findings are positive, dissection is not ruled out! Proximal dissections may sever or occlude the coronary arteries, resulting in myocardial ischemia and possible sudden death.

What are the findings on physical exam?

Weak or absent peripheral pulses (variable, depending on the site of dissection); different blood pressure in the upper extremities

In addition to MI, what are other potential sequelae of dissection, and what signs are associated with each?

1. Cardiac tamponade (if the ascending aorta ruptures proximal to the pericardial reflection): Beck triad (hypotension, distended neck veins, and muffled heart sounds)
2. Acute aortic insufficiency (because of dilation of the aorta annulus and resultant CHF): diastolic murmur, hypotension, and rales
3. Occlusion or shearing of the branches of the aorta to the brain, extremities, and viscera: unequal pulses and signs of ischemia in these regions
4. Rupture of the aorta: presentation depends on the severity and site of rupture

What is the most common site of rupture?

Proximal ascending aorta, because the adventitia of the intrapericardial aorta is thin. Tamponade is a frequent cause of death.

What is the most common finding on CXR?

Normal CXR

What CXR findings suggest contained rupture of the aortic dissection?

Wide mediastinum (especially if > 8 cm); loss or blurring of the aortic knob shadow; depression of the left main-stem bronchus, elevation of the right main-stem bronchus, and tracheal and esophageal deviation to the right. If the aorta is ruptured, left pleural effusion or pleural cap may be seen.

What percentage of patients with contained rupture have a normal CXR?

Only 10% (i.e., it is a sensitive screening test)

What diagnostic studies are used to visualize an aortic dissection?

CT scan with contrast, MRI, aortogram, or transesophageal echocardiography

What additional study is recommended in elderly patients preoperatively?

Coronary angiogram

How are the different types of dissection USUALLY managed?

1. Type A (or I and II): Managed **surgically** because of the risk of occlusion of coronary or cerebral circulation, aortic insufficiency, and pericardial tamponade
2. Type B (or III): Managed **medically** if uncomplicated

What are the indications for surgical treatment of type B dissection?

Continued pain, inability to control blood pressure, evidence of arterial occlusion (carotid, renal, mesenteric, or extremity), rupture or expansion of the aneurysm. (Unlike most centers, the Stanford group now recommends early surgical intervention, even for uncomplicated type B dissection.)

What is the initial acute management of aortic dissection?

Bed rest; close monitoring with telemetry, arterial pressure catheter (radial artery + femoral artery), central venous pressure catheter, and Foley catheter; antihypertensive therapy; sedation. The primary initial goal is to convert the acute dissection to a subacute or chronic one to reduce the morbidity and mortality of surgery.

What is the primary purpose of antihypertensive therapy?

Prevention of the progression of dissection by controlling blood pressure **and** reducing myocardial contractility (shear forces)

Which antihypertensive agents are most commonly used?

IV nitroprusside and esmolol (or propranolol)

What is the surgical procedure for ascending dissection?

Tube graft replacement of the involved segment of the aorta, including the original intimal tear, to direct blood into the true aortic lumen and obliterate the false lumen, ± aortic valve replacement (Bentall procedure) or valve repair (resuspension of valve leaflets). The procedure requires CPB ± hypothermic circulatory arrest.

What type of incision is used for ascending dissection?	Median sternotomy
What procedure is used for descending dissection?	Tube graft replacement, as in ascending dissection; CPB is required
What type of incision is used for descending dissection?	Left posterolateral thoracotomy
What is the critical feature of repair of any dissection?	Graft replacement of the region of the aorta at the site of the intimal tear
What is the most common cause of intraoperative death?	Hemorrhage from suture lines because of the poor quality of the diseased aorta and intraoperative anticoagulation
What is the cornerstone of postoperative management?	Meticulous control of blood pressure (e.g., β-blockers, hydralazine)
What is the duration of this treatment, and why?	Lifelong. Surgery controls life-threatening complications, but does not cure dissection.
What is the primary reason for close long-term follow-up?	High risk of future dissection or aneurysm in any residual aorta

See the Trauma to the Heart and Great Vessels section for a discussion of traumatic aneurysms of the thoracic aorta.

SUPERIOR VENA CAVA SYNDROME

What is superior vena cava syndrome?	Complex of signs and symptoms caused by occlusion or stenosis of the superior vena cava
What is the primary collateral for blood around the superior vena cava occlusion?	Azygous vein, which eventually empties into the inferior vena cava below the diaphragm
What are the two most common etiologies?	1. Bronchogenic carcinoma (65%–80%) 2. Malignant lymphoma (5%–15%) Malignancy accounts for 80% to 90% of cases.

What is the most common benign etiology?	Chronic fibrosing mediastinitis
What are the symptoms?	Headache, shortness of breath, confusion, and dizziness
What are the associated signs?	Venous distension of the chest, head, and neck; facial edema and plethora; and hoarseness and dyspnea as a result of edema of the vocal cords and larynx
What other conditions are included in the differential diagnosis?	Constrictive pericarditis, CHF, and angioneurotic edema
What is the usual cause of death in acute complete obstruction?	Cerebral edema
What is the diagnostic study of choice?	CT scan with contrast (or MRI) **plus** percutaneous needle biopsy for tissue diagnosis. In the occasional case of surgical intervention, a venogram provides additional detail of the venous anatomy.
What is the treatment of malignant superior vena cava obstruction?	Diuretics, fluid restriction, and upright positioning, ± corticosteroids to reduce cerebral edema, **plus** radiation therapy (70%), chemotherapy (25%–30%), or surgical bypass of the obstruction with spiral vein graft (< 1%)
What is the most effective acute treatment for a patient in extremis?	Emergency radiation therapy (1000–1500 rads)
What is the treatment of benign superior vena cava obstruction?	Diuretics, fluid restriction, and upright positioning. Treatment is usually necessary only temporarily until sufficient collaterals develop. In some cases of incomplete obstruction, surgical resection of the compressive mass is indicated.

What is the usual length of survival of patients with superior vena cava syndrome because of lung malignancy?	6 to 8 months

HEART TRANSPLANTATION

What are the indications for heart transplantation?	Ischemic cardiomyopathy ("end-stage" CAD), idiopathic (primary) cardiomyopathy (i.e., dilated, restrictive), secondary cardiomyopathy (i.e., viral, alcoholic, infiltrative, toxic, metabolic), some types of congenital heart disease, and retransplantation for severe acute or chronic rejection
What are the absolute contraindications to transplantation?	Pulmonary hypertension (> 6 Wood units and uncontrollable with oral pharmacologic therapy), active infection, active malignancy, irreversible hepatic disease, irreversible renal disease (if renal transplant is not possible), and age > 65 years old (age criteria are institution-dependent)
What is the major limiting factor in the number of heart transplants currently performed?	Scarcity of donor cardiac allografts
What are the potential future alternatives to allograft transplantation?	Long-term LV assist devices (LVAD), xenotransplants (the use of animal hearts), and artificial hearts

Preoperative Period and Procedure

What interventions are used to support the patient who is awaiting transplantation?	Pharmacologic treatment to reduce volume overload and maintain CO (i.e., diuretics, digoxin, dopamine, dobutamine, amrinone), IABP, and mechanical circulatory assist devices (LVAD or biventricular assist devices; the "bridges to transplantation")
What criteria are used to match donors and recipients for heart transplantation?	ABO compatibility (because of the shortage of donors and the limits of myocardial preservation, HLA matching is not feasible) and cytomegalovirus

(CMV) status. In adults, size matching plays a minor role.

What is the accepted limit of ex vivo ischemic time for the donor heart?

Only 4 to 6 hours!

What are the two types of heart transplantation?

1. Orthotopic: Removal of the recipient ventricles (accounts for > 95% of transplants performed)
2. Heterotopic: Piggybacking of the donor heart onto the recipient heart

How is the recipient heart excised?

The patient is place on cardiopulmonary bypass and the aorta is cross-clamped. The aorta and pulmonary artery are transected, and a circumferential incision is made proximal to the AV groove, leaving most of the left and right atria in the recipient.

Effects of donor heart denervation

What does "denervation" of donor heart refer to?

Harvesting of a donor heart necessitates transection of its innervating fibers.

What are the important physiologic results of denervation?

1. Baseline tachycardia (90–110 beats/min) because of the loss of parasympathetic tone that normally inhibits the sinoatrial node
2. Delayed myocardial response to stress because of the exclusive dependence on circulating catecholamines from distant noncardiac sites for positive chronotropic and inotropic effects

What standard cardiac therapeutic interventions are ineffective with loss of autonomic innervation?

Atropine, digoxin, carotid sinus massage, and the Valsalva maneuver

How does denervation complicate the presentation of MI?

Heart transplant recipients do **not** have angina because of the lack of afferent sensory fibers. Several years after transplantation, a few patients apparently have reinnervation of the donor heart and experience angina, but these are rare and unpredictable exceptions.

Early postoperative hemodynamic complications

What is the usual etiology of early postoperative low CO?

The newly transplanted heart is noncompliant and stiff because of the injury associated with harvesting, cooling, and ischemia. Fortunately, this dysfunction usually resolves during the first 3 days.

What is the treatment of early low CO?

Volume (to optimize preload in the noncompliant ventricles), isoproterenol (to maintain the heart rate at 100–125 beats/min), ± additional inotropic support with dobutamine

What are two additional complications and their first-line treatment?

1. RV failure: Isoproterenol
2. Sinus bradycardia and junctional rhythms: Isoproterenol, **not** atropine

A patient moves to a chair on postoperative day 2 and promptly loses consciousness. What is the most likely etiology?

Orthostatic hypotension because of the loss of normal reflex tachycardia as well as a great dependence on preload.

What is the most common cause of death in the first year?

Infection

What is the most common cause of death after the first year?

Rejection

Infectious complications

What is the most common site of infections in heart transplant recipients?

Lungs

These patients are at risk for opportunistic infections in addition to the usual spectrum of bacterial pathogens encountered in surgery. When is each type of infection most prevalent?

Bacterial: Acute infections (< 1 month postoperatively)
Opportunistic: Subacute infections (> 1 month, especially 1–4 months)

What are the most common organisms in acute infections?

Gram-negative bacilli (*Pseudomonas, Escherichia coli,* and *Klebsiella*)

What are the most common organisms in subacute infections?

CMV, although some groups report *Pneumocystis* as the most prevalent

What are the four types of opportunistic infection?

1. Intracellular: *Listeria, Mycobacterium, Salmonella*
2. Fungal: *Candida, Aspergillus*
3. Viral: Herpes simplex, CMV
4. Protozoal: *Pneumocystis, Toxoplasma*

What drug is given if a CMV-positive heart is transplanted into a CMV-negative recipient (CMV mismatch)?

Ganciclovir (also used to treat serious CMV infection)

What is the standard immunosuppressive maintenance regimen for heart transplantation?

Triple therapy: Cyclosporine, prednisone, and azathioprine (Imuran)

What is the most common type of rejection?

Acute rejection (days to months postoperatively). The highest incidence of rejection occurs in the first 3 months.

What percentage of patients have a rejection episode during the first few months?

80%!

What is the classic manifestation of chronic rejection (controversial)?

Accelerated coronary artery disease (ACAD). Some theorize that there are nonrejection etiologies for ACAD (e.g., CMV).

What is the most common presentation of rejection?

Usually asymptomatic, unless severe

What are the classic signs?

Fever; if severe, signs of RV and/or LV dysfunction (e.g., S3, S4, JVD, hepatomegaly and arrhythmias)

What is the most reliable way to diagnose rejection?	Endomyocardial biopsy of the RV septum with a percutaneous bioptome
What is the most common treatment of rejection?	Corticosteroids: Short course of IV methylprednisolone (Solu-Medrol) on an outpatient basis, requiring a daily visit to the hospital **or** increased dose of oral prednisone, if rejection is mild
What is the main complication of this treatment?	Increased risk of opportunistic infection. Over the last several years, the threshold for treatment of rejection has become steadily higher to avoid the more dangerous infectious complications of additional immunosuppression.
What additional immunosuppressive agents may be used if steroids fail?	The monoclonal antibody OKT3 or ATG (antithymocyte globulin)
What is the most common reason for retransplantation?	Chronic rejection (ACAD), which accounts for 66% of cases
What are the most common neoplasms seen in heart transplant recipients?	Carcinoma of the skin and lip (i.e., squamous cell carcinoma); non-Hodgkin lymphoma
What are the survival rates at 1 and 5 years?	1 year: 80% to 90%; 5 years: 50% to 60%

CARDIOPULMONARY BYPASS

What are the functions of CPB?	Perfusion of the body with blood, gas exchange (oxygen added and carbon dioxide removed from the blood), alterations of core temperature (decrease in temperature during surgery to reduce the metabolic rate)
Compare total CPB with partial CPB.	Total CPB: All venous blood is bypassed to the pump Partial CPB: Some venous blood passes through the lungs

What are the components of the basic CPB circuit?

Venous cannula(e) from the RA (or superior and inferior vena cava); heart–lung machine with pump apparatus, heat exchanger, and oxygenator; arterial filter; arterial cannula into the ascending aorta. (The femoral artery and vein occasionally are used for cannulation sites.)

How is the heart arrested so that surgery can be performed safely?

Infusion of a cold, high-potassium solution (i.e., cardioplegia) into the aortic root or directly into the coronary arteries after cross-clamping of the ascending aorta. Topical cold saline (4°C) helps to maintain myocardial temperature at ≈ 15°C.

To what temperature is the patient usually cooled for a standard cardiac procedure?

28° to 32°C (mild hypothermia)

What is deep, or profound, hypothermia?

< 18°C

How low may pump rate be reduced during profound hypothermia?

Pump may be turned off (i.e., hypothermic circulatory arrest)

For what procedures is profound hypothermia indicated?

Aortic arch surgery and complex congenital cardiac surgery

What step is necessary to prevent thrombosis in the pump?

Patient must be anticoagulated with heparin (activated clotting time is monitored intraoperatively)

A patient is not weaning from CPB (i.e., as the pump rate is decreased, the patient cannot maintain blood pressure). What steps are taken to permit successful discontinuation of CPB?

1. Intravascular volume (crystalloid or blood) is increased
2. Vasopressor and inotropic support (infusions of dopamine, dobutamine, or epinephrine) is provided
3. ± IABP is placed
4. ± Left and/or right ventricular assist device is placed
5. Very rarely, heart transplant is performed.

Shortly after the discontinuation of CPB, severe pulmonary hypertension suddenly develops. What is the most likely etiology?

Protamine reaction. Protamine sulfate is used to reverse the activity of heparin after the completion of CPB.

What features of the patient history suggest the potential for protamine reaction?

Diabetes (protamine in insulin); allergies to iodine or seafood; patient or family history of protamine reaction

What is "postperfusion syndrome" (PPS)?

End-organ effects of the "whole-body inflammatory reaction" associated with CPB, manifested as postoperative pulmonary insufficiency, renal failure, bleeding disorder, and/or myocardial dysfunction.

What is the etiology of PPS?

Uncertain. Current evidence suggests that contact with the synthetic surfaces of the extracorporeal circuit activates the humoral (i.e., complement) and cellular (i.e., neutrophil) cascades of the acute inflammatory response, resulting in endothelial injury

Which factor is activated at the onset of CPB and appears to initiate the various humoral cascades?

Factor XII (Hageman factor)

Which complement anaphylatoxins appear intimately involved in PPS?

C3a and C5a

What is the treatment of PPS?

Supportive therapy (e.g., ventilator, dialysis) until the patient recovers

POSTOPERATIVE INTENSIVE CARE MANAGEMENT

CARDIAC OUTPUT

What are the physiologic determinants of CO?

1. **Heart rate** (HR)
2. **Preload** (end-diastolic volume of the ventricle)
3. **Compliance** (tendency of the ventricle to permit distension with blood

4. **Afterload** (the force opposing ventricular ejection)
5. **Contractility** (intrinsic contractile performance, independent of the other determinants of CO) CO = SV x HR

What is the cardiac index (CI)?

CO per body surface area expressed in meters squared

What are the normal values for CO and CI?

CO = 4 to 8 L/min, CI = 2.5 to 4 L/min/m²

What is the Frank-Starling relation?

Relation between the resting muscle length (determined by preload) and the tension achieved by the contracting muscle. Up to a point defined by the Frank-Starling curve of the ventricle, increases in preload augment stroke volume and thus CO.

What is the key determinant of CO in a heart with normal versus reduced compliance?

Normal compliance: Preload
Reduced compliance: Afterload

Why is blood pressure an INSENSITIVE index of myocardial performance?

Blood pressure is the product of systemic vascular resistance and CO. If CO decreases, blood pressure is maintained initially by compensatory arterial vasoconstriction because of reflex sympathetic discharge; thus, a decrease in blood pressure is often a late sign of reduced myocardial performance.

Low Cardiac Output Syndrome (LCOS)

What is the presentation of LCOS?

Cool, clammy skin; slow capillary refill; oliguria (< 0.5 ml/kg/hr); restlessness; depressed mental status; tachypnea, metabolic acidosis

What are the etiologies of LCOS in the postoperative period?

Hypovolemia (third spacing, diuresis, bleeding, or relative hypovolemia because of the reflex vasodilation associated with postoperative warming); elevated systemic vascular resistance (hypothermia, circulating catecholamines); myocardial dysfunction (ischemia, hypothermia, volume overload); pericardial tamponade; dysrhythmia; and increased intrathoracic pressure [positive end-expiratory pressure (PEEP), tension pneumothorax]

In what order are these determinants of CO addressed to improve CO?

1. Heart rate (and arrhythmias)
2. Preload
3. Afterload
4. Contractility

For each determinant, what disturbance usually causes LCOS, and what are the therapeutic options and management?

Bradycardia: Atropine, isoproterenol, temporary pacer

Tachycardia: Fluids, oxygen, anxiolytics, morphine, esmolol (rarely)

Inadequate preload: Fluids, control of mediastinal bleeding (and rule out tamponade)

Elevated afterload: Warming lights or blanket, fluids, vasodilator therapy

Reduced contractility: Inotropic therapy, mechanical assist device (and rule out myocardial ischemia; see the Postoperative Myocardial Ischemia section)

What are the first-line inotropic agents?

Dopamine and dobutamine

What are the second-line agents (e.g., used if the first-line agents are ineffective)?

Epinephrine and amrinone (rarely used)

If LCOS persists despite second-line inotropic therapy, and all other determinants of CO are optimized, what mechanical assist is initiated?

IABP and/or ventricular assist device

What is the primary benefit of each mechanical assist device?

IABP: can be placed percutaneously (ventricular assist device requires open-chest surgery)

VAD: Completely **replaces** the pumping function of the heart (IABP only **augments** existing cardiac function)

POSTOPERATIVE MYOCARDIAL ISCHEMIA

What is the incidence of postoperative MI following cardiac surgery?	3% to 15%
When in the postoperative period is the patient at greatest risk of myocardial ischemia?	First 6 hours
What are the sequelae of myocardial ischemia?	MI, LCOS, arrhythmias, RV failure, acute mitral regurgitation, acute ventricular septal defect, and acute ventricular free wall rupture ($\pm$ pericardial tamponade)
What are the treatment goals, and how are they achieved?	1. Alleviation of myocardial ischemia: Oxygen, nitrates, $\pm$ surgery 2. Treatment of ventricular dysfunction: According to the LCOS treatment regimen 3. Prevention or treatment of arrhythmias: Correction of electrolyte disturbances, administration of lidocaine or procainamide
When is surgery indicated for myocardial ischemia after cardiac surgery?	1. Patients who are hemodynamically or electrically unstable because of significant myocardial ischemia 2. Mechanical complications of ischemia (i.e., acute MR or VSD). See the Acquired Coronary Artery Disease section for a discussion of these mechanical complications.
What is the treatment of RV failure?	1. **Volume expansion** (the foundation of treatment of RV failure) 2. Dobutamine, the overall pharmacologic agent of choice because it reduces pulmonary afterload **and** provides inotropic support.

POSTOPERATIVE HYPERTENSION

What are the etiologies of postoperative hypertension?	Pain or anxiety, hypothermia, hypoxia, hypercarbia, LCOS (with reflex vasoconstriction), and hyperdynamic myocardium syndrome

What are the sequelae?

Myocardial ischemia, LCOS, cerebrovascular accident, increased postoperative bleeding, and aortic dissection

What is the goal of treatment?

Reduction of blood pressure while maintaining adequate visceral perfusion, especially coronary and cerebral. The target mean arterial pressure is 60 to 85 mm Hg (variable depending on patient's baseline blood pressure).

What hemodynamic parameter MUST be optimized before a vasodilator is initiated?

Preload. To avoid severe hypotension caused by the relative intravascular hypotension that occurs with vasodilation

What is the first-line parenteral agent for vasodilation?

Sodium nitroprusside

What is the first-line oral agent for vasodilation?

Nifedipine

POSTOPERATIVE HYPOTENSION

What are the most common etiologies in the postoperative cardiac surgery patient?

Hypovolemia, myocardial ischemia or infarction, cardiac tamponade, arrhythmias, and tension pneumothorax

What is shock?

Inadequate perfusion pressures to preserve visceral function (**not** hypotension per se)

What are the etiologies of cardiogenic shock?

Large MI (> 30%–40% of LV), acute mitral regurgitation, acute ventricular septal defect, RV failure

What is the mortality rate associated with cardiogenic shock?

75%

HYPERDYNAMIC MYOCARDIUM SYNDROME

What is hyperdynamic myocardium syndrome?

Elevated cardiac output caused by increased myocardial contractility ± tachycardia. The mechanism is uncertain, but may involve circulating catecholamines.

Which patients are at greatest risk for hyperdynamic myocardium syndrome?	Patients with compensatory hypertrophy of the LV because of preoperative systemic hypertension, AS, or idiopathic subaortic stenosis
What is the indication for treatment?	Significant tachycardia with untoward effects on diastolic ventricular filling or myocardial oxygen demand
What is the pharmacologic intervention of choice?	Esmolol (parenteral β-blocker with a short half-life)

POSTOPERATIVE HEMORRHAGE

What is the medical management?	Increased PEEP on the ventilator, vasodilators for hypertension, protamine sulfate, fresh-frozen plasma (if prothrombin time or partial thromboplastin time is elevated), and platelets (if platelet count < 100,000). Desmopressin acetate (DDAVP) is rarely used today.
When is cryoprecipitate indicated?	Fibrinogen < 100 mg/dl
What are the indications for re-exploration?	Bleeding rate from chest tubes of 200 ml/hr for 4 to 6 hours (> 1500 ml over 12 hours), evidence of pericardial tamponade, or sudden significant increase in chest tube output (300–500 ml)

Pericardial tamponade

How does pericardial tamponade reduce CO?	Preload reduction: Low pressure of venous return has difficulty overcoming the intrapericardial pressure gradient formed by the tamponade
What is the usual presentation of tamponade?	Tachycardia, hypotension, distended neck veins, and pulsus paradoxus, often in a patient with bleeding from the chest tube that is initially heavy and suddenly stops; however, freely draining chest tubes and tamponade are not mutually exclusive

What is the classic finding on Swan-Ganz catheter readings?

Equalization of diastolic pressures in the heart [central venous pressure (CVP), RV end-diastolic pressure, pulmonary diastolic pressure, and PCWP], usually 18 to 22 mm Hg

What is the treatment?

Volume loading, inotropes, and elevation of the feet until an OR is available for re-exploration of the mediastinum. If the patient becomes unstable before surgery despite the conservative measures, emergent **bedside** re-exploration is performed.

MISCELLANEOUS ICU TOPICS

Swan-Ganz Catheter

What are the three most useful parameters for hemodynamic management with a Swan-Ganz catheter?

CO, systemic vascular resistance (SVR), and PCWP

How is SVR calculated?

$$SVR = \frac{MAP - CVP}{CO} \times 80$$

How is pulmonary vascular resistance (PVR) calculated?

$$PVR = \frac{Mean\ pulmonary\ artery\ pressure - PCWP}{CO} \times 80$$

What are the units of this calculation?

Dynes/sec/cm^2

How is PVR calculated in Wood units?

$$PVR = \frac{Mean\ pulmonary\ artery\ pressure - PCWP}{CO}$$

What is the standard criterion for irreversible pulmonary hypertension?

6 Wood units

What are the normal values for the following parameters:

1. CO and CI?

1. CO = 4 to 8 L/min; CI = 2.5 to 4 L/min/m^2

2. CVP?

2. CVP = 0 to 4 mm Hg

3. PCWP?

3. PCWP = 12 to 15 mm Hg

4. SVR?

4. SVR = 900 to 1400 dynes/sec/cm^2

5. PVR?

5. PVR = 150 to 250 dynes/sec/cm^2

In patient management, **trends,** rather than absolute numbers, are key, but these values are guidelines.

What is the general management regimen for each of the following classic clinical scenarios:

1. Decreased CO, decreased PCWP, increased or decreased SVR?

1. Volume (i.e., crystalloid, blood)

2. Normal or increased CO, but decreased BP, normal PCWP, decreased SVR?

2. Vasopressor (i.e., phenylephrine)

3. Decreased CO, increased PCWP, normal or decreased SVR?

3. Inotrope (i.e., dopamine, dobutamine)

4. Decreased CO, increased PCWP, increased SVR?

4. Vasodilator (i.e., sodium nitroprusside) + IABP if blood pressure is too low for vasodilator therapy alone

What measurement is performed to evaluate oxygen delivery and the adequacy of tissue perfusion?

Mixed venous oxygen saturation. A sample is drawn slowly through the distal port of the Swan-Ganz catheter (the site of the most deoxygenated blood in the body, the pulmonary artery).

What is a normal value of this measurement?

65% to 75% saturation. A low saturation value warrants further evaluation, but a normal value does not guarantee adequate visceral perfusion.

What does an increase in oxygen saturation between the proximal port of the Swan-Ganz catheter (in the RA) and the distal port (in the PA) suggest?	Intracardiac shunt (i.e., VSD)

Cardiovascular Drugs

What cardiovascular drug is associated with:

1. **Splanchnic vasodilation?**
2. **Methemoglobinemia?**
3. **Lupus-like syndrome?**
4. **Sudden death if abruptly withdrawn?**
5. **Coronary steal phenomenon?**
6. **Cyanide (thiocyanate) toxicity?**

1. Dopamine

2. NTG
3. Hydralazine
4. β-blockers (e.g., atenolol)

5. Sodium nitroprusside

6. Sodium nitroprusside

How do patients with cyanide toxicity present initially?	Decreased contractility and CO
What are the classic LATE findings of toxicity?	Dilated pupils, headache, absent reflexes, nausea, mental status changes ± coma, death

TRAUMA TO THE HEART AND GREAT VESSELS

PENETRATING CARDIAC TRAUMA

Wounds to what region of the anterior chest are considered to involve the heart until proven otherwise?	Below the clavicles, above the costal margin, and between the midclavicular lines. Some include the epigastrium in this region of cardiac risk. Cardiac injury also is possible in patients with posterior thoracic injuries above the lumbar curve.
What are the relative frequencies of injury to each cardiac chamber?	RV: 40% to 45% LV: 30% to 35% RA: 15% LA: 5%

What are the two most common presentations, and what is the usual mechanism of injury for each?

1. Pericardial tamponade: 80% caused by stab wounds
2. Hemorrhagic shock: 80% caused by gunshot wounds. Stab wounds tend to seal more readily than the gaping wound of a bullet.

What is the most common cause of distended neck veins in the patient with thoracic trauma?

Tension pneumothorax, not tamponade

Why is neck vein distension often absent on arrival at the emergency room, even in the setting of an injury that classically causes it?

Patients are often severely intravascularly hypovolemic. With successful volume resuscitation, neck vein distension becomes apparent.

What triad of findings on physical exam suggests pericardial tamponade?

Beck triad (hypotension; muffled heart sounds, which are difficult to determine in a noisy emergency room; and distended neck veins), seen in 10% to 60% of patients with pericardial tamponade

How much blood in the pericardial sac can cause tamponade?

As little as 60 to 100 ml

Why is CXR often not helpful in the diagnosis of traumatic tamponade?

Acute tamponade infrequently causes significant distension of the relatively inelastic pericardium.

What are the indications for limited probing of the wound (e.g., with a cotton swab) to determine its depth within the cardiac risk region?

None. Probing may cause life-threatening bleeding with suboptimal options for control of the hemorrhage.

What are the current indications for echocardiography in cardiac trauma?

Stable patient with a low suspicion of cardiac trauma. As echocardiography becomes more available in the trauma suite, it may eventually be used as a rapid screen for all patients. In most centers, it is now too time-consuming for even mildly unstable patients.

What is the most important aspect of emergent therapy of cardiac trauma, regardless of injury, and why?

Rapid volume resuscitation. Increasing the intravascular volume causes increased cardiac filling pressures (the best temporizing therapy to counteract the effects of tamponade) and begins to restore adequate tissue perfusion in patients with hemorrhagic shock.

What is the initial procedure of choice in the relatively stable patient?

Subxiphoid pericardial window, which is often both diagnostic and therapeutic

Why should this procedure be done in the OR, not the emergency room (ER)?

Pericardial tamponade is often **lifesaving** because it can prevent further cardiac bleeding. A pericardial window can cause exsanguinating hemorrhage if the physician is not prepared to proceed immediately with median sternotomy if necessary.

What is the initial procedure of choice in the profoundly hypotensive patient?

Emergent (ER) left anterolateral thoracotomy

What is the sequence of steps taken after the thoracotomy incision is made?

The pericardium is incised longitudinally, anterior to the phrenic nerve, to relieve tamponade and expose the heart. The descending aorta is clamped to improve coronary and cerebral perfusion, and bleeding is controlled with digital pressure or a Foley catheter inserted into the cardiac wound and inflated.

When is pericardiocentesis indicated?

When no surgeon or OR is available. Despite frequent recommendations in emergency medicine texts, performing this procedure is unreliable and complicated in inexperienced hands. Pericardiocentesis is rarely indicated in trauma.

What is the standard technique for repair of a cardiac laceration or gunshot wound?

Bleeding is controlled with digital pressure or a Foley catheter, and cardiorrhaphy is performed with interrupted pledgeted horizontal mattress sutures.

A superficial cardiac injury is repaired, and the patient is now in cardiac failure. What is the likely problem?

Unrecognized valvular or septal injury

What is the treatment of coronary artery injury?

The artery is ligated proximal and distal to the injury, ± CABG **if** the injury is located in the proximal two-thirds of the artery.

When is CPB indicated in penetrating cardiac injury?

Complex cardiac injuries, including trauma to valve, proximal coronary artery, septum, or extensive ventricular wall defect; occasionally, posterior cardiac injuries because of impaired venous return when the heart is lifted for repair

What is the mortality rate of a stab wound versus a gunshot wound to the heart in patients who undergo surgery?

Stab wound: 10%
Gunshot wound: 40% to 50% (85%–90% of patients with gunshot wounds to the heart die in the field)

BLUNT CARDIAC TRAUMA

What is the most common cardiac injury caused by blunt chest trauma?

Myocardial contusion. Cardiac laceration or rupture as a result of blunt trauma is rare, but pericardial tamponade **is** possible with blunt trauma.

What chamber is most often injured?

Right ventricle

What are the acute sequelae of myocardial contusion?

Arrhythmias, low CO ± cardiogenic shock, and valve injury + CHF

What screening studies are performed on all patients with potentially significant blunt trauma to the precordium?

EKG and creatinine phosphokinase (CPK)-MB level. The reliability of cardiac isoenzyme levels is controversial, but monitoring them is currently the standard of care.

What are the findings on EKG?

Nonspecific ST-T wave changes, ventricular ectopy, and right bundle branch block

What is the most useful adjunctive diagnostic study?

Echocardiogram. (99mTc is unreliable, and MUGA radionuclide angiogram is too expensive and impractical for trauma use.)

Which patients should receive this study?

Any patient who has hemodynamic instability, a significant increase in CPK-MB level, or significant ventricular ectopy

What is the management of patients with myocardial contusion?

Monitored bed for observation, continuous telemetry (EKG), supplemental oxygen, serial EKG studies and CPK-MB levels every 6 hours. Management is similar to that of acute MI because the injury is similar and infarction may develop within the contusion.

What additional therapy may be necessary if the patient becomes unstable because of the contusion?

Inotropic support and IABP

How long is the patient closely observed and monitored with telemetry?

Patients with a mechanism of injury that might result in myocardial contusion are monitored for at least 24 hours. (If no evidence of ventricular irritability is seen within the first 24 hours, arrhythmia is unlikely.)

If EKG findings are abnormal, CPK-MB level is significantly increased (usually 5%, but the level is controversial), or the patient shows clinical evidence of cardiac injury (i.e., ventricular irritability, low CO), the patient is monitored for at least 48 to 72 hours.

If echocardiogram findings confirm myocardial contusion (i.e., hypokinetic or akinetic region), the patient is monitored for 1 to 3 weeks or more, depending on the clinical course.

What percentage of patients with myocardial contusion have permanent reduction in ventricular function?

< 10%

What is the primary concern about pericardial injury caused by blunt trauma?	Potential for herniation of the heart through a pericardial tear, with obstruction of venous return

TRAUMATIC ANEURYSMS OF THE THORACIC AORTA

What is the claim to fame of traumatic aneurysms of the thoracic aorta?	Most common cause of immediate death in blunt trauma (e.g., motor vehicle accident, fall)
What is the mechanism by which these aneurysms develop?	Rapid deceleration injury
What are the most common sites of intimal tear?	Aortic isthmus, opposite the insertion of the ligamentum arteriosus, just distal to the left subclavian artery (75%); proximal to the innominate artery in the ascending aorta
What factor usually determines survival?	Continuity of the relatively strong adventitial layer, which can sometimes contain the hematoma, even in the setting of complete transection of the aorta (i.e., false aneurysm)
What is the overall acute survival rate?	2% to 5%
What is the usual presentation?	Wide spectrum that ranges from asymptomatic patients with no evidence of external injury to hypotensive patients with gross evidence of thoracic injury. **The key to diagnosis is a high index of suspicion!**
What are the classic findings on physical exam?	Upper extremity hypertension and absent or weak femoral pulses
What are the usual findings on CXR?	Wide mediastinum (especially if > 8 cm); loss or blurring of the aortic knob shadow; depression of the left main-stem bronchus; elevation of the right main-stem bronchus; and tracheal and esophageal deviation to the right. If the aorta is ruptured, left pleural effusion or pleural cap may be seen.

What is the current diagnostic study of choice?

MRI; the second choice is spiral CT scan with contrast

When is an aortogram performed?

Stable patients with suspected aortic injury

What medical therapy is crucial?

Prevention of hypertension with potent antihypertensive agents (nitroprusside) and sedation. The goal mean arterial pressure is $\approx$ 80 mm Hg.

What is the standard surgical procedure?

Interposition Dacron tube graft replacement of the involved segment of the aorta, usually performed with partial CPB (left atriofemoral or femorofemoral)

What modification is usually reserved for unstable patients or those with massive hemorrhage on chest entry?

"Cross-clamp and sew," without CPB

What modification is usually reserved for patients with contraindications to the systemic heparinization required for CPB?

Heparin-bonded Gott or TDMAC shunt (aortoaortic or aortofemoral), without CPB

What is the maximal safe normothermic cross-clamp time?

30 minutes; less than 20 minutes is preferred

What type of incision is used?

Left posterolateral thoracotomy for an intimal tear at the ligamentum ductus; median sternotomy for a tear proximal to the innominate artery

What is the most common cause of intraoperative death?

Uncontrollable hemorrhage caused by rupture of the false aneurysm before proximal clamping is performed or from the bypass or shunt cannulation site

What are the associated complications?	Paraplegia caused by spinal ischemia; myocardial ischemia caused by LV strain associated with proximal aortic clamping. These complications are particularly common with the clamp and sew technique.
What is the mortality rate for patients who survive to undergo surgery?	< 10%. Most of these deaths are caused by associated injuries, not the dissection.

See the Thoracic Trauma section in the Thoracic Surgery chapter.

ADDITIONAL CARDIAC SURGERY TOPICS

POSTPERICARDIOTOMY SYNDROME

What is postpericardiotomy syndrome?	Aseptic pericarditis after pericardiotomy (etiology unknown)
What analogous syndrome occurs after MI?	Dressler syndrome
What is the usual presentation?	Fever, chest pain, malaise, pericardial friction rub, and normal white blood cell count
When in the postoperative period does it usually develop?	2 to 4 weeks, but may be as long as 12 weeks after surgery
What are the classic EKG changes?	ST segment elevation in all leads, except V1 and AVR
What is the treatment?	NSAIDs (e.g., indomethacin, ibuprofen), aspirin, or steroids (rarely); rest

INTRA-AORTIC BALLOON PUMP

What are the indications for IABP?	1. Refractory LV failure after CPB (e.g., inability to wean from bypass pump) 2. Unstable angina refractory to medical treatment 3. Congestive heart failure in a patient awaiting surgery (i.e., acute mitral regurgitation or VSD, transplant candidate) 4. Cardiogenic shock caused by MI (now rare, unless the patient is a candidate for CABG or PTCA)

What are the contraindications to IABP?

1. Aortic aneurysm or synthetic thoracic aortic graft (may rupture with balloon inflation)
2. Moderate or severe aortic regurgitation (IABP may worsen regurgitation)

What is the usual route of insertion?

Femoral artery, but the pump can be placed directly into the aorta at the time of median sternotomy if severe peripheral atherosclerosis precludes a femoral approach

Where does the balloon reside in the aorta?

Between the left subclavian artery and the diaphragm

What complication occurs if the balloon migrates?

Intermittent ischemia in territories supplied by vessels that are intermittently occluded by the inflated balloon (e.g., carotid, subclavian, renal, celiac)

How does the IABP work?

Balloon **inflates** during **diastole,** increasing pressure inside the aorta which increases coronary and visceral perfusion; the balloon **deflates** during **systole,** reducing afterload, which decreases cardiac work

What is the key benefit of IABP over medical treatment of hypotension or decreased CO?

No increase in oxygen consumption or demand, unlike α- or β-agonists, which cause increased cardiac work because of increased afterload or HR and contractility, respectively

What are the complications of IABP?

1. Lower extremity ischemia because of occlusion of the femoral artery. It is **imperative** that distal pulses be monitored.
2. Emboli caused by thrombosis around the balloon
3. Bowel infarction, renal failure, and paraplegia caused by migration of the balloon
4. Mechanical damage to formed components of the blood (i.e., "blood trauma")

LEFT VENTRICULAR ASSIST DEVICE

What are the indications for LVAD?	1. Intraoperative MI to reduce LV work temporarily and allow the heart to recover more quickly 2. "Bridge" for heart transplant candidates until a donor is available
What are the differences between current short-term (< 1 week) and long-term LVAD?	Short-term (i.e., centrifugal): Device is external, cannulae are smaller, inflow source is the LA Long-term (i.e., Novacor, Heartmate): Device is internal, cannulae are larger (less blood trauma), inflow source is the LV apex. Both systems have outflow into the ascending aorta.
Why is LVAD not true cardiopulmonary bypass?	Only a perfusion device, with no oxygenator in the circuit
How is the LVAD fundamentally different from the IABP?	LVAD provides "flow" and can fully replace the pumping function of the heart; IABP provides "pressure assistance" and only augments existing cardiac function.
How is the LVAD different from extracorporeal membrane oxygenation (ECMO)?	ECMO includes a membrane lung apparatus and can also provide support for respiratory insufficiency; the inflow source is the RA

AUTOMATIC IMPLANTABLE CARDIOVERTER DEFIBRILLATOR (AICD)

What are the three components of the AICD?	1. Sensory leads to detect arrhythmia 2. Anode–cathode titanium patches around the heart 3. Pulse generator to terminate arrhythmia Newer devices also have pacing capability for bradycardia and asystole.
What is the indication for AICD?	Malignant ventricular arrhythmia refractory to medical therapy
What are the 1-year survival rates in treated patients and untreated historical control subjects?	AICD: 95% to 98% Untreated: 30% to 40%. These patients are at high risk for sudden death syndrome.

Why is pharmacologic therapy necessary after AICD placement?

Episodes of nonsustained ventricular tachycardia and atrial fibrillation can cause inappropriate discharge of the AICD.

CARDIAC TUMORS

What is the most common type of cardiac tumor?

Metastatic neoplasm (lung, breast, melanoma, and lymphoma), which accounts for 65% to 70% of all malignant cardiac tumors.

What is the most common complication associated with this type of tumor?

Pericardial tamponade from bloody pericardial effusion

What are the two most common primary malignant cardiac tumors?

1. Sarcoma (i.e., rhabdomyosarcoma, angiosarcoma): 15% to 20% of all malignant cardiac tumors
2. Melanoma: 5% to 10%

How do these tumors differ grossly from myxoma?

Intramural rather than intraluminal; thus, almost always unresectable. Transplantation is not a treatment option.

What is the most common cardiac tumor in children?

Rhabdomyoma (benign)

What is the most common primary tumor of the pericardium?

Mesothelioma

What aspect of the surgical intervention reduces the incidence of recurrence?

Resection of the origin of the stalk (part of the septal wall)

Benign Cardiac Tumors

What is the most common benign cardiac tumor?

Myxoma, which is also the most common primary cardiac tumor, accounting for 60% to 80% of all primary cardiac tumors

This tumor occurs most frequently in which chamber?

LA: 75% (>95% in atria)

What is the classic gross feature?

Pedunculated (stalk attached to the atrial septal wall)

What complications are associated with this tumor?

LA outflow obstruction ("ball valve") and emboli (from the friable surface of the myxoma). Acute vascular obstruction in patients with no heart disease, especially if young, suggests this source.

46

Vascular Surgery

Kirk J. Fleischer, MD

ARTERIAL OCCLUSIVE DISEASE

ACUTE ARTERIAL OCCLUSION

What are the etiologies of acute arterial occlusion?	1. Embolus 2. Thrombosis 3. Trauma
How long after occlusion does ischemic necrosis develop?	4 to 8 hours
Which tissue types in limb are most sensitive to anoxia?	Peripheral nerve > skeletal muscle
What are the classic signs and symptoms?	The 6 Ps: pain, pallor, pulselessness, paresthesia, paralysis, and poikilothermia
What percentage of patients have sudden, severe pain?	80%
Why may pain be mild or absent?	Adequate collateral flow, rapid onset of paresthesia, or presence of diabetic neuropathy
What is the progression of cutaneous changes with arterial occlusion?	Initial pallor followed by mottled cyanosis (marbling) after several hours
What is the progression of neurologic deficit with arterial occlusion?	Loss of light touch sensation, then complete anesthesia (pain, pressure, and temperature) and, finally, loss of motor function

Which signs and symptoms are the best predictors of the development of gangrene, and why?

Paralysis and paresthesia. Because nervous tissue is the most sensitive to ischemia, gangrene is **unlikely** to develop if motor and, to a lesser extent, sensory function is intact.

Why does motor function of the digits often remain intact, even with prolonged distal occlusion?

Most muscle bellies for movement of the digits are located in the forearm and leg, not the hand and foot.

How reliable is a palpable pulse for detecting occlusion?

Not reliable. An intimal flap, transmission of pulse through a clot, and more distal occlusion can permit palpation of a pulse.

How is arterial occlusion distinguished clinically from phlegmasia cerulea dolens in a limb?

Although venous obstruction may present as a pulseless, painful limb, the extremity appears frankly cyanotic, not palloric, and often edematous in phlegmasia cerulea dolens.

What is the medical treatment of acute arterial occlusion?

1. IV heparin is begun immediately to prevent further propagation of the thrombus in vessels distal to the occlusion if no contraindications to anticoagulation are present.
2. Fluid and electrolyte abnormalities are corrected.

In which patients should a preoperative arteriogram be performed?

Patients with normal or minimally impaired musculosensory function. Otherwise, most surgeons forgo this time-consuming procedure and proceed immediately to surgery. (Some surgeons attempt a trial of thrombolytic therapy despite the presence of neurologic deficits).

What are the surgical options?

1. Thromboembolectomy
2. Endarterectomy
3. Bypass procedure
(Regardless of the procedure performed, a complete arteriogram is performed before the patient leaves the OR.)

The role of thrombolytic therapy in acute arterial occlusion is unclear. What are some of the drawbacks of this type of therapy?	It is expensive and leads to increased risk of hemorrhage, delayed restoration of arterial flow (compared with immediate surgery), reduced long-term patency, and the potential risk of emboli because of partial lysis of mural thrombi in the heart.
For which type of embolus is thrombolytic therapy ineffective?	Embolic fragments from atherosclerotic plaques and atrial myxoma

Complications of Reperfusion of Ischemic Limbs

What are the classic complications?	1. Hypotension "reperfusion shock" 2. Arrhythmias 3. Acute tubular necrosis 4. Compartment syndrome
What is the etiology of the cardiovascular instability?	Metabolic acidosis and hyperkalemia caused by anoxia and resultant cell death in the limb
What is the treatment?	1. Sodium bicarbonate 2. Glucose and insulin for hyperkalemia 3. Vasopressor support
What is the etiology of the renal failure?	Myoglobinuria (with precipitation of myoglobin in the renal tubules) associated with lysis of necrotic muscle cells
What is the treatment?	1. Hydration 2. Diuresis with mannitol 3. Alkalinization of urine with sodium bicarbonate to increase the solubility of myoglobin

ARTERIAL EMBOLUS

What is the most common source of arterial embolus?	Heart (90%)
What specific conditions predispose patients to emboli?	1. Atrial fibrillation (most common) 2. Mural thrombus secondary to myocardial infarction 3. Mitral stenosis 4. Any valvular disease with vegetations 5. Atrial myxoma

What are the other major sources of emboli?

1. Ulcerated plaques in the aorta and iliac arteries
2. Mural thrombi in aneurysms

What is a paradoxic embolus?

A venous embolus that occludes a systemic artery

How does this occlusion occur?

The embolus traverses a communication between the right and left sides of the heart (patent foramen ovale, atrial septal defect, ventricular septal defect).

What is the most common source of paradoxic emboli?

Deep venous thrombus in a lower extremity showers emboli to the lung, causing pulmonary hypertension and increasing right atrial pressure and flow across the intracardiac shunt, usually a patent foramen ovale.

What are the most common regions of embolic occlusion?

1. Lower extremity (70%)
2. Cerebral circulation (25%)

What are the four most commonly occluded vessels?

1. Common femoral artery (35%)
2. Common iliac artery (15%)
3. Popliteal artery (15%)
4. Aorta (10%)
(Occlusion is common at bifurcations.)

What is the characteristic feature of an embolus?

Sudden onset

How is an embolus initially distinguished from arterial thrombosis?

Patient history. Patients with thrombosis have a history of chronic arterial insufficiency (e.g., claudication).

What are the classic angiographic findings?

Abrupt cutoff of a normal-appearing artery without well-developed collaterals in the region of obstruction. Collaterals are more suggestive of thrombosis.

What additional studies are performed?

1. Electrocardiogram (EKG)
2. Echocardiogram
3. Abdominal x-ray (e.g., for calcifications in the aorta)

What is the medical treatment?	IV heparin to prevent the propagation of thrombi and provide prophylaxis against additional emboli
What is the surgical treatment?	Thromboembolectomy with a Fogarty catheter
What additional procedure may be required?	Endarterectomy or bypass procedure if a significant thrombotic component is present (stenosis). If the patient is elderly or unstable, this definitive procedure is delayed until the patient recovers from the acute injury.
Why are the embolic fragments sent to the pathology department?	To exclude myxoma as a source. This etiology is common in young patients with acute arterial occlusion.
What are the two critical components of the postoperative management of patients with emboli?	1. Determination and correction, if possible, of the embolic source 2. Anticoagulation with heparin initially, then warfarin (Coumadin) **as long as the source of embolus is present**
What is the risk of limb loss?	10% with the first embolus, 20% with the second, and 50% with the third

What are the most important features influencing:
1. Success of surgery in salvaging the limb?

1. Viability of the limb on presentation and the time until arterial flow is restored

2. Long-term patency of the artery?

2. Correction of the source of the embolus

ACUTE ARTERIAL THROMBOSIS

What is the most common etiology?	Arterial stenosis as a result of atherosclerosis
What are the other etiologies?	1. Low flow states as a result of hypotension, dehydration, or reduced cardiac output 2. Trauma 3. Hypercoagulable states 4. Acute **venous** outflow obstruction

What is the treatment?   Depends on the etiology, but for atherosclerotic stenoses, the options are bypass procedure, endarterectomy, and percutaneous angioplasty.

ARTERIAL TRAUMA

See the Vascular Trauma section for a complete discussion of arterial trauma.

CHRONIC ARTERIAL OCCLUSIVE DISEASE

What is the etiology?   Atherosclerosis. (There are also several rare nonatherosclerotic etiologies, such as popliteal entrapment syndrome and Buerger disease.)

What is the basic sequence of events in the current theory of atherosclerosis?   Repetitive endothelial injury, followed by progressive subintimal lipid infiltration, smooth muscle migration, and proliferation and, finally, plaque formation

What are the risk factors?
1. Advanced age
2. Male gender
3. Tobacco abuse
4. Hypertension
5. Diabetes
6. Hyperlipidemia
7. Family history of atherosclerosis

What is a "critical" arterial stenosis?
1. **Symptomatic** arterial stenosis
2. Arteriographic criterion: diameter of vessel reduced by > 50% (correlates with a reduction in the cross-sectional area of the vessel by > 75%; area = $3.14 \times radius^2$)

What is the most important hemodynamic factor responsible for the decrease in pressure across a stenosis?   Turbulence. It also causes poststenotic dilation and endothelial damage.

What two adaptive processes does the body use to maintain distal perfusion in the face of progressive arterial stenosis?	Dilation of the stenotic artery (limited); dilation of collateral vessels
What are the characteristic changes in the appearance of the chronically ischemic leg?	Dry, shiny skin with little subcutaneous tissue, thick nails, and paucity of hair (trophic changes); muscle atrophy
How well does the intensity of an auscultated bruit correlate with the severity of stenosis?	No consistent correlation
What are the three progressive clinical stages of chronic peripheral arterial insufficiency?	1. Intermittent claudication 2. Ischemic rest pain 3. Ischemic necrosis (gangrene and ulcers) (Stages 2 and 3 are classified as threatened "limb loss.")
What is claudication?	Extremity pain (in some cases, fatigue) induced by exertion **and relieved by short periods of rest** (5–10 minutes)
What is the character of the pain?	Ache or cramp (in some cases, severe fatigue)
What is the most common site of pain?	Calf
What percentage of patients with claudication progress to gangrene?	Only 2% to 3% yearly
What conditions most frequently mimic claudication?	Lumbar spinal stenosis (caused by narrowing by osteophytes) and osteoarthritis of the knee or hip
What is the character of ischemic rest pain?	Severe, burning pain
What is the most common site of pain?	Metatarsal heads

When does pain characteristically occur?

At night (frequently awakens the patient from sleep)

What condition often mimics ischemic rest pain?

Diabetic neuropathy

What feature of ischemic rest pain distinguishes it from most other etiologies of leg pain?

Pain is exacerbated by elevation and relieved by a dependent position. Many patients sleep with the affected leg hanging over the side of the bed to prevent the pain.

What are the two usual distributions of occlusive disease seen in patients with ischemic rest pain?

1. Combined aortoiliac and superficial femoral artery disease
2. Combined femoropopliteal and distal tibial disease

What is the gross appearance of an ischemic ulcer?

Pale, "punched-out" ulcer with surrounding rubor

Is the ulcer painful?

Yes, unless concurrent diabetic neuropathy is present

Compare the sites of ulcers in arterial versus venous insufficiency of the lower extremity.

1. Arterial: Toes or plantar surface of the foot
2. Venous: Over the medial malleolus

Describe the appearance of the two general types of gangrene.

1. Wet: Poorly demarcated, violet-red, foul-smelling, and "wet" (blebs, bullae, often oozing)
2. Dry: Sharply demarcated, black-brown, often odorless, and dry (eschar)

What accounts for the difference between the types of gangrene?

Wet gangrene is **infected;** dry is aseptic

Without surgery, what percentage of patients with ischemic rest pain or necrosis lose the extremity?

100% (i.e., threatened limb loss)

What is the simplest screening test to evaluate the lower extremities for arterial occlusive disease?

Ankle:brachial index (ABI) = systolic blood pressure (SBP) of the ankle divided by the SBP of the arm. This test is most accurately performed with bedside Doppler ultrasonography.

What is an abnormal value for this test?

ABI < 0.95

What are the ranges of ABI values for each clinical stage of chronic arterial insufficiency?

1. Claudication: 0.5 to 0.9
2. Rest pain: 0.2 to 0.5
3. Necrosis: < 0.3
These are rough guidelines; there is considerable overlap.

What is the most common etiology of a falsely elevated ABI?

Diabetes (arterial walls become less compliant because of the calcifications of medial calcinosis). Diabetes is suspected if ABI > 1.20.

What are the three major studies of the noninvasive vascular laboratory? What does each study evaluate?

1. Doppler waveform analysis: Evaluates the change in arterial waveform along the course of the arterial tree
2. Plethysmography: Evaluates the change in extremity volume during the cardiac cycle
3. Duplex ultrasound: Evaluates the change in blood velocities during the cardiac cycle

What are the basic changes seen in each of these studies in the setting of arterial stenosis?

1. Doppler: Loss of the normal triphasic pattern and eventual blunting or flattening of the systolic upstroke of the waveform
2. Plethysmography: Reduction in extremity volume changes with systole
3. Duplex: Jets and turbulence caused by stenosis; elevated velocity

Which study most accurately localizes and characterizes the arterial stenosis?

Duplex ultrasound

What adjunctive technique assists in the evaluation of a patient with less severe disease (i.e., mild claudication)?

Exercise testing

With this technique, what is the finding in a patient with stenosis, and why?

Reduction in ankle pressure with exercise (normally unchanged). Exercise causes vasodilation, but the stenosis prevents sufficient blood flow to the distal extremity to maintain local blood pressure.

What is the key concept regarding arteriograms and the diagnosis of significant arterial insufficiency?

Arteriograms can show the anatomic lesion, but the diagnosis of its "severity" depends on the patient's symptoms and the results of the vascular laboratory's hemodynamic studies. Arteriography is performed only **after** the patient is identified as a candidate for surgery.

What are the basic limitations of arteriography in the evaluation of arterial occlusive disease?

1. Arteriography often **under**estimates the amount of disease in the patent vessel.
2. Nonvisualization of a vessel does not necessarily confirm occlusion.

What laboratory test is performed before arteriography?

Serum blood urea nitrogen and creatinine values are obtained to evaluate renal function. Acute renal failure may result from the standard dye load in patients with impaired renal function.

What is done to reduce the dye load in patients with known renal insufficiency?

Digital subtraction arteriography (digitization of x-ray signals followed by enhancement of the image with a computer subtraction technique)

What is the best way to reduce the risk of contrast-induced renal failure?

Presence of a normal intravascular volume. The patient must be hydrated before and after the arteriogram!

Because of the diffuse nature of atherosclerosis, what additional evaluations are undertaken preoperatively?

Significant coronary artery or cerebrovascular disease is excluded. Myocardial infarction and stroke are the leading causes of death.

What are the indications for medical treatment?

Medical treatment is tried in **virtually all** patients with claudication alone for at least 6 to 12 months before surgery is attempted (unless acute occlusion occurs).

What are the cornerstones of medical therapy?

1. Exercise to the point of claudication (increases collaterals)
2. Cessation of smoking
3. Weight reduction and low-fat diet that may include lipid-reducing drugs
4. Antiplatelet drugs (e.g., aspirin)

What percentage of patients treated medically require amputation?

Only 5% to 10%

What are the indications for surgical treatment?

1. Limb-threatening ischemia as evidenced by ischemic rest pain, gangrene, or nonhealing ulcers
2. Distal emboli from ulcerated plaques
3. Severe claudication
4. Claudication that decreases the patient's usual quality of life or ability to perform occupational tasks

(Surgery in patients with mild claudication is controversial.)

What objective findings suggest sufficient arterial insufficiency to warrant surgery?

1. Absent pulses by Doppler ultrasound
2. Ankle pressure ≤ 60 mm Hg
3. Flat pulse volume recording at the ankle

What are the surgical options?

1. Arterial reconstruction or bypass procedure
2. Endarterectomy
3. Balloon angioplasty
4. Amputation

Regardless of the procedure performed, what is always done before wound closure?

Completion arteriogram to confirm adequate inflow, runoff, and, in the case of in situ saphenous bypass, the absence of residual arteriovenous (AV) fistula

What are the indications for postoperative IV heparin?

1. Precarious distal lower extremity bypass
2. Chronic arterial stenosis complicated by embolic events

In patients with inoperable disease, what palliative procedure may provide some (usually transient) relief from ischemic pain?

Lumbar sympathectomy, which causes vasodilation and provides some pain relief in 50% of patients

What are the early postoperative complications?	1. Hemorrhage 2. Thrombosis 3. Graft infection
What is the usual etiology of hemorrhage after day 5?	Infection (weakening of the anastomosis)
What percentage of grafts remain patent after an episode of early thrombosis?	Only 20%, even if flow is successfully restored through the graft
What are the late postoperative complications?	1. Thrombosis 2. Anastomotic pseudoaneurysm 3. Graft infection
What is the best way to prevent thrombosis?	Frequent reevaluation (every 3–6 months) of the patient with ABI to identify progressive stenotic lesions before thrombosis. If the lesion is detected before thrombosis, the graft can be salvaged > 80% of the time.

CHRONIC ARTERIAL OCCLUSIVE DISEASE OF THE LOWER EXTREMITY

What are the three major regions of subdiaphragmatic occlusive atherosclerotic disease?	1. Aortoiliac 2. Femoropopliteal 3. Tibioperoneal
What percentage of patients have significant lesions in more than one region?	> 33%
Which region has the highest incidence of disease?	Femoropopliteal (50% of cases)
What is the most common site of occlusion in the lower extremity?	Superficial femoral artery (SFA) within the adductor (Hunter) canal
Which territory is the most challenging to manage?	Tibioperoneal

See the Chronic Arterial Occlusive Disease section for a general discussion of the presentation, diagnosis, and treatment of chronic arterial insufficiency.

Aortoiliac Occlusive Disease

What is the most common presentation?

Claudication in the thigh or buttock

What are the three types?

1. Type I: Confined to the distal abdominal aorta and common iliac arteries
2. Type II: Extending down to the internal and external iliac arteries
3. Type III: Diffuse, with extension below the inguinal ligaments

What two classic syndromes are associated with aortoiliac disease?

1. Blue toe syndrome
2. Leriche syndrome

Describe each syndrome.

1. Blue toe syndrome ("trash foot"): Painful, necrotic toe lesions caused by digital artery occlusion by microemboli from ulcerative aortoiliac plaques
2. Leriche syndrome: Triad of absent femoral pulses, intermittent buttock or hip claudication, and impotence because of the gradual occlusion of the distal aorta

What does the occurrence of blue toe syndrome indicate about the vasculature of the lower limb?

A major arterial pathway is patent! Otherwise, microemboli could not reach the toe.

What is the etiology of the impotence of Leriche syndrome?

Reduced blood flow through both **internal** iliac arteries

What named collateral path provides arterial flow to the lower extremity in the setting of complete aortoiliac occlusion?

Collaterals of Winslow, which connect the subclavian arteries with the external iliac arteries through the internal mammary and inferior epigastric arteries

What are the standard treatment options?

1. Aortobifemoral bypass with bifurcated prosthetic graft (most common)
2. Aortoiliac endarterectomy (± patch angioplasty of the common iliac arteries)
3. Percutaneous balloon angioplasty

What are additional surgical options for the high-risk patient?

Extra-anatomic bypass (femorofemoral or axillobifemoral bypass). Can be performed under local anesthesia. Laparotomy is not required.

What are the other indications for extra-anatomic bypass?

1. Intra-abdominal infection (e.g., infected aortic graft)
2. History of multiple abdominal procedures (with resultant adhesions; "hostile" abdomen)

Why is aortoiliac bypass no longer the procedure of choice?

Aortobifemoral bypass is technically easier.

What is done if the profunda femoris artery is stenosed?

Patch profundaplasty, either as a separate procedure or as part of the femoral limb anastomosis. This situation is the most common indication for profundaplasty disease, especially in cases of concurrent SFA occlusion.

What is the treatment of choice for iliac lesions?

Balloon angioplasty with stent if the stenosis is < 5 cm. If the stenosis is > 5 cm, the long-term patency is reduced.

What surgical procedure is performed for the patient with symptomatic unilateral iliac artery occlusion?

Femorofemoral bypass. (Controversial in low-risk patients because of reports of better patency rates with direct aortofemoral or iliofemoral bypass.)

What are the 5-year patency rates for:
1. Aortobifemoral bypass?

1. 85% to 90%. (Rates are reduced by 15% to 20% if there is concurrent distal occlusive disease because patent outflow is crucial for long-term graft patency.)

2. Axillobifemoral bypass?
3. Femorofemoral bypass?
4. Percutaneous iliac artery angioplasty?

2. 70% to 75%
3. 80% to 85%
4. 80% to 90%

See the Aneurysms section for a complete discussion of the surgical and postoperative management of abdominal aortic lesions.

Femoropopliteal Occlusive Disease

What is the most common presentation of femoropopliteal occlusive disease?

Claudication in the calf

What is the usual route by which blood reaches the foot in cases of SFA occlusion?

The profunda femoris artery collateralizes through the genicular artery to the popliteal artery.

What are the indications for surgery?

1. Limb salvage
2. Lifestyle-limiting claudication

What are the surgical options?

1. Femoropopliteal bypass
2. Profundaplasty
3. Endarterectomy

Why are prosthetic grafts avoided for bypass below the knee?

Reduced long-term patency. (It is no longer recommended to save the saphenous vein for future coronary artery bypass graft. The best possible bypass should be performed with the conduits available at the time of the procedure.)

What percentage of patients with combined aortoiliac and femoropopliteal occlusive disease require a more distal revascularization procedure after an aortobifemoral bypass?

20%. The more proximal occlusion is always corrected first, with distal progress as needed.

What is the 5-year patency rate for femoropopliteal bypass?

Saphenous vein graft: 70% to 80%
Polytetrafluoroethylene [PTFE (i.e., Gore-tex)] graft: 60% to 70%

Tibioperoneal Occlusive Disease

What patients are at increased risk for tibioperoneal occlusive disease?

Patients with diabetes or Buerger disease

Why are these lesions more limb-threatening than more proximal disease?

Less abundant collateral pathways

What are the indications for surgery?

Limb salvage and ischemic ulcers only. (Because of the difficulty of successful bypass, the threshold for surgery in the patient with tibioperoneal occlusion is elevated.)

What are the surgical options?

1. Femorotibial or femoropopliteal bypass
2. Multiple short distal–distal grafts for multisegmental occlusions

What are the conduit options if insufficient vein is available for femorodistal bypass?

1. Composite graft: Proximal segment of PTFE and distal segment of saphenous vein
2. Venoveno grafts: Anastomosis of short segments of available veins

Avoid using prosthetic grafts below the knee!

How is a patient with preoperative forefoot necrosis managed?

Débridement and drainage ± limited amputation and IV antibiotics. Once infection clears, distal bypass is performed.

How is a patient with preoperative heel or posterior arch necrosis managed?

Extension of necrosis proximal to the forefoot rarely permits successful distal bypass. A below-the-knee amputation is usually indicated.

What is the 5-year patency rate for femorodistal bypass?

50%

Name the labeled arteries of the lower extremity.

1. **External iliac artery**
2. Deep circumflex iliac artery
3. Superficial circumflex iliac artery
4. Profunda femoris artery
5. Lateral circumflex femoral artery
6. Perforating arteries
7. **Popliteal artery**
8. Superior lateral genicular artery
9. Inferior lateral genicular artery
10. Perforating branch of peroneal (fibular) artery
11. Lateral malleolar artery
12. Lateral tarsal artery
13. Arcuate artery
14. Dorsal digital artery
15. Deep plantar branch
16. Medial tarsal artery
17. **Dorsalis pedis artery**
18. Medial malleolar artery
19. **Anterior tibial artery**
20. Anterior tibial recurrent artery
21. Inferior medial genicular artery
22. Superior medial genicular artery
23. Descending genicular artery
24. **Superficial femoral artery**
25. Medial circumflex femoral artery
26. Obturator artery
27. External pudendal artery
28. **Common femoral artery**
29. Inferior epigastric artery
30. **Internal iliac artery**
31. **Common iliac artery**
32. Superior gluteal artery
33. Inferior gluteal artery
34. Medial circumflex femoral artery
35. **Profunda femoris artery**
36. **Superficial femoral artery**
37. **Popliteal artery**
38. Genicular arteries (originate from the popliteal artery)
39. **Posterior tibial artery**
40. Medial plantar artery
41. Deep branch of dorsalis pedis artery
42. Plantar arch
43. Lateral plantar artery
44. **Peroneal (fibular) artery**
45. **Anterior tibial artery**

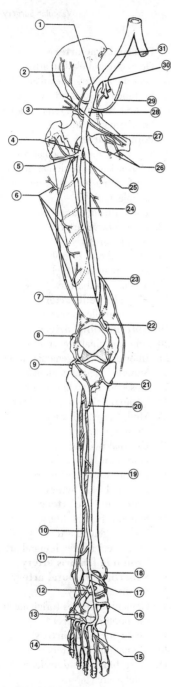
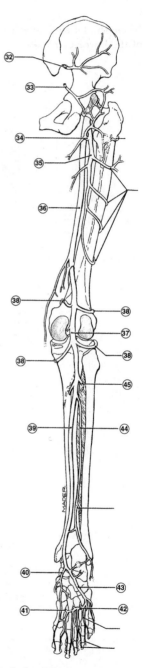

A, Anterior view

B, Posterior view

ARTERIAL OCCLUSIVE DISEASE OF THE UPPER EXTREMITY

Arterial occlusive disease of the upper extremity accounts for what percentage of cases of extremity ischemia?

5%

What are the etiologies?

Diverse, including atherosclerosis, embolism, trauma, thoracic outlet syndrome, arteritis (e.g., Buerger and Takayasu diseases), and vasospastic disorders (e.g., Raynaud syndrome)

Why are proximal occlusions usually asymptomatic?

Extensive arterial collaterals around the shoulder girdle

What clinical test is performed to evaluate the patency of ulnar and radial arteries?

Allen test

How are atherosclerotic lesions of the upper extremity different from those of the lower extremity?

Significantly increased incidence of atheroembolization

What is the most common site of stenosis?

Subclavian artery (75% occur on the left)

What are the treatment options?

Endarterectomy, bypass procedure or, occasionally, percutaneous balloon angioplasty

What is the procedure of choice for subclavian artery stenosis?

Common carotid to subclavian artery bypass with a PTFE conduit. To avoid the use of prosthetic material, an end-to-side anastomosis can be performed by transecting the subclavian artery and transposing the distal end.

Name the labeled arteries of the upper extremity.
(see following page)

1. **Subclavian artery**
2. Suprascapular artery
3. **Axillary artery**
4. Thoracoacromial artery
5. Posterior circumflex humeral artery
6. Anterior circumflex humeral artery
7. Profunda brachii artery
8. Radial recurrent artery
9. **Radial artery**
10. **Superficial palmar arch**
11. **Deep palmar arch**
12. Anterior interosseous artery
13. **Ulnar artery**
14. Common interosseous artery
15. Anterior and posterior ulnar recurrent arteries
16. Inferior ulnar collateral artery
17. Superior ulnar collateral artery
18. **Brachial artery**
19. Subscapular artery
20. Lateral thoracic artery
21. Internal mammary artery
22. **Aorta**
23. **Brachiocephalic trunk**
24. **Common carotid arteries**
25. **Vertebral artery**
26. Thyrocervical trunk
27. Transverse cervical artery

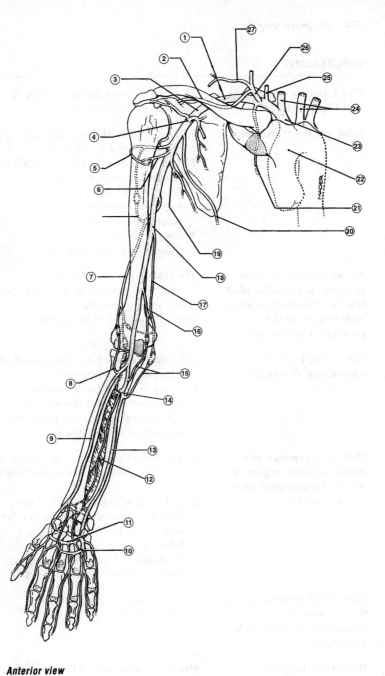

Anterior view

AMPUTATIONS

Which patient population is at highest risk?

Diabetics (account for 50% to 60% of nontraumatic amputations).

What are the indications?

1. Gangrene, usually secondary to chronic arterial insufficiency
2. Ischemic extremity pain as a result of inoperable vascular disease
3. Infection that is not resolved by aggressive débridement and parenteral antibiotics
4. Trauma (crush)
5. Tumors (soft tissue or bone)

As the amputation level proceeds proximally, what two key trends are seen with respect to the postoperative course?

The healing rate improves, but rehabilitation potential decreases. These factors must be considered when determining the level of amputation.

How is the level of amputation determined?

1. Clinical judgment (e.g., appearance of skin, pulses, capillary refill)
2. Measurement of transcutaneous oxygen tension, skin clearance of ^{133}Xe, or high-energy phosphates by magnetic resonance imaging

How does preoperative infection in the region of planned amputation alter management?

1. The definitive procedure is delayed until the infection is resolved with IV antibiotics.
2. If the trial of antibiotics fails, open guillotine amputation (as distal on the limb as possible) is performed, followed by continuation of IV antibiotics and frequent dressing changes until the infection clears.

With which amputations is this preoperative management particularly important?

Distal amputations (toe or ray) in diabetic patients

What basic surgical principles are important for successful amputation?

Minimal manipulation of the marginally vascularized distal tissue; tension-free closure of the amputation site; meticulous hemostasis; avoidance of the use of drains; sufficient viable soft tissue flaps to cover the stump

How should transection of the nerves be performed, and why?

Ligation and transection with gentle traction. The nerve retracts into the stump and reduces the risk of painful neuroma.

What is the best intraoperative indicator to guide the decision about the level of amputation?

Amount of bleeding at the proposed amputation site. For the wound to heal, adequate blood flow is essential. Amputation is performed until the level at which tissue bleeds well is reached.

Lower Extremity Amputations

What are the standard lower extremity amputations?

Above-the-knee (AKA), below-the-knee (BKA), transmetatarsal, ray, and toe amputations

What is the level of amputation of the infrequently used Syme and Lisfranc procedures?

Syme: Just proximal to the articular surfaces of the tibia and fibula
Lisfranc: Between the tarsals and metatarsals

For an AKA, what type of incision is used?

Circular or fishmouth (short anterior and posterior flaps)

Where is the bone divided?

At the junction between the middle and distal thirds of the femur

What procedure may be performed for failed AKA?

Hip disarticulation

For a BKA, what type of incision is used?

Anterior incision: 1 to 2 cm distal to the site of bone division
Posterior incision: Allowing a sufficient flap of skin, gastrocnemius, and soleus to cover the stump

Where is the bone divided?

Tibia: 8 to 12 cm distal to the tibial tuberosity
Fibula: As proximal as possible to reduce the risk of injury to the flap when the patient bears weight

For a transmetatarsal amputation, what type of incision is used?

Anterior incision (no flap): Midmetatarsal region
Posterior incision: Just proximal to the crease of the metatarsophalangeal joint. (Viability of the posterior flap is **essential** for the success of this amputation.)

What is ray amputation?

Amputation of the toe and part (or all) of its metatarsal

What is done if amputation of the toe extends to the metatarsophalangeal joint?

The cartilage is removed from the metatarsal head, or a ray amputation is performed. The presence of the cartilage does not permit adequate healing.

What are the mortality rates for hip disarticulation, AKA, and BKA?

Hip disarticulation: 80%
AKA: 15% to 40%
BKA: 5% to 15%

How are these rates altered by the presence of diabetes?

No difference, except that long-term survival is reduced in the diabetic patient

What are the independent (prosthetic) ambulation rates after:
1. BKA?
2. AKA?
3. Bilateral BKA?
4. Bilateral AKA?

1. 66% to 80%
2. 35% to 50%
3. 45%
4. 10%

What are the etiologies of failure of the stump to heal?

1. Arterial insufficiency to the stump because of inadequate amputation
2. Mechanical injury to marginal tissue intraoperatively
3. Infection
4. Hematoma caused by suboptimal intraoperative hemostasis
5. Postoperative trauma

What are the healing rates for AKA and BKA?

AKA: 95%
BKA: 70%

What are the etiologies of postoperative pain?

1. Infection
2. Normal postoperative pain
3. Phantom pain

What is the treatment for a patient who falls and ruptures open an amputation site in the early postoperative period?

Emergent surgery for sterile reclosure

Why is physical therapy initiated early?

To reduce the risk of flexion contracture and DVT (seen in 10%–15% of amputees)

What is the overall survival rate at 1, 3, and 5 years after lower extremity amputation?

1 year: 75%
3 year: 50%
5 year: 35%
Because of associated atherosclerotic lesions elsewhere (e.g., heart)

EXTRACRANIAL CEREBROVASCULAR DISEASE

Anatomy

What are the origins of the carotid arteries?

Right: Innominate artery
Left: Aorta

What are the origins of the vertebral arteries?

Respective subclavian arteries

What is the classic collateral connection between the carotid and vertebral circulations?

Circle of Willis: Paired anterior and posterior communicating cerebral arteries connect the two arterial circulations. Up to 50% of patients have an incomplete circle.

What territories are supplied by the vertebral arteries?

1. Posteroinferior cerebral hemisphere
2. Cerebellum
3. Brain stem

What is the most frequently diseased region in the carotid artery?

Carotid bifurcation

What is the most frequently diseased region in the vertebral artery?

Origin

Etiology

What are the general mechanisms for cerebrovascular ischemia?	1. Embolism 2. Thrombosis 3. Intracranial hemorrhage 4. Hypoperfusion caused by arterial stenosis or systemic hypotension
What are the specific etiologies of reduced cerebrovascular blood flow?	1. Atherosclerosis, causing cerebrovascular stenosis or ulceration with emboli 2. Fibromuscular dysplasia 3. Aortic dissection, with resultant occlusion of the carotid or vertebral arteries 4. Obliterative arteritis (Takayasu)
What is the mechanism of acute stenosis or plaque fragmentation in the atherosclerotic artery?	Intramural and subplaque hemorrhage (the most common pathologic finding in the carotid artery)
When does stenosis usually compromise flow?	> 75% loss of cross-sectional area (50% loss of diameter)

Classic Ischemic Neurologic Events

Define TIA.	Transient ischemic attack. Neurologic deficit lasting < 24 hours (usually < 5 minutes).
What are the classic ocular symptoms of TIAs?	Amaurosis fugax (transient monocular blindness)
What is the mechanism of this ocular symptom?	Emboli to the ophthalmic artery. Hollenhorst cholesterol plaques are seen on retinal exam.
What percentage of TIAs are caused by extracranial cerebrovascular disease?	Only 50%. The rest are caused by cardiac thromboemboli **and intra**cranial vascular disease.
What percentage of strokes are preceded by a TIA?	> 50%

What percentage of patients with TIAs progress to stroke at 1, 3, and 5 years?	1 year: 25% 3 years: 35% 5 years: 45%
Define RIND.	Resolving ischemic neurologic deficit: Neurologic deficit of 24- to 72-hour duration, with complete resolution
Define CVA.	Cerebrovascular accident: Neurologic deficit of > 24-hour duration without complete resolution

Compare:

1. Crescendo TIA	1. Repeated neurologic events, with return to baseline status between events
2. Stroke in evolution	2. Repeated events with actively deteriorating neurologic status
3. Completed stroke	3. Leveling off of the rate of neurologic loss at a new, lower baseline level

Carotid vs. Vertebrobasilar Disease

How do the plaques in carotid disease differ from those in vertebrobasilar disease?	Carotid: High incidence of ulcerated plaques Vertebral: Usually a smooth intimal surface
Which type is usually associated with unilateral versus bilateral neurologic deficits?	Carotid: Usually unilateral Vertebral: Often bilateral
Where is the bruit auscultated in each type?	Carotid: Anterior border of the sternocleidomastoid muscle near the angle of the mandible Vertebral: Supraclavicular fossa
In which situation are "drop attacks" common?	Vertebrobasilar disease. The patient suddenly falls to the ground because of bilateral lower extremity motor deficit ($\pm$ loss of consciousness with rapid recovery).

Presentation and Diagnosis

What is the most common presentation?	Painless, abrupt loss of focal neurologic function, usually with maximal deficit at the time of presentation (completed stroke)

What signs and symptoms suggest vertebrobasilar insufficiency?

Dizziness, vertigo, tinnitus, syncope, dysarthria, and homonymous hemianopsia

What signs and symptoms suggest intracerebral hemorrhage?

Pain (headache) and progression of neurologic deficits (stroke in evolution, progressing stroke)

What are the three common presentations of asymptomatic carotid disease?

1. Asymptomatic cervical bruit
2. Asymptomatic carotid lesion contralateral to a symptomatic lesion
3. Asymptomatic carotid lesion discovered during preoperative screening for another procedure (usually a cardiac or another vascular procedure)

What screening studies are performed?

1. Duplex ultrasound of the extracranial carotid arteries (study of choice)
2. Transcranial Doppler ultrasound of the intracranial carotid and vertebrobasilar arteries
3. Oculoplethysmography (evaluates flow through the ophthalmic artery)

What are the two diagnostic components of duplex scanning?

1. B-mode: To identify the region of arterial stenosis
2. Pulse Doppler: To evaluate the pulse wave and flow characteristics

What are the sensitivity and specificity of duplex scanning?

Both > 90%

Is a computed tomography (CT) scan necessary, and why?

Yes.
1. For all patients, CT scan is used to exclude other causes of symptoms (neoplasm, subdural hematoma, AV malformation) and document the presence of any baseline (preoperative) cerebral infarction.
2. For patients with evidence of recent stroke, CT scan is used to distinguish between hemorrhagic and ischemic stroke. Surgery is avoided in hemorrhagic stroke because of the increased risk of further hemorrhage.

What additional study is used to further define the anatomic lesion before surgery?	Conventional (four-vessel) angiogram for detailed evaluation of the cerebrovascular anatomy

Treatment

Is medical or surgical treatment the management of choice to reduce the risk of stroke?	Depends on the severity of arterial stenosis 1. For stenoses ≥ 60%, surgery is the choice. 2. For those < 40%, either modality is used, and medical therapy is usually chosen. 3. For those between 40% and 60%, prospective studies are ongoing (i.e., NASCET study).
What is the medical treatment?	Aspirin ± dipyridamole or ticlopidine (antiplatelet therapy). (Medical treatment reduces the risk of stroke only in **symptomatic** patients!)
What are the indications for surgical treatment?	1. Symptomatic patients with extracranial cerebrovascular disease 2. Asymptomatic patients with carotid stenosis ≥ 80% 3. Asymptomatic patients with complex ulcerated plaques (The indications are still controversial and are evolving.)
Which patients with evolving stroke are considered for surgery?	Only patients with accessible cerebrovascular lesion, "nonmassive" stroke, **intact** mental status, **and no** intracranial hemorrhage
How is the brain protected from ischemia intraoperatively?	1. Adequate blood pressure is maintained. Manipulation of the carotid body often results in labile blood pressure. 2. Manipulation of the artery is minimized to reduce the risk of embolic events. 3. A carotid shunt is placed in some patients to permit continued arterial flow through the carotid system that is undergoing surgery.

What are the indications for shunt placement (controversial)?

1. Complete carotid occlusion on the contralateral side
2. Intraoperative measures of marginal cerebral perfusion: Carotid stump pressure < 40 to 50 mm Hg, electroencephalogram wave slowing, or loss of normal β waves with clamping of the carotid artery
3. Neurologic dysfunction while the carotid artery is occluded under local anesthesia

In the surgical treatment of carotid artery disease, what is the most commonly performed procedure?

Carotid endarterectomy (CEA)

What is the standard incision?

Longitudinal incision along the anterior border of the sternocleidomastoid muscle

What vein is divided to provide better exposure of the carotid bifurcation?

Facial vein

What are the two possible planes of dissection used in CEA, and what is the benefit of each?

1. Through the **internal** elastic lamina (between the intima and media): Permits an easier transition to the intima at the edges of the CEA
2. Through the **external** elastic lamina: Removes surface irregularities of the circular smooth muscle layer of the media

Which nerves neighboring the carotid artery may be injured intraoperatively, and what defects are noted postoperatively?

1. Mandibular branch of the facial nerve (CN VII): Inability to raise the corner of the mouth (smile)
2. Glossopharyngeal nerve (CN IX): Horner syndrome, decreased gag reflex
3. Vagus nerve (CN X): hoarseness (recurrent laryngeal nerve), voice fatigability (superior laryngeal nerve)
4. Hypoglossal nerve (CN XII): Deviation of the tongue to the side of the injury

What is the long-term prognosis of the injured nerve?

Function is usually regained in 2 to 6 months because injury is often caused by retraction rather than transection of the nerve.

Name the labeled structures of a right CEA.

1. Hypoglossal nerve (CN XII)
2. Internal carotid artery
3. Ligated facial vein
4. Sternocleidomastoid muscle
5. Internal jugular vein
6. Superior thyroid vein
7. Common carotid artery
8. Ansa cervicalis
9. Superior thyroid artery
10. External carotid artery
11. Lingual artery
12. Vagus nerve

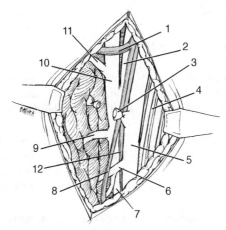

What are the most common causes of abnormality on intraoperative Doppler ultrasound or angiogram at the completion of CEA?

Intimal flap or platelet aggregates at the edge of the CEA. A flap requires tacking sutures to prevent further dissection and occlusion.

What are the most commonly performed surgical procedures in the treatment of vertebral artery disease?

1. Trans-subclavian endarterectomy of the vertebral artery origin
2. Vertebral–carotid transposition (end-to-side implantation of a normal distal vertebral artery into the ipsilateral common carotid artery)

What is the usual treatment for complete occlusion of the internal or common carotid artery?	Antiplatelet therapy
When is surgery indicated in this setting?	When symptoms recur during medical therapy
What are the surgical options for complete occlusion?	1. Extracranial–intracranial bypass (neurosurgery) 2. CEA plus repair of the blind internal carotid artery stump to reduce the incidence of embolus
What is the incidence of supratentorial neurologic deficits in the early postoperative period?	1% to 4 %
What is the usual etiology?	Embolus
What percentage of patients have hypertension postoperatively, and why?	20%; often as a result of denervation of the carotid sinus baroreceptors (located in the carotid bifurcation)
What is the treatment?	IV sodium nitroprusside. The systolic blood pressure is maintained at < 160 to 180 mm Hg to reduce the risk of blowout of the arteriotomy.
What is the recommended treatment of a new neurologic deficit in the early postoperative period?	Immediate reexploration to examine the carotid or vertebral artery directly
What is the usual etiology of acute airway compromise in the early postoperative period?	Neck hematoma
What is the key point to remember about the management of this complication?	The wound is opened immediately **at the bedside** to relieve compartment pressure. The patient then goes emergently to the OR.

What is the mortality rate of CEA?	1%
What is the most common cause of death after CEA?	Myocardial infarction
What is the most common late complication?	Recurrent carotid artery stenosis
What are the risk factors of this late complication?	1. Small diameter (< 4–5 mm) internal carotid artery 2. Female sex (likely because of smaller size) 3. Primary CEA arteriotomy closure (rather than patch closure) 4. Hyperlipidemia 5. Continued tobacco abuse
What percentage of patients are symptomatic versus asymptomatic because of recurrent stenosis?	Symptomatic: 1% to 3% Asymptomatic: 10% to 15%

ANATOMY OF THE VISCERAL BRANCHES OF THE AORTA

MESENTERIC ARTERIES

What are the three main mesenteric arteries and the territory of bowel that each supplies?	1. Celiac artery: Stomach to ampulla of Vater (middle of the second portion of the duodenum) 2. Superior mesenteric artery (SMA): To the splenic flexure of the colon 3. Inferior mesenteric artery: To the rectum
What is the key "watershed" area?	Splenic flexure of the colon (often has a break in the continuity of the marginal artery of Drummond)
What are the branches of the celiac artery?	1. Left gastric artery 2. Splenic artery 3. Hepatic artery
What are the first two branches of the SMA?	1. Inferior pancreaticoduodenal (PD) artery 2. Middle colic artery

What are the branches of the inferior mesenteric artery (IMA)?	1. Left colic artery 2. Sigmoid arteries 3. Superior hemorrhoidal artery
What is the major arterial collateral path between the celiac artery and the SMA?	Celiac artery → Hepatic artery → Gastroduodenal artery → Superior PD artery → Inferior PD artery → SMA
What is the major arterial collateral path between the SMA and the IMA?	Arch of Riolan: SMA → Middle colic artery (left branch) → Left colic artery (ascending branch) → IMA
What is the "meandering mesenteric artery"?	The tortuous, enlarged, and dilated arch of Riolan that results with increased blood flow through this collateral

RENAL ARTERIES

Renal arteries are located at what lumbar level?	L1 to L2
Is the right renal artery anterior or posterior to the IVC?	Posterior
How is the right renal artery exposed intraoperatively?	Kocher maneuver (medial mobilization of the hepatic flexure of the colon and the third portion of the duodenum) ± retraction of the inferior vena cava (IVC) for exposure of the most proximal portion of the renal artery
What is the most common anatomic "anomaly" of the renal artery?	Accessory renal arteries (seen in 20%–25% of the population)

VISCERAL ISCHEMIC SYNDROMES

ACUTE MESENTERIC ISCHEMIA

What are the etiologies?	1. Embolus 2. Thrombosis 3. Nonocclusive etiologies (i.e., vasospasm associated with low cardiac output, venous thrombosis)

What is the most common surgically treatable cause?	Arterial embolism
What is the most common site of embolism?	Proximal SMA (at the SMA origin or at the takeoff of the middle colic artery)
Why do emboli tend to enter this vessel?	The SMA is large, and its takeoff from the aorta is at an acute angle versus the more perpendicular celiac, IMA, and renal origins.
What are the symptoms?	Early: Severe abdominal pain with fairly **benign** abdominal findings. Pain is classically "out of proportion to the signs" on physical exam. Later: Fever, tachycardia, hypotension, vomiting, diarrhea (often heme positive), abdominal distension, peritonitis
What is the character of the bowel sounds?	Early: Hyperactive Later: Absent
What is the general presentation of embolus versus thrombosis?	Embolus: Acute, rapidly progressive symptoms Thrombosis: More insidious. Patients usually have a history consistent with chronic mesenteric ischemia (see the Chronic Mesenteric Ischemia section).
What are the laboratory findings?	1. Severe leukocytosis (often > 20,000 if infarcted) 2. Metabolic acidosis (later in the course) 3. Elevated amylase and lactate values (nonspecific, but helpful)
Which patients often do not have leukocytosis?	Elderly patients
What are the abdominal x-ray findings?	Distended loops of bowel, air–fluid levels, and edematous bowel wall. In the setting of infarction, gas may be seen in the bowel wall or portal venous tree.
What is the diagnostic study of choice?	Angiogram. (Duplex ultrasound is gaining popularity in larger centers.)

Which view is most helpful, and why?

The lateral view because it facilitates visualization of the classic atherosclerotic ostial lesions.

What are the classic angiographic findings for embolus, thrombosis, and nonocclusive etiologies?

1. Embolus: Abrupt occlusion with a "meniscus sign," usually 5 to 8 cm from the origin of the SMA
2. Thrombosis: Occlusion of the origin itself or a very proximal region of the mesenteric arteries
3. Nonocclusive: Smooth, gradual tapering of more distal branches (because of vasospasm)

What is the preoperative preparation?

1. Volume resuscitation. Significant intravascular hypovolemia often develops as a result of third spacing of fluid into the bowel.
2. Swan-Ganz catheter placement to optimize cardiovascular status
3. Broad-spectrum IV antibiotics
4. Correction of electrolyte disturbances and acidosis

What are the procedures of choice for embolus, thrombosis, and nonocclusive etiologies?

1. Revascularization procedure:
   a. Embolism: Embolectomy with a Fogarty catheter through transverse arteriotomy
   b. Thrombosis: Aortovisceral bypass, preferably with autologous vein, or thromboendarterectomy
   c. Nonocclusive: Selective intra-arterial infusion of a vasodilator (papaverine) and IV heparin
2. Resection of nonviable bowel

When is bowel nonviability determined?

After the revascularization procedure

How is bowel viability assessed intraoperatively?

1. Gross examination: Palpable pulses, pink color, visible peristalsis
2. Wood lamp inspection after IV fluorescein
3. Doppler ultrasound of the mesentery artery adjacent to the bowel in question

When is the decision made to perform a second-look laparotomy?	**At the time of the original surgery!** No postoperative clinical findings or diagnostic tests (except direct visualization) are reliable for the assessment of bowel viability.
How is bowel viability assessed postoperatively?	1. Colonoscopic inspection of the colonic mucosa 2. Second-look laparotomy (6–24 hours later)
What do the terms "antegrade" and "retrograde" refer to in describing aortovisceral bypass?	The site of aortic anastomosis with respect to the origin of the mesenteric vessel being bypassed (e.g., antegrade is proximal to the origin)
Which site is usually preferred, and why?	Antegrade because it offers better long-term patency
What is the mortality rate for acute mesenteric ischemia?	55% to 85%
What factor accounts for much of this high mortality rate?	Delayed diagnosis

CHRONIC MESENTERIC ISCHEMIA

What is the etiology?	Atherosclerosis
How is the extent of disease different from acute mesenteric ischemia?	Disease involves two or all three major mesenteric vessels, rather than one.
Why?	Collateral formation that accompanies chronic changes protects against ischemia.
Which patients are the exception to this rule?	Patients who have had abdominal surgery with transection of potential collateral pathways (i.e., partial colectomy)

What are the symptoms?

1. Postprandial abdominal pain ("intestinal angina," colicky pain)
2. Weight loss, primarily caused by loss of desire to eat because of pain and, to a lesser extent, malabsorption. An alternative diagnosis should be considered in patients with no significant weight loss.

What other abdominal pathology may present in a similar fashion?

1. Partial bowel obstruction
2. Carcinoma (stomach, pancreas, or colon)

(These etiologies are much more common than chronic mesenteric ischemia.)

What does constant pain BETWEEN meals suggest in a patient with chronic mesenteric ischemia?

Mesenteric infarction

What is a common finding on physical exam of the abdomen?

Epigastric bruit

What is the treatment for chronic mesenteric ischemia?

1. Aortovisceral bypass graft
2. Thromboendarterectomy

What are the most common causes of acute mesenteric ischemia in a patient with chronic mesenteric ischemia?

Low cardiac output because of congestive heart failure, acute myocardial infarction, or arrhythmia

What is the celiac artery compression syndrome?

Compression of the celiac artery by the crura of the diaphragm. It is usually asymptomatic, but occasionally causes symptoms similar to those of chronic mesenteric ischemia.

RENOVASCULAR HYPERTENSION

What is the general vascular lesion, and how does it result in hypertension (HTN)?

Stenosis of the renal artery. Renin is released by juxta-glomerular apparatus in response to decreased pressure in the renal arterioles (because of stenosis). Renin is involved in the synthesis of angiotensin II, resulting in vasoconstriction and increased production of aldosterone with resultant sodium retention and increased total intravascular volume.

Renovascular hypertension accounts for what percentage of all cases of HTN?

5%. It is the most common type of surgically correctable HTN.

In what percentage of patients with HTN and renal artery stenosis is the stenosis solely responsible for the patient's HTN?

Only 50%

What features of the patient history suggest renal artery stenosis as the cause of HTN?

1. New onset of HTN in patient < 30 years old or > 60 years old
2. Abrupt onset of HTN or difficult to control HTN at any age
3. No family history of HTN

What are the most common etiologies?

1. Renal artery atherosclerosis (70%–80%)
2. Fibromuscular dysplasia (FMD; 15%–20 %)

Less common etiologies include renal artery trauma, dissection, and embolus.

In atherosclerosis versus FMD:
1. What is the gender predominance?
2. What side is normally affected?
3. Which segment of the renal artery is usually affected?
4. What is the frequency of bilateral involvement?

1. Atherosclerosis: Male; FMD: Female
2. Atherosclerosis: Left; FMD: Right
3. Atherosclerosis: Ostia and proximal third; FMD: Middle and distal thirds
4. Atherosclerosis: 25% to 33%; FMD: > 50%

Which type of FMD is most common?

Medial fibrodysplasia accounts for 85% of cases.

What is the classic finding on physical exam?

Epigastric or abdominal bruit (50%–80%)

What screening studies are performed to exclude primary renal lesions?

1. IV pyelogram
2. Renal isotope scan

What screening study is performed to detect renal artery stenosis?	Duplex scan (nearly 100% sensitivity)
What is the diagnostic study for definitive diagnosis?	Aortogram or selective renal angiogram. (Intra-arterial digital subtraction angiogram is no longer recommended because of lack of sensitivity.)
What is the classic finding with this study in the setting of FMD?	A "string of beads" appearance because of multiple microaneurysms (alternating stenoses and dilations) along the course of the artery
What study is used to evaluate the FUNCTIONAL significance of the renal artery stenosis?	Selective renal vein renin assay ± captopril stimulation
What finding is diagnostic of renovascular HTN?	Renin ratio between the kidneys > 1.48 (or 1.5). The ischemic kidney produces more renin, especially with captopril stimulation.
What is the most common cause of false-negative results?	Bilateral renal artery stenosis (e.g., both kidneys produce increased amounts of renin)
What is the medical treatment?	1. Angiotensin-converting enzyme (ACE) inhibitors (e.g., captopril) are the most effective agents. 2. Calcium channel blockers and beta blockers also have some success. (Medical therapy is reserved for patients whose condition is not amenable to surgery.)
Which agents cause deterioration of renal function, and which patients are at highest risk?	ACE inhibitors; patients with **bilateral** renal artery stenosis
What are the basic indications for surgery?	1. Hypertension 2. Declining renal function (The exact criteria are controversial.)

What are the surgical options?

1. Aortorenal bypass (procedure of choice)
2. Transaortic endarterectomy
3. Percutaneous transluminal angioplasty (PTA)
4. Ex vivo repair with autotransplantation
5. Nephrectomy (last resort to eliminate the source of elevated renin levels)

Which surgical option is usually not helpful in atherosclerosis versus FMD?

PTA: atherosclerosis
Endarterectomy: FMD

In aortorenal bypass, compare the conduit used in the adult versus the conduit used in the child.

Adult: Saphenous vein graft (occasionally a prosthetic graft)
Child: Internal iliac artery graft (vein grafts tend to become aneurysmal in pediatric patients)

Why is it important to minimize perirenal dissection?

Enlarged collaterals increase the risk of significant bleeding.

What are the surgical options for a patient with a severely diseased infrarenal aorta?

1. Aortic reconstruction (i.e., aortoiliac bypass) combined with aortorenal bypass
2. Extra-anatomic renal artery bypass, usually through the saphenous vein graft from splenic, hepatic, or gastroduodenal arteries (if the patient is too high risk for aortic reconstruction)

When is ex vivo ("bench") repair indicated?

For complex renal lesions that cause renal HTN (i.e., intraparenchymal stenoses)

When is nephrectomy indicated for renal HTN?

Blood pressure uncontrolled by medical therapy in the setting of:
1. Atrophic kidney (< 6–7 cm)
2. Inoperative disease (i.e., severe arteriolar nephrosclerosis)
3. Complete renal artery occlusion **with infarction.** When occlusion is very gradual, arterial collaterals may prevent ischemia.

What percentage of patients require nephrectomy?	< 10 %
In atherosclerosis versus FMD, what percentage of patients are cured?	Atherosclerosis: 25% to 40% FMD: 55% to 75%
What percentage of patients show improvement, but are not cured?	Atherosclerosis: 50% to 60% FMD: 20% to 40%

ANEURYSMS

What is the general criterion for "aneurysm"?	Increase in arterial diameter by ≥ 50%
What feature distinguishes true aneurysms from false aneurysms?	True: Involves all layers of the vessel wall False: Lesion in an inner layer permits dissection within the wall (i.e., only the outer layers are dilated)
Why is the vessel lumen frequently not increased on an arteriogram of an aneurysm?	True: Mural thrombus deposits are seen within the aneurysmal dilation (caused by stagnant flow and eddy currents). False: The intima is frequently not dilated (hematoma within vessel wall increases the diameter of the vessel).

ABDOMINAL AORTIC ANEURYSM (AAA)

What vertebral levels correspond to the origin and bifurcation of the abdominal aorta?	Origin: T12 (aortic hiatus of the diaphragm) Bifurcation: L4
What is the approximate site of bifurcation with respect to external landmarks?	Level of the umbilicus
What is the mean normal diameter of the aorta?	2 cm (1.8 cm in women, 2.2 cm in men)

What is the incidence of AAA in patients with peripheral vascular disease versus the general population?	20% versus 2% (10-fold increased risk)
What is the key factor determining the risk of AAA rupture?	Size of the aneurysm
What is the incidence of rupture at 5 years?	If < 6 cm: 20% If ≥ 6 cm: 40% to 60%
What is the average growth of AAA diameter annually?	4 to 5 mm annual increase in diameter. This expansion is not linear over time. Spurts occur intermittently over the course of a year.
What is the most common location of AAAs?	Infrarenal
What are the gross characteristics?	Fusiform; true aneurysm (95%)
What percentage involve renal arteries?	2%
What are the etiologies of AAA?	1. Atherosclerosis (> 90%) 2. "Inflammatory" causes (5%) 3. "Mycotic" causes (does not imply fungal)
What underlying defect is common to all types?	Vessel wall weakness caused by destruction of the tunica media (loss of elastin)
What is the characteristic gross appearance of inflammatory AAAs?	Dense, white, fibrotic inflammatory reaction that covers the aorta and adjacent abdominal structures (e.g., duodenum, ureters)
What are the most common etiologies of mycotic AAAs?	1. *Staphylococcus epidermidis* and *Staphylococcus aureus* 2. *Salmonella* ("Mycotic" does not imply fungal causes in AAAs.)

Presentation and Diagnosis

What is the most common presentation?	Palpable pulsatile mass in an **asymptomatic** patient

What does pain usually suggest?

1. Rapidly enlarging AAA
2. Ruptured, leaking AAA

What is the classic presentation triad of ruptured AAA?

1. Abdominal, back, or flank pain
2. Hypotension
3. Pulsatile abdominal mass

What is the presentation of inflammatory AAA?

1. Chronic abdominal pain
2. Weight loss
3. Increased erythrocyte sedimentation rate

What is the classic finding on x-ray?

"Eggshell" calcification of the vessel wall, especially on the lateral view

What is the diagnostic study of choice in the emergency room?

CT scan

What is the definitive diagnostic study of choice?

CT scan

What are the benefits of this study?

1. Shows the true diameter of the AAA, unlike an aortogram, which often shows a falsely decreased diameter due to the intra-aneurysmal thrombus
2. Detects retroperitoneal leak or rupture
3. Accurately locates the level of the AAA
4. Detects structural anomalies that complicate the repair of AAAs
5. Diagnoses inflammatory AAAs

What are examples of the structural anomalies shown on CT scan?

1. Retroaortic left renal vein. There is a risk of injury to this vein with aortic cross-clamp.
2. Horseshoe kidney

What additional information may an aortogram provide?

Detection of visceral arterial stenoses (celiac, SMA, IMA, renal), suprarenal extension of AAA, iliofemoral stenoses or aneurysms, and other arterial anomalies (i.e., accessory renal arteries). Overall, however, many believe it is a low-yield study.

When is ultrasound the diagnostic test of choice?

1. Long-term follow-up of poor surgical candidates or patients with small AAAs
2. In emergency rooms, as a quick screen in patients with acute symptoms

What study is performed if a rupture is suspected?

None! The best place to diagnose a ruptured AAA is the OR!

What is the most common cause of death?

Myocardial infarction

What is the most common site of rupture?

2 to 4 cm infrarenal in the left posterolateral wall (i.e., retroperitoneal)

What is the classic finding on physical exam?

Ecchymosis in the inguinal and groin region (tracking of blood around the abdominal wall from the retroperitoneum)

What complication is common in inflammatory AAAs?

Ureteral obstruction. Inflammatory reaction results in fibrotic attachments with ureters, IVC, etc.

Treatment

What are the indications for elective repair of AAA?

1. Diameter ≥ 5 to 5.5 cm
2. Growth in diameter > 5 mm annually (These criteria are evolving.)

What is the indication for emergent repair?

A symptomatic patient with known or suspected AAA

What surgical procedure is used?

"Resection" of AAA. This term is a misnomer because the AAA is usually merely filleted open. Aortic continuity is restored with a prosthetic tube or bifurcation graft (aortoaortic, aortoiliac, or aortofemoral bypass).

What is the graft material of choice?

Dacron (woven or knitted, ± collagen impregnation). The second choice is PTFE.

What are the two surgical approaches?

1. Transabdominal approach through a midline laparotomy incision
2. Retroperitoneal approach through a left flank incision

What are the benefits of each approach?

1. Transabdominal:
   a. Permits concurrent exploratory laparotomy (e.g., to confirm bowel viability)
   b. Provides easier access to the right renal artery and distal right iliac artery
2. Retroperitoneal
   a. Does not require entry into the abdominal cavity (the approach of choice in patients with a "hostile" abdomen (e.g., adhesions, obesity, ascites)
   b. Offers decreased postoperative ileus
   c. Is better tolerated by patients with poor pulmonary reserve
   d. Provides easier proximal control, especially of the suprarenal aorta

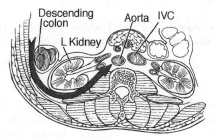

Path of retroperitoneal dissection to abdominal aorta.

In a patient with a ruptured AAA, what is the first step after midline laparotomy?

Immediate compression of the supraceliac aorta against the vertebral bodies

What are the next steps?

The left crus of the diaphragm is divided, the supraceliac aorta is clamped, the neck of the AAA (usually infrarenal) is exposed and clamped, the supraceliac clamp is removed, and the graft is placed.

What frequently obstructs access to the neck of the AAA in the transabdominal approach?

Left renal vein

What is done if retraction does not provide adequate exposure?

The left renal vein is ligated and divided as close to the IVC as possible.
Adequate collateral drainage is provided through the left gonadal and adrenal veins.

The origin of which anterior vessel lies in the middle of most AAAs?

IMA

What are the indications for reimplantation of this artery into an aortic graft?

1. Poor back-bleeding of the IMA, or IMA stump pressure $\leq$ 40 to 50 mm Hg, suggesting insufficient collateral arterial flow
2. Stenotic lesions in the celiac artery or SMA
3. Previous left colonic surgery with disruption of arterial collaterals

What is done to prevent pelvic ischemia after AAA repairs?

At least one internal iliac (hypogastric) artery is preserved.

What common complication occurs at the time of declamping of the aorta at the end of the procedure?

Declamping shock as a result of myocardiodepressive anaerobic by-products from the lower extremities or hypoxic vasodilation

What is the most common reason for an absent lower extremity pulse at the end of the procedure?

Arterial occlusion by emboli dislodged from the AAA because of intraoperative manipulation

What is the treatment?

Embolectomy with a Fogarty catheter until brisk back-bleeding from the iliac arteries is seen and the pulse is restored. Untreatable microemboli are common and are responsible for the classic "trash foot."

With a transabdominal approach, carcinoma of the colon is found intraoperatively. What procedure should be performed?

1. If AAA repair is **elective** and the bowel is prepared, the carcinoma is resected and the AAA is repaired later. If the bowel is not prepared, the incision is closed and the carcinoma resected after the bowel is prepared.
2. If AAA repair is **emergent,** the AAA is repaired and the carcinoma is resected

later to avoid placement of a prosthetic graft in a field that is contaminated by colectomy on an unprepared bowel.

With a transabdominal approach, cholelithiasis is found intraoperatively. What should be done?

Controversial. Most studies show no increased morbidity or mortality rates when a combined cholecystectomy and vascular procedure is performed. Many centers perform cholecystectomy after the vascular procedure is complete and the retroperitoneum is closed.

Postoperative Complications

What are the early postoperative complications?

1. Myocardial infarction
2. Colonic ischemia
3. Acute renal failure
4. Graft infection
5. Spinal ischemia (rare)

What are the late complications?

1. Aortoenteric fistula
2. Aortocaval fistula
3. Graft infection
4. Anastomotic pseudoaneurysm

How does colonic ischemia present?

Abdominal pain, diarrhea, and heme-positive stools. If the patient has a bowel movement < 24 to 48 hours postoperatively (especially if heme-positive), the diagnosis is mesenteric ischemia until it has been ruled out.

What are the etiologies of colonic ischemia in the setting of AAA?

1. Low flow because of perioperative hypotension
2. Ligation of the IMA in the setting of marginal collateral mesenteric flow

What region of the bowel is at highest risk?

Sigmoid colon and rectum (IMA territory)

How is the risk of colonic ischemia reduced?

The IMA is reimplanted or circulation is preserved through at least one internal iliac artery.

How long after myocardial infarction is elective AAA repair performed?

6 months

How is the risk of acute renal failure reduced?

1. Intraoperative volume loading to maintain renal perfusion pressure
2. Brisk diuresis with mannitol (Lasix) at the time of aortic cross-clamping

What other genitourinary complications are common postoperatively, and why?

1. Retrograde ejaculation (> 50%) because of disruption of the sympathetic plexus covering the aorta
2. Impotence (33%) because of decreased blood flow to the pelvis associated with ligation of the internal iliac arteries

When does aortoenteric fistula usually present?

> 4 to 6 months postoperatively

What is the usual presentation?

Herald bleed that resolves spontaneously, followed by exsanguinating bleed (one of the rare lesions that cause concurrent hematemesis **and** bright red rectal bleeding). Fewer than 33% of patients have abdominal pain.

What is the mechanism?

Proximal suture line erosion

What is the most common site?

The third or fourth portion of the duodenum

What is done at the time of the original repair to reduce the risk of aortoenteric fistula?

Native AAA wall is wrapped around the prosthetic graft.

What is the treatment?

The infected graft is removed, the bowel is repaired, IV antibiotics are given, and one of the following is performed:
1. Extra-anatomic bypass (axillobifemoral bypass)
2. Homograft aorta transplantation
3. Prosthetic graft replacement (controversial)

What is the presentation of aortocaval fistula?

High-output congestive heart failure, hypotension, cyanosis, venous distension of the lower extremities, abdominal bruit, and palpable abdominal thrill

What is the treatment?	The fistula is closed: achieve proximal and distal control of the aorta and IVC, an incision is made in the aortic graft, the fistula is repaired from **within** graft with large suture bites, and the aortic graft is closed.
What is excluded in the setting of pseudoaneurysm?	Graft infection
In graft infection, what is the most common organism?	*Staphylococcus* species
What are the CT findings?	Perigraft fluid collection ± gas
What is the treatment?	1. The **entire** infected graft is excised. Focal resection of grafts is usually unsuccessful, except for the occasional femoral anastomosis pseudoaneurysm. 2. Extra-anatomic bypass, homograft aorta, transplant, or graft replacement is performed. 3. IV antibiotics are given.
What is the mortality rate for elective AAA repair?	3% to 5%
What is the most common cause of death?	Myocardial infarction
What is the mortality rate for emergent AAA repair for rupture?	30% to 80%, depending on patient comorbidity factors, the interval between rupture and repair, the presence of retroperitoneal versus free rupture, and the experience of the surgical team

PERIPHERAL ARTERY ANEURYSM

What is the most common etiology of true peripheral aneurysm?	Atherosclerosis
What are the most common etiologies of false peripheral aneurysm?	1. Vascular bypass procedures 2. Trauma

What are the most common locations of true aneurysms?

1. Popliteal artery (70%)
2. Femoral artery (15%–20%)

What diagnostic study is performed in patients with true peripheral artery aneurysms, and why?

Complete arteriogram of the abdominal aorta and its branches to the lower extremity. Between 75% and 85% of these patients have an additional aneurysm elsewhere.

What is the most common complication of true aneurysms?

Distal arterial occlusion caused by emboli from a mural thrombus within the aneurysm. Rupture is rare.

What percentage of true aneurysms are bilateral?

60% to 75%

What are the indications for surgery?

1. Symptoms caused by embolic events or local compression
2. Aneurysm > 2 cm

What is the surgical procedure?

Excision or exclusion (proximal and distal ligation) of the aneurysm (to prevent further embolic events) plus a bypass procedure

Popliteal Artery Aneurysm

Most commonly associated with what other vascular lesion?

AAA (present in 35%–65%). (Only 3% to 5% of patients with AAA have popliteal artery aneurysm.)

What nonvascular lesion also occurs as a mass in the popliteal fossa?

Baker cyst (midline popliteal extension of the synovial sac or bursa of the knee)

Is aneurysm excision or exclusion the procedure of choice in popliteal artery, and why?

Exclusion by proximal and distal ligation. Attempts to excise the aneurysm "invariably" cause popliteal vein injury.

VISCERAL ARTERY ANEURYSM

What is the etiology?

Medial degeneration of the arterial wall

What are the most common locations?

1. Splenic artery (60%)
2. Hepatic artery (20%)

What is the presentation?

Vague upper quadrant or epigastric pain is occasionally present, but most patients are asymptomatic.

What is the most common complication?

Rupture

What is the incidence of rupture?

Splenic artery: 2%
Hepatic artery: 20%

What is the classic sequence of events in splenic artery aneurysm rupture?

"Double rupture": Herald bleed occurs into the lesser omental sac (± transient hypotension); then rupture occurs into the peritoneal cavity (± exsanguination).

What factor significantly increases the risk of rupture in patients with splenic artery aneurysm?

Pregnancy

What is the mortality rate if rupture occurs in the pregnant patient?

> 70%

What are the indications for treatment?

1. Symptomatic patient
2. Aneurysm > 2 cm
3. Splenic artery aneurysm in a patient who is pregnant or plans to become pregnant

What surgical procedure is performed?

1. Excision or exclusion of aneurysm ± bypass procedure
2. Splenectomy is sometimes performed.
3. For intrahepatic aneurysms, hepatic resection may be indicated.

Which sites do not require bypass graft, and why?

1. Splenic artery: Collateral arterial flow can occur through the short gastric arteries from the left gastroepiploic artery
2. **Proximal** common hepatic artery: Collateral flow through the gastroduodenal and right gastric arteries

NONATHEROSCLEROTIC VASCULAR DISEASE

What feature common to these disorders may facilitate their diagnosis?	Symptoms of limb ischemia in a **pre**atherosclerotic age-group of patients

THROMBOANGIITIS OBLITERANS (Buerger disease)

What is the target patient population?	Young men (20–35 years old) who are heavy tobacco abusers
What are the classic histologic findings?	Nonnecrotizing, segmental panarteritis with fibrous obliteration of the arterial lumen on healing; intraluminal thrombosis
How does TAO differ from atherosclerotic disease?	1. Involves all three layers of artery 2. Involves more peripheral vessels (small and medium arteries) 3. As many as 40% of patients have symptomatic upper extremity involvement
What is the etiology?	Uncertain, but believed to be autoimmune (possible association with HLA antigens A9 and B5)
What are the symptoms?	1. Excruciating rest pain 2. **Tender,** bilateral digital ulceration and gangrene 3. Occasionally, claudication (but much less frequently than with atherosclerotic occlusive disease)
What are the classic arteriographic findings?	Uninvolved large vessels with abrupt occlusion in medium and small arteries; "corkscrew" or "tree root" appearance (thought to be caused by dilated vasa vasorum collaterals around the occlusion)
What treatment is most effective?	Abstinence from tobacco (disease usually goes into remission)
What is the surgical treatment?	1. Sympathectomy (for vasodilation; yields transient improvement in symptoms) 2. Digital amputation for gangrene

Why is surgical bypass rarely possible?	Diffuse distal disease (i.e., no target for bypass)

POPLITEAL ENTRAPMENT SYNDROMES

What is the target patient population?	Young men (< 40 years old)
What is the etiology?	Congenital anomaly in the development of the popliteal artery or neighboring muscles, resulting in arterial compression
What structure is most often responsible for compression?	Medial head of the gastrocnemius muscle (> 80%)
Is involvement usually unilateral or bilateral?	Unilateral (75%)
What is the most common symptom?	Intermittent claudication of the leg or foot. Rest pain or gangrene is rare.
What is the classic finding on physical examination?	Loss of pedal pulses with ankle flexion or knee extension (contraction of the gastrocnemius muscle)
What diagnostic study is performed?	Arteriogram taken with the leg in various positions to show intermittent occlusion
What is the treatment?	1. Myotomy to divide the entrapping muscle 2. ± Femorodistal popliteal bypass (frequently necessary because of popliteal stenosis or aneurysm)
What disorder mimics popliteal entrapment syndrome?	Adventitial cystic degeneration of the popliteal artery (enlarging, subadventitial mucin-containing cysts causing obstruction)
How is this disorder distinguished from popliteal entrapment?	Arteriogram of adventitial cystic degeneration shows the pathognomonic "scimitar sign" (external compression of the popliteal lumen by expanding cysts).

TAKAYASU'S ARTERITIS

What is the target patient population?	Young women (< 30 years old), often with Asian ancestry
What vessels are most commonly involved?	1. Thoracic aorta ± arch vessels (Types I–IV) 2. Abdominal aorta (Types II and III) 3. Occasionally, the pulmonary arteries (Type IV)
What are the early symptoms?	Fever, arthralgia, myalgia, and anorexia
What is the medical treatment?	High-dose steroids
What is the surgical treatment?	Bypass procedures for stenoses. Endarterectomy fails in this disorder.
What is the relative contraindication to surgery?	Active arteritis. The vascular inflammation must be reduced with a course of steroids before a bypass procedure is attempted.
What are the complications?	1. Stroke 2. Hypertension (usually caused by renal artery stenosis) 3. Congestive heart failure

VENOUS AND LYMPHATIC DISEASE

VENOUS ANATOMY AND PHYSIOLOGY

What is the basic gross anatomy of the venous circulation?	The superficial venous system is connected to the deep venous system by perforating veins that pass through the fascial layer of the extremity. The perforating veins have valves that are oriented to permit flow to pass only from the superficial to the deep system (except in the foot, where the reverse is true).
What are the two main superficial veins of the lower extremity and the deep veins they feed?	1. Greater saphenous vein: Empties into the common femoral vein 2. Lesser saphenous vein: Empties into the popliteal vein

What is the main
mechanism by which blood
is returned to the heart?

Pumping action of the muscles of the
leg, especially the calf muscles. Venous
pressure normally decreases to less than
half its resting level with exercise.

What are the sinusoids?

Thin-walled venous cavities within the
muscles of the lower extremity. They
play an essential role in the
musculovenous pump.

DIAGNOSIS OF VENOUS INSUFFICIENCY

What three basic lesions
lead to venous
hypertension in the lower
extremity?

1. Venous obstruction
2. Valvular incompetence
3. Ineffective musculovenous pump

What two clinical tests are
used to evaluate the
venous system of the lower
extremity?

1. Trendelenburg test
2. Perthes test

Describe how each test is
performed.

1. Trendelenburg test: The leg is raised
   to drain the venous system, and a
   venous tourniquet is applied over the
   saphenofemoral junction. The patient
   then stands.
2. Perthes test: A venous tourniquet is
   applied proximal to varicoses or
   suspected incompetent perforators.
   Then the patient ambulates.

What is the purpose of
each test?

1. Trendelenburg test: To exclude
   saphenofemoral and perforator
   valvular incompetence
2. Perthes test: To exclude perforator
   valvular incompetence and deep
   venous occlusion

What do the following
observations suggest?
1. Trendelenburg test
   a. Slow filling of
      varicosities before the
      tourniquet is
      released?

1. Trendelenburg test
   a. Competent perforators (if filling is
      rapid, incompetent)

b. **Rapid filling of varicosities when the tourniquet is released?**

b. Incompetent saphenofemoral valve

2. **Perthes test**

   a. **Increase in varicosities with exercise?**

   b. **Decrease in varicosities with exercise?**

2. Perthes test

   a. Deep venous thrombosis

   b. Normal deep venous system and competent perforators

What is the diagnostic study of choice for venous disease, and why?

Duplex ultrasound: Clearly shows the two basic pathologic venous lesions (valvular incompetence and venous occlusion)

LOWER EXTREMITY VARICOSITIES

What is the claim to fame of lower extremity varicosities?

Most common lower extremity vascular disorder, affecting 10% to 20% of the population

What are the "types" and their main etiologies?

1. Primary varicosities: Genetic predisposition (exact mechanism is uncertain)
2. Secondary varicosities: Deep venous thrombosis, resulting in shunting of blood through incompetent perforators to the superficial system

What are the symptoms?

Fatigue, heaviness, or aching of the limb, especially when standing erect

What is the conservative therapy?

Elastic support stockings; elevation of the affected extremity when sitting

What are the indications for surgery?

1. Cosmetic
2. Symptomatic (e.g., aching)
3. Occasionally, complications of chronic venous insufficiency (e.g., recurrent superficial thrombophlebitis, ulcer)

What is the most frequently performed procedure?

Simple sclerotherapy (injection of a sclerosing agent into the varicose veins)

What agent is used?	Sodium tetradecyl sulfate
What is the contraindication to this therapy?	Incompetent saphenofemoral or saphenopopliteal valves. Sclerotherapy alone invariably fails.
What is the procedure of choice if simple sclerotherapy is contraindicated?	1. Proximal ligation and division of the greater saphenous vein at the saphenofemoral junction 2. Sclerotherapy or vein stripping (either of these ablation techniques is satisfactory)
What is the contraindication to proximal ligation or vein stripping?	Deep venous thrombosis, which results in venous drainage, primarily through the superficial system
What is done to reduce the risk of recurrence as a result of neovascularization?	Several centimeters of the greater saphenous vein are **excised** at the saphenofemoral junction. Even with this procedure, the recurrence rate is 30%.
What are the other surgical options?	Procedures typically used for chronic venous insufficiency (e.g., subfascial ligation of perforators, valve transplant). These procedures are rarely indicated for simple varicose veins.

SUPERFICIAL THROMBOPHLEBITIS

What are the most common etiologies?	Intravenous catheter, varicose veins, intravenous drug abuse, and trauma
What is Mondor disease?	Superficial thrombophlebitis of the thoracoepigastric veins of the anterior chest wall or breast
What condition is most commonly associated with migratory thrombophlebitis?	Carcinoma of the pancreas
What is the presentation of superficial thrombophlebitis?	1. Fever 2. Tender, indurated subcutaneous venous "cord" with accompanying local erythema 3. No significant edema

What percentage of cases are complicated by concurrent deep venous thrombosis?	10% to 15%
What is the treatment of uncomplicated superficial thrombophlebitis?	1. Mild cases require only mild analgesic and Ace wrap. Ambulation is encouraged. 2. More severe cases require elevation of the extremity, **bed rest,** and warm compresses.
What is the treatment of septic thrombophlebitis?	1. IV antibiotics 2. Removal of the IV catheter
What additional therapy is necessary for suppurative thrombophlebitis?	If purulent drainage is expressed from the vein, the vein is excised and the wound packed open.
What is the treatment of Mondor disease?	It is self-limiting.

CHRONIC VENOUS INSUFFICIENCY

What are the etiologies?	1. Valvular venous incompetence (90%) 2. Venous obstruction (10%) secondary to postphlebitic syndrome
What is the primary physiologic derangement?	Chronic venous hypertension
What is the result?	Local hypertension causes reduced capillary perfusion and interstitial accumulation of hemosiderin and fibrin (through dilated endothelial pores). Oxygen transport to tissue is reduced.
What are the clinical manifestations of this reduced tissue oxygenation?	Poor healing of cutaneous traumatic lesions, eventually followed by spontaneous breakdown of the skin
What are the classic cutaneous changes of chronic venous insufficiency?	1. Brawny edema, hyperpigmentation, stasis dermatitis 2. Liposclerosis (thick, hardened subcutaneous tissue because of fibrin deposits) 3. Venous ulceration

What is the classic location of venous ulcers?

Superior and posterior to the medial malleolus, the site of five to six perforators from the greater saphenous vein of the superficial venous system to the deep posterior tibial vein

Are these ulcers painful or painless?

Usually painless unless infected

What are the most common organisms associated with infected venous ulcers?

1. *Staphylococcus aureus*
2. *Streptococcus faecalis*
3. *Klebsiella*

What is Marjolin ulcer?

Malignant transformation of a chronic venous ulcer

What is the conservative management of chronic venous insufficiency?

Meticulous skin care, limb elevation, elastic compression stockings, and hydrophobic dressing

What additional therapy is useful in the management of venous ulcer?

Unna boot (gauze with calamine, zinc oxide, and gelatin firmly wrapped around the foot or lower leg, and changed every week for 6–12 weeks)

When is this therapeutic adjunct contraindicated?

Patients with concurrent arterial occlusive disease

How successful is conservative therapy?

90% to 95%

What are the indications for surgery?

Persistent venous ulcer in:
1. Relatively young, **active** patients. The repetitive calf muscle contraction usually prevents healing with conservative therapy alone.
2. **Compliant** patients despite aggressive conservative management. If the patient is noncompliant, surgery inevitably fails.

What are the surgical options for incompetent valves?

1. Subfascial ligation of incompetent perforators (Linton procedure)
2. Correction of incompetence of deep venous valves by suture plication of the cusps (valvuloplasty)
3. Venous segment transposition, valve transplant, or valve banding

What is the procedure for venous obstruction?	Saphenous vein venous bypass procedure
What is the surgical management of venous ulcers?	Excision or débridement, followed by coverage with split-thickness skin graft

DEEP VENOUS THROMBOSIS (DVT): LOWER EXTREMITY

What are the three classic mechanisms associated with DVT?	Virchow triad: 1. Venous stasis 2. Endothelial damage 3. Hypercoagulability
Where is the usual nidus of a DVT?	The relatively stagnant blood behind the cusp of the venous valves (the venous sinus)
What are the risk factors for DVT?	1. > 40 years old 2. Obesity 3. Malignancy 4. Pregnancy 5. History of DVT or pulmonary embolism (PE) 6. Prolonged bed rest 7. Estrogen therapy 8. Varicose veins 9. Heart failure 10. Trauma
What surgical procedures have an increased risk of DVT?	1. Hip surgery 2. Knee surgery 3. Prostatectomy 4. Gynecologic surgery 5. General abdominal surgery
What is the usual presentation?	Acute pain and swelling of the calf or thigh. Pain on rapid dorsiflexion of the foot (Homan sign) is unreliable.
What percentage of patients are correctly diagnosed on physical exam alone?	Only 50%

What are the complications of DVT?	1. Post-phlebitic syndrome (5%–10%) 2. Pulmonary embolus (< 1%) 3. Limb loss secondary to venous gangrene (phlegmasia cerulea dolens, which is rare)
Which general type of DVT is at low risk for PE?	Those confined to the calf
Compare phlegmasia cerulea dolens and phlegmasia alba dolens.	Both are the result of iliofemoral venous thrombosis. Phlegmasia alba dolens is the earlier condition, in which the leg appears pale and the pulses are reduced because of arterial spasm. Later, the limb becomes massively edematous and cyanotic (phlegmasia cerulea dolens), and venous gangrene is imminent.
What are the noninvasive diagnostic studies for DVT?	Doppler ultrasound, impedance plethysmography, duplex ultrasound, fibrinogen ^{125}I scanning
Which study is the best for the detection of calf DVT?	Fibrinogen ^{125}I scan. (The worst study for distal DVT is Doppler ultrasound.)
What are the sensitivity and specificity of each of the remaining studies in the detection of proximal DVT?	1. Doppler: Sensitivity 80% to 90%; Specificity 50% to 75% 2. Plethysmography: Sensitivity 85% to 95%; Specificity 70% to 80% 3. Duplex: Sensitivity 90% to 95%; Specificity 90% to 95%
What is the standard therapy for DVT?	1. Anticoagulation: Heparin IV for 5 to 7 days followed by 3- to 6-month course of Coumadin. Coumadin is given soon after heparin is initiated so that the dose is therapeutic by day 5 to 7. 2. Bed rest with leg elevation
What is the purpose of the use of these anticoagulants?	To prevent extension of the thrombus, thus permitting the body's thrombolytic system to lyse the clot (i.e., neither heparin nor Coumadin actively promotes lysis of the clot)
How long is strict bed rest enforced for proximal DVT, and why?	5 to 7 days, the time required for the thrombus to firmly adhere to the wall of the vein, thus reducing the risk of PE

In some patients with DVT, anticoagulation is contraindicated. What is the alternative management?	Vena caval filter for prophylaxis against pulmonary embolus
What is the classic hematologic complication associated with heparin use?	Thrombocytopenia caused by the development of antiplatelet antibodies. Paradoxic clotting may also eventually occur.
What is the treatment?	1. Heparin is discontinued. 2. If Coumadin is not yet therapeutic, a venacaval filter may be placed.
In which DVT risk group is Coumadin contraindicated, and what is the therapy of choice?	Pregnancy, because Coumadin is teratogenic. Subcutaneous heparin is given on an outpatient basis.
What is the therapy for phlegmasia cerulea dolens?	1. Surgical thrombectomy or thrombolytic therapy 2. Fasciotomies for compartment syndrome
What is the standard perioperative prophylaxis against DVT?	1. Low-dose subcutaneous heparin (5000 units every 8–12 hours) 2. Elastic compression stockings and an intermittent pneumatic compression device to mimic the action of a musculovenous pump 3. Early ambulation postoperatively
What is the reduction in the incidence of DVT and PE with the use of low-dose heparin?	Incidence of DVT reduced by 70% and of PE by 50%

DEEP VENOUS THROMBOSIS: UPPER EXTREMITY

What are the most common etiologies?	1. Effort-induced thrombosis (Paget-von Schroetter syndrome) 2. Subclavian thrombosis caused by a central IV catheter
What is the usual presentation?	Edema, mild cyanosis, pain, and heavy sensation of the arm

Why is massive thrombosis rare?	Extensive venous collaterals around the shoulder girdle
What is the incidence of pulmonary embolus?	10% to 15% (higher than previously believed)
What is the treatment of effort-induced thrombosis?	Regional thrombolytic therapy urokinase; correction of thoracic outlet obstruction (if present)
What is the treatment of catheter-related thrombosis?	The catheter is removed if possible, and systemic heparinization is followed by 1 to 2 months of Coumadin therapy
Why are these etiologies managed differently?	Effort-induced thrombi occur in young, healthy individuals who are at low risk for hemorrhage. In an ill or elderly patient with a central venous catheter, thrombolytic therapy is more likely to cause bleeding.
What is the prognosis?	Only 15% to 30% of patients have complete resolution of symptoms.

PULMONARY THROMBOEMBOLISM (PE)

What is the most common source of thrombus?	Proximal lower extremity and pelvic veins
What is the criterion for massive PE?	Occlusion of > 2 lobar arteries or > 50% occlusion of pulmonary vasculature
What is the usual presentation?	Dyspnea, tachypnea, chest pain, hypotension, hemoptysis, and, occasionally, cyanosis
What initial diagnostic studies are performed immediately if PE is suspected?	Arterial blood gas, chest x-ray, and EKG
What are the usual arterial blood gas findings?	Hypoxia (because of shunt caused by PE) and hypocarbia (because of hyperventilation)
What percentage of patients are not hypoxic?	10%

What is the usual finding on chest x-ray?	Normal
What is the classic finding on x-ray with PE?	Westermark sign (paucity of pulmonary vascular markings in the region of the embolus)
What is the usual finding on EKG?	Sinus tachycardia. Less common, but more suggestive of PE, is the new onset of atrial fibrillation in a patient without a history of heart disease.
What is the classic EKG finding with PE?	Right heart strain pattern of $S_1 Q_3 T_3$
What is the first diagnostic study obtained after the initial evaluation if suspect PE?	Radioisotope ventilation and perfusion (V/Q) scan
Compare the results of this scan in PE versus pulmonary parenchymal disease.	PE: Perfusion defect in the region of embolic occlusion without an accompanying ventilation defect (V/Q mismatch) Parenchymal disease: Matched perfusion and ventilation defects (i.e., in the same region of the lung)
What is the likelihood of PE if the results of the scan are normal, low probability, and high probability?	Normal: 0%. (Unfortunately, the result is never reported as normal.) Low probability: 15% High probability: > 85%
What additional study should be performed in cases of indeterminate or intermediate probability?	Pulmonary arteriogram or a noninvasive study to confirm the presence of proximal DVT
What are the primary indications for arteriogram?	1. Whenever confirmation of PE is essential (e.g., a patient with increased risk of hemorrhage) 2. When a surgical procedure related to PE is planned (e.g., vena caval filter) 3. When a patient is not responding to medical therapy

What is the medical treatment?

1. Cardiovascular resuscitation
2. Monitored bed
3. Supplemental oxygen ± intubation
4. IV heparin for 5 to 10 days followed by Coumadin for 6 weeks to 6 months (duration controversial)

What additional medical therapy is considered in patients with massive PE?

Thrombolytic therapy. Some centers are liberalizing the criteria for the use of thrombolytics to include patients with less hemodynamically significant emboli.

What is the management of a patient who has recurrent emboli while receiving anticoagulant therapy?

Placement of a vena caval filter. There is increasing literature on possible first use of filter in proven cases.

What is the indication for emergency pulmonary embolectomy?

Refractory hypotension despite maximal resuscitation (fluids, inotropes, vasopressors) in the setting of **angiographically** documented **massive** PE in a patient with an absolute contraindication to thrombolytic therapy (i.e., rarely indicated)

What is the mortality rate for operative embolectomy?

30% to 50%

LYMPHEDEMA

What are the etiologies?

1. Primary lymphedema: Congenital hypoplasia of lymphatics
2. Secondary lymphedema: *Wuchereria bancrofti* (filaria) infection, iatrogenic destruction of lymphatics with surgery (axillary lymph node dissection) or radiation, and malignancy

What diagnostic studies are performed to visualize the lymphatics?

1. Lymphangiogram with oil-soluble contrast (Lipiodol)
2. Lymphoscintigraphy with ^{99m}Tc antimony sulfide

What potential complications are associated with lymphangiogram?	Contrast material may cause pulmonary edema or lymphangitis, exacerbating the lymphedema.
What is the conservative treatment?	Meticulous skin care, elastic and pneumatic compression stockings, and extremity elevation
What percentage of patients undergo surgery?	15%
What are the indications for surgery?	1. Recurrent infections 2. Progressive extremity edema
What are the basic surgical options?	1. Excision of excess skin and subcutaneous tissue and coverage of the unaffected subfascial tissues with full-thickness skin grafts (i.e., Charles procedure) 2. Transfer of the tissue flap with normal lymphatics to the area of lymphedema (i.e., Thompson procedure)

VASCULAR TRAUMA

What determines the prognosis for limb salvage?	Degree of muscular necrosis and soft tissue or bone trauma. It rarely depends on the arterial trauma because most arterial lesions can be repaired or bypassed.
What steps are taken in the case of grossly contaminated wounds?	1. Débridement and copious irrigation 2. Muscles are approximated over vascular repairs or exposed bone 3. Wound is left open for delayed primary closure in 7 to 14 days
Which vascular injuries (arterial or venous) are easier to repair?	Arterial. Meticulous technique is essential for successful venous repair.

ARTERIAL INJURY

What are the two basic complications of arterial injury?	Ischemia and hemorrhage (and hypovolemic shock)

Compare the tendency to bleed in completely and partially severed arteries.

Complete: Bleeding often stops spontaneously because of the retraction of the ends into the surrounding tissue.
Partial: Vascular wounds tend to gape and often cause significant bleeding.

What are the late sequelae of partially severed arteries?

1. False aneurysm
2. Arteriovenous fistula (if a neighboring vein is also injured)

What are the etiologies of arterial occlusion in a nonsevered (intact) artery?

1. Intramural hematoma
2. Intimal tear with thrombosis because of the attraction of platelets and fibrin
3. Intimal flap

What are the classic "hard" (overt) signs of extremity arterial injury?

1. Massive bleeding
2. Expanding hematoma
3. Palpable thrill
4. Bruit
5. Any of the signs of arterial ischemia (pulselessness, pain, pallor, paresthesia, paralysis, or poikilothermia)

What are the "soft" signs of arterial injury?

1. Small, nonexpanding, nonpulsatile hematoma
2. Reduced pulse
3. Proximity of the cutaneous wound to the artery
4. History of suspected arterial bleeding at the scene
5. Anemia
6. Neurologic extremity deficit
7. Hypotension

What percentage of patients with soft signs have a lesion on arteriogram?

3% to 10 %

What is the most common lesion associated with a soft sign?

Nonocclusive intimal defect

What percentage of arterial injuries associated only with soft signs heal without surgical repair?	> 90%
What arterial lesion is associated with bruit?	AV fistula or intimal flap
What are the indications for angiogram?	1. Suspected injury with soft signs 2. Injury with hard signs, but uncertain location of injury in a stable patient 3. Wide mediastinum 4. Cervical injuries in zone I or III
What are the angiographic findings?	1. Lateral (partial) filling defect because of intramural hematoma or partial transection 2. Abrupt end to the contrast column ± extravasation (because of complete transection)
How is Doppler ultrasound helpful in the initial evaluation of extremity trauma?	If SBP is > 60 mm Hg distally (radial, posterior tibial, or dorsal pedis arteries), collateral flow is sufficient to prevent ischemia. This information is helpful in prioritizing injuries in a patient with multiple injuries.
How is arterial bleeding from an extremity controlled in an emergency room?	Direct pressure is applied over the wound and on the proximal arterial pressure point. A blood pressure cuff is placed over the proximal part of the limb for temporary emergent occlusion when necessary.
What are the indications for surgery?	1. Hard sign of arterial injury 2. Documented lesion on arteriogram
What are the key points concerning operative preparation and draping?	1. **WIDE** preparation and draping to provide ample access for proximal control of the injured artery 2. Preparation of one or both saphenous veins for possible autogenous graft harvest
What is the first operative goal in arterial injury?	Obtain control of the arteries proximal **and** distal to the injury

What are the surgical options for arterial injury?	1. Lateral arteriorrhaphy ± vein patch 2. Segmental arterial resection with end-to-end anastomosis or interposition graft (if a segment > 1–2 cm is resected)
What is the graft material of choice?	Autogenous saphenous vein
What steps are taken to minimize postoperative arterial occlusion as a result of intraoperative thrombosis while the injured artery is clamped for repair?	1. Systemic or "regional" heparinization (regional technique involves injection of heparin proximally and distally in the injured artery) 2. Embolectomy maneuver with a Fogarty catheter before the anastomosis is completed 3. Arteriogram after the repair is completed
What is done to reduce the risk of graft rupture postoperatively?	All vascular repairs are covered with autogenous tissue (e.g., muscle) before skin closure to reduce the risk of desiccation and infection
What is the standard postoperative management?	1. Monitoring of distal pulses (by palpation or Doppler ultrasound) 2. Maintenance of adequate intravascular volume status and blood pressure
What is the classic early postoperative complication associated with delayed arterial repair?	Compartment syndrome (see the Other Vascular Topics section)
What postoperative anticoagulation is indicated?	None. Anticoagulation provides little antithrombotic benefit, but carries a significant risk of bleeding.
What is the nonoperative management of stable patients with soft signs?	Close observation with serial examinations of pulses

Selected Arterial Injuries

In what type of cervical arterial injury is preoperative angiogram indicated?	Injuries to cervical zones I (base of neck) and III (cephalad to the angle of the mandible) if the patient is stable

What is the standard incision for carotid artery versus vertebral artery injury?

Carotid artery: Anterior border of the sternocleidomastoid muscle
Vertebral artery: Supraclavicular incision (vertebral artery is the first branch off of the subclavian artery)

What is done if proximal control of the carotid artery cannot be achieved?

The neck incision is extended to a median sternotomy.

In what setting is a carotid artery injury not repaired, and why (controversial)?

Complete carotid artery transection or thrombosis (i.e., no prograde flow) with major, fixed neurologic deficit. Restoration of flow may exacerbate brain edema; thus, many surgeons merely ligate the carotid artery in this setting.

In thoracic arterial injury, what incision is normally used for repair of injury to:
1. **Ascending aorta?**
2. **Innominate artery?**
3. **Proximal third of the subclavian artery?**
4. **Distal two-thirds of the subclavian artery?**
5. **Descending thoracic aorta?**

1. Median sternotomy
2. Median sternotomy
3. On the right: median sternotomy; on the left: left anterolateral thoracotomy
4. Supraclavicular incision ± resection of the clavicle
5. Left posterolateral thoracotomy

For additional questions on thoracic vascular injury, see the Aortic Dissection section in Chapter 48 and the Thoracic Trauma section in Chapter 55.

In a patient with abdominal arterial injury, a midline laparotomy incision is made, and blood pressure suddenly drops. What is initially done?

1. The aorta is compressed or clamped just below the diaphragm.
2. Aggressive fluid resuscitation is provided.
3. Absorptive packs are placed in the abdomen to identify the sites of hemorrhage.

How is exposure of the abdominal aorta achieved?

1. Lateral attachments of the left colon, kidney, and spleen are divided.
2. These viscera are mobilized medially.

Which abdominal hematomas are explored?

1. Enlarging, pulsatile, or ruptured hematomas caused by blunt injury (other hematomas from blunt trauma are often observed)
2. All hematomas caused by penetrating injury, except **stable retrohepatic** hematomas (in **stable** patients)

VENOUS INJURY

What are the surgical options for treatment of venous injury (in order of preference)?

1. Ligation (most common)
2. Lateral phleborrhaphy
3. End-to-end anastomosis
4. Autogenous venous patch or replacement graft

(Synthetic grafts are avoided unless they are necessary for repair of the SVC or IVC.)

Which veins should not be ligated?

1. Right renal vein
2. Suprarenal IVC
3. Bilateral internal jugular veins
4. Popliteal vein
5. SVC, except in life-threatening situations in which the SVC is ligated **distal** to the azygous vein

Venous repairs are at higher risk of what complications compared with arterial repairs?

Thrombosis and stricture. Despite early concerns, studies show no increased risk of pulmonary embolism in the setting of venous repair.

What suture technique is used to reduce the incidence of thrombosis?

Everting suture technique (so that only the intima is in contact with blood)

What is the primary goal of the postoperative management of extremity venous injury?

Limb edema is minimized through elevation of the extremity while the patient is supine or the use of elastic support hose while the patient is ambulatory.

What are the most common surgical options for inferior vena caval injury?

1. Lateral phleborrhaphy
2. Ligation (if injury is **infrarenal**)

In infrahepatic IVC injury, how is exposure of the infrahepatic IVC achieved?

1. Lateral attachments of the right colon, duodenum, and terminal ileum are divided.
2. Bowel is mobilized to the left.

How is bleeding controlled to permit IVC repair?

1. IVC is compressed proximal and distal to the injury with sponge sticks.
   ± Additional medial and lateral compression is performed to occlude the lumbar veins.

2. If necessary, a side-biting or tangential vascular clamp (Satinsky) is used.

Why is the use of clamps avoided?

Increased risk of tearing the thin IVC wall

Care is taken not to occlude which renal vein, and why?

Right vein. Few collaterals are available for drainage, unlike the left renal vein, which drains through the gonadal or adrenal veins.

What is the claim to fame of retrohepatic IVC or hepatic vein injury?

Most inaccessible venous injury in the body

How is bleeding initially controlled to evaluate the injury?

Perihepatic region is packed, and Pringle maneuver is performed (occlusion of the portal triad)

If bleeding is still profuse, what other techniques are attempted to control bleeding?

1. Vascular clamps or tourniquets are applied to the suprahepatic and infrahepatic IVC and to the portal triad.The abdominal aorta is clamped just below the diaphragm.
2. Atriocaval shunt. The liver is "bypassed" with a thoracostomy tube or endotracheal tube (with a side hole for atrial inflow) inserted through the atrial appendage and advanced down into the abdominal IVC. The shunt is secured in place with vascular tourniquets around the IVC above and below the liver.

(see following page)

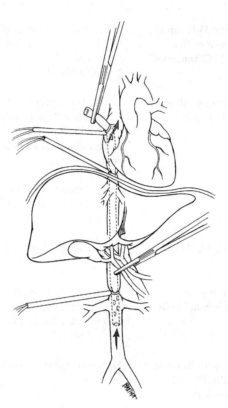

How long can the portal triad be safely clamped in the normothermic patient?

Traditionally, 20 to 30 minutes, but the warm ischemic time has been extended to 60 minutes with satisfactory results.

How is exposure of the retrohepatic region achieved?

The right lobe of the liver is mobilized cephalad after the coronary ligaments are divided.

What is the management of stable retrohepatic hematoma?

Close observation. Surgery is performed if the patient becomes unstable.

VASCULAR ACCESS FOR HEMODIALYSIS (HD)

What is the minimal flow rate required to drive the hemodialysis process?

150 ml/min

TEMPORARY ACCESS FOR ACUTE HEMODIALYSIS

What are the types of temporary access?

Central venous double-lumen catheters placed percutaneously with the Seldinger technique (Shiley catheter) or subcutaneously with an open procedure (Permacath or Hickman catheter)

What are the sites for catheter placement (in the usual order of preference)?

1. Femoral vein (first choice in a bedridden patient)
   Right internal jugular vein (first choice in an ambulatory patient)
2. Left subclavian vein
3. Right subclavian vein (difficult because of the angle with the SVC)
4. Left internal jugular vein (difficult because of the tortuous route to the SVC)

What are the benefits of the subcutaneous types?

1. Reduced risk of infection
2. Increased catheter life span

What additional type of hemodialysis is used for patients who are too unstable to tolerate the hemodynamic changes associated with standard hemodialysis?

Continuous venoveno hemofiltration or hemodialysis (dialysis driven by IV pumps)

ACCESS FOR CHRONIC HEMODIALYSIS

What are the two general types of chronic access procedures?

1. Autogenous fistula: Direct anastomosis of artery to vein
2. Interposition AV fistula: Interposition of a prosthetic graft between artery and vein

Which specific type is the preferred first operation, and why?

Brescia-Cimino autogenous fistula: Radial artery to cephalic vein. Autogenous fistulas are associated with improved long-term patency and reduced risk of infection; further, the Brescia-Cimino fistula requires minimal, superficial dissection.

What percentage of patients are candidates for an autogenous fistula?

15% to 20% because these patients, who often have a long history of illness, have few patent upper extremity veins

What is the prosthetic material of choice for interposition AV fistula?

PTFE

What is the most common site used?

Forearm of the nondominant hand: PTFE loop between the radial (or brachial) artery and the antebrachial region vein (e.g., cephalic, basilic)

Compare the postoperative waiting period required before the use of autogenous and interposition AV fistulas, and explain the rationale for these waiting periods.

Autogenous: 3 to 6 weeks to allow the fistula to mature. The vein must hypertrophy and arterialize to permit repeated punctures with the large HD needle.

Interposition: 2 weeks. The prosthetic material will be the site of needle puncture, but a fibrous scar must develop around the graft so that hematomas will not develop at the puncture sites. Hematomas predispose patients to infection.

What is the most common cause of failure of an AV fistula?

Thrombosis as a result of poor venous outflow (acutely because of technical error, chronically because of neointimal hyperplasia)

What are the treatment options for thrombosis?

1. Thrombectomy (first-line procedure)
2. Percutaneous balloon angioplasty
3. Thrombolytic (urokinase) therapy
4. Operative revision of fistula (e.g., patch angioplasty, new venous anastomosis)

[Revision (or replacement) is eventually required in almost all patients.]

In a patient who has distal extremity pain, what must be ruled out?

Arterial steal syndrome (ischemia distal to a fistula caused by retrograde flow through the distal artery)

What is the treatment?

Acutely, pressure is applied to the fistula to restore antegrade flow to the limb. Banding or ligation of the fistula or revision of arterial anastomosis is then performed. The AV fistula often thromboses when firm pressure is applied for 15 to 20 minutes; if it does not, surgery cannot be delayed for elective repair.

What are the other complications of AV fistula?

1. Venous aneurysmal dilation caused by needle puncture
2. Limb edema caused by venous hypertension distal to the fistula
3. Pseudoaneurysm at the anastomosis or needle puncture site
4. Infection
5. Rarely, high-output cardiac failure caused by AV shunting

Compare the 1-year and 5-year patency rates between autogenous and interposition AV fistulas.

1 year: Autogenous 65% to 80%; Interposition: 75% to 80%
5 year: Autogenous 65% to 80%; Interposition: 40% to 50%

OTHER VASCULAR TOPICS

Compartment Syndrome

Define compartment syndrome.

Increased pressure within a fascial compartment resulting in decreased arterial flow, neuromuscular deficits, and tissue ischemia

What are the two basic etiologic mechanisms?

1. Increased volume of compartment contents
2. Decreased compartment size

What are the specific etiologies?

Trauma (most common), revascularization procedures for arterial insufficiency, phlegmasia cerulea dolens or deep venous thrombosis, external pressure (compression dressing, cast), snake bite, bleeding disorder or anticoagulant therapy, and cardiopulmonary bypass

What are the four compartments of the leg and the nerves within each?

1. Anterior compartment: Deep peroneal nerve
2. Lateral compartment: Superficial peroneal nerve
3. Deep posterior compartment: Tibial nerve

4. Superficial posterior compartment: Sural nerve

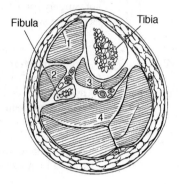

What is the most commonly affected compartment?

Anterior compartment of the lower leg

What is the first and most dominant symptom?

Pain that is out of proportion to signs and is exacerbated by passive stretching of the extremity

What is the most reliable sign?

Palpable tenseness of the compartment

What are the classic neurologic deficits in compartment syndrome of the leg?

Weak toe dorsiflexion and decreased sensation between the first and second toes on the dorsum of the foot (supplied by the deep peroneal nerve, which traverses the anterior compartment)

How is the diagnosis confirmed?

Direct measurement of compartment pressure with a basic needle catheter–manometry setup or a commercially available device (e.g., Stryker)

What is a normal compartment pressure?

< 10 mm Hg

What is considered an abnormal compartment pressure?

> 40 to 50 mm Hg. (The patient's arterial diastolic pressure must be considered. Lower systemic pressure increases the risk of ischemia; thus, a compartment pressure of 30 mm Hg may require treatment if the patient is hypotensive.)

At what level is the extremity positioned relative to the heart?	At the level of the heart. **Elevation of the extremity must be avoided.**
Is surgery indicated in a patient who has strongly palpable pulses in a crushed extremity?	This decision cannot be made with the information provided. Loss of pulses is a **late** finding, and ischemia within the compartment is often ongoing, even in the setting of palpable pulses.
What is the surgical management?	Fasciotomy and débridement of any necrotic tissue. Wounds are left open and covered with moist dressing for 5 to 10 days. Delayed primary closure or split-thickness skin grafting is performed to close the defects.

Thoracic Outlet Syndrome

Define.	Syndrome of diverse signs and symptoms caused by a variety of anatomic abnormalities (muscular, fibrosis, and bony) causing compression of the neurovascular bundle of the arm
What structures compose this neurovascular bundle?	Subclavian artery, subclavian vein, and brachial plexus
What structure is most frequently compressed?	Brachial plexus (> 90%)
What bony anomaly can cause the syndrome?	Cervical rib
What is the incidence of this anomaly in the general population?	0.5% to 1%
What percentage of patients are symptomatic?	Only 10%
What is the most common age-group and gender?	Women 35 to 55 years old
What are the symptoms in the upper extremity?	Pain, weakness, paresthesia, claudication, coldness, edema, "heaviness," and cyanosis

What signs are positive on physical exam?	Adson sign: When the arm is abducted and the head is rotated to the contralateral side, the radial pulse weakens. Tinsel sign: Percussion of the supraclavicular fossa reproduces the neurologic symptoms.
What other signs may be found on physical exam?	Supraclavicular fossa bruit, edema or varicosities, weak arterial pulse, and muscle atrophy (especially thenar muscles)
What is the usual cause of distal ischemia?	Emboli from the mural thrombus in a subclavian aneurysm (poststenotic dilation caused by turbulence)
What diagnostic studies are performed?	1. Cervical and chest x-rays 2. Doppler studies with the arm in multiple positions 3. Electromyography and nerve conduction studies (reliable in < 50%), somatosensory evoked potentials (SEPs) 4. Arteriogram (only if occlusion, aneurysm, or distal embolic events are suspected) 5. Rarely, venograms
What is the conservative treatment?	1. Exercises for improving posture 2. Weight reduction
How long is conservative treatment used before surgery is considered?	3 to 6 months
What are the indications for surgery?	1. Failure of conservative treatment 2. Arterial insufficiency 3. Venous insufficiency
What percentage of patients require surgery?	15% to 20%
What are the surgical approaches?	1. Supraclavicular incision 2. Transaxillary incision

What are the surgical options?	1. Resection of the first rib, cervical rib and, rarely, medial clavicle
	2. Anterior (± middle) scalenectomy
	3. Resection and bypass of the subclavian aneurysm
	(Although venous thrombectomy is occasionally indicated, most cases recannulize with anticoagulant ± thrombolytic therapy after correction of the anatomic abnormality).

SUBCLAVIAN STEAL SYNDROME

What are the anatomic lesion and the resultant hemodynamic disturbance in subclavian steal syndrome?	Subclavian (or occasionally, brachiocephalic) artery stenosis or occlusion proximal to the origin of the vertebral artery, which predisposes the patient to episodic retrograde blood flow down the ipsilateral vertebral artery
This syndrome occurs most frequently on which side?	Left (70%)
What is the presentation?	1. Upper extremity claudication
	2. Symptoms referable to vertebrobasilar insufficiency (e.g., dizziness, syncope, vertigo, drop attack, tinnitus)
	(Contrary to popular belief, although the claudication is associated with upper extremity activity, the vertebrobasilar insufficiency usually is not.)
What percentage of patients are symptomatic?	Only 30%. This syndrome is probably uncommon because many patients have good collaterals.
How is the lesion usually discovered?	Blood pressure discrepancy on the arms on routine exam (usually a difference of > 20–30 mm Hg)
What is the treatment?	Carotid and subclavian artery bypass, either with PTFE anastomosed end-to-side to each vessel or with direct end-to-side bypass subclavian artery transposition

DIABETIC VASCULAR DISEASE

How does atherosclerosis differ in diabetic and nondiabetic patients?

Diabetic atherosclerosis develops earlier in life, progresses more rapidly, and involves more distal vessels (including diabetic microangiopathy).

In addition to atherosclerosis, what sequelae of diabetes put the lower extremity at further risk of future amputation?

1. Diabetic neuropathy
2. Increased risk of infection (e.g., because of impaired leukocyte function)

What is the most common diabetic foot lesion?

Neurotrophic (mal perforans) ulcer

What are the gross appearance and usual location of this lesion?

Sharply demarcated, **painless** ulcer surrounded by dense callus with communication to the underlying joint space; located on pressure points on the plantar surface of the foot, usually under the first and third metatarsal heads. In addition to neurotrophic ulcers, diabetic patients may have painful ischemic ulcers.

What is the concurrent orthopedic lesion?

Charcot joint (neurogenic arthropathy): Extensive degenerative joint disease caused by impairment of pain sensation and proprioception (neuropathy), with resultant loss of joint protective reflexes. It is likely the primary etiology of the neurotrophic ulcer.

What is the treatment of neurotrophic ulcer?

Although a conservative trial of débridement, local wound care, and non–weight-bearing ambulation is warranted, most require resection of the involved joint (i.e., ray amputation).

What are the key points regarding the management of diabetic foot infection?

1. Prompt, aggressive surgical débridement
2. Early, broad-spectrum antibiotics until the specific organisms are identified. Diabetic infections are **poly**microbial.

CAROTID BODY TUMOR

What is the origin?	Afferent ganglion of the glossopharyngeal nerve
What are the gross characteristics?	Well encapsulated and tightly adherent to the adventitial surface of the carotid arteries
What is the presentation?	Asymptomatic mass at the angle of the jaw
What is the classic finding on physical exam?	Mass that is mobile in the horizontal axis (anteriorly and posteriorly), but fixed in the vertical axis
What is the classic radiographic finding?	Splaying of the bifurcation of the carotid artery. The carotid body rests in the crotch of the bifurcation.
What is the treatment?	1. Preoperative embolization to reduce blood loss at the time of surgery (very vascular tumors); usually reserved for masses > 3 cm
	2. Excision of tumor ± carotid reconstruction
What is the incidence of metastasis?	5 %

PHYSICS OF BLOOD FLOW

In the Poiseuille equation, blood flow (Q) through a stenotic lesion is:	
1. **Inversely proportional to?**	1. Length of the stenosis and viscosity of the blood
2. **Directly proportional to?**	2. Radius of the arterial lumen at the stenosis
What is the Reynolds number?	Dimensionless quantity that defines the point at which laminar (streamlined) flow becomes turbulent
What is the usual critical threshold for turbulence?	≈ 2000

VASCULAR SURGICAL PROCEDURES

VASCULAR BYPASS

What are the types of bypass conduits?

1. Autograft (e.g., greater saphenous vein)
2. Prosthetic graft (e.g., PTFE, Dacron)
3. Allograft (e.g., umbilical vein)

What are the most common mechanisms for long-term bypass graft failure?

1. Atherosclerotic disease developing in the vein graft
2. Progression of atherosclerotic disease in the native artery
3. Neointimal hyperplasia at proximal and distal anastomotic sites

What are the treatment options for long-term graft failure?

1. Thromboembolectomy
2. Balloon angioplasty
3. Revision of bypass at the stenotic anastomotic site
4. "Jump graft" from the patent segment of the graft to the patent native artery (to bypass the stenosis)

What are two ways that the saphenous vein is used for bypass?

"Reversed": Harvest and reimplantation in the reverse direction to permit flow through the valve

"In situ": No harvest, but valvulotomy to destroy the valves and permit retrograde flow. All venous tributaries are ligated.

Why is a meticulous search for patent venous tributaries essential for in situ bypass?

If the tributaries are not ligated, an AV fistula will develop and ultimately may affect long-term patency by reducing flow through the distal graft.

What are the potential disadvantages of each technique?

Reversed:
1. Compliance mismatch because of anastomosis of the small end of the vein to the large femoral artery. Increased myointimal hyperplasia may occur.
2. Size mismatch in proximal anastomosis, which results in:
   a. Technically more difficult anastomosis
   b. Reduced vein utilization

3. Devitalization of vein graft (loss of native nutrient supply)

In situ:
1. Intimal damage with valvulotome
2. Incomplete lysis of valves
3. AV fistula

Which technique has the best long-term patency?

No difference

What are the rare noncardiac indications for the use of arterial autograft?

1. Use of the internal iliac artery autograft for reconstruction of the renal artery in children
2. Use of an arterial autograft to span an infected surgical field

What are the types of Dacron grafts and the basic benefits of each?

1. Woven: Low porosity (minimal leak, even if the graft is not preclotted with blood)
2. Knitted: high porosity (permits ingrowth of the neointima along the length of the graft, but preclotting is required and more bleeding may occur)

What recent advancement precludes preclotting of some knitted grafts?

Collagen-impregnated grafts (i.e., Hemashield)

What are the key benefits of Dacron over PTFE?

1. Dacron is crimped to allow increased flexibility or stretching and maneuvering of curves without kinking.
2. Less bleeding occurs from the needle holes.

What is the primary complication associated with prosthetic grafts?

Graft infection

What are the most common bacterial etiologies?

1. *Staphylococcus aureus* and *Staphylococcus epidermidis*
2. *Escherichia coli*

What is the primary complication associated with umbilical vein autografts?

Aneurysmal dilation, even when a standard Dacron sleeve is used

ENDARTERECTOMY

How is the procedure performed?	Blunt spoons and arterial wire loop strippers are used to remove the thrombus and intima. This procedure is technically more difficult than most bypasses.
Why might acute occlusion develop at the restoration of blood flow?	Blood may dissect under the free edge of the intima, forming an occlusive intimal flap
What technique decreases the incidence of stenosis occlusion associated with long arteriotomies?	Closure with a roof patch (vein or prosthetic)
How does the patency of endarterectomy compare with that of bypass?	Similar

BALLOON ANGIOPLASTY

What lesions are most amenable to angioplastic dilation?	Short (< 5 cm), concentric stenoses. Complete occlusion is not a contraindication to angioplasty. If the segment is short, a guidewire may be passed through the occlusion.
What is the most common noncoronary vessel for which angioplasty is used?	Common iliac artery
What is the usual indication?	Angioplasty is often performed on the common iliac artery before a more distal bypass is performed to ensure adequate inflow and improve the patency rate of the distal bypass.
For which visceral vascular lesion is angioplasty used most frequently?	Fibromuscular dysplasia of the renal artery
What are the complications of percutaneous angioplasty?	1. Arterial rupture 2. Distal emboli 3. Hematoma at the groin puncture site 4. Complete occlusion of a previous stenotic lesion because of intimal dissection or, rarely, thrombosis

What percentage of   1% to 10%
patients require immediate
surgical intervention for
these complications?

47

Pediatric Surgery

Cynthia A. Gingalewski, M.D.
Peter Mattei, M.D.

PEDIATRIC HEAD AND NECK DISORDERS

THYROGLOSSAL DUCT CYST

What is a thyroglossal duct cyst?	A lesion of the neck, typically located at or near the midline. It arises from the tissue of the thyroglossal duct tract that remains after the embryologic migration of the thyroid from its origin at the foramen cecum of the tongue.
What is the usual presentation?	Midline cervical nontender nodule noted in older infants or young children. The cysts may become acutely infected and present with a tender nodule and stigmata of infection.
What is included in the differential diagnosis?	1. Dermoid cyst 2. Lymph node 3. Aberrant thyroid tissue (in rare cases, this tissue is the patient's only functioning thyroid tissue)
When is surgical resection indicated, and why?	In all cases, because of the risk of infection and the malignant potential if thyroid tissue is present in the cyst
What surgical procedure is performed?	Sistrunk procedure: Excision of the duct, including the entire tract to the foramen cecum. The central portion of the hyoid bone must be included because the tract passes through it.
When is a thyroid scan performed?	When thyroid tissue is found in the surgical specimen

What is the recurrence rate?	< 10% if the entire tract is completely excised; ≈ 90% if the central portion of the hyoid bone is not excised

BRANCHIAL CLEFT REMNANTS

What are branchial cleft remnants?	Remnants of the first, second, or third branchial cleft
What are the potential anatomic anomalies?	1. Cleft 2. Fistula 3. Cyst
What is the usual location of each type?	First: From the cartilage of the external auditory canal to the skin of the neck, beneath the center of the body of the mandible Second: From the tonsillar fossa to the skin anterior to the sternocleidomastoid muscle Third: Extending between the bellies of the sternocleidomastoid muscle, above the clavicle
What percentage of cases are bilateral?	10%
What is the usual treatment?	1. Antibiotics for infection 2. Surgical excision
What is the surgical procedure?	Small elliptic skin incision at the site of the external opening of the sinus and careful excision of the tract with traction and blunt dissection
What structures are at risk for injury during surgery for: **1. First cleft fistula?** **2. Second cleft fistula?**	1. Facial nerve 2. Hypoglossal and glossopharyngeal nerves; bifurcation of the carotid artery

CYSTIC HYGROMA

What is a cystic hygroma?	Lymphangioma with dilated cystic lymph channels that arise from the jugular lymph sacs that are present in infancy. They vary in size from small cysts to massive disfiguring tumors.

What is the usual location?	Primarily the neck, but also within the mediastinum, axilla, or mesentery
Why are they life-threatening?	Rapid enlargement may cause airway obstruction.
What is the usual treatment?	Early surgical excision. Complete excision is required to prevent recurrence.
Why are multiple resections sometimes required?	Although not malignant, cystic hygromas may involve adjacent tissues and vital structures, making complete excision impossible or dangerous. They are unroofed and drained, but recur.

PEDIATRIC THORACIC DISORDERS

PECTUS EXCAVATUM

What is pectus excavatum?	Deformity of the chest wall in which the sternum is displaced posteriorly (and to the left), most severely at the xiphoid and, to a varying degree, above the xiphoid
What is the usual etiology?	Congenital malformation, apparently caused by a deformity of the costal cartilages (fifth through eighth), which develop abnormally in a concave manner, pushing the sternum posteriorly
What are the usual indications for surgery?	1. Cosmetic reasons (primary indication). Although it is usually present at birth, the deformity is most prominent during adolescence, when the psychologic effect can be enormous. 2. Cardiorespiratory compromise in patients with Marfan syndrome (uncommon)
What are the usual clinical manifestations?	Controversial and difficult to document objectively, they include limitations in cardiopulmonary reserve and exercise tolerance. Physical compression and displacement of the heart may be shown by computed tomography (CT) scan, and depressed cardiac function is seen in some studies.

**What are the key features
of surgical treatment?**

1. Inframammary transverse incision for
   better cosmetic outcome
2. Osteotomy of the sternum to displace
   it anteriorly
3. Subperichondrial resection of the
   costal cartilages usually involved (fifth
   through eighth, bilaterally)
4. Physical maintenance of the new
   sternal position with a metal or
   plastic strut, overlapping costal
   cartilages, or a free cartilage graft to
   the osteotomy site

ESOPHAGEAL ATRESIA AND TRACHEOESOPHAGEAL (TE) FISTULA

**What are esophageal
atresia and TE fistula?**

Series of malformations in which
abnormal growth and differentiation of
the esophagus and trachea cause
incomplete esophagus, TE fistula, or both

What are the five types?

1. Type A: Esophageal atresia **without**
   TE fistula
2. Type B: Esophageal atresia with
   proximal TE fistula
3. Type C: Esophageal atresia with
   distal TE fistula
4. Type D: Esophageal atresia with both
   proximal and distal TE fistulas
5. Type E: "H-type" TE fistula without
   esophageal atresia

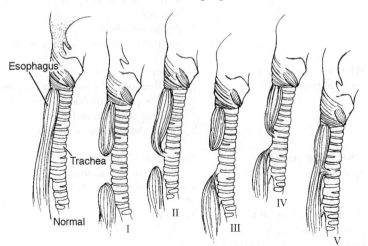

What is the relative incidence of each type?	Type A: 8% Type B: 1% Type C: 85% Type D: 2% Type E: 4%
What are the usual symptoms?	1. Excessive salivation 2. Inability to take feedings 3. Respiratory distress caused by aspiration
Which type usually presents at an older age?	Type E (H-type)
How is the presence of the following confirmed: **1. Esophageal atresia?** **2. TE fistula?** **3. H-type TE fistula?**	1. Inability to pass a nasogastric tube beyond the blind proximal pouch 2. Air present in the distal GI tract on x-ray 3. Bronchoscopy
What are the associated anomalies?	30% to 50% have associated anomalies: skeletal, cardiac, or GI (especially imperforate anus); VATER syndrome includes vertebral, anal, TE, radial, and renal anomalies
What is the initial treatment?	1. Suction of the pouch with a Replogle tube 2. Maintenance of an upright position at all times 3. Prophylactic antibiotics 4. Gastrostomy if the infant is unstable
What are the basic steps of surgical treatment?	1. Closure of the fistula 2. Mobilization of the esophageal ends by dissection into the neck and circular myotomy (Livaditis technique) 3. Primary anastomosis of the esophagus
What is the surgical approach?	Types A, B, C, and D: Right extrapleural thoracotomy Type E: Right cervical incision
What vein is ligated to permit intraoperative exposure of the TE fistula?	Azygous vein

FOREIGN BODIES: TRACHEA

What age-group is affected most often?	2 to 4 years of age
What is the usual presentation?	1. Cough, wheezing, dyspnea, inspiratory and expiratory stridor, and/or fever 2. Unilateral diminished breath sounds or wheezing
A tracheal foreign body is often confused with what other diagnosis?	Severe asthma
How is the diagnosis made?	Neck and chest plain x-ray may show a radiopaque foreign body, a hyperinflated lobe or segment, or an atelectatic lobe or segment.
What are the indications for intervention?	Highly suggestive signs and symptoms with confirmatory x-rays or a suspicious history in a toddler
What is the usual treatment?	Rigid bronchoscopy with forceps retrieval of the foreign body

FOREIGN BODIES: ESOPHAGUS

What are the common esophageal levels of lodgment?	Sites of esophageal narrowing: 1. Cricopharyngeal muscle 2. Arch of the aorta (level of carina) 3. Gastroesophageal junction
What is the usual presentation?	Drooling, dysphagia, and pain
What is the life-threatening sequela of a long-standing untreated esophageal foreign body?	Mediastinitis after erosion through the esophageal wall
How is the diagnosis made?	Plain x-ray showing radiopaque objects

What is the usual treatment?	1. At the level of the cricopharyngeus and carina: Rigid or flexible esophagoscopy with mechanical retrieval by forceps
	2. At the gastroesophageal junction: Observation
	Most surgeons discourage the use of a Fogarty balloon catheter to retrieve esophageal foreign bodies.
What are the risks of treatment?	1. Esophageal perforation
	2. Aspiration, which is prevented by placing the patient in the prone position

CONGENITAL DIAPHRAGMATIC HERNIA

What are the two types and the general location of each?	1. Bochdalek: Posterolateral, left > right
	2. Morgagni: Anterior parasternal position
Which type is rare?	Morgagni (< 5%)
Which type is usually asymptomatic?	Morgagni
How are most congenital diaphragmatic hernias diagnosed?	Fetal ultrasound
What is the usual presentation?	1. Respiratory distress, tachypnea, and cyanosis
	2. Scaphoid abdomen
	3. Diminished bowel sounds in the abdomen; bowel sounds in the chest
How is the diagnosis confirmed?	Plain x-ray showing bowel in the chest
What factors determine the prognosis?	Extent of pulmonary hypoplasia and associated malformations
Which infants generally do well with surgical repair?	Those who are asymptomatic **or** who present after 24 hours of life (10%–15%)

What is the usual preoperative management?	1. Intubation 2. Nasogastric decompression 3. Vasodilators to decrease pulmonary artery hypertension and right to left shunt; vasopressors may also be needed
What may severely unstable infants require for cardiopulmonary support before surgery?	Extracorporeal membrane oxygenator (ECMO)
What are the steps in surgical repair?	1. Transabdominal approach through the left subcostal incision 2. Reduction of the hernia, excluding the peritoneal sac in the hemithorax 3. Suture repair of small defects; flap or mesh repair of large defects
Where is residual diaphragmatic muscle found?	In the retroperitoneum, above the adrenal glands
What is the overall survival rate?	≈ 50%

EVENTRATION OF THE DIAPHRAGM

What are the two types and the etiology of each?	1. Congenital: Embryologic muscular defect 2. Acquired: Usually caused by phrenic nerve injury
What is the usual presentation?	Varies from asymptomatic to respiratory distress, especially in infants
What diagnostic study is performed?	Fluoroscopy, which shows paradoxic motion of the diaphragm
What is the usual treatment?	1. Asymptomatic patient: None 2. Symptomatic patient: Plication and stabilization of the diaphragm in the expiratory position

CONGENITAL PULMONARY CYSTIC DISEASES

What are the four types?

1. Cystic adenomatoid malformation (CAM)
2. Pulmonary sequestration
3. Bronchogenic cysts
4. Congenital lobar overinflation

Describe each type.

1. CAM: Cystic and solid masses of immature lung tissue that communicate with the normal airway
2. Pulmonary sequestration: Collection of abnormal lung tissue with systemic venous drainage
3. Bronchogenic cyst: Extrapulmonary cysts, formed from immature bronchial tissue separated from the lung during early embryonic development, lined with ciliated columnar epithelium, and surrounded by a fibrous wall that contains cartilage
4. Congenital lobar overinflation: Normal lung tissue with abnormally formed bronchus that causes air trapping and overinflation

What is the usual presentation?

1. Respiratory distress caused by compression of a normal lung in the newborn
2. Recurrent infections in the older child

Bronchogenic cysts and extrapulmonary sequestrations are usually asymptomatic.

What diagnostic studies are performed?

1. Chest CT scan (study of choice)
2. Ultrasound
3. Esophagoscopy for patients with dysphagia
4. Magnetic resonance imaging (MRI) and aortography, which can show systemic vasculature in sequestration

What is the usual treatment?

1. Bronchogenic cysts are excised.
2. Lobectomy is the treatment of choice for other congenital cystic diseases of the lung. It is well tolerated in infants, the complication rate is lower

than that for segmental resections, and the lung parenchyma is still growing in small children, with resultant formation of new alveoli.

PEDIATRIC GASTROINTESTINAL DISORDERS

What are the components of preoperative preparation for nearly all pediatric GI disorders?

1. IV hydration
2. Nasogastric or orogastric suction
3. Correction of electrolyte abnormalities if necessary

GASTROSCHISIS

What is gastroschisis?

Full-thickness abdominal wall defect with no peritoneal sac

What is the usual location?

Just to the right of the umbilicus, with herniated uncovered intestine that is often malrotated and shortened

What is the typical size of these lesions?

2 to 3 cm

What is the associated anomaly?

Rarely, intestinal stenosis or atresia

What is the usual preoperative management?

1. Transport with a bowel bag to keep the bowel moist and protected
2. Maintenance of normothermia with warm saline-soaked gauze over the bowel in a warmed environment
3. Nasogastric suction
4. Aggressive IV fluid management with $D_{10}LR$ and albumin
5. Broad-spectrum IV antibiotics
6. Total parenteral nutrition, which may be needed for weeks **after** closure

What is the surgical treatment?

Primary closure of the abdominal wall defect

What may be used if the bowel is not initially reducible?

Silastic silo for successive reduction over several days

| What are the long-term complications? | 1. Transmural inflammation, which causes malabsorption and motility disorders
2. Hepatotoxicity by total parenteral nutrition
3. Necrotizing enterocolitis
4. Gastroesophageal reflux |

OMPHALOCELE

What is omphalocele?	Abdominal wall defect at the umbilicus, with herniated bowel, which is covered by a membrane (amnion) derived from the peritoneum
What is the usual size?	2 to 15 cm
Are associated anomalies common?	Yes (50%–60%)
What organ systems are often anomalous?	GI, cardiovascular, urologic, and neurologic systems; complications may be severe and life-threatening
What is the prognosis?	Excellent for small omphaloceles, but the mortality rate is high after surgery for defects > 8 cm
What is the initial treatment?	Similar to that for gastroschisis (nasogastric suction, IV fluids, warm saline-soaked gauze over the defect, and antibiotics). The patient is also evaluated for associated anomalies.
What is the usual surgical treatment?	1. Surgical closure of the defect. Staged repairs with a Silastic silo are sometimes necessary. 2. Many advise nonoperative management for defects > 8 cm to allow the defect to eschar over and the edges to contract together.

UMBILICAL HERNIA

| What is an umbilical hernia? | Abdominal wall fascial defect at the umbilicus covered with normal skin |

What is the incidence of this defect?	5% to 10% in whites; 25% to 50% in blacks
What is the primary risk factor?	Prematurity (> 60% occur in premature infants)
What is the natural history?	Most close spontaneously in the first 3 years of life. An omphalomesenteric duct remnant may inhibit closure.
What are the indications for surgery?	1. Incarceration of the abdominal viscera 2. Pain or other symptoms 3. Cosmetic concerns 4. Failure to close by 2 to 3 years of age
What technical points should be considered for an optimal surgical result?	The omphalomesenteric duct remnant is divided.

INGUINAL HERNIA

What is an indirect inguinal hernia?	Abnormal protrusion of the peritoneum, through the internal inguinal ring, along the path of the processus vaginalis
What is the usual presentation?	Abnormal bulge in the inguinal region that is usually intermittent and increases with intra-abdominal pressure
What are the primary complications?	Incarceration, strangulation, obstruction, or infarction of the bowel. The bladder and ovaries may also herniate through the defect.
What is the usual treatment?	1. Reducible hernias: Elective surgical repair 2. Incarcerated hernias: IV hydration and emergent exploration
What patients usually undergo contralateral exploration for occult hernia?	Boys < 1 year old and girls < 6 years old

What technical points should be considered for an optimal surgical result?	1. High ligation of the hernia 2. Preservation of the blood supply to the vas deferens in males 3. Separation of the sac (medial) from cord structures (lateral) by blunt dissection to minimize the risk of injury to the cord 4. If the internal ring is large, internal inguinal ring surgery in males; closure of the internal inguinal ring in girls

HYDROCELE

What is a hydrocele?	Collection of fluid within the tunica vaginalis of the scrotum
What is the key diagnostic finding?	Transillumination with light
What are the types?	1. Communicating: Patent processus vaginalis, with filling and emptying of the tunica vaginalis with peritoneal fluid, depending on the infant's position 2. Noncommunicating: Fluid in the tunica vaginalis, with obliterated processus vaginalis
Which type usually resolves spontaneously?	Noncommunicating (often by 1 year of age)
What is the usual surgical treatment?	Evagination or excision of the tunica vaginalis ± repair of any associated inguinal hernia

HYPERTROPHIC PYLORIC STENOSIS (HPS)

What is HPS?	Gastric outlet obstruction caused by muscular hypertrophy of the pylorus
What is the usual presentation?	Nonbilious projectile vomiting
What is the usual patient population?	1. Usually males, especially firstborns (may be familial) 2. Typical age is 4 to 8 weeks, but may occur between 2 weeks and 3 months

How is the diagnosis made?	1. Most often by physical exam alone ("olive" is palpable in the epigastrium or right upper quadrant) 2. Ultrasound 3. Upper GI series if HPS is suspected, but there is no palpable olive
What other lesions are included in the differential diagnosis?	Reflux, web, and malrotation
What electrolyte and acid-base abnormalities are characteristic?	Hypokalemic, hypochloremic metabolic alkalosis
What other laboratory abnormality is seen in 1% to 2% of patients?	Indirect hyperbilirubinemia
What is the usual treatment?	Ramstedt-Friedet pyloromyotomy, which is safe and effective, with a minimal morbidity rate. Surgery is performed when hypovolemia, hypokalemia, and hypochloremia are corrected.
What is the surgical procedure?	1. Muscle of the pylorus is divided longitudinally from the stomach to the duodenum. All muscle fibers must be divided, to prevent recurrence (which usually occurs on the stomach side). 2. Any mucosal injury is repaired to prevent postoperative leak.
When does feeding begin postoperatively?	After 6 to 12 hours

DUODENAL OBSTRUCTION IN THE NEWBORN

What are the causes of duodenal obstruction in the newborn?	1. Duodenal stenosis 2. Duodenal atresia 3. Duodenal web 4. Annular pancreas
What are the usual locations?	90% occur distal to the ampulla of Vater; 10% occur proximal to the ampulla

What is the usual presentation?	1. Feeding intolerance and bilious vomiting in the first 24 to 48 hours of life 2. Distended stomach with an otherwise scaphoid abdomen
Are associated anomalies common?	Yes
What is the most common anomaly?	20% to 40% also have trisomy 21 (Down syndrome); congenital heart defects are also seen
What is the classic finding on x-ray?	Plain x-rays may show a "double bubble" (air-distended stomach and duodenum).
What additional study may be performed, and why?	Upper GI series if the diagnosis is in doubt **or** malrotation is suspected
Why is surgery performed promptly?	Lethal malrotation is often included in the differential diagnosis.
What is the usual surgical treatment?	1. Duodenoduodenostomy (primary or bypass) 2. Duodenojejunostomy if distal duodenal obstruction is present
What procedure is usually performed for duodenal webs?	Web resection with longitudinal duodenotomy

INTESTINAL ATRESIA

What is intestinal atresia?	Intestinal obstruction from stenosis or atresia of the jejunum, ileum, or colon thought to be caused by a vascular accident in utero or by intrauterine volvulus, hernia, intussusception, or malrotation
What are the types?	Type I: Intraluminal diaphragm or web Type II: Fibrous cord connecting two blind ends, with the mesentery intact Type IIIa: Discontinuous bowel with a V-shaped mesenteric defect (most common type) Type IIIb: Apple peel deformity Type IV: Multiple atretic segments separated by relatively normal bowel

What is the usual presentation?	1. Antenatal polyhydramnios 2. Bilious vomiting 3. Abdominal distension 4. Failure to pass meconium
What contrast study is performed to aid diagnosis?	Contrast enema. Upper GI is often unnecessary and may complicate surgery.
What type of bowel biopsy may be performed during the evaluation?	Suction rectal biopsy
Why is this biopsy performed?	To rule out Hirschsprung disease
What is the usual surgical treatment?	Resection of the affected bowel with primary anastomosis
What technical points should be considered for an optimal surgical result?	1. Preservation of bowel length, regardless of the number of anastomoses needed 2. Tapering of the dilated proximal end to reduce the size discrepancy 3. Preservation of the ileocecal valve

MECONIUM ILEUS

What is meconium ileus?	Distal ileal obstruction caused by thick, inspissated meconium in neonates
What disease is often associated with it?	Cystic fibrosis (CF)
What is the usual presentation?	1. Abdominal distension 2. Bilious vomiting 3. Failure to pass meconium
What are the usual findings on plain abdominal x-ray?	1. Dilated loops of bowel 2. Soap bubble or Neuhauser sign: Ground-glass appearance of meconium mixed with air in the right lower quadrant
What is the appearance on contrast enema?	Microcolon (small diameter)

What is the initial treatment?	Nonoperative therapy is successful in 60% to 70% of cases. It includes enemas with saline irrigation, meglumine diatrizoate (Gastrografin), or 1% N-acetylcysteine (Mucomyst).
What is the usual surgical treatment?	If enemas are unsuccessful, enterotomy and manual clearance of meconium from the bowel are used.
What intestinal complications often occur?	One-third of cases are complicated by segmental volvulus, bowel ischemia, stenosis, atresia, or perforation. These patients usually need resection and primary anastomosis.
What complicates the postoperative management of many patients?	Respiratory compromise caused by CF

INTESTINAL MALROTATION

What is intestinal malrotation?	Abnormal intestinal anatomy caused by improper or incomplete rotation of the midgut during embryologic development
What is the normal rotation of the midgut?	Rotates counterclockwise 270° on the axis of the superior mesenteric artery
What are the types of malrotation?	1. Nonrotation: Colon is on the left, small intestine is on the right, cecum is at the midline, and duodenum does not cross the midline 2. Incomplete rotation: Colon is on the left, small intestine is mostly on the right, cecum is in the left upper quadrant, and duodenum does not cross the midline 3. Mesocolic hernia: Incomplete rotation of the small or large bowel with failure of fusion of the right or left mesocolon to the posterior abdominal wall, with subsequent potential space for a hernia to develop

What are Ladd bands?

Dense, fibrous bands that form from the cecum to the posterior body wall, typically in the right upper quadrant. They often pass anterior to the duodenum, jejunum, and colon in malrotation.

What is the usual presentation?

Bilious vomiting, usually in the neonate. Most present by 1 year of age.

What causes this presentation?

Duodenal obstruction caused by Ladd bands, or midgut volvulus

What is the gold standard for diagnosis?

Upper GI contrast study in the acute setting

What finding on this study rules out malrotation?

Duodenum crosses the vertebral column, ascends to the greater curvature of the stomach, and then descends

What is the usual surgical treatment?

1. **Emergent** laparotomy with counterclockwise detorsion of the midgut. Because of the concern about midgut volvulus, this procedure is one of the few truly emergent pediatric surgical procedures.
2. Division of the Ladd bands
3. Passage of a Foley catheter to rule out duodenal obstruction
4. Placement of the cecum in the **left** upper quadrant and the duodenum in the **right** upper quadrant
5. Appendectomy

HIRSCHSPRUNG DISEASE

What is Hirschsprung disease?

Congenital failure of distal migration of the intestinal ganglion cells in the myenteric (Auerbach) and submucosal (Meissner) plexuses, resulting in functional intestinal obstruction; also called congenital aganglionosis coli

What is the classic triad of presentation?

1. Bilious emesis
2. Abdominal distension
3. Constipation

What finding suggests this diagnosis in the neonate?

Delayed passage of meconium

What are the steps in the evaluation of a patient suspected of having Hirschsprung disease?

1. Rectal exam to rule out anorectal anomalies and confirm the presence of normal meconium
2. Abdominal x-ray to rule out other forms of obstruction
3. Barium enema to identify the transition zone and rule out other forms of colonic obstruction
4. Suction rectal biopsy to look for ganglion cells

What is included in the differential diagnosis?

1. Necrotizing enterocolitis
2. Meconium plug syndrome
3. Meconium ileus
4. Intestinal dysmotility syndrome
5. Functional constipation
6. Hypothyroidism
7. Neuronal intestinal dysplasia
8. Magnesium sulfate tocolysis therapy

What are the stages of surgical treatment?

Three stages, depending on the status of the infant (i.e., enterocolitis, associated anomalies):
1. Colostomy proximal to the transition zone (established by barium enema or exploratory laparotomy) immediately
2. Definitive procedure (discussed later) after 6 to 12 months
3. Colostomy closure 1 to 3 months after the definitive procedure

What three definitive procedures are performed?

1. Swenson procedure: Distal ileorectal anastomosis
2. Duhamel-Martin procedure: Ileorectal anastomosis with aganglionic bowel placed anteriorly and normal bowel placed posteriorly
3. Soave-Boley procedure: Mucosal proctectomy with endorectal pull-through

NECROTIZING ENTEROCOLITIS (NEC)

What characterizes enterocolitis as NEC?

Mucosal ischemia, which can progress to full-thickness necrosis

What is the usual age at presentation?

Newborn period, most commonly the first 2 weeks of life

What are the risk factors?

Prematurity, hypoxia, hypotension, jaundice, anemia, polycythemia, sepsis, exchange transfusions, hyperosmolar feedings, intracranial bleeding, and maternal use of cocaine

What is the usual clinical presentation?

Nonspecific findings in a neonate at risk: Abdominal distension, vomiting or high gastric residuals, diarrhea, or hematochezia. Lethargy, apnea, and signs of poor peripheral perfusion can also occur.

What is the etiology of NEC?

Unknown. Current theories include:
1. Mesenteric ischemia leading to patchy bowel injury
2. Infectious: *Clostridium difficile*, viral causes, *Escherichia coli*, or *Klebsiella pneumoniae*
3. Toxicologic: Methylxanthines, vitamin E, indomethacin, or maternal cocaine use

What is the usual treatment?

1. NPO and nasogastric suction
2. IV hydration and hyperalimentation
3. IV antibiotics and enteral vancomycin
4. Surgical resection of any necrotic bowel

What is the prognosis for NEC?

Overall, excellent (> 90% survival rate; > 95% continence rate)

INTUSSUSCEPTION

What is intussusception?

Invagination of a portion of the bowel into itself, resulting in bowel obstruction

What is the most common anatomic location?

Ileocolic intussusception: A portion of the terminal ileum is drawn into the colon across the ileocecal valve

What is the etiology?

Unknown. A "lead point" is thought to be present, but is identified in only 5% of cases. Other cases are thought to be caused by intramural lesions or thickening as a result of lymphoid hyperplasia (viral infections), Meckel diverticulum, polyps, or lymphoma. In older children with CF, inspissated feces are thought to be the cause.

What is the primary danger associated with intussusception?

Prolonged intussusception leads to edema and ischemia of the proximal portion, causing infarction, gangrene, and perforation.

What is the usual age at presentation?

Between 5 and 10 months of age, but it can occur in any age-group. The average age of patients with CF and intussusception is 9 years.

What is the usual clinical presentation?

1. Colicky abdominal pain with asymptomatic intervals
2. Vomiting that becomes bilious
3. Abdominal distension

What are the classic findings on physical exam?

1. Sausage-shaped abdominal mass, typically in the right lower quadrant
2. "Currant jelly" (bloody, mucoid) stools on rectal exam
3. Occasionally, the Dance sign (empty right lower quadrant if the ileocecal region has intussuscepted distally)

What is the diagnostic procedure of choice?

Contrast enema is both diagnostic and therapeutic. Plain films are typically nondiagnostic.

What is the classic finding of this study?

Coiled-spring sign

What alternative diagnostic test is used at some centers?

Ultrasound examination (typically used when clinical suspicion is low)

What nonoperative techniques are routinely used?

1. Hydrostatic reduction: Barium enema; fluid column of no more than 3 feet for 10 minutes at a time
2. Pneumatic reduction: Air contrast enema; 80 mm Hg for small infants, ≤ 120 mm Hg for older infants

What is the success rate for each technique?	1. Hydrostatic reduction: 40% to 80% 2. Pneumatic reduction: 90%
What is the management in the period immediately after enema?	Hospitalization, IV hydration, observation, and resumption of the usual diet
What are the indications for surgery?	1. Signs of peritonitis or shock 2. Failure of nonoperative methods
What is the operative procedure?	1. Incision in the right lower quadrant 2. Reduction by massaging distally to proximally (never by pulling apart) 3. Resection for inability to reduce, gangrene, or a worrisome lead point (e.g., Meckel diverticulum or a suspicious lesion); primary end-to-end anastomosis 4. Appendectomy (because the incision is in the right lower quadrant)
What is the recurrence rate?	≤ 12%
What is the treatment of choice for a recurrence?	Repeat enema
What is the exception to this choice of treatment, and why?	Older children with recurrence are more likely to have a tumor or polyp as the lead point. Exploratory surgery is warranted.

IMPERFORATE ANUS

What is the incidence of imperforate anus?	1:4000 to 1:5000 newborns
What is the classification system?	Anatomically characterized as high or low (above or below the levator ani or puborectalis muscle), but these are not prognostic or therapeutic groupings. Therefore, many group them as to whether a colostomy is required (high) or is not required (low).
What finding on physical exam is usually seen with the low type?	Perineal meconium fistula. High types often have a fistula to the urethra, vagina, or bladder.

What type of x-ray helps to distinguish the high type from the low type?

Pelvic x-ray with the infant held upside down. The x-ray is performed several hours after birth to permit swallowed air to reach the distal colon.

What are the most common associated anomalies?

1. Sacral deformities (i.e., missing sacral vertebrae, hemivertebrae, hemisacrum)
2. Urogenital defects (20%–54%), which are more common with high malformations. Complications of these defects are major sources of morbidity and mortality (i.e., hydronephrosis, urosepsis, metabolic acidosis).

What is the surgical treatment of each type?

1. Low type: Usually repaired primarily with a perineal approach
2. High type: Diverting colostomy in infancy; later, the distal colon is brought to the perineal surface and the previous colostomy is taken down

APPENDICITIS

What percentage of appendixes rupture before surgery?

33%

What is the most important factor in the pathogenesis of appendicitis?

Luminal obstruction

What are the etiologies?

1. Fecalith (most common)
2. Lymphoid hyperplasia (in the prodromal stage of measles)
3. Pinworms (*Enterobius vermicularis*)
4. Carcinoid tumor

What is the classification system?

Staging reflects the clinicopathologic stage: simple, suppurative, gangrenous, ruptured (usually at the antimesenteric border), and abscessed (right iliac fossa, retrocecal, pelvic).

What organisms are usually involved in infectious complications?	1. *Escherichia coli* 2. *Bacteroides* 3. *Streptococcus*
What are the usual symptoms?	Abdominal pain (periumbilical shifting to the right lower quadrant) followed by anorexia, nausea, and vomiting. Unusual anatomic locations cause variations in symptoms (e.g., retrocecal: flank or back pain; pelvic: urinary symptoms). An inflamed tip resting against the ureter may cause inguinal or testicular pain. Regardless of the location of the appendix, pain is usually initially periumbilical.
What is the psoas sign?	Pain with hyperextension of the right hip. Iliopsoas rigidity indicates a retrocecal location.
What is the Rovsing sign?	Pain in the right lower quadrant when pressure is applied to the opposite side of the abdomen
How often is fecalith seen on abdominal x-ray?	Only 20% of cases; a patient with right lower quadrant pain and fecalith virtually always has appendicitis
What other findings on abdominal x-ray suggest appendicitis?	Abnormal gas pattern in the right lower quadrant, scoliosis to the right, and soft tissue mass. These findings are helpful in infants.
What other imaging studies are used?	1. CT scan 2. Ultrasound
What is included in the differential diagnosis?	Gastroenteritis, genitourinary infection, mesenteric adenitis, Meckel diverticulitis, pelvic inflammatory disease, pneumonia of the right lower lobe, intussusception, measles, and mittelschmerz. Rarer causes with a similar presentation include sickle cell crisis, twisted ovarian cysts, omental infarct, and cholecystitis.

What key feature of the history distinguishes appendicitis from gastroenteritis?

Gastroenteritis usually causes vomiting before pain.

What feature of the history suggests mesenteric adenitis?

Accompanying or recent respiratory infection

What is the surgical treatment?

Appendectomy

What technical points should be considered for an optimal surgical result?

1. Right lower quadrant muscle-splitting incision
2. No need for stump inversion if it is cauterized
3. Peritoneal lavage (≥3 L) if the appendix is ruptured
4. Primary skin closure in most cases; delayed closure if the appendix is ruptured with gross wound contamination

When is placement of a drain considered?

Only if there is a well-localized abscess cavity

How long is antibiotic administration continued?

24 hours in uncomplicated cases; 3 to 5 days or longer if the appendix is gangrenous or ruptured

When is incidental appendectomy considered in children?

Prophylactic removal whenever feasible in the course of other abdominal procedures in children, particularly if a right lower quadrant incision is used

What is the incidence of appendicitis in infants and neonates?

< 2% in infants; extremely rare in neonates

Is the rate of rupture higher or lower in infants and neonates than in older children?

Higher (difficult exam)

What are the usual symptoms?

Usually, vomiting and irritability. Pain is indicated by drawing up of the legs. Anorexia, lethargy, fever, and mass are present in 50% of patients. Abdominal distension is common.

Appendiceal rupture may be a manifestation of what disorders in these patients?	1. NEC 2. Hirschsprung disease 3. Meconium plug syndrome

MECKEL DIVERTICULUM

What is Meckel diverticulum?	Persistence of the vitelline duct (omphalomesenteric duct), creating an ileal diverticulum
Where is it located?	Arises on the antimesenteric border of the ileum within 2 feet of the ileocecal valve
What is the incidence?	2% of the population
What percentage of patients are symptomatic?	Classically, part of the "2s" of Meckel diverticulum (2% are symptomatic)
What is the claim to fame of Meckel diverticulum?	Most common cause of lower GI bleeding in children
What complications are associated with Meckel diverticulum?	1. Lower GI bleeding 2. Intestinal obstruction 3. Intestinal perforation 4. Chronic abdominal pain 5. Intussusception 6. Volvulus
What is the etiology of intestinal hemorrhage?	Ectopic gastric mucosa is seen in 50% of these diverticula (development of peptic ulceration).
What other pediatric disorder may present with GI bleed secondary to ectopic gastric mucosa?	Enteric duplication
What other heterotopic tissue is seen in 5% of patients with Meckel diverticulum?	Pancreatic tissue
What is the diagnostic study of choice?	"Meckel scan": Scintigraphy with a pertechnetate isotope (taken up by gastric mucosa). Contrast studies are rarely helpful.

How sensitive is this study?   ≈ 80%

What are the causes of false-positive results?   Disorders that cause mucosal hyperemia or bleeding, including enteric duplication, intussusception, bowel obstruction, ulcer, arteriovenous malformation, urinary tract abnormalities, and intestinal duplication

What step is taken if the scan findings are negative?   Repeat scan if clinical suspicion is high

What are the indications for surgical treatment?
1. Symptoms or complications
2. Incidental finding of Meckel diverticulum in an infant or young child

What is the surgical procedure?   Diverticulectomy with transverse closure of the enterotomy

GASTROINTESTINAL HEMANGIOMAS

What is the usual location?   Any segment of the GI tract

What is the most common complication?   Bleeding (characteristically chronic and intermittent)

What four syndromes are associated with GI hemangiomas?
1. Osler-Weber-Rendu syndrome
2. Klippel-Trenaunay syndrome
3. Turner syndrome
4. von Hippel-Lindau syndrome

What radiologic studies are usually performed?
1. Barium enema or enteroclysis to show mucosal filling defects or pseudopolyps
2. Selective angiography to show large aberrant vessels, dilated small vessels, rapid venous filling, or vascular tufts

What is the usual surgical treatment?   Careful cautery, laser, or ligature ablation of lesions. If multiple lesions are present, bowel length is conserved by careful harvesting and segmental resection of clustered lesions.

PEDIATRIC HEPATOBILIARY AND PANCREATIC DISORDERS

HEPATIC NEOPLASMS

Hemangioma

What is the usual location of hemangiomas?

Multicentric origin; therefore, often confused with metastasis

What is the claim to fame of hemangiomas?

Most common benign liver tumor (> 50%)

What is the most common symptom?

Upper abdominal discomfort

What diagnostic studies are performed?

Doppler ultrasound, dynamic CT, MRI, angiography, and tagged red blood cell scan (^{99m}Tc)

What are the associated complications?

1. Intraperitoneal bleeding
2. Chronic or subacute heart failure secondary to arteriovenous shunting through the tumor vasculature
3. Thrombocytopenia and angiopathic anemia secondary to platelet or red blood cell trapping within the tumor vasculature

What is the usual treatment?

1. Usually can be watched if the tumor is small (< 4 cm) and asymptomatic
2. Surgical resection or embolization (interventional radiology) if complications (discussed earlier) occur

Hepatic Hamartomas

What is a hepatic hamartoma?

Benign tumor secondary to new growth of normal epithelial tissues (e.g., fluid-filled cysts) in the liver

What is the usual treatment?

Catheter drainage of cyst acutely; later, complete excision (lobectomy is frequently not necessary)

Hepatoblastoma

Is hepatoblastoma benign or malignant?

Malignant

What is the average age at diagnosis?	1 year
What laboratory value is frequently elevated?	α-Fetoprotein (in > 90%)
Hepatoblastoma is associated with what: 1. Orthopedic abnormalities, and why? 2. Genitourinary abnormalities, and why?	1. Multiple pathologic fractures caused by abnormal calcium metabolism 2. Isosexual precocity, with genital enlargement and pubic hair secondary to human chorionic gonadotropin (hCG) production (10% of males)
What is the usual treatment?	Surgical resection and chemotherapy (doxorubicin, cisplatin)

Hepatocellular Carcinoma

How is hepatocellular carcinoma histologically distinguished from the adult form?	Histologically indistinguishable: Invasive, multicentric, and frequently bile-stained (unlike hepatoblastoma)
What are the usual sites of metastatic spread?	Spread to regional nodes, lung, and bone is common at diagnosis.
What is the average age at diagnosis?	9 to 10 years
What is the usual clinical presentation?	Abdominal pain, anorexia, and weight loss are common. Jaundice is seen in 20% of patients.
What laboratory values are frequently elevated?	1. a-Fetoprotein (in 50%); levels are lower than in hepatoblastoma 2. Liver enzymes and alkaline phosphatase
What is the usual treatment?	Same as hepatoblastoma (i.e., combination of surgical resection and chemotherapy), but chemotherapy is not as effective

BILIARY ATRESIA

What is biliary atresia?

Obstructive condition of the bile ducts caused by progressive obliteration and sclerosis and resulting in neonatal jaundice

What is the claim to fame of biliary atresia?

Most common cause of jaundice requiring surgery in infants

What is the etiology?

Unknown

What is the incidence?

1:15,000 live births

What are the two general types?

1. Extrahepatic biliary atresia
2. Intrahepatic biliary atresia

Which type is rare?

Intrahepatic biliary atresia

What are the associated histopathologic changes?

Evidence of cholestasis and progressive portal and periportal fibrosis, followed by bile duct proliferation with inspissated bile plugs and, eventually, cirrhosis

What feature of the history suggests biliary atresia?

Infantile jaundice that lasts > 2 weeks.

What diagnostic studies are performed?

1. Percutaneous liver biopsy
2. HIDA (lidofenin) scan: Rapid uptake by hepatocytes, with no excretion into the bowel
3. Ultrasound: Increased echogenicity of the liver; small, shrunken gallbladder; and biliary dilation (with the extrahepatic type)

What is the usual surgical treatment?

Two-stage procedure:
1. Diagnostic procedure: Operative cholangiogram through the gallbladder; open liver biopsy
2. Kasai portoenterostomy: Removal of the obliterated extrahepatic ducts; single-layer anastomosis of an intestinal conduit (Roux-en-Y hepaticojejunostomy) to the transected ducts at the liver hilum. Level of transection is determined by frozen section of proximal end.

Why is the intestinal conduit exteriorized during the early postoperative period?

1. To reduce postoperative cholangitis
2. To monitor bile flow

What is the most common postoperative complication?

Cholangitis. Despite this, prophylactic antibiotics have no role in management.

What three other complications occur, and how are they treated?

1. Cessation of bile flow (often associated with cholangitis); treated with steroids (methylprednisolone 10 mg/kg) tapered over 3 to 5 days
2. Fat malnutrition and fat-soluble vitamin deficiency (vitamins A, D, E, and K); treated with medium chain triglycerides
3. Portal hypertension secondary to continued fibrosis, despite successful Kasai procedure; treated with liver transplantation. Transplantation is usually reserved for patients who have an unsuccessful Kasai procedure.

What are the 5- and 10-year survival rates?

5-year rate: 50%; 10-year rate: 25% to 30%

CHOLEDOCHAL CYSTS

What are choledochal cysts?

Congenital malformation of the bile ducts causing cystic dilations

What are the five types?

Type I: Dilation of the common bile duct
Type II: Diverticulum of the common bile duct
Type III: Choledochocele
Type IV: Multiple intrahepatic and extrahepatic choledochocysts
Type V: Single or multiple intrahepatic cysts (Caroli disease)

Which type is the most common?

Type I

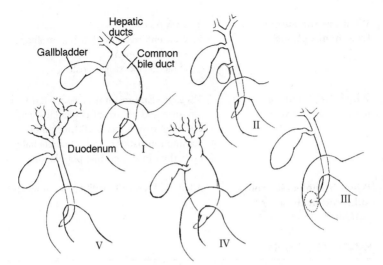

Which country has the highest incidence?	Japan

What is the sex predilection?

Female (3:1)

What is the classic triad of presentation?

1. Recurrent abdominal pain
2. Mild episodic jaundice
3. Right upper quadrant mass

Is this presentation seen more frequently with younger or older children?

Older

What are the usual complications?

Cholangitis, pancreatitis, cholelithiasis, cirrhosis, portal hypertension, hepatic abscess, biliary carcinoma, and rupture, with bile peritonitis

What is the initial diagnostic study?

Ultrasound

What other diagnostic studies are performed?

1. Hepatobiliary scintigraphy to detect associated intrahepatic cystic disease or obstruction
2. Endoscopic retrograde cholangiopancreatography (ERCP)
3. Percutaneous transhepatic cholangiography

What are the surgical treatment options?	1. Cyst excision 2. Cyst enterostomy: Internal drainage with Roux-en-Y choledochocystojejunostomy
Which treatment option is preferred, and why?	Excision. Enterostomy is associated with stricture and recurrent cholangitis, and bile duct carcinoma is 20 times more common in patients with choledochal cysts than in the normal population.
When is cholecystectomy indicated in these patients?	All should have the gallbladder removed.

PANCREAS DIVISUM

What is pancreas divisum?	Anatomic variant that occurs when the dorsal and ventral duct structures of the pancreas do not fuse during embryologic development
What is the main pancreatic duct?	Duct of Wirsung
What duct persists in pancreas divisum?	Duct of Santorini
What is the incidence?	10% of the population
What is the diagnostic study of choice?	ERCP
What is the most common complication?	Repeated bouts of pancreatitis
What is the most common indication for surgery?	Documented recurrent acute pancreatitis
What is the procedure of choice?	Open dorsal duct sphincteroplasty
What procedure is performed in a patient with chronic pancreatitis and a dilated dorsal duct?	Anterior longitudinal pancreaticojejunostomy with a Roux-en-Y loop

PEDIATRIC GENITOURINARY DISORDERS

HORSESHOE KIDNEY

What is a horseshoe kidney?	Renal fusion anomaly in which the lower poles of two distinct renal masses are joined by renal parenchyma or fibrous tissue (isthmus of the kidney)
What is the claim to fame of horseshoe kidney?	Most common renal fusion anomaly
What is the incidence?	1:300 to 1:1800
What causes most complications?	Collecting system anomalies that result in hydronephrosis, infection, and renal stones
Affected individuals are at increased risk for what tumors?	Hydronephromas, Wilms tumor, and a variety of collecting system and parenchymal tumors

INFANTILE POLYCYSTIC KIDNEY DISEASE

What is the claim to fame of infantile polycystic kidney disease?	Although rare, it is the most common genetically determined cystic disease of the kidney in childhood.
What is the route of genetic transmission?	Autosomal recessive
What is the finding on physical exam?	Palpable, often visible, massively enlarged hard flank masses at birth
What is included in the differential diagnosis?	1. Hydronephrosis 2. Renal neoplasm 3. Renal vein thrombosis
What diagnostic tests are performed?	1. Excretory urography: Radial streams of contrast material from the medulla to the surface of the cortex, with alternating radiolucent and radiodense areas (sun ray effect) 2. Ultrasound: Hyperechogenic masses and disseminated small cysts

What other organ is also diseased in these patients?	Liver: Proliferation and dilation of the bile ducts, with varying amounts of periportal fibrosis and, occasionally, portal hypertension
What is the prognosis for these patients?	Poor. Death usually occurs in the first several months of life.

URETEROPELVIC JUNCTION (UPJ) OBSTRUCTION

What is UPJ obstruction?	Fibrosis or interruption of smooth muscle continuity across the UPJ, leading to interruption of the orderly transmission of peristaltic waves
What are the associated complications?	1. Hydronephrosis 2. Urinary tract infection (UTI) 3. If uncorrected, renal failure
What diagnostic studies are performed?	1. Ultrasound: Renal pelvic dilation 2. Renal scintigraphy if ultrasound shows persistent hydronephrosis. Persistence of the radioactive label in the renal pelvis suggests UPJ obstruction.
What additional study is included to rule out vesicoureteral reflux?	Voiding cystourethrogram (VCUG)
What is the surgical treatment?	Pyeloplasty to enlarge the UPJ
When is antenatal intervention considered?	Only if ultrasound shows significant oligohydramnios, no cystic changes of the kidneys, bilateral hydronephrosis, and impending pulmonary hypoplasia

VESICOURETERAL REFLUX

What is vesicoureteral reflux?	Retrograde passage of urine from the bladder into the ureter
What is the sex predilection?	Girls account for 85% of cases.

What are the complications?	1. UTI 2. Renal failure
What is the usual treatment?	Nonoperative management (including suppression antibiotics and close follow-up with urine cultures, cystourethrograms, and measurement of serum creatinine values) is successful in most patients.
What are the indications for surgery?	1. Recurrent UTI 2. Progressive renal injury 3. Noncompliance 4. Severe reflux
What is the surgical treatment?	Ureteral reimplantation with a long segment of the intravesicular ureter

URETHRAL VALVES

What are urethral valves?	Exaggerated forms of the normal small fold in the male urethra
What is the usual presentation?	UTI, bed-wetting, poor urinary stream, urinary frequency, hematuria, and acute urinary retention
What is the diagnostic study of choice?	VCUG
What is the surgical treatment?	Endoscopic valve resection. If the infant is too small to permit use of the scope, temporary vesicostomy is performed until the infant is several months old.

EXSTROPHY OF THE BLADDER

What is exstrophy of the bladder?	Defect in the ventral coverage of at least part of the bladder, with pubic diastasis
Males have a 10-fold increased risk of what disorder?	Cryptorchidism
If untreated, all patients are at increased risk for what disorder?	Bladder carcinoma

What is the surgical treatment?	Multistage procedure:

What is the surgical treatment?

Multistage procedure:
1. Primary bladder closure (accompanied by herniorrhaphy and orchidopexy, if indicated), which causes incontinence
2. Epispadias repair during the next 3 to 5 years as the bladder enlarges (≥ 60 ml capacity is needed for continent surgery); bladder neck reconstruction to achieve continence

HYPOSPADIAS

What is hypospadias?

Anomaly in which the urethral meatus opens onto the ventral surface of the penis, proximal to the end of the glans

What is the incidence?

1:300 live male births

What is the etiology?

Defect in androgen stimulation of the developing penis, precluding complete formation of the urethra and its surrounding structures

What are the indications for surgical treatment?

All patients are offered surgical treatment for psychological reasons.

What is the timing of surgery?

Within the first year of life

What are the primary goals of surgery?

Straightening the penis and placing the meatus at the tip of the glans

PRUNE BELLY SYNDROME

What is the triad of physical findings?

1. Congenital absence or hypoplasia of the abdominal wall musculature
2. Urinary tract abnormalities, with a large hypotonic bladder, dilated ureters, and a dilated prostatic urethra
3. Bilateral cryptorchidism

What is another name for this syndrome?

Eagle-Barrett syndrome

TESTICULAR TORSION

What is the claim to fame of testicular torsion?	Most common genitourinary tract emergency of childhood
What is the peak age-group?	14 to 15 years
What is included in the differential diagnosis?	1. Appendicular or epididymal torsion 2. Epididymo-orchitis 3. Incarcerated inguinal hernia
What is the most common symptom?	Scrotal pain that is **abrupt** in onset, with radiation of pain upward into the groin
How do the other disorders included in the differential diagnosis differ in their presentation?	Pain is usually gradual over > 12 hours.
What is the "blue dot" sign?	With torsion of the appendix, testes, or epididymis, the necrotic appendage is visualized as a blue dot.
What diagnostic tests are performed?	1. Duplex Doppler ultrasound 2. Nuclear testicular scintigraphy (^{99m}Tc), which shows decreased blood flow to the affected testes or a halo of mildly increased activity surrounding a cold center
What is the management of an acute scrotum with positive or equivocal study results?	Immediate scrotal exploration and bilateral orchidopexy if testicular torsion is present
What factor determines the testicular salvage rate?	Time to surgery: If < 6 hours, > 85% are salvaged If > 24 hours, < 10% are salvaged

PEDIATRIC ONCOLOGY

NEUROBLASTOMA

What is neuroblastoma?	Tumor arising from the sympathetic nervous tissue

What is the most common location?

Adrenal gland

What is the claim to fame of neuroblastoma?

Most common tumor in children < 1 year of age; overall, the third most common childhood cancer (after leukemia and brain tumor)

What favorable evolution in the tumor may occur?

Tumor may spontaneously regress or mature into a ganglioneuroblastoma or ganglioneuroma (benign). Patients < 1 year of age have a much better prognosis than older children.

What percentage of tumors are biologically active?

> 90%

What substances do they secrete?

1. Vanillylmandelic acid (from norepinephrine)
2. Homovanillic acid (from dopamine)
3. Acetylcholine

Do more differentiated tumors produce more or less vanillylmandelic acid than less differentiated tumors?

More because of increased norepinephrine production

The level of what substance is elevated in almost all patients with metastases?

Neuron-specific enolase (NSE)

Genetic abnormalities are seen in what percentage of patients? Provide two examples.

80% of patients, including:
1. Deletions in the short arm of chromosome 1 (1p-)
2. Amplification of the n-*myc* oncogene

What triad is associated with myoclonus-opsoclonus syndrome?

Polymyoclonia, cerebellar ataxia with gait disturbances, and opsoclonus; 50% of patients with this syndrome have primary tumor in the thorax

What scan best defines the location of the neuroblastoma tumor?

MIBG scan. Metaiodobenzylguanidine, which resembles norepinephrine, is labeled with ^{131}I, or ^{123}I binds to norepinephrine.

What is a "dumbbell" tumor?

Extension of a neuroblastoma through the neuroforamina

What is the staging system?

Stage 1: Localized to the site of origin, complete excision ± microscopic residual disease, and negative nodes

Stage 2A: Unilateral tumor, incomplete excision, and negative nodes

Stage 2B: Unilateral tumor ± complete excision, positive ipsilateral nodes, and negative contralateral nodes

Stage 3: Tumor crossing the midline ± node involvement, unilateral tumor with contralateral node involvement, or midline tumor with bilateral node involvement

Stage 4: Tumor dissemination to distant nodes, bone, bone marrow, liver, or other organs

Stage 4S: Localized primary tumor as defined for Stage 1, 2A, or 2B, with metastases limited to the liver, skin, or bone marrow

What is the survival rate for each stage?

Stage 1: 100%
Stages 2A and 2B: 78%
Stage 3: 43%
Stage 4: 15%
Stage 4S: 70%

What is the usual treatment?

Multimodal therapy:
1. Surgery: Complete excision (if possible), lymph node sampling, and liver biopsy. If the tumor is unresectable, the patient is given chemotherapy and radiation therapy and returned to the OR for resection of residual tumor.
2. Chemotherapy: Used if resection is incomplete. Multiple agents (e.g., ifosfamide, carboplatin, and iproplatin) are more successful than single agents.
3. Radiation therapy: Tumor is radiosensitive. However, when the tumor is localized, radiation therapy offers little benefit beyond surgery

and chemotherapy, **except** in patients
with Stage 3 disease and > 1 year old.

When is second-look surgery indicated after chemotherapy?	When the tumor is located in the abdomen or pelvis, not the neck or chest
Which age-group has a limited response to chemotherapy?	> 1 year old
What other treatment is under investigation?	Bone marrow transplant after melphalan administration and total body irradiation

WILMS TUMOR

What is the claim to fame of Wilms tumor?	Most common renal malignancy of childhood
What is another name for this tumor?	Nephroblastoma
How frequently is it bilateral?	5% to 7% of cases
The familial form is caused by a deletion on what chromosome?	11p
What are the associated congenital anomalies?	Cryptorchidism, hemihypertrophy, hypospadias, aniridia, and Wiedemann-Beckwith syndrome
What abdominal finding on physical exam distinguishes Wilms tumor from neuroblastoma?	Abdominal mass usually crosses the midline in neuroblastoma, but **not** in Wilms tumor
What condition may cause congestive heart failure in patients with Wilms tumor?	Hypertension
Compare the findings on plain x-ray in Wilms tumor versus neuroblastoma.	Wilms tumor: Linear calcifications Neuroblastoma: Fine-stippled calcifications

What vascular complication is well recognized in Wilms tumor?

Propensity for venous extension. The patency of the inferior vena cava and extension into the right atrium are documented preoperatively. Cardiac surgery may be necessary.

What is the staging system for Wilms tumor?

Stage I: Limited to the kidney and completely excised

Stage II: Extending beyond the kidney, but completely excised

Stage III: Residual nonhematogenous tumor remaining within the abdomen, including nodal metastases, peritoneal implants, and incompletely resected tumor

Stage IV: Hematogenous spread

Stage V: Bilateral disease at presentation

What is the single most important prognostic factor?

Histopathology. Anaplastic and sarcomatous lesions have the most unfavorable prognosis (60% mortality rate).

What factor is another important predictor of poor outcome?

Race. Black and Hispanic patients have a greater incidence of unfavorable histology than white patients.

What is the usual treatment?

Multimodal therapy:
1. Immediate unilateral nephroureterectomy with lymph node dissection
2. Chemotherapy for all patients (dactinomycin, vincristine, ± doxorubicin)
3. Radiation therapy to the tumor bed for patients with Stage III or IV disease and for patients with Stage II disease with unfavorable histology

What is the management of a solitary hepatic or pulmonary metastasis?

Resection

What is the overall cure rate?

> 80%

What is nephroblastomatosis?

Persistent metanephric tissue in the kidney after the thirty-sixth week of gestation

What is the incidence of nephroblastomatosis in patients with Wilms tumor?	25% to 40% of children with Wilms tumor
What is Drash syndrome?	Pseudohermaphroditism, Wilms tumor, and degenerative renal disease in male infants
What is the usual course?	Progressive end-stage renal disease (ESRD) within the first year of life
What is the usual treatment?	Prophylactic nephrectomy soon after the development of ESRD

TERATOMAS

What are teratomas?	Germ cell tumors containing elements of all three layers (endoderm, mesoderm, and ectoderm). They contain tissue foreign to the anatomic location (formed from tissue that could not have resulted from metaplasia of the cells normally found there).
What are the common components?	1. Skin 2. Teeth 3. Central nervous system tissue 4. Respiratory and alimentary mucosa 5. Cartilage and bone
Why do they cause symptoms?	Obstruction or compression of viscera
What are the tumor markers?	1. Chorionic gonadotropin (hCG): Choriocarcinoma 2. α-Fetoprotein: Tumors containing yolk sac carcinoma and embryonal carcinoma; teratoma containing immature tissue 3. Lactate dehydrogenase isoenzyme 1: Yolk sac tumors (not specific)
Which type of: 1. **Teratoma is most common in neonates?** 2. **Teratoma is most common in adolescents?** 3. **Teratoma presents as a suprapubic mass?**	1. Sacrococcygeal 2. Ovarian 3. Ovarian

4. Extragonadal teratoma is seen only in males?

4. Gastric

5. Teratoma is the most common extragonadal type?

5. Sacrococcygeal

What is the characteristic appearance of the sacrococcygeal type?

Protruding from the space between the anus and coccyx and usually covered with normal intact skin

What is included in the differential diagnosis of sacrococcygeal teratoma?

1. Myelomeningocele
2. Pilonidal cyst

What is the treatment of sacrococcygeal teratoma?

1. Surgical excision in continuity with excision of the coccyx. Formation of an anatomically normal gluteal crease is dependent on suturing the perianal sphincter to the presacral space.
2. If benign, close perineal and rectal follow-up and excision of any recurrences
3. If malignant, aggressive chemotherapy. Recurrence after excision of malignant teratoma is associated with a high mortality rate. (Another indication for chemotherapy is tumor containing immature tissue with an increase in the α-fetoprotein level.)

What is the usual presentation of gastric teratoma?

Palpable epigastric mass and/or GI bleed

What is the treatment of gastric teratoma?

Surgical excision

What is the prognosis for gastric teratoma?

If excised completely, no additional therapy is required because these tumors are benign.

Which teratoma is often called a "dermoid" tumor?

Ovarian

What is the source of pain from this teratoma?

Volvulus of the ovarian pedicle

What must be included in the differential diagnosis?	Pregnancy
What is the treatment of ovarian teratoma?	Surgical excision, leaving functional ovarian tissue only if the tumor is clearly benign

PEDIATRIC TRAUMA

What are the important considerations in children?	1. Maintenance of body temperature 2. Accurate determination of body weight (e.g., for medications) 3. Child abuse (must be ruled out)
What are the most common mechanisms of injury?	80% are secondary to blunt trauma, motor vehicle–pedestrian accidents, or falls
What are the airway considerations?	1. If intubation is necessary, an **uncuffed** endotracheal tube is used. The size should approximate the width of the fingernail of the fifth digit or can be calculated as (age + 16) divided by 4. 2. Cricothyroidotomy is **not** performed in young children; needle cricothyroidotomy is preferred (14 g).
What is the most reliable indication of hypovolemia in the child, and why?	Tachycardia is the most reliable indicator. Children maintain normal blood pressure (BP) in the presence of progressing hypovolemia secondary to increases in peripheral vascular resistance because of adrenergic constriction of medium to small arteries (decreased ability with increasing age to constrict the peripheral vasculature effectively).
What are the normal values for BP and pulse in children?	

Age	BP	HR
Neonate	70/40	120–160
3–12 months	90/50	90–140
1–6 years	95/60	80–110
6–12 years	100/70	70–100
> 12 years	120/70	60–90

What are the intravenous access sites, in order of preference?

1. Greater saphenous vein at the ankle
2. Median cephalic vein at the elbow
3. Main cephalic vein in the arm
4. External jugular vein
5. Intraosseous sites (anterior tibial plateau, 2–3 cm below the tuberosity)
6. Subclavian vein

Which patients are candidates for the interosseous route?

< 6 years old

What is the fluid resuscitation regimen for the hypotensive patient?

1. Bolus with normal saline or lactated Ringer solution (20 ml/kg)
2. Bolus repeated once if the patient remains hypotensive
3. If the patient is still hypotensive, transfusion of 10 ml/kg packed red blood cells is provided, and the patient is prepared for surgical exploration.

What is a normal blood volume?

80 ml/kg

Why is multisystem injury the rule rather than the exception in children?

1. Less body fat
2. Less elastic connective tissue
3. Closer proximity of multiple organs

What organ system is usually injured?

Neurologic. (Cushing reflex may not be present if the cranial sutures are not fused.)

Are rib fractures more common in children or adults, and what is the significance of the difference?

Adults, because the ribs are pliable in children. Rib fracture in children implies a significant force and increased suspicion for serious injury. Bronchial injuries and diaphragmatic rupture occur frequently.

What facilitates abdominal exam?

Early insertion of a nasogastric tube

What are the steps in the management of splenic and liver injuries?

1. Monitoring in the pediatric intensive care unit
2. Serial hematocrit determinations
3. Laparotomy only if the patient becomes hemodynamically unstable

or requires transfusion of > 50% of blood volume

What is the risk of postsplenectomy sepsis and the mortality rate if it develops?

1.5%; 50% mortality rate

What additional x-rays are performed in pediatric trauma patients, but are not necessary in adults?

X-ray of the asymptomatic contralateral uninjured extremity to avoid confusion about growth plates and ossification centers

PEDIATRIC FLUID AND ELECTROLYTE MANAGEMENT

What changes in body fluid compartments occur between the first trimester and age 2 years?

1. Total body water accounts for 95% of body weight during the first trimester, 78% at term, and 60% at 2 years of age.
2. Extracellular fluid volume decreases from 60% during the second trimester to 45% at birth and 20% over the next 2 years.

What is the renal function in the child, and what is its significance?

Glomerular filtration rate is 25% of the adult value. The rate reaches the adult value at 2 years of age. Therefore, renal concentrating ability is significantly reduced (500–600 mOsm maximum in children).

What are the daily water requirements in the first week, second week, and thereafter?

1. ≈ 60 ml/kg/24 hr for the first week of life
2. 72 ml/kg/24 hr during the second week of life
3. 84 ml/kg/24 hr thereafter (urine output 2.5 ml/kg/hr)

What is the calculation for the rate of maintenance intravenous fluids?

4 ml/kg/hr for the first 10 kg
2 ml/kg/hr for the second 10 kg
1 ml/kg/hr for each kg > 20 kg

What is the daily sodium requirement?

2 mEq/kg/24 hr

What is the daily potassium requirement?

2 mEq/kg/24 hr after the first 2 to 3 days of life

What is the initial fluid of choice pre- and postoperatively in the pediatric population?

D_5 or D_{10} 0.25NS (at 100–150 ml/kg/24 hr)

48

Orthopedic Surgery

Michael E. Tjarksen, M.D.

ANATOMY AND BIOLOGY

Name the labeled areas.

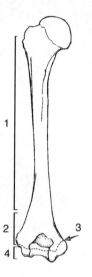

1. Diaphysis
2. Metaphysis
3. Physis (growth plate)
4. Epiphysis

What type of bone formation results in:
1. Long bones?
2. Flat bones?

1. Endochondral ossification
2. Intramembranous ossification

What type of bone growth determines long bone:
1. Length?
2. Width?

1. Interstitial
2. Appositional

What cell type:
1. Produces osteoid?
2. Resorbs bone?

1. Osteoblasts
2. Osteoclasts

What type of collagen predominates in:
1. Bone?
2. Articular cartilage?

1. Type I
2. Type II

What is the composition of articular cartilage?

1. Water (65%)
2. Collagen, type II (20%)
3. Proteoglycan (10%)
4. Chondrocytes (5%)

What are the systemic effects of:
1. Parathyroid hormone?

1. Parathyroid hormone
   a. Bone: Mobilizes calcium (Ca^{2+}) and phosphorus (Po_4^{2-})
   b. Kidney: Resorbs Ca^{2+}, excretes Po_4^{2-}, and increases vitamin D level
   c. Gut: Increases absorption of Ca^{2+} and Po_4^{2-} (through vitamin D)
   d. Overall effect: Increases plasma Ca^{2+} level
2. Vitamin D

2. Vitamin D?

   a. Bone: Mobilizes Ca^{2+}
   b. Kidney: Resorbs Po_4^{2-}
   c. Gut: Promotes Ca^{2+} and Po_4^{2-} absorption
   d. Overall effect: Increases plasma Ca^{2+} and Po_4^{2-} levels
3. Calcitonin

3. Calcitonin?

   a. Bone: Decreases mobilization of Ca^{2+} and Po_4^{2-}
   b. Kidney: Decreases resorption of Ca^{2+} and Po_4^{2-}
   c. Gut: Increases electrolyte secretion
   d. Overall effect: Decreases plasma Ca^{2+} level

What are the two primary components of a sarcomere?

1. Thick filament: Myosin
2. Thin filament: Actin

FRACTURE HEALING

What are the three stages of fracture healing?

1. Inflammation: Infiltration of hematopoietic cells and osteogenic precursors
2. Repair (2 weeks): Callus, cartilage, and woven bone formation

3. Remodeling: Lamellar bone formation, development of normal shape and configuration, and repopulation of marrow

What type of bone formation occurs in fractures treated with a cast?

Endochondral ossification

What is the usual appearance on x-ray?

Fracture callus

What type of bone formation occurs in fractures treated with open reduction and internal fixation?

Primary bone formation

What is the usual appearance on x-ray?

Blurring of fracture line; no callus

TRAUMA

A patient comes to the emergency room after a motor vehicle accident. She has an obviously deformed leg. What is the first step in management?

Airway, breathing, and circulation: ABCs of the advanced trauma life support (ATLS) protocol

In a patient who has had trauma, after the ABCs are established, how are the following elements of the musculoskeletal survey addressed:
1. Observation?

1. Cervical spine immobilization is maintained until cleared; the patient is examined for any obvious deformities, abrasions, or open wounds

2. Palpation?

2. All long bones, even uninjured, nontender segments

3. Function?

3. Range of all joints is determined, ligaments are stressed, an obviously fractured pelvis is not stressed, and neurologic and vascular evaluation is performed

What x-rays are mandatory in a patient with trauma?

Anteroposterior (AP) and lateral x-rays of the cervical spine, AP x-ray of the chest, and AP x-ray of the pelvis

For a traumatized extremity, what x-rays are obtained?

AP and lateral views of the affected long bone **plus** an evaluation of the joints proximal and distal to the long bone

What is the initial treatment of a traumatized extremity?

1. Splinting
2. Reduction of deformities (i.e., restoration of the normal alignment of the bone or joint)
3. Irrigation of any open wounds and application of a sterile dressing

What are the general indications for open (surgical) reduction?

1. Failed closed reduction
2. Intra-articular fractures
3. Extremity function requiring perfect reduction
4. Multiple trauma
5. Advanced age (i.e., long nonambulatory period increases the morbidity rate)

How does orthopedic surgery help to prevent pulmonary complications in patients with multisystem trauma?

1. Early mobilization of the patient with operative fixation of fractures allows upright posture.
2. Surgery reduces the incidence of adult respiratory distress syndrome secondary to fat embolism in patients with long bone fractures.

Which fractured bone is most commonly associated with a fat embolism?

Femur

How does a fat embolism present?

Shortness of breath and petechiae across the chest and in the axilla 48 hours after injury

In an extremity that is deformed because of fracture or dislocation, what assessments are performed before reduction is attempted?

1. Vascular status
2. Neurologic status
3. Identification of open wounds

What treatment is performed emergently on a deformed extremity with vascular compromise?

Correction of the deformity by gentle traction in-line of the injured bone; splinting

What procedure is performed on a pulseless extremity whose pulses do not return after reduction?

Immediate operative exploration with intraoperative arteriogram to identify the level of vascular injury

What areas are incorporated into a splint?

The joints proximal and distal to the injured bone are immobilized.

What is the treatment of an extremity whose neurologic function was compromised before reduction and remains compromised after reduction?

Observation

What is the treatment if the neurologic function is compromised only after reduction?

Surgical exploration

ORTHOPEDIC EMERGENCIES

What are the classic orthopedic emergencies?

1. Unstable pelvic fracture
2. Unstable spine fracture
3. Open fracture
4. Septic joint
5. Septic osteomyelitis
6. Displaced long bone fracture with neurovascular compromise
7. Compartment syndrome
8. Dislocation

FRACTURES

What features on clinical examination are used to describe a fracture?

1. Open (i.e., break in the skin integrity near the fracture) versus closed
2. Location along the length of the bone
3. Pattern of the fracture (i.e., comminuted, spiral)
4. Degree of angulation

Define the following types of fracture:

1. Comminuted?

1. Fracture with more than two fragments

2. Pathologic?

2. Fracture through a bone weakened by tumor, osteoporosis, or other bony abnormalities

3. Torus?

3. Cortex buckled, but not disrupted, because of impaction injury; seen in children

4. Greenstick?

4. Incomplete fracture with disruption of the cortex on only one side; seen in children

OPEN FRACTURES

What is an open fracture?

Fracture with communication with the external environment

What is the primary complication associated with these fractures?

Infection

What is the Gustillo classification for open fractures?

Grade I: Wound < 1 cm; minimal contamination and soft tissue injury; simple or minimal comminuted fracture

Grade II: Wound 1 to 10 cm; moderate contamination; soft tissue injury; fracture comminution

Grade III: Wound > 10 cm; gross contamination; severe soft tissue injury; fracture comminution

What additional features classify an open fracture as grade III, regardless of the size of the cutaneous lesion?

1. Soil contamination
2. Vascular injury
3. Close-range shotgun injury

What are the subgroups of grade III lesions?

Grade IIIA: Soft tissue adequate for coverage of the wound

Grade IIIB: Soft tissue loss that mandates flap coverage of the wound

Grade IIIC: Concurrent vascular injury requiring repair

What is the incidence of infection for grades I, II, and III?	Grade I: 0% to 2% Grade II: 2% to 7% Grade III: 10% to 50%
What is the treatment of an open fracture?	1. Operative irrigation and débridement within 6 hours; repeat débridement or irrigation may be needed in 24 to 72 hours 2. IV antibiotics 3. Tetanus inoculation 4. Open reduction and stabilization of the fracture
What is the antibiotic regimen for each grade?	Grade I: First-generation cephalosporin (i.e., cephazolin) for 48 hours Grades II and III: Gram-negative coverage (i.e., gentamicin) for at least 72 hours For soil contamination, penicillin is provided for clostridial coverage.
What are the options for stabilizing open fractures?	1. Internal fixation 2. External fixation Casting, splinting, and traction generally are **not** used for open fractures.
What are the benefits of external fixation?	1. No need for additional dissection of the injured soft tissue 2. Placement of the fixator out of the region of injury 3. Easy access to the wound for observation and wound care
When is wound closure performed?	At 3 to 7 days **if** there is no evidence of infection
What are the relative indications for primary amputation in a mangled extremity?	1. Increased age 2. Untreated shock 3. > 6 hours of ischemia 4. Severe soft tissue injury

SPRAIN AND STRAINS

What is a sprain?	Ligament tear
What is the usual presentation?	Swelling and tenderness over the ligament; increased pain on stretching of the ligament

How are sprains graded?

Grade I: Minor incomplete tear; no laxity compared with the contralateral ligament

Grade II: Significant incomplete tear; increased laxity; significant swelling and ecchymosis

Grade III: Complete tear of the ligament; no end point felt when stress is applied to the ligament. Diagnosis may be missed because of muscle spasm and pain that prevent adequate examination of the ligament.

What is strain?

Partial tear of the musculotendinous unit

CLAVICLE FRACTURE

What is the most common site of clavicular fracture?

Central one-third: 80%
Distal one-third: 12% to 15%
Proximal one-third: 5%

What is the usual treatment of this fracture?

Sling or figure-of-eight shoulder harness for 6 to 8 weeks; orthopedic referral in 3 to 5 days

What clavicle fractures require surgical fixation?

1. Concurrent vascular injury
2. Displaced distal clavicle fracture
3. Fracture end embedded in or piercing the trapezius muscle
4. Fracture end tenting the skin
5. Open fracture

What type of fixation is used for a clavicle fracture?

Plates and screws, not pins, because pins may migrate into the chest and erode into the chest cavities

What vascular structure is located directly beneath the clavicle?

Subclavian vein. Vascular injuries are rare.

SCAPULA FRACTURE

What is the significance of scapula fracture?

Indicates significant injury. The patient must be thoroughly evaluated for life-threatening lesions (i.e., pneumothorax, aortic dissection, pelvic fracture).

What is the usual treatment?	Conservative management

SHOULDER JOINT

Shoulder Sprain

What shoulder joint is most commonly sprained?	Acromioclavicular (AC) joint
What ligaments stabilize the AC joint?	1. AC ligaments 2. Coracoclavicular (CC) ligaments (conoid and trapezoid)
What is the usual mechanism of ligament injury?	Fall on the side of the shoulder
How are these injuries evaluated?	AP x-ray taken with weight (10 lb) hanging from the arm and compared with the contralateral side
How are ligamentous sprains graded?	Grade I: Ligament continuity; no joint opening Grade II: Ligament continuity; joint opening Grade III: No ligament continuity; complete tear of AC and CC ligaments
What is the usual treatment?	Sling for comfort for all grades with early range of motion. Orthopedic referral in 3 to 5 days for grades I and II and immediately for grade III because surgery may be indicated.

Shoulder Dislocation

What is the most common direction of shoulder dislocation?	Anterior inferior
What is the usual presentation?	Pain and reduced shoulder mobility, with the injured arm held by the contralateral arm in slight abduction; prominent acromion

What x-ray views are included in a shoulder trauma series?

AP, lateral Y, and axillary views

What nerve is most commonly injured during shoulder dislocation?

Axillary nerve (almost always a neurapraxia)

What are the usual findings on physical exam if this nerve is injured?

Decreased sensation in the region of the lateral shoulder; decreased deltoid strength

What is the usual technique for reduction of anterior shoulder dislocation?

The patient lies prone with the affected arm hanging over the side of the stretcher. A 5- to 10-lb weight is hung from the wrist. The patient is given muscle relaxant and medication for pain relief. After reduction, the arm is immobilized with a sling or swathe.

What step is important after reduction?

Reevaluation of the neurovascular status of the limb

What factor is most predictive of a recurrent shoulder dislocation?

Younger age at first dislocation increases the risk of recurrence. Anterior shoulder reconstruction may be required.

What structure is at increased risk for injury during shoulder dislocation in the elderly?

Axillary artery

How does shoulder dislocation usually present?

Rapid axillary swelling and discoloration; pulses may still be intact distally.

What is the usual presentation of posterior shoulder dislocation?

Arm is held adducted and internally rotated; the posterior shoulder is more prominent. Until proved otherwise, if the patient cannot externally rotate the shoulder beyond the neutral position or cannot supinate the hand, a posterior dislocation is present. These dislocations are frequently missed!

What are common mechanisms for posterior dislocation of the shoulder?	Seizure and electrocution
What is the usual treatment?	Closed reduction

Rotator Cuff Pathology

How does rotator cuff tendinitis usually present?	Middle-aged man (40s) with gradually increasing pain in the shoulder and difficulty raising the arms above the head
What clinical findings support the diagnosis of rotator cuff tendinitis?	Passive internal rotation, flexion, and abduction of the shoulder cause severe pain.
What are the muscles of the rotator cuff?	SITS acronym: 1. Supraspinatus muscle 2. Infraspinatus muscle 3. Teres minor muscle 4. Subscapularis muscle
Which muscle tendon is usually affected by tendinitis?	Supraspinatus muscle
What factors contribute to rotator cuff tendinitis?	1. Impingement from bone spur of the acromion or AC joint 2. Vascular watershed of the tendon 3. Repetitive trauma from overhead activities
What is the end-stage condition of rotator cuff impingement?	Rotator cuff tear with eventual proximal migration of the humerus; severe pain
What is the usual presentation of acute tear of the rotator cuff?	Acute onset of pain and inability to raise the arm over the head after a traumatic event
What radiographic studies are used to diagnose rotator cuff tears?	Magnetic resonance imaging (MRI) or arthrogram

What is the usual medical treatment?	1. Physical therapy 2. Nonsteroidal anti-inflammatory drug (NSAID) 3. Steroid injection
What is the usual surgical treatment of severe impingement or rotator cuff tear?	1. Removal of the bony spurs (acromioplasty) 2. Repair of the rotator cuff

HUMERUS FRACTURE

What are the four anatomic parts that can be displaced in a proximal humerus fracture?	1. Head 2. Shaft 3. Greater tuberosity 4. Lesser tuberosity
What muscle inserts on the: **1. Greater tuberosity?** **2. Lesser tuberosity?**	1. Supraspinatus muscle 2. Subscapularis muscle
What x-rays are mandatory for a proximal humerus fracture?	AP, Y, and axillary view
What nerve is at risk for injury in a humerus shaft fracture?	Radial nerve
What is the incidence of injury to this nerve?	5% to 10% of humerus shaft fractures
What muscles are innervated by the radial nerve distal to the shaft of the humerus?	Extensors of the wrist and fingers
What is the usual treatment of nondisplaced fractures of the proximal humerus?	Sling for comfort, with gentle range of motion begun as soon as the proximal humerus can move as a unit
What is the usual treatment of displaced proximal humerus fractures?	Open reduction, internal fixation, or hemiarthroplasty (replacement of the proximal humerus only), with repair of the rotator cuff tear

Should a humerus fracture with 30° angulation be corrected, and why?	No. The mobility of the shoulder joint allows the extremity to remain functional.
What is the usual treatment of humerus shaft fractures?	Coaptation or "U" splint and sling as long as there is bony opposition
What are the usual indications for surgical fixation of shaft fracture?	1. Segmental fracture 2. Distal fracture 3. Pathologic fracture 4. Concurrent forearm fracture (floating elbow) 5. Radial nerve injury incurred during reduction

ELBOW

Elbow Dislocations

What is the most common direction of an elbow dislocation?	Posterior (radius and ulna posterior to the humerus); others are rare
What nerves are most commonly injured with an elbow dislocation?	Median and ulnar nerves
What muscles does the median nerve innervate distal to the elbow?	Radial wrist flexor (flexor carpi radialis) and deep flexor of the thumb, index, and long finger, and all superficial flexors
What muscles does the ulnar nerve innervate distal to the elbow?	Ulnar wrist flexor (flexor carpi ulnaris), deep flexors to the ring and small fingers, and intrinsic muscles to the hand
What artery may be injured?	Brachial artery
What is the usual treatment of elbow dislocation?	Closed reduction with splinting; splinting should last no more than 3 weeks to prevent joint contractures
What are the indications for open reduction?	1. Irreducible dislocation 2. Incongruent reduction

Elbow Fractures

What is a Monteggia fracture?
Proximal ulna fracture **plus** radial head dislocation

What nerve may be injured with this fracture?
Posterior interosseous nerve (PIN; distal radial nerve)

What muscles does the PIN innervate?
Extensor carpi ulnaris; finger and thumb extensors

What is a Galeazzi fracture?
Radial fracture at the junction of the middle and distal thirds **plus** subluxation of the radioulnar joint

What classic x-ray finding suggests occult elbow fracture?
"Sail sign": Fat anterior to the distal humerus has a triangular appearance because of joint capsule distension

What is the usual treatment of elbow fracture?
Open reduction and internal fixation; precise alignment is needed for upper extremity function

Nursemaids' Elbow

What is nursemaids' elbow?
Subluxation of the radial head because of a sudden tug on a child's arm while it is pronated and extended

What is the usual presentation?
Local tenderness, limited use of the arm, but no swelling or x-ray abnormalities

What is the usual treatment?
Closed reduction by the supinating arm; no immobilization is necessary

FOREARM FRACTURES

What is a Colles fracture?
Fracture of the distal radius with **dorsal** carpal displacement

What is a Smith fracture?
Fracture of the distal radius with **volar** carpal displacement

What is the usual treatment of displaced midshaft radius fractures?
Open reduction with internal fixation

What is the usual treatment of displaced distal radius fractures?
Closed reduction with splinting

Why are distal radius fractures splinted initially?	Casts do not allow for swelling.
What joints are immobilized when a distal radius fracture is splinted?	Elbow and wrist
What postreduction parameters determine whether surgical intervention is warranted for a distal radius fracture?	1. Articular congruency 2. Radial length 3. Lack of volar tilt (in the AP plane)
What injury to the carpus is commonly missed with a distal radius fracture?	Scapholunate dissociation
What does "snuff-box" tenderness usually indicate?	Scaphoid (or navicular) bone fracture

PELVIS

Pelvic Fractures

What bones are included in the pelvic ring?	Ilium, ischium, and pubis
What ligaments connect the: **1. Sacrum to the ilium?** **2. Sacrum to the ischium?**	1. Anterior and posterior sacroiliac ligaments and interosseous ligaments 2. Sacrotuberous ligament and sacrospinous ligament

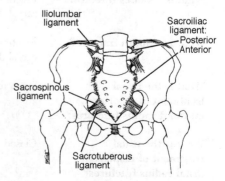

Iliolumbar ligament

Sacroiliac ligament:
Posterior
Anterior

Sacrospinous ligament

Sacrotuberous ligament

What ligament joins the ring anteriorly?

Pubic symphysis

What x-rays are necessary to evaluate a pelvic fracture?

1. AP, inlet, and outlet
2. Computed tomography (CT) scan if the patient is hemodynamically stable

Describe a pelvis fracture classification by mechanism, including the feature that classifies each type as unstable:
1. Type I?

2. Type II?

3. Type III?

1. Lateral compression: Unstable when the posterior ligamentous or bony structure is disrupted
2. AP compression: Unstable when the pubic diastasis is > 2.5 cm, which indicates that the posterior ligamentous or bony structure is disrupted
3. Vertical shear: Unstable by definition

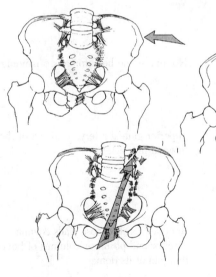

What aspect of a physical exam is mandatory before a Foley catheter is inserted?

Rectal exam (for high-riding prostate) and inspection for blood at the urethral meatus because of the risk of urethral disruption with pelvic fracture

What percentage of patients with major pelvic fracture:

1. Have concurrent intra-abdominal injury?
2. Require blood transfusion?
3. Have injury to a major pelvic vessel?

1. 10% to 20%
2. 40%
3. 2%

What are the usual applications for CT scan?

1. Evaluation of the posterior ligaments
2. Evaluation of the acetabulum
3. Identification of a pelvic hematoma or liver or splenic injury

What is the quickest form of surgical treatment of a hemodynamically unstable patient with an unstable pelvic fracture?

External fixation, with pins placed through the skin and into the iliac wings and connected to a bar externally

Is external fixation done before exploratory laparotomy?

Yes

Is a pelvic hematoma explored during laparotomy for internal injuries?

No, unless the hematoma is expanding

What vessel is at risk for injury for a pelvic fracture through the greater sciatic notch?

Superior gluteal artery, a branch of the internal iliac artery

Acetabulum Fractures

What is the basic anatomy of the acetabulum?

Rounded cavity whose walls contain anterior and posterior columns of bone that join at its dome

Which fractures do not require surgical treatment?

1. < 2 mm displacement
2. Satisfactory joint congruity

If surgery is necessary, when are these fractures usually repaired?

3 to 10 days after trauma to reduce the risk of hemorrhage

What complications are associated with acetabular fractures?	1. Sciatic nerve palsy 2. Posttraumatic arthritis 3. Heterotopic ossification that may limit hip motion

HIP

Hip Dislocation

What is the most common mechanism of injury?	Motor vehicle accident (75%)
What is the most common type of hip dislocation?	Posterior
What is the usual presentation of an anterior hip dislocation?	Externally rotated extremity with anterior hip fullness
What vascular structure can be injured with anterior dislocation?	Femoral artery
What is the usual presentation of posterior hip dislocation?	Internally rotated extremity with posterior fullness
What neurologic structure can be injured with posterior dislocation?	Sciatic nerve
What is the usual incidence of this injury?	10%
What is the usual treatment of hip dislocation?	Attempted closed reduction followed by open reduction if the dislocation is irreducible. Hip dislocation is an orthopedic emergency!
Why is closed reduction best performed in the OR?	More complete muscle relaxation can be achieved to reduce the risk of injury to the articular cartilage during closed reduction.
How is the stability of reduction assessed?	Hip is flexed to 90° in neutral rotation. If the hip redislocates, it is considered unstable.

| What are the usual indications for open reduction? | 1. Failed closed reduction
2. Incongruent reduction
3. Intra-articular debris
4. Unstable reduction |

| What intervention is sometimes needed to prevent acute redislocation? | Traction |

| What follow-up study is necessary after reduction, and why? | X-ray (or, ideally, CT scan) to evaluate for:
1. Congruency of reduction
2. Presence of intra-articular bodies, which must be surgically removed |

| What are the usual late complications after hip dislocation? | 1. Avascular necrosis (osteonecrosis) of the femoral head
2. Post-traumatic arthritis |

| What is the usual incidence of each complication? | 1. Avascular necrosis: 15% to 20% in posterior dislocation; 5% to 10% in anterior dislocation
2. Arthritis: 25% to 60% in both |

Hip Fracture

| Describe a hip fracture classification by location. | 1. Femoral neck fracture
2. Intertrochanteric fracture (fracture traverses the metaphyseal region from the greater to the lesser trochanter)
3. Subtrochanteric fracture (fracture extends in the shaft of the femur below the lesser trochanter) |

| What is the usual position of the leg of a fractured hip? | Shortened and externally rotated |

| What is the usual treatment? | Closed reduction with internal fixation. In the elderly, traction is often the first line of therapy. |

| Describe a classification of femoral neck fractures. | Garden classification:
Type I: Incomplete; valgus impaction
Type II: Complete; undisplaced
Type III: Complete; partially displaced
Type IV: Complete, totally displaced |

What is the usual treatment of Garden type I and type II fractures?	Closed reduction with internal fixation
What is the usual treatment of Garden type III and type IV fractures?	Hip replacement
What is a common complication of femoral neck fractures?	Avascular necrosis (AVN) of the femoral head
Why?	Blood supply is interrupted as it travels distally to proximally.
What factors correlate most closely with the risk of AVN in femoral neck fractures?	Closeness of the fracture to the femoral head Degree of displacement at the time of injury
What is the usual mortality rate after hip fractures: **1. In-hospital?** **2. At 1 year?**	1. 10% 2. 35%

FEMORAL SHAFT FRACTURES

What fracture commonly occurs at the same time as a femoral shaft fracture?	Ipsilateral femoral neck fracture
What is the usual treatment of adult femoral shaft fractures?	Closed intramedullary nailing (with locking screws)
What is the usual treatment of pediatric femoral shaft fractures?	Hip spica cast

KNEE INJURIES

Name the labeled structures (patella and patella tendon removed).

1. Medial collateral ligament
2. Lateral collateral ligament
3. Anterior cruciate ligament
4. Posterior cruciate ligament
5. Medial meniscus
6. Lateral meniscus

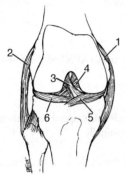

Knee Dislocations

What neurovascular structures are most commonly injured during knee dislocations?

1. Popliteal artery
2. Peroneal nerve

What is the usual incidence of injury of each structure?

Popliteal artery: 20% to 40%
Peroneal nerve: 15%

What is the usual treatment?

Closed reduction is attempted; however, open reduction may be necessary.

What study is performed after reduction?

Arteriogram to evaluate the popliteal artery

In which direction does the patella most commonly dislocate?

Laterally

What is the usual treatment?

Closed reduction by knee extension and manipulation. The dislocation often reduces spontaneously.

Why is a postreduction x-ray necessary?

To identify osteochondral fractures that require surgical repair

Knee Ligament Surgery

What is a common mechanism for rupturing the anterior cruciate ligament (ACL)?

Changing direction at high speed on a planted foot

What is the most common finding on knee aspiration after an ACL rupture?

Hemarthrosis (blood); 70% of patients with hemarthrosis and **stable** ligamentous findings actually have an ACL injury

What physical findings are consistent with ACL deficiency?

1. Increased anterior translation of the tibia on the femur with the knee in 90° flexion (**anterior drawer** test)
2. Increased translation of the tibia on the femur with the knee in 20° to 30° flexion (**Lachman** test)

What study best evaluates intra-articular abnormalities of the knee?

MRI

What intra-articular structure is most commonly injured with a traumatic ACL rupture?

Lateral meniscus

What physical finding is consistent with a medial collateral ligament rupture?

Increased pain and medial joint opening with the knee in slight flexion and valgus stress applied

What physical finding is consistent with a lateral collateral ligament rupture?

Lateral joint opening with the knee in slight flexion and valgus stress applied

What is the most sensitive physical finding that suggests an acute posterior cruciate ligament rupture?

Quadriceps active test: Increased anterior translation of the tibia on the femur from a posteriorly displaced position when the knee is actively extended against gravity from a position of flexion

What is the usual conservative therapy?

Ice, elevation, compression, immobilization, non–weight-bearing with crutches, and physical therapy

What is the usual surgical therapy?	Reconstruction of the ligament with arthroscopic assistance, using the patella tendon or a hamstring autograft

Patellar Fractures

What is a bipartite patella?	Patella with a well-defined superior-lateral secondary ossification center that is often mistaken for a fracture
What is the usual treatment of nondisplaced patellar fracture?	Cylinder cast
What is the usual indication for surgical repair of a patellar fracture?	> 3 mm of displacement or loss of the extensor mechanism

TIBIAL SHAFT FRACTURES

What complications often affect patients with tibial fractures?	1. Open fracture 2. Compartment syndrome
Why are tibial fractures prone to open wounds?	Subcutaneous position
What flap can be used for coverage of an open fracture wound in the:	
1. **Proximal one-third of the tibia?**	1. Gastrocnemius muscle
2. **Middle one-third of the tibia?**	2. Soleus muscle
3. **Distal one-third of the tibia?**	3. Free flap
What fracture configuration is most amenable to:	
1. **Intramedullary rod fixation?**	1. Transverse
2. **External fixation?**	2. Open, comminuted
3. **Casting?**	3. Spiral, nondisplaced

ANKLE AND FOOT INJURIES

What x-rays are mandatory in evaluating an ankle fracture?	AP, lateral, and mortise views

What does the mortise view evaluate?

Articular congruency (medially, superiorly, and laterally) and competency of the tibiofibular interosseous membrane

What ligament is most commonly injured in an ankle sprain?

Anterior talofibular ligament

What is the most common mechanism of ankle fracture?

Externally rotated leg on a supinated foot

What are the indications for surgery for ankle fractures?

1. Unstable ankle fractures (lateral and medial malleolus fracture or ligamentous disruption)
2. Incongruent joint after closed reduction
3. Syndesmotic rupture (disruption of the distal tibiofibular ligamentous complex)

Where does the talus usually fracture?

Talar neck

What are the complications of talus fractures?

AVN of the body or dome; severe soft tissue injury

What is the usual mechanism of injury for calcaneus fractures?

Axial load (fall from a height)

What other fracture is common with a calcaneus fracture?

Lumbar spine fracture (10%)

What is the goal of treatment of a calcaneus fracture?

1. Prevent widened heel so that the foot can fit into a shoe
2. Maintain subtalar joint congruency to minimize the risk of post-traumatic arthritis

What is a Lisfranc fracture or dislocation?

Fracture or dislocation of the base of the second metatarsal-cuneiform joint

What is the usual treatment?	Displaced injuries require anatomic reduction (open or closed) and fixation (percutaneous pin or screw).
What tendon is responsible for avulsion injuries to the base of the fifth metatarsal?	Peroneus brevis
What is the usual treatment?	Hard-soled shoe or cast for 2 to 3 weeks

COMPARTMENT SYNDROME

What injuries are particularly susceptible to compartment syndrome?	1. Tibial shaft fractures 2. Extremity vascular injuries 3. Burn injuries (thermal or electric) 4. Supracondylar elbow fractures in children
What are the most reliable symptoms of compartment syndrome?	Pain out of proportion to the expected injury
What physical findings strongly suggest compartment syndrome?	Tense or firm compartments with pain on passive stretching of the involved compartments
When are compartment pressures measured?	When exam findings are equivocal or the patient is uncooperative (e.g., head injury, intoxication)
What is the normal pressure of a compartment?	0 to 5 mm Hg
What pressure suggests compartment syndrome?	> 30 mm Hg
What is the usual treatment of compartment syndrome?	Open fasciotomy

What are the muscular and neurovascular contents of the following compartments of the leg:

1. Anterior compartment?

1. **Muscles:** Anterior tibialis, extensor hallucis longus, extensor digitorum longus, and peroneus tertius; **Nerve:** Deep peroneal; **Artery:** Anterior tibial

2. Lateral compartment?

2. **Muscles:** Peroneus longus and peroneus brevis; **Nerve:** Superficial peroneal

3. Superficial posterior compartment?

3. **Muscles:** Gastrocnemius, soleus, and plantaris

4. Deep posterior compartment?

4. **Muscles:** Posterior tibialis, flexor hallucis longus, and flexor digitorum longus; **Nerve:** Tibial; **Arteries:** Posterior tibial and peroneal

What is the sequela of compartment syndrome that is not decompressed within 4 to 6 hours?

Muscle ischemia and necrosis resulting in contracture

PEDIATRIC ORTHOPEDIC SURGERY

Name and describe the classification used for pediatric fractures.

Salter classification of fractures involving the physis (growth plate):
  I. Through the growth plate only
  II. Through the metaphysis and growth plate
  III. Through the epiphysis and growth plate
  IV. Through the epiphysis, growth plate, and metaphysis
  V. Crushed growth plate
Most "ligamentous" injuries in children are actually fractures involving the physis.

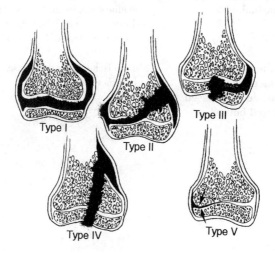

What are the undesirable effects of growth plate injuries?

Angular deformity and growth arrest with limb length discrepancy

What possibility should be investigated in children with spiral or oblique fractures?

Child abuse

What is the most commonly fractured bone in childhood?

Clavicle

LEG LENGTH DISCREPANCY

What leg length discrepancy goes unnoticed by patients?	≤ 1 cm
What leg length discrepancy can be treated with a shoe lift?	≤ 2.5 cm
What leg length discrepancy is generally treated by epiphysiodesis (i.e., limb shortening)?	2.5 to 5 cm (discrepancy > 5 cm is generally treated with limb lengthening)

HIP DISORDERS

How do hip abnormalities commonly present in children?	Knee pain referred from the hip
What nerve is responsible for this referred hip pain?	Obturator nerve
What is the differential diagnosis for a child with hip or knee pain and a waddling gait?	1. Late developmentally dysplastic hip 2. Perthes disease 3. Slipped capital femoral epiphysis
What is the usual presentation of developmentally dysplastic hips?	1. Hip "click" detected by newborn screening 2. Asymmetric skinfolds and thigh lengths in newborns Most common in girls, firstborns, and infants presenting in the breech position
What physical maneuver is used to screen a newborn's hips?	**Barlow test:** Hip is dislocated by adducting the leg while driving the hip posteriorly **Ortolani test:** Hip is reduced by abducting the leg while pulling the hip anteriorly
What is the usual treatment in a child 0 to 6 months old?	Pavlik harness (straps that hold the hips flexed and slightly abducted)

What is the usual treatment in a child > 6 months old?	Traction or surgery

Legg-Calvé-Perthes Disease

What is Legg-Calvé-Perthes disease?	Osteochondritis of the capital femoral epiphysis
What is the usual presentation?	Painless limp in a child 4 to 8 years old; knee pain
What is the differential diagnosis?	Hypothyroidism, infection, and epiphyseal dysplasia
What are the principles of treatment for Perthes disease?	1. Maintain the range of motion of the hip 2. Contain the softened revascularizing femoral head in the acetabulum during remodeling
How are these goals achieved?	Bilateral walking long leg casts fixed together with transverse bars until x-rays show that mature bone has replaced the avascular epiphysis (usually 18 months)

Slipped Capital Femoral Epiphysis

What is the usual presentation of slipped capital femoral epiphysis (SCFE)?	Painful, waddling gait in an adolescent; most common in black, obese males
What is the classic physical finding?	Obligatory external rotation with hip flexion
How is SCFE quantified?	Degree or percentage of translation of the capital femoral epiphysis in relation to the femoral neck as seen on a lateral (frog leg) hip x-ray
What steps are mandatory in the evaluation of a patient diagnosed with SCFE?	1. Evaluation of the contralateral hip ($\approx$ 25% are bilateral) 2. Endocrine evaluation to rule out hypothyroidism
What is the usual treatment?	Mandatory admission with strict non–weight-bearing until operative pinning is performed; some deformities require an osteotomy

What maneuver is avoided during the treatment of SCFE?	Forceful reduction of the hip

SCOLIOSIS

What is scoliosis?	Lateral curvature of a segment of the spine
What are the two general types?	1. Structural: Does not correct with positional changes 2. Nonstructural: Corrects with positional changes
What is the most common form of scoliosis?	Adolescent idiopathic scoliosis
What is the usual presentation?	Adolescent girl with painless curvature or asymmetric shoulders, pelvis, or rib hump (seen with forward bending)
What is the differential diagnosis?	Congenital vertebral malformation, neuromuscular disorders, tumors, or spinal dysraphism
What is the most common direction and location of adolescent idiopathic scoliosis?	Convexity to the right in the thoracic spine
What findings require further evaluation with MRI or bone scan?	1. Pain 2. Left thoracic curve 3. Neurologic compromise
Which adolescent idiopathic scoliotic curves require treatment?	Curves that are likely to progress or those that show progression. Others need serial observation until the patient reaches maturity.
How is adolescent idiopathic scoliosis treated in skeletally immature patients?	1. Bracing for curves that are 25° to 30° and show progression of 5° to 10° 2. Bracing for any curve that is 30° to 40° 3. Surgical fusion for curves > 40°
What degree of scoliosis is likely to progress in skeletally mature patients?	> 50°

What degree of curvature is associated with cardiopulmonary compromise?

> 90°

CEREBRAL PALSY (CP)

What is CP?

Nonprogressive, neuromuscular disease secondary to injury of the immature brain

What types of movement characterize CP?

Spasticity, athetosis, ataxic, and mixed

What are the patterns of movement of the extremities?

Hemiplegic (upper and lower extremities on the same side), diplegic (both lower extremities), and totally involved

What is the most common type of CP?

Spastic and diplegic

Which type has the worst prognosis for ambulation?

Totally involved

Which type has the best prognosis for ambulation?

Hemiplegic

What is the usual treatment?

Physical therapy and orthotics. Surgery is not commonly used, but may be necessary for lengthening or transplantation of the tendons, arthrodesis of the joints, or correction of limb length inequality.

MYELODYSPLASIA (SPINAL DYSRAPHISM)

What is myelodysplasia?

Defect of spinal cord closure ranging from only the posterior vertebral arch (spina bifida occulta) to exposed neural elements (rachischisis)

Compare meningocele and myelomeningocele.

Meningocele: Exposed sac protruding into the defect **without** neural elements
Myelomeningocele: Protruding sac containing neural elements

What factors determine the functional prognosis in myelodysplasia?	Level of defect and extent of neurologic injury
What is the highest level of myelodysplasia that allows ambulation?	Fourth lumbar
What muscle group is innervated by the fourth lumbar nerve roots?	Quadriceps by L2, L3, and L4
What are the usual orthopedic manifestations of myelodysplasia?	Scoliosis, dislocated hips (from unopposed flexion and adduction at the level of L3 to L4), lower extremity contraction and fractures

DUCHENNE MUSCULAR DYSTROPHY (DMD)

What is DMD?	X-linked recessive, noninflammatory disorder of progressive muscle weakness affecting young males
What is the usual presentation?	Young male with clumsiness, lumbar lordosis, and calf pseudohypertrophy
What is the Gower sign?	Child stands from the recumbent position by walking his hands up his legs.
What laboratory value supports the diagnosis of DMD?	Highly elevated creatinine phosphokinase level
What are the orthopedic manifestations of DMD?	Flexion contractures of the joints and neuromuscular scoliosis
What is the usual prognosis?	Most patients die by 20 years of age as a result of cardiopulmonary complications.

TOEING-IN

What is the differential diagnosis for pigeon toe (toeing-in gait) in a child?	1. Metatarsus adductus 2. Tibial torsion 3. Excessive femoral anteversion
Which type is the most common?	Tibial torsion

What is metatarsus adductus?	Adducted forefoot
What is the most commonly affected age-group?	First year of life
What is the usual treatment?	If flexible, stretching; if inflexible, osteotomy
What is tibial torsion?	Rotational deformity of the tibia proximally to distally
What is the most commonly affected age-group?	2 years of age
What is the usual treatment?	None. Spontaneous resolution is the norm.
What is femoral anteversion?	Increased internal rotation of the femur in relation to the femoral neck and head
What is the most commonly affected age-group?	3 to 6 years of age
What is the usual treatment?	Spontaneous resolution by 10 years of age is the norm.

SEPTIC ARTHRITIS

What is the usual presentation?	Progressive hip pain, inability to hold weight on the affected leg, and recent history of upper respiratory infection
What percentage of septic joints have positive culture findings on aspiration?	Only 50%; therefore, blood cultures are mandatory
What is the usual treatment?	Operative incision and drainage; IV antibiotics

JOINT RECONSTRUCTION

What three forms of arthritis commonly require joint replacement?	1. Osteoarthritis 2. Rheumatoid arthritis 3. AVN

What are the radiographic hallmarks of osteoarthritis?

Loss of joint space, periarticular osteophytes, subchondral sclerosis, and subchondral cyst formation

What are the radiographic hallmarks of rheumatoid arthritis?

Periarticular erosions and osteopenia

What are the radiographic hallmarks of AVN of the femoral head?

Stage I: Normal x-ray findings; decreased signal by MRI

Stage II: Femoral head that has subchondral radiodensity or radiolucency, but no collapse

Stage III: Femoral head that has collapse, with a "crescent sign" and no acetabular involvement

Stage IV: Femoral head involvement with acetabular involvement

Describe the ideal candidate for joint replacement surgery.

Elderly patient with debilitating pain localized to a joint and radiographic evidence of arthritis; failed nonoperative treatment

What are the classic nonoperative treatment modalities?

Unloading of joints through weight loss or a cane; support of joints through muscle strengthening or bracing; and relief of symptoms with an NSAID or joint injections with anesthetics and steroids

What are the contraindications to joint replacement surgery?

1. Active infection
2. Neurologic compromise
3. Young, active patient

What surgical options are available for the young patient with debilitating arthritis?

1. Osteotomy: Controlled fracture of the bone and fixation to correct the alignment
2. Arthrodesis: Joint fusion

What are the major complications after total hip arthroplasty (replacement) and the incidence of each?

1. Deep venous thrombosis: 70% (by venogram)
2. Infection: 1%
3. Dislocation: 1% to 5%

What structures are at risk because of screw penetration of the inner wall of the acetabulum during total hip arthroplasty?	1. External iliac artery and vein in the anterior superior quadrant 2. Obturator nerve artery and vein in the anterior inferior quadrant

FOOT

DIABETIC FOOT

What two entities in patients with diabetes cause deformity and radiographic obliteration of the affected joints?	1. Infection 2. Neuropathic joint (Charcot joint)
How do these two entities differ?	Charcot joint presents with a swollen, warm, relatively painless deformed foot with no systemic fever and a low WBC count.
What is the usual treatment of Charcot joint?	Immobilization in a cast until the inflammation resolves

FLATFOOT

What is the differential diagnosis for flatfoot in adulthood?	1. Posterior tibial tendon rupture 2. Talonavicular arthritis 3. Neuropathic arthritis
What is the differential diagnosis for rigid flatfoot in childhood?	1. Tarsal coalition 2. Congenital vertical talus
When is treatment of flatfoot indicated?	When it becomes painful
What is the usual treatment?	Flexible flatfoot is generally treated with orthotics (arch supports). Rigid flatfoot requires surgical correction.

TOE ABNORMALITIES

What is a claw toe?	Extended metatarsal phalangeal (MTP) joint and flexed proximal interphalangeal (PIP) and distal interphalangeal (DIP) joints

What is a hammer toe?	Flexed PIP joint ± extended MTP joint
What is a mallet toe?	Flexed DIP joint
What is the most common cause of deformed toes?	Narrow toe box of shoes

SPINE

LOW BACK PAIN

What is the most common cause of low back pain in children?	Spondylolysis
What are the common intrinsic spine disorders of children with back pain?	Congenital, developmental, and infectious disorders; tumors
What are the common intrinsic spine disorders of young adults with back pain?	Disk disease, spondylolisthesis, and acute fractures
What are the common intrinsic spine disorders of older adults with back pain?	Spinal stenosis, metastatic disease, and osteoporotic compression fractures
What percentage of the population shows evidence of herniated nucleus pulposus by MRI?	≈ 30%; most are asymptomatic

SPONDYLOLYSIS

What is spondylolysis?	Bony defect in the pars interarticularis, usually caused by a fatigue fracture
What x-ray views best show spondylolysis?	Oblique lumbar spine views, which show a break in the neck of the "Scottie dog"
What is the usual treatment of spondylolysis?	Asymptomatic spondylolysis is not treated. Symptomatic cases are treated with activity restrictions and, rarely, fusion.

SPONDYLOLISTHESIS

What is spondylolisthesis?	Slippage of one vertebra on another
What are the causes of spondylolisthesis?	Congenital, elongation of the pars interarticularis, degenerative, traumatic, pathologic, and postsurgical
What is the usual presentation of childhood spondylolisthesis?	Tight hamstrings, low back pain
At what level does childhood spondylolisthesis typically occur?	L5 to S1
At what level does adult degenerative spondylolisthesis usually occur?	L4 to L5
What is the usual treatment of spondylolisthesis?	Mild slips are treated with activity restriction until symptoms disappear. Severe slips are treated with fusion.

INFECTIONS

What is Pott disease?	Tuberculosis infection of the spine
What is the usual presentation?	Back pain, ± fever and weight loss, in an exposed or immunocompromised patient
What is the usual treatment?	Immobilization and IV antibiotics; if this treatment fails, then surgical débridement and stabilization
How is pyogenic vertebral osteomyelitis differentiated radiographically from tumor?	Infection often involves the disk space; tumor commonly spares the disk space.

TUMORS

What is the usual treatment for extremity tumors?	Wide excision or amputation; adjunctive chemotherapy or radiation therapy

SOFT TISSUE TUMORS

What is the most common soft tissue sarcoma of late adulthood?

Malignant fibrous histiocytoma

What is the most common soft tissue mesenchymal tumor?

Lipoma

What is the most common soft tissue sarcoma of childhood?

Rhabdomyosarcoma

What is the most common sarcoma of the hand?

Epithelioid sarcoma

BONE TUMORS

What is the most common malignancy of bone?

Metastatic disease

What is the most common tumor of the spine?

Metastatic disease

What primary malignancies commonly metastasize to bone in adults?

Breast, lung, prostate, kidney, and thyroid carcinoma

What primary malignancies commonly metastasize to bone in children?

Neuroblastoma and Wilms tumor (hypernephroma)

What is the usual treatment of metastatic disease to the bone?

Radiation therapy and, in some cases, prophylactic fixation

What is the most common benign primary bone tumor?

Nonossifying fibroma

Primary Bone Malignancies

What is the most common primary bone malignancy in adults?

Multiple myeloma

What are the most common primary bone malignancies in children and adolescents?	1. Osteosarcoma 2. Ewing sarcoma
What is the most common location for each type?	Both are usually found in the region of the knee (distal knee, proximal tibia).
What are the classic radiographic findings for each type?	1. Osteosarcoma: Sunburst pattern 2. Ewing sarcoma: "Onion skinning" pattern
What is the usual treatment?	1. Osteosarcoma: Wide or radical excision with multiagent chemotherapy 2. Ewing sarcoma: Chemotherapy with wide excision or radiation therapy

Unicameral Bone Cyst

What is a unicameral bone cyst?	Benign fluid-filled cyst found in bone
What is the most common location?	Proximal humerus
What is the most common age-group?	5 to 15 years
What is the usual presentation?	Pain or pathologic fracture
What is the usual treatment?	Steroid injections

INFECTION

SEPTIC ARTHRITIS

What is the most common route of infection that causes a septic joint?	Hematogenous
What is the usual presentation of bacterial septic arthritis?	Localized joint pain, erythema, warmth, swelling with pain on active and passive range of motion, inability to bear weight, ± fever

**What are the components
of the diagnostic
evaluation?**

X-ray (to rule out osteomyelitis),
erythrocyte sedimentation rate, WBC
count, blood cultures, and aspirate

**What findings on aspirate
are diagnostic of infection?**

1. WBC > 80,000; > 90% neutrophils
2. Protein level > 4.4 gm/dl
3. Glucose level significantly < blood
   glucose level
4. No crystals
5. Positive gram stain results

**What is the most common
organism that causes
septic arthritis?**

Staphylococcus aureus

**What other organism must
be considered in a sexually
active patient?**

Neisseria gonorrhoeae

**What is the usual
treatment of septic
arthritis?**

1. Hip joint is emergently decompressed
   and drained surgically; other joints
   may be serially aspirated
2. IV antibiotics

OSTEOMYELITIS

**What is the usual
presentation of
osteomyelitis?**

Localized extremity pain, ± fever, 1 to 2
weeks after respiratory infection or
infection at another nonbony site

**What is the most common
organism in the
bacteriology of
osteomyelitis?**

S. aureus

**Which patients are
susceptible to gram-
negative organisms?**

Neonates and immunocompromised
patients

**Which additional organism
is common in patients with
sickle cell disease?**

Salmonella

**What classic radiographic
findings are associated
with osteomyelitis?**

Lytic, eccentrically located serpiginous
lesion involving the cortex

What other studies confirm the diagnosis?	Blood cultures, aspirate cultures, erythrocyte sedimentation rate, leukocytosis, and increased uptake on bone scan
What other organism must be considered when osteomyelitis occurs in a child < 5 years old?	*Haemophilus influenzae*
What organisms must be considered in the IV drug abuser?	Gram-negative organisms and *Pseudomonas aeruginosa*
What organism must be considered in the patient with sickle cell disease?	*Salmonella typhi*
What organism must be considered in patients with foot puncture wounds?	*Pseudomonas*
What is the usual treatment of osteomyelitis?	Surgical decortication and drainage; IV antibiotics

MISCELLANEOUS ORTHOPEDIC TOPICS

COMMONLY MISSED ORTHOPEDIC INJURIES

List some commonly missed orthopedic injuries.	1. Carpal bone injuries, especially scaphoid 2. Radial head fractures 3. Posterior dislocation of the shoulder 4. Patellar tendon tears 5. Compartment syndrome 6. Rotational deformities of metacarpal and phalangeal fractures 7. Tendon injuries of the hand 8. Femoral neck fractures in the elderly
How should potential injuries in these regions be managed by the nonorthopedist?	1. Immobilization 2. Repeat x-rays in 7 to 10 days An orthopedic surgeon should be consulted if there is any doubt.

COMMON EPONYMS

Name the following fractures or overuse injuries:

1. **Distal radial fracture with dorsal displacement?**

   1. Colles, which usually occurs secondary to a fall on an outstretched hand

2. **Lunate fracture?**

   2. Kienböck

3. **Radial fracture at the junction of the middle and distal thirds, with distal radial–ulnar dislocation?**

   3. Galeazzi

4. **Avulsion of the anterior glenoid labrum?**

   4. Bankart

5. **Tarsal–metatarsal fracture or dislocation?**

   5. Lisfranc

6. **Fifth metatarsal shaft fracture?**

   6. Jones

7. **Radial head subluxation in a child?**

   7. Nursemaid's elbow

8. **Tibial tuberosity osteochondrosis?**

   8. Osgood-Schlatter

9. **Osteochondrosis of the navicular bone?**

   9. Kohler

10. **Fracture of the distal fibula?**

    10. Pott

11. **Fracture of the spinous process of C7?**

    11. Clay shoveler's

12. **Fracture of the pedicles of C2?**

    12. Hangman's

13. **Fracture of the metacarpal neck?**

    13. Boxer's; classically, the fifth digit

BIOMECHANICS

What is stress?	Force per unit area
What is strain?	Change in length divided by the original length
What is the Wolfe law?	Bone is formed along the lines of stress and resorbed from areas without stress.
What is stress shielding?	A rigid implant removes the stress from an area of bone, and the bone weakens as a response to the Wolfe law.

Which of the following common orthopedic materials most closely matches the rigidity of bone: stainless steel, titanium, polymethyl methacrylate (PMMA; cement), or polyethylene?	PMMA
What type of force does bone most strongly resist?	Compression
What type of force does ligament or tendon most strongly resist?	Tension

GAIT ANALYSIS

Where is the center of gravity for the human body?	Just anterior to sacral vertebra 2
How far does the center of gravity move during gait?	Horizontal and vertical oscillation of 5 cm
What is a concentric contraction?	Muscle fires while shortening (e.g., a person is about to jump)
What is an eccentric contraction?	Muscle fires while lengthening (e.g., a person is landing from a jump)
Are most muscles of the lower extremity most active during concentric or eccentric contraction?	Eccentric
What percentage of gait is spent in stance?	≈ 60%
What is the increased energy expenditure during gait with: 1. Unilateral below-the-knee amputation? 2. Bilateral below-the-knee amputation? 3. Unilateral above-the-knee amputation?	1. 25% 2. 40% 3. 60%

PERIPHERAL MOTOR NERVE INJURY

For each listed nerve, identify the contributing spinal levels and the motor test used to evaluate motor function:

1. **Axillary nerve?**
2. **Musculocutaneous nerve?**
3. **Radial nerve?**
4. **Median nerve?**

5. **Ulnar nerve?**

6. **Femoral nerve?**
7. **Obturator nerve?**
8. **Superior gluteal nerve?**
9. **Inferior gluteal nerve?**
10. **Tibial nerve (sciatic nerve)?**
11. **Deep peroneal nerve (sciatic nerve)?**

1. C5 to C6; abduction of the shoulder
2. C5 to C6; flexion of the elbow

3. C6 to C8; extension of the thumb
4. C6 to T1; flexion of the thumb interphalangeal joint
5. C7 to T1; abduction of the index finger

6. L2 to L4; extension of the knee
7. L2 to L4; adduction of the hip
8. L5; abduction of the hip
9. S1; extension of the hip
10. L4 to S3; plantar flexion of the toe and ankle
11. L4 to S2; dorsiflexion of the toe

DEFINITIONS

Define the following terms:

1. **Valgus?**
2. **Varus?**

3. **Dislocation?**

4. **Subluxation?**

5. **Osteotomy?**
6. **Arthrodesis?**

7. **Arthrometer?**

8. **Arthroplasty?**
9. **Volkmann contracture?**

10. **Dupuytren contracture?**

1. Turned inward (toward the midline)
2. Turned outward (away from the midline)
3. Complete loss of congruity between the articular surfaces of a joint
4. Partial loss of congruity between the articular surfaces
5. Cutting of bone for realignment
6. Surgical immobilization or fusion of a joint
7. Instrument to measure the degree of movement of a joint
8. Joint replacement or reconstruction
9. Contractures of the forearm flexors (because of compartment syndrome)
10. Contracture (thickening) of the palmar fascia

49

Otolaryngology Head and Neck Surgery

Brian Romaneschi, MD
Philip Pollice, MD

SALIVARY GLANDS

ANATOMY

What are the major salivary glands?

1. Parotid
2. Submandibular
3. Sublingual

Where are the minor salivary glands?

The entire oral cavity and upper aerodigestive tract (600–1000 glands)

What is the general location for each major salivary gland duct?

1. Parotid—Stensen's (at 2nd maxillary molar)
2. Submandibular—Wharton's (in floor of mouth)
3. Sublingual—multiple ducts (in floor of mouth)

What are the primary secretory cell types for each major salivary gland?

1. Parotid—Serous
2. Submandibular—Both serous and mucous
3. Sublingual—Mucous

Which intraoperative technique is most frequently used to find the facial nerve within the parotid gland?

Identification of the nerve at the stylomastoid foramen where it exits the skull and trace distally. Alternatively, a branch may be identified peripherally and traced proximally.

What are the motor branches of the facial nerve?

1. Temporal
2. Zygomatic
3. Buccal
4. Mandibular
5. Cervical
(CN VII supplies innervation to all muscles of facial expression.)

Which three nerves are in close proximity to the submandibular gland?	1. Marginal mandibular nerve (CN VII)→Superficial 2. Lingual nerve (CN V)→Deep and superior 3. Hypoglossal nerve (CN XII)→Deep to anterior belly of digastric muscle

SALIVARY GLAND TRAUMA

How is traumatic disruption of the extratemporal facial nerve managed?	Immediate primary repair
Which disruptive extratemporal facial nerve injuries do NOT require repair, and why?	Those lying medial to a vertical line through the lateral canthus or involving the cervical branch. The nerve will regenerate spontaneously.
Which surgical principles improve reinnervation following facial nerve repair?	Use of operating microscope to align fascicles, anastomosis with fresh, sharp nerve edges, atraumatic nerve handling, minimal number of sutures (usually four 8–0 to 10–0 monofilament), and avoidance of tension or crowding
How is traumatic facial nerve paresis managed?	Expectantly, because function usually returns with time
Which structures are likely to be injured by a vertical laceration near the anterior border of the masseter muscle?	1. Stensen's duct 2. Buccal branch of CN VII
How is duct injury managed?	Repair over polyethylene stent (6–0 to 7–0 monofilament); leave stent in place for 10 days
What are the complications of salivary gland duct injury?	1. Stricture 2. Obstruction 3. Sialoceles (stones) 4. Fistulas

ONCOLOGIC LESIONS OF THE SALIVARY GLANDS

What percentage of head and neck tumors are salivary gland tumors?	Only 5%

What is the most common site of salivary gland tumor?

Parotid gland (80%). (Tumors in the submandibular gland account for 10%–15%, and those in the sublingual or minor glands account for the remaining 5%–10%.)

What are the relative incidences of benign versus malignant tumors for each salivary gland?

1. Parotid: **80% benign;** 20% malignant
2. Submandibular: 50% benign; **50% malignant**
3. Sublingual: 40% benign; 60% malignant
4. Minor salivary: 25% benign; **75% malignant**

(The **smaller** the gland, the **higher** the incidence of malignancy.)

Which benign neoplasms are most common?

1. Pleomorphic (benign mixed) adenoma—70%
2. Warthin's tumor (papillary cystadenoma lymphomatosum, adenolymphoma)

Which malignant neoplasms are most common?

1. Mucoepidermoid carcinoma
2. Adenoid cystic carcinoma (cylindroma)

Which histologic types are considered low-grade malignancies?

1. Low-grade mucoepidermoid carcinoma
2. Acinic-cell carcinoma

Which histologic types are considered high-grade malignancies?

1. High-grade mucoepidermoid carcinoma
2. Adenoid cystic carcinoma (cylindroma)
3. Squamous cell carcinoma
4. Adenocarcinoma
5. Undifferentiated carcinoma
6. Ex-mixed tumor

Which childhood salivary gland neoplasm is the most common?

Hemangioma (Capillary hemangiomas tend to occur in infancy, whereas cavernous hemangiomas are seen in older children.)

What are the physical signs of parotid malignancy?

1. Facial nerve paralysis
2. Lymphadenopathy
3. Skin changes
4. Pain (associated but **not** diagnostic for malignancy)

How is salivary gland tumor stage determined?

Tumor size

What is the diagnostic workup for a parotid mass?

Fine-needle aspiration (FNA), superficial parotidectomy (resection of parotid superficial to facial nerve), or both. Open incisional biopsies are not indicated.

What important information can CT scan or MRI provide?

Tumor extension into deep lobe of parotid gland, presence of parapharyngeal extension, nodal involvement, extension into skull, or carotid encasement

What is the basic TMN staging system for salivary gland tumors?

T1: Tumor < 2 cm
T2: Tumor 2 to 4 cm
T3: Tumor > 4 cm
N0: No regional nodal involvement
N1: Palpable nodes
M0: No distant metastasis
M1: Distant metastasis

What is the management of benign or low-grade malignant neoplasms?

1. Parotid→Superficial parotidectomy
2. Submandibular→Excision of mass (with rim of normal gland)
3. Sublingual→Excision

What is the surgical management of high-grade malignant neoplasms?

1. Parotid→Total parotidectomy with excision of involved facial nerve branches
2. Submandibular→Excision including involved surrounding tissue
3. Sublingual→Excision including involved surrounding tissue

What are the indications for radical neck dissection?

1. Enlarged, palpable lymph nodes
2. Any large or rapidly growing tumors
3. Small tumors of selected histologic types, including squamous cell, adenoid cystic, malignant mixed tumor, or high-grade mucoepidermoid carcinoma

What are the indications for postoperative radiation (XRT)?

1. High-grade malignancies
2. Residual disease
3. Recurrent disease
4. Invasion of adjacent structures
5. T3 or T4 parotid malignancies

What are the indications for chemotherapy?
Currently, no successful chemotherapeutic regimen is available.

What is the 5-year survival rate from mucoepidermoid carcinoma?
Low grade (85%–95%); high grade (30%–45%)

SIALADENITIS

What is sialadenitis?
Inflammation of the salivary gland

What causes sialadenitis?
1. Infection
2. Obstruction of duct by calculi, stricture, or mucus plug

Infectious Sialadenitis

How does infectious sialadenitis present?
Unilateral gland pain, fever, swelling, pus from duct orifice, and leukocytosis

What are the causes of infectious sialadenitis?
1. Viral (CMV, coxsackie virus, and mumps)
2. Bacterial (Anaerobes, *Escherichia coli, Haemophilus influenzae, Staphylococcus aureus,* and *Streptococcus*)

Which of these infectious etiologies are most common?
1. Mumps
2. *Staphylococcus aureus*

What is the treatment of infectious sialadenitis?
1. Hydration, massage, sialogogues (agents that stimulate secretion of saliva, such as lemon juice), and warm compresses for symptomatic relief
2. Antibiotics for bacterial etiologies
3. Failure of antibiotics after 1 week of therapy; recurrences and multiple stones may mandate surgical excision of gland

What is the most common cause of acute suppurative parotiditis?
Staphylococcus aureus

Which group of patients is at risk for acute suppurative parotiditis?
Debilitated patients who have a tendency toward dehydration and do not maintain good oral hygiene

What is the treatment of acute suppurative parotiditis?	Same as that of sialadenitis. Surgical drainage may be required if abscess develops.

Sialolithiasis

Which salivary gland is most commonly affected by calculi?	Submandibular—80% (versus parotid only 20%)
What percentage of salivary gland calculi are radiopaque?	Depends on the location (90% of calculi in the submandibular gland versus only 10% in the parotid gland). Overall, approximately 75% are radiopaque.
What are the symptoms?	Recurrent swelling and pain associated with eating
How is the condition diagnosed?	Plain films, sialography (injection of contrast dye through duct orifice), ultrasound, or CT scan
What is the initial treatment?	Conservative. Oral hydration (to stimulate salivary flow) and sialagogues
What is the treatment of chronic sialadenitis?	1. Stone removal (if distal) via duct papillotomy or excision of papilla 2. Gland excision (if proximal)

LARYNX

ANATOMY

What are the anatomic borders of the larynx?	Inferior: Inferior border of cricoid cartilage Superior: Tip of epiglottis and aryepiglottic folds Anterior: Thyroid cartilage Posterior: Posterior cricoid, arytenoid cartilages, and interarytenoid tissue
What are the three anatomic regions of the larynx?	1. Glottis: From between the true and false cords to 1 cm inferior to the vocal folds 2. Supraglottis: From the superior glottis to the tip of epiglottis and superior border of hyoid 3. Subglottis: From the inferior glottis to the inferior edge of cricoid

What are the cartilaginous components of the larynx?

1. Thyroid cartilage
2. Cricoid cartilage
3. Arytenoid (and corniculate) cartilages
4. Epiglottic cartilage

What are the numbered structures in this midsagittal view of the right larynx?

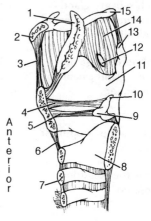

1. Epiglottis
2. Body of hyoid bone
3. Median thyrohyoid ligament
4. Vestibular ligament
5. Vocal ligament
6. Cricoid membrane
7. Tracheal ring
8. Cricothyroid cartilage
9. Arytenoid cartilage
10. Corniculate cartilage
11. Thyroid cartilage
12. Foramen for superior laryngeal nerve and artery
13. Superior horn of thyroid cartilage
14. Thyrohyoid membrane
15. Greater horn of hyoid bone

Which nerves innervate the larynx?

Superior and inferior laryngeal nerves from vagus nerve

Which sensory regions and muscles do these nerves innervate?

Superior laryngeal nerve
1. Sensory to supraglottis
2. Motor to cricothyroid muscle (external branch of superior laryngeal nerve)

Inferior laryngeal nerve
1. Sensory to glottis and subglottis
2. Motor to all other intrinsic laryngeal muscles

What is the arterial supply to the larynx?

1. Superior laryngeal artery (Branch of superior thyroid artery from external carotid artery)
2. Inferior laryngeal artery (Branch of inferior thyroid artery from thyrocervical trunk)

In order of importance, what are the three basic functions of the larynx?

1. Airway protection
2. Respiration
3. Vocalization

CONGENITAL LARYNGEAL DISEASE

What is the classic sign of upper airway obstruction?

Stridor (audible noise produced by turbulence)

How can the "phase" of stridor be used to localize the site of obstruction?

1. Supraglottic (Inspiratory)
2. Glottic (Biphasic)
3. Subglottic (Expiratory)

What is the most common cause of CHRONIC pediatric stridor?

Laryngomalacia (Self-limited disorder worsening from birth to 6 months and resolving spontaneously by 12 to 18 months of age)

What are the fiberoptic exam findings in laryngomalacia?

Inspiratory collapse of aryepiglottic folds and arytenoid cartilages

What are other causes of congenital stridor?

Subglottic stenosis, hemangioma, laryngeal papilloma, vocal fold paralysis, and vascular anomalies

What is the most common benign pediatric laryngeal tumor?

Papilloma

What is the etiology of this tumor?

Human papilloma virus (HPV)

What is the natural course of laryngeal papilloma after excision?

Recurrence (repeated CO_2 laser excisions are the rule with timing based on obstructive symptoms)

What is the treatment of hemangioma?

Observation. These lesions typically regress spontaneously. However, airway involvement may require tracheostomy, CO_2 laser, XRT, steroids, embolization, or other surgery.

What is the treatment of lymphangioma?

Resection. Lymphangiomas are unlikely to regress.

What are the most common causes of recurrent laryngeal nerve paralysis in children?

1. Cardiac surgery (injury to recurrent laryngeal nerve)
2. Central lesions (hydrocephalus and Arnold-Chiari malformation)

Which vascular anomalies cause tracheal compression?

1. Anomalous innominate artery
2. Vascular rings

LARYNGEAL TRAUMA

What are the symptoms of acute laryngeal trauma?

Hoarseness, pain, dyspnea, and dysphagia

What are the signs of acute laryngeal trauma?

Stridor, hemoptysis, subcutaneous emphysema, loss of laryngeal prominence, and palpable interruption of laryngeal cartilage

What is the FIRST step in the evaluation and management of the patient with acute laryngeal trauma?

Stabilization of the airway (observation versus tracheotomy or cautious intubation)

In the setting of a stable airway, what is the next diagnostic step?

Fiberoptic exam. If abnormal, CT scan may help determine whether surgical intervention is needed.

What is the management of impending airway obstruction?

Tracheostomy versus intubation followed by direct laryngoscopy and esophagoscopy (with findings determining necessity for open surgical repair). Note: Less experienced surgeons should perform cricothyrotomy instead of tracheostomy in the emergent setting because it is easier and safer.

What is the management of impending airway obstruction in children?	Tracheostomy after stabilizing the airway using a ventilating bronchoscope
What is the most common injury to the larynx?	Vertical fracture of thyroid cartilage $\pm$ cricoid cartilage
Which laryngeal injuries can be managed expectantly?	Laryngeal edema, small hematomas with intact mucosa, small lacerations without exposed cartilage, and single nondisplaced thyroid cartilage fractures
What is the conservative therapy for laryngeal injury?	Cool humidified oxygen, IV fluids, $\pm$ penicillin, $\pm$ corticosteroids
What are the indications for surgical management?	Comminuted laryngeal fracture, exposed cartilage, large mucosal laceration, vocal fold immobility, arytenoid dislocation, or disruption of the anterior commissure
What should be done intraoperatively if a high tracheostomy or cricothyrotomy is performed emergently, and why?	Revise as soon as possible to tracheostomy at third or fourth tracheal ring. Reduces incidence of vocal cord paralysis or subglottic stenosis.

ONCOLOGICAL LESIONS OF THE LARYNX

What percentage of head and neck tumors are laryngeal tumors?	Only 2% to 3%
What is the classic symptom of laryngeal cancer?	Voice change (hoarseness)
What other symptoms may be present?	Dyspnea, stridor, hemoptysis, odynophagia, dysphagia, otalgia, neck masses, and weight loss
What are the risk factors?	Tobacco abuse raises risk ($\approx$ 10 times); higher risk also with alcohol abuse, radiation, and certain occupations (nickel- and woodworkers)

Which laryngeal region is most commonly involved?	Glottis (66%) > supraglottis
Specifically, what is the most common site?	Anterior portion of true cords
What is the predominant histologic type?	Squamous cell carcinoma (> 90%)
How is tumor stage determined?	Site of involvement; with advanced cancer, tumor fixes the cords, extends beyond the larynx, invades cartilage, or a combination of these conditions.
What does the workup include?	Laryngoscopy, bronchoscopy, esophagoscopy and biopsy, CT scan, CXR, liver function tests and barium swallow
What are the metastatic sites?	Neck (Distant metastases are unusual but involve lung and mediastinum.)
Are metastases more common with glottic or supraglottic tumors?	Supraglottic
What is the treatment?	1. Radiation therapy is most useful for early lesions. 2. Surgery is useful for early to advanced cancers. Options include endoscopic tumor excision off the cord, supraglottic laryngectomy, hemilaryngectomy, or total laryngectomy. 3. Combination therapy improves survival with advanced disease.
What are the indications for neck dissection?	Clinically evident neck nodes by physical exam or CT scan. (Note: N0 neck dissection is controversial.)
What are the indications for chemotherapy?	Currently, no successful chemotherapeutic regimen is available.

LARYNGEAL INFECTIONS

What are the most common infectious causes of acute stridor in children?	1. Laryngotracheobronchitis 2. Croup

Croup

What is croup?	Viral inflammation of subglottis and larynx
What is the usual etiology?	Parainfluenza virus
Which age-group is at risk?	Usually ages 6 months to 3 years
What is the classic presentation of croup?	Barking cough (seal-like), biphasic stridor, and low-grade fever
What is the classic x-ray finding?	Steeple sign on the AP neck films (caused by subglottic narrowing)
How is uncomplicated croup managed?	At home without medication
How is croup with respiratory distress managed?	Hospitalization, aerosolized racemic epinephrine, cool humidification, ± steroids. Keep child calm. Rarely, tracheostomy is necessary.
What is the usual course of croup?	Resolves in 3 to 4 days
To what other infection may croup progress?	Bacterial tracheitis (*Staphylococcus* or *Streptococcus*)
How does bacterial tracheitis present?	Respiratory distress and high fevers
What are the diagnosis and treatment of bacterial tracheitis?	1. Endoscopy is both diagnostic and therapeutic; may require intubation. 2. IV antibiotics

Epiglottitis

What is epiglottitis?	Rapidly progressive infection of epiglottis
What is its usual etiology?	*Haemophilus influenzae* type B (HIB)

Which age-group is at risk?	Usually 1 to 5 year olds
How does epiglottitis present?	Upper respiratory infection progressing to high fever (40° C), severe throat pain, and respiratory distress. Child assumes sitting position, *leans forward*, drooling, and has severe inspiratory stridor.
What are the classic x-ray findings?	"Thumbprint" sign on lateral neck film (caused by epiglottic swelling)
What is the treatment of epiglottitis?	1. Immediately to the OR for intubation or tracheostomy. Do not attempt to visualize in the ER because laryngospasm and acute airway obstruction may occur! 2. IV antibiotics (second- or third-generation cephalosporins) 3. ± Steroids

Laryngitis

What is the most common infectious etiology of laryngitis?	Rhinovirus. (Note: *Streptococcus* and *Haemophilus* may also cause laryngitis.)
What is the treatment?	Usually self-limited. Voice rest and humidification. ± antibiotics (amoxicillin) if bacterial etiology is suspected

RECONSTRUCTIVE AND REHABILITATIVE LARYNGEAL SURGERY

What are the common non-neoplastic causes of hoarseness in adults?	Vocal cord (VC) nodules and polyps
What is the cause of VC nodules?	Voice abuse
What is the cause of VC polyps?	Smoking, gastroesophageal reflux, and voice abuse
What is the histologic appearance of VC nodules?	Epithelial hyperplasia and submucosal connective tissue fibrosis

What is the histologic appearance of VC polyps?	Subepithelial edema

What is the treatment of nodules and polyps?	Medical: Removal of offending agents, voice therapy Surgical: Microsurgical excision

What is the result of unilateral VC immobility?	1. Voice disturbance 2. Airway protective deficits

What is the rehabilitative therapy for these entities?	1. Vocal cord injections (temporary medialization possible with Gelfoam) 2. Medialization thyroplasty

NOSE, PARANASAL SINUSES, AND FACE

ANATOMY

What are the paranasal sinuses?	1. Maxillary sinuses 2. Ethmoid (anterior and posterior) sinuses 3. Frontal sinuses 4. Sphenoid sinus

What is the first sinus to develop?	Maxillary

At what age do the sinuses reach their final size?	Maxillary: Present at birth; biphasic growth age 3 and 7 to 18 Ethmoid: Present at birth; full size by age 12 Frontal: Rarely demonstrable radiographically before age 2; full size by 16 to 19 Sphenoid: Pneumatizes at age 4 to 5; full size by age 12 to 15

Which sinus is aplastic in > 5% of patients?	Frontal

Where is each paranasal sinus ostia located?	Maxillary: Middle meatus Anterior ethmoid: Middle meatus Posterior ethmoid: Superior meatus Frontal: Middle meatus Sphenoid: Sphenoethmoidal recess

Where is the lacrimal gland ostium located?	Inferior meatus
What are the components of the cartilaginous framework of the nose?	Upper lateral cartilages, lower lateral cartilages, cartilaginous septum, and sesamoid cartilages
What structures contribute to formation of the nasal septum?	Quadrangular cartilage, perpendicular plate of the ethmoid, vomer, maxillary crest, and palatine bone

What is the arterial supply of the nose and their sources?

1. Anterior and posterior ethmoid arteries (Branches of the ophthalmic artery from the internal carotid artery)
2. Sphenopalatine and greater palatine arteries (Branches of the internal maxillary artery from the external carotid artery)
3. Superior labial artery (Branch of the facial artery from the exterior carotid artery)

Why are the veins of the face likely to propagate septic emboli to the brain?	Facial veins are valveless.

CONGENITAL LESIONS TO THE FACE

Which condition is likely to be present in a newborn with cyclic respiratory distress relieved by crying and opening the mouth?	Bilateral choanal atresia—Bony or membranous obstruction of the posterior nasal passageway (Note: Atresia is usually unilateral with no respiratory distress.)
Why does bilateral atresia cause respiratory distress?	Infants are obligate nose breathers.
How is choanal atresia diagnosed?	Inability to pass a catheter beyond 32 mm past the nares. CT scan is confirmatory.
What is the treatment of choanal atresia?	Transnasal or transpalatal repair with stenting

What are the congenital midline nasal lesions?

1. Dermoid
2. Encephaloceles
3. Gliomas

What are the clinical findings of each type of congenital midline nasal lesion?	1. Dermoids→A pit or fistulous tract [epithelium-lined] between glabella and nasal tip; hair and sebaceous contents 2. Encephaloceles→Soft pulsatile mass that enlarges with straining; direct herniation through fonticulus of dura and brain 3. Gliomas→Intra- or extranasal firm mass that does not change size with straining; contains brain tissue and probably represents an encephalocele that is separated from brain by bony closure
Which condition has the highest risk of meningitis?	Encephaloceles
What is the incidence of CNS attachment for each type?	1. Dermoids: rare 2. Encephaloceles: 100% 3. Gliomas: 15%

FACIAL TRAUMA

Epistaxis

What is the most common site of spontaneous nasal hemorrhage or epistaxis?	Erosion of superficial blood vessel in Kiesselbach's plexus (a confluence of vessels at the anterior nasal septum (contributing vessels include greater palatine, sphenopalatine, anterior ethmoid, and superior labial arteries)
What is the most common source of posterior epistaxis?	Sphenopalatine arteries
What are the causes of epistaxis?	Trauma, inflammation, foreign bodies, hypertension, Osler-Weber-Rendu (hereditary hemorrhagic telangiectasia), arteriosclerosis, blood dsycrasias, and renal failure
What tumor must be ruled out in pubescent males with epistaxis?	Juvenile angiofibroma→purplish polypoid mass that is nonmetastasizing but locally aggressive
What is the treatment of this tumor?	Excision after pre-op embolization

What is the management for epistaxis?	1. Upright position, local pressure, cool compresses, control of hypertension, fluid/blood resuscitation 2. Anterior or posterior packing; silver nitrate cauterization; balloon (30-cc Foley) tamponade; arterial embolization, endoscopic cauterization, or both
What surgical intervention is indicated if these measures fail?	Internal maxillary artery ± anterior/posterior ethmoid arteries ligations via Caldwell-Luc approach

Nasal Bone Fractures

What are the indications for reduction of nasal bone fractures?	Unsatisfactory external appearance or functional deficits
What is the ideal timing for repair?	Within 3 to 7 days (i.e., does not require urgent repair)

Traumatic Septal Hematoma

What is the treatment of traumatic septal hematoma?	Urgent incision and drainage (may use Penrose drain and nasal packing)
Why?	To prevent cartilage necrosis and resulting saddle-nose deformity

For a discussion of facial fractures, see Plastic Surgery Chapter.

ONCOLOGIC LESIONS OF THE FACE AND SINUSES

Neoplasms of nose and paranasal sinuses account for what percentage of head and neck tumors?	< 1%

Benign Neoplasms

What is the most common benign neoplasm of the nose and paranasal sinuses?	Papilloma
How does inverting papilloma present?	Unilateral polypoid intranasal mass that is locally aggressive

What is the incidence of malignant transformation?	10% (to squamous cell carcinoma, SCC)
What is the treatment?	Surgical excision (no adjuvant radiotherapy because tumor is radioresistent). Due to the high recurrence rate, more radical surgery is often required, including lateral rhinotomy and medial maxillectomy.

Malignant Neoplasms

What is the most common malignant neoplasm?	Squamous cell carcinoma (80%)
How is tumor stage determined?	Site
What are the symptoms?	Unilateral nasal obstruction, facial or dental pain, epistaxis. As disease spreads to adjacent structures, symptoms include diplopia, visual loss, blood-tinged mucus, epiphora, facial swelling, trismus, malocclusion, and facial numbness.
What are the risk factors?	Industrial fumes and wood dust
Which sinus is most commonly involved?	Maxillary (66%)
What diagnostic studies are used?	Endoscopic exam and CT scan; MRI is useful for delineation of soft tissue and intraorbital extent.
Where does the tumor metastasize?	Metastatic disease is uncommon even in advanced stages.
What is the treatment of SCC?	1. Radical excision for most tumors, ± radical neck dissection 2. XRT as adjuvant treatment for advanced tumors and as primary treatment for poor surgical candidate
What are the indications for chemotherapy?	Currently, no successful chemotherapeutic regimen is available.
What is the second most common malignant neoplasm of nose and paranasal sinuses?	Adenoid cystic and adenocarcinoma (10% of cases)

What is the most common malignant lesion of the nasal dorsum or vestibule?

Basal cell carcinoma (BCC); predilection for sun-exposed regions

What is the classic appearance of BCC?

Solitary ulcerated nodules with smooth raised borders

What is the treatment of BCC?

Mohs' micrographic surgery; wide local excision

What are the signs of malignant melanoma in a pigmented lesion?

Irregular borders, ulceration, bleeding, rapid growth, or characteristic colors (red, white, blue)

How is tumor stage of melanoma determined?

Depth of melanoma penetration

What other factors influence prognosis of melanoma?

Location (with scalp lesions having poor outcome), ulceration, and nodal metastases

What are the two staging systems for melanoma?

1. **Clark's staging** is based on level of invasion.
   Level I—Epidermis
   Level II—Through the basal lamina
   Level III—Into papillary dermis
   Level IV—Into reticular dermis
   Level V—Subcutaneous spread
2. **Breslow's staging** is based on depth of penetration: epidermis < 0.75 mm, papillary dermis 0.75 to 1.5 mm, reticular dermis 1.5 to 4.0 mm, and subcutaneous > 4.0 mm.

How are diagnosis and staging of melanoma determined?

Punch biopsy (shave or curettage biopsy contraindicated). Some prefer to perform a simple excision with narrow margins (2 mm) and reexcise the scar after diagnosis and microstaging.

What is the treatment of melanoma?

1. Surgical excision (1–2-cm margins)
2. Neck dissection indicated with evidence of nodal metastasis or intermediate depth lesions (stages II and III)

INFECTIOUS LESIONS OF THE FACE AND SINUSES

Sinusitis

What is its claim to fame?

Most common health care complaint in the United States (affects nearly 31 million people yearly with a cost of $150 million in 1989)

How is sinusitis classified?

1. Acute→1 day to 4 weeks
2. Subacute→4 weeks to 3 months
3. Chronic→greater than 3 months

What are the risk factors for sinusitis?

Allergy, nasal polyposis, blockage of the sinus outflow passages, immune compromise, upper respiratory infection, and apical dental infections

How does acute sinusitis present?

Headache, facial pain, periorbital swelling, nasal obstruction or crusting, mucopurulent drainage, ear popping or fullness, diffuse dental pain, fetid breath, hoarseness, fever, lethargy, cough

How does chronic sinusitis present?

Many of the previously listed signs, but generally without fevers and with less prominent facial or headache pain

What are the common bacterial pathogens in sinusitis?

1. Acute→*Streptococcus*, *Staphylococcus*, *Haemophilus influenzae*, and *Moraxella* (Note: Many cases of acute sinusitis are felt to have a viral origin followed by superinfection with a bacterial organism.)
2. Chronic→Anaerobes and *Staphylococcus*

What additional pathogen is more common in ICU and immunocompromised patients?

Fungus

How is sinusitis diagnosed?

1. History and physical examination (Note: Facial x-ray series cost nearly as much as CT scan.)
2. CT scan is generally obtained after failure of medical therapy (earlier in immunodeficient hosts).

What are the classic CT scan findings with sinusitis?

Acute: Air–fluid levels in the sinus
Chronic: Mucoperiosteal thickening (±
   bone sclerosis)
Fungal: Hyperdense concretions in the
   sinus

What is the role of MRI in diagnosing sinusitis?

MRI is useful in evaluating soft tissue densities, fungal infections, and orbital or intracranial extension of sinus pathology.

What are the indications for a sinus tap or irrigation?

1. Mucopurulent fluid in an immunocompromised host with radiographic findings of sinus air–fluid levels
2. Patients with air–fluid levels who have failed aggressive medical therapy especially if poor surgical candidate

What is the best treatment of acute sinusitis?

Empiric therapy with antibiotics for 14 days (commonly used agents including amoxicillin ± clavulanate, trimethoprim-sulfamethoxazole, cefuroxime, erythromycin sulfate, or loracarbef), decongestants, saline nasal irrigation, humidification, and mucolytics

What is the management of chronic sinusitis that is unresponsive to medical therapy?

Endoscopic sinus surgery (e.g., nasal polypectomy, intranasal antrotomy)

Which complications of sinusitis warrant emergent surgical intervention?

1. Extension of infection to orbit (orbital abscess)
2. Extension of infection intracranially
   a. Frontal lobe, epidural, or subdural abscess
   b. Meningitis
   c. Cavernous sinus thrombosis

Adenoiditis

Which bacterial pathogens are common in adenoiditis?

1. *Streptococcus*
2. *Haemophilus influenzae*
3. *Moraxella*

What is the initial treatment of adenoiditis?

Antibiotics

What are the indications for adenoidectomy?	Nasal obstruction from adenoid hyperplasia, obstructive sleep apnea, recurrent or chronic adenoiditis, recurrent otitis media with effusions, chronic otitis media, or suspected neoplasm

Facial Cellulitis

What is the treatment of facial cellulitis?	Hospital admission, IV antibiotics, and close observation
Why is this treatment chosen?	To facilitate early detection of intracranial propagation of bacteria via valveless facial veins

FACIAL PLASTICS AND RECONSTRUCTIVE SURGERY

What are the indications for septal reconstruction?	1. Nasal obstruction due to significant nasal septal deviation 2. External cosmetic defects related to nasal septal anatomy
How is septal reconstruction accomplished?	1. Intranasal resection of deformed septal cartilage and bone 2. Replacement of straightened cartilage within the mucoperichondrial envelope
What are the aesthetic nasal subunits?	Nasal dorsum, sidewall, tip–columella, alar lobule, supra-alar facet depressions
How are external nasal defects managed?	Resection and replacement of the entire nasal subunit with skin of similar texture and color
What advantages are offered by local flaps in facial defect repair?	Superior tissue match, single stage, no disruption of muscle or nerve function
What are the three patterns of blood supply to local flaps?	1. Random (Dermal and subdermal plexus) 2. Axial (Cutaneous named artery and vein paralleling the axis of the flap) 3. Myocutaneous (Segmental artery and vein giving off perforators to overlying muscle and skin)

What are the common donor sites for bony nasal or facial repair?	Rib, tibia, iliac crest, scapula, and calvarium
Which site is often favored for its low donor site morbidity and ease of harvest?	Calvarium

ORAL CAVITY AND OROPHARYNX

ANATOMY

What is the oral cavity?	The region extending from the vermilion border of the lips to the hard–soft palate junction superiorly and the circumvallate papillae inferiorly. Structures include the lips, buccal mucosa, alveolar ridges (upper and lower), retromolar trigones, hard palate, teeth, anterior two-thirds of tongue, and floor of mouth.
What is the oropharynx?	The region bordered anteriorly by the circumvallate papillae of the tongue, laterally by the tonsillar fossae and lateral pharyngeal walls, inferiorly by an axial plane through the vallecula, superiorly by an axial plane through the soft palate, and posteriorly by the posterior pharynx

CONGENITAL LESIONS OF THE OROPHARYNX

Cleft Lip and Palate

What is the claim to fame of these defects?	Most common congenital malformation of the head and neck (second most common overall malformation after clubfoot)
What is the incidence?	Cleft lip with or without cleft palate: 1 in 1000 Cleft palate alone: 1 in 2000
When is cleft lip repair generally performed?	"Rule of tens": 10 weeks old, weight of 10 pounds, Hgb > 10 g

When is cleft palate repair generally performed?

Controversial. Generally 10 to 18 months of age. Early closure provides velopharyngeal competence for speech and deglutition, but may adversely alter maxillofacial growth.

Apnea
What is apnea?

Absence of respiration for 10 or more seconds

What are the three types of apnea?

1. Obstructive (Lack of airflow with continued effort)
2. Central (Absence of effort)
3. Mixed (Both)

In obstructive sleep apnea (OSA) patients, what is the predominant site of obstruction?

Oropharynx. Obstruction can result from tongue, soft palate, tonsillar, adenoid, and pharyngeal wall.

How is OSA diagnosed?

1. History (Loud snoring, restless sleep, periods of apnea, and daytime somnolence)
2. Physical exam (Associated with obesity, macroglossia, micrognathia, retrognathia, adenotonsillar hypertrophy, shallow palatal arch, large palate, or both)
3. Diagnostic study (Sleep study [polysomnogram])

What is the treatment of pediatric OSA?

Adenotonsillectomy

What is the treatment of OSA in adults?

1. Medical therapy (continuous positive airway pressure [CPAP]) masks, weight loss, avoidance of CNS depressants, and protriptyline
2. Surgery therapy (May include tonsillectomy and adenoidectomy, uvulopalatopharyngoplasty and tracheotomy, midline glossectomy, mandibular advancements or osteotomy, and hyoid advancement)

What malformations are found in Pierre-Robin syndrome?

1. Glossoptosis
2. Micrognathia
3. Cleft palate
These children often present with inadequate oral intake and aspiration

that may require tracheostomy and gastrostomy tube.

What malformations are found in Apert's syndrome?

Midface hypoplasia with a small retrodisplaced maxilla, orbital hypertelorism, and a short widened skull

ONCOLOGIC LESIONS OF THE OROPHARYNX

Benign Neoplasms

What is the most common benign tumor of oropharynx?

Juvenile angiofibroma

What is the target population?

Male patients between 7 and 21 years of age

What is the most common presentation?

Epistaxis (highly vascular, locally invasive tumor)

What is the treatment?

1. Preoperative embolization of tumor (primary blood supply is the internal maxillary A.) ± estrogen therapy ± XRT to decrease blood loss at time of surgery
2. Surgical excision (under hypotensive anesthesia)

Malignant Neoplasms

What is the most common histologic type of malignant neoplasm?

Squamous cell carcinoma (95%)

What are the other types of malignant neoplasms of the oropharynx?

Lymphoma, melanoma, and minor salivary gland tumors

What are the most common sites?

1. Tongue
2. Lip

How is tumor stage determined?

Size

What are the signs and symptoms?

Pain, bleeding, dysphagia, trismus, tooth loss or pain, odynophagia, otalgia, nonhealing ulcer, or mass

What are the risk factors?

1. Smoking or chewing tobacco
2. Alcohol abuse

Where does this tumor metastasize?	1. Neck (common even with early lesions) 2. Bone 3. Lung
What is the incidence of a second primary tumor?	Up to 40%
What are the treatment options?	1. Wide local excision is the choice for easily accessible tumors. 2. Larger or inaccessible tumors may be treated with combination surgery and XRT. 3. Again, no successful chemotherapeutic regimen is available.

INFECTIONS OF THE OROPHARYNX

Tonsillitis

What are the most common bacterial causes of tonsillitis?	1. *Streptococcus* 2. *Haemophilus influenzae* 3. *Moraxella* (Note: Mononucleosis is an infrequent viral cause)
What is acute management of tonsillitis?	Antibiotics (usually penicillin)
What agents may be useful for chronic infection?	1. Clindamycin 2. Augmentin (amoxicillin–clavulanic acid)
What are the indications for tonsillectomy?	Tonsillar hyperplasia with obstructive sleep apnea, failure to thrive, swallowing abnormalities, airway narrowing, recurrent or chronic infection, tonsillitis with peritonsillar abscess, cervical node abscess, cardiac valve disease, or suspected neoplasm

Peritonsillar Abscess

What is the etiology of peritonsillar abscess?	Incompletely treated or chronic tonsillitis
What is the location?	Fascial (potential) space between pharyngeal constrictor muscles and tonsillar capsule

What are the symptoms?	Painful swollen throat, trismus, otalgia, and dysphagia
What are the signs?	Uvula deviation and erythematous unilateral palatal swelling, drooling, fever, and a "hot potato" voice
What is the acute treatment of peritonsillar abscess?	1. Assurance of airway patency 2. Rehydration 3. Drainage (using either incision and drainage or aspiration techniques) 4. IV antibiotics
What are the indications for hospital admission?	1. Immunocompromised, debilitated, dehydrated, or septic patient 2. Airway instability
What is the subacute treatment of peritonsillar abscess?	Tonsillectomy > 1 month after resolution of infection

Ludwig's Angina

What is Ludwig's angina?	The spread of an infectious process into the sublingual, submandibular, and submental spaces
What is the most concerning complication?	Rapid progression of airway compromise (with floor of mouth edema displacing tongue posteriorly)
What are the signs and symptoms?	Limited movement of tongue, swelling of floor of mouth and submental region, fluctuance, and pain on movement of tongue
What is the most common source?	Dental infection (especially mandibular)
What are the most common pathogens?	Mixed oral flora
What is the treatment?	Same as for peritonsillar abscess

Other Oropharyngeal Abscesses

What is the location of a parapharyngeal abscess?	Fascial space between pharyngeal constrictor muscles and superficial layer of deep cervical fascia
What is the location of a retropharyngeal abscess?	Fascial space between posterior pharyngeal wall and prevertebral fascia

What are the complications?	1. Airway obstruction 2. Hemorrhage due to erosion into vessels of neck (e.g., carotid) 3. Intracranial infections 4. Aspiration 5. Spread to thoracic cavity (mediastinitis or empyema)
What is the treatment?	IV antibiotics, incision, and drainage
Should the procedure be performed under local or general anesthesia?	**Local.** General anesthesia can be dangerous with these abscesses because of sudden airway obstruction. Even with local anesthesia, the surgeon must be prepared to perform tracheostomy.

OROPHARYNGEAL TRAUMA

How are penetrating wounds of the oral cavity managed?	1. Always address the ABC's of ATLS first, particularly when securing the airway in these injuries. 2. Small well-aligned mucosal tears may be left to heal by second intention. 3. Larger tears should be débrided and closed loosely (in selected cases, split-thickness skin graft or local flap closure indicated)

EARS

ANATOMY

What are the labeled landmarks of the external ear or auricle?	1. Helix 2. Scaphoid fossa 3. Triangular fossa 4. Concha 5. Antihelix 6. Tragus 7. Antitragus 8. Intertragic incisure 9. Lobule

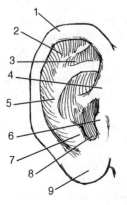

Which two components form the external canal?	Lateral cartilaginous and medial bony components
Which nerves travel within the internal auditory canal (IAC)?	Vestibulocochlear and facial nerves
What are the anatomic relationships within the middle ear?	Anterior: Eustachian tube and carotid Inferior: Jugular bulb Superior: Tegmen (floor of middle cranial fossa) Posterior: Mastoid wall Medial: Cochlea (anterior), vestibular apparatus (posterior) Lateral: Tympanic membrane ossicles that lie within the middle ear, running from the tympanic membrane to the medial wall (oval window) in the posterior/superior quadrant

CONGENITAL LESIONS OF THE EAR

Which lesions are examples of minor malformations of the ear?	Preauricular tags and pits
What is the treatment?	Excision for isolated tags; excision of entire tract for pits (if symptomatic)
What lesions are examples of major malformations?	1. Microtia (rudimentary pinna) 2. Atresia (lack of formation of external auditory canal with bony plate) (Note: Microtia and atresia often occur in concert.)
What is the treatment?	Repair of atresia follows repair of microtia. Microtia (Staged auricular reconstruction begins with contralateral costochondral cartilage.) Atresia (Once conchal position is established with microtia repair, the atretic canal can be drilled out.)

ACQUIRED NONINFECTIOUS LESIONS

Otosclerosis

What is otosclerosis?	Development of new spongy bone around the stapes footplate causing ankylosis (fixation) of the footplate

What is the cause?	Autosomal dominant; more frequently seen in white patients and women.
What are the symptoms?	Conductive hearing loss (painless). It is the most common cause of progressive conductive hearing loss.
What is the treatment?	Stapedectomy (removal of stapes), then reconstruction with a metallic prosthesis

Cholesteatoma

What is cholesteatoma?	An epidermal inclusion cyst composed of desquamated keratin debris; located in the middle ear or mastoid, and has a pearly appearance
What are the complications associated with cholesteatoma?	1. Conductive hearing loss due to ossicular erosion 2. Sensorineural hearing loss and vertigo due to local invasion
What is the treatment?	Excision of cyst, ± reconstruction of ossicles

EAR TRAUMA

Injury to auricle

How are auricular hematomas managed?	Incision and drainage with application of bolster
What process is this treatment aimed to prevent?	Cartilaginous necrosis leading to cauliflower ear
How are the following injuries to the auricle repaired:	
Simple lacerations to the skin?	Closed primarily with small (6-0) monofilament nonabsorbable suture.
Lacerations involving cartilage?	Closed primarily in layers, with loose approximation of cartilage with absorbable sutures.

Partial and total avulsion?	Preserving and reapproximating attached tissue (no matter how small the pedicle).
Complete avulsion of auricle?	Reimplantation or de-epithelialization and burial in postauricular pocket

Tympanic Membrane Perforation

What are the common mechanisms of tympanic membrane perforation?	1. Barotrauma 2. Blast injury 3. Foreign body
What are the symptoms?	1. Pain 2. Conductive hearing loss 3. Tinnitus
What is the treatment?	1. Expectant management initially 2. Surgical repair for persistent perforation
What should be used for irrigation if foreign bodies in the ear and tympanic membrane perforation are suspected?	Warm oil or 95% alcohol (not water)

Temporal Bone Fractures

What are the two general configurations of temporal bone fractures?	Longitudinal (70%) and transverse (20%), whereas 10% follow no distinct pattern.
Which configuration is commonly associated with injury to:	
Tympanic membrane and hemotympanum?	Longitudinal
Internal auditory canal?	Transverse
External auditory canal?	Longitudinal
Facial nerve?	Transverse
Cochlea?	Transverse
Ossicles?	Longitudinal
What is the study of choice to diagnose temporal bone fractures?	CT scan with fine cuts in the axial and coronal planes

What is the treatment?	1. IV antibiotics (penicillin!) because of potential risk of meningitis 2. If progressive facial nerve paralysis develops, immediate neuronal decompression indicated

ONCOLOGIC LESIONS OF THE EAR

What are the most common malignant neoplasms of the external ear?	1. Squamous cell carcinoma 2. Basal cell carcinoma
Why is the auricle at increased risk for skin malignancies?	High exposure to ultraviolet radiation of the sun
What is the treatment?	1. Simple wedge resection if tumor isolated to auricle 2. Partial resection of temporal bone if extension into the canal or middle ear

INFECTIONS OF THE EAR

Acute Otitis Externa (Swimmer's Ear)

What is the cause?	Bacterial infection of the ear canal resulting from a break in the cerumen–skin protective barrier
What are the signs and symptoms?	Pain (especially on pinna movement), decreased hearing, pruritis, aural fullness, exudative drainage, edema, and erythema
What are the predisposing factors?	1. Trauma to canal 2. Diabetes 3. Any immune suppression 4. Persistent canal moisture
What are the most common pathogens?	1. *Pseudomonas* (most common) 2. *Proteus* 3. *Staphylococcus* 4. *Streptococcus* 5. Occasionally, fungus

What is the treatment?	1. Thorough cleaning, topical antibiotic drops (± hydrocortisone). Oto-wick may be required if infection is severely edematous. 2. Severe cases may require systemic antibiotics.
What is malignant or necrotizing otitis externa?	A severe otitis externa extending to surrounding tissue, with **granulation tissue** in the canal
Which patients are at highest risk for malignant otitis externa?	Poorly controlled diabetics
What is the treatment?	Control of diabetes, hospitalization, IV antibiotics, and débridement

Acute Otitis Media

What is acute otitis media?	Initial 3 weeks of an inflammatory process of the middle ear
What are the signs and symptoms?	Pain, otorrhea, fever, conductive hearing loss, irritability, tugging on ears, bulging red tympanic membrane (TM), with decreased mobility, and purulent fluid in middle ear
What are the predisposing factors?	Cleft palate, craniofacial anomalies, day care, immune deficiencies, ciliary dyskinesias, nasogastric tube, prolonged nasotracheal intubation, any obstruction or dysfunction of eustachian tube
What are the most common pathogens?	1. *Streptococcus* (most common) 2. *Haemophilius influenzae* 3. *Moraxella catarrhalis* 4. *Staphylococcus*
What are the findings on otoscopy?	TM redness, followed by bulging of TM (with loss of normal TM landmarks), then impaired TM mobility (pneumatic otoscopy)
What is the initial treatment?	Oral antibiotics for 10 days. Amoxicillin is the agent of choice.

What is the treatment of patients who fail medical therapy?	Placement of pressure equalization (PE) tubes
What are the indications for PE tubes?	1. Recurrent acute otitis media 2. Otitis media with effusion for greater than 6 months, with a hearing loss

Acute Mastoiditis

What is acute mastoiditis?	Infection of the mastoid space that may lead to coalescence and suppuration
What is the usual presentation?	Pain, fever, otorrhea, protruding ear; postauricular erythema, fluctuance, and edema
What are the predisposing factors?	Untreated or unresponsive acute otitis media
What are the most common pathogens?	Same as those for otitis media **plus** anaerobes
What is the treatment?	1. PE tube placement (or myringotomy) 2. IV antibiotics 3. Cortical mastoidectomy for bony involvement
What are the complications?	1. Labyrinthitis 2. Sigmoid sinus thrombophlebitis 3. Epidural, subdural, or brain abscess 4. Meningitis 5. Facial nerve paralysis

Bullous Myringitis

What is bullous myringitis?	Vesicular infection of uncertain etiology (viral versus *Mycoplasma*) involving the TM and deep canal
What is the treatment?	Topical analgesics, ± PO antibiotics (erythromycin for *Mycoplasma*). Usually resolves in 1 to 2 days.

RECONSTRUCTIVE SURGERY OF THE EAR

How is protruding ear diagnosed?	By visualization. Objective measures include the distance or angle from skull to helical rim (abnormal: > 2 cm or > 30°)
What are the responsible anatomic defects?	Overdeveloped concha, poorly developed antihelical fold, or both

What is the treatment?   Otoplasty (often involving modification of the concha, antihelical fold, or both)

NECK

ANATOMY

Major Muscular Structures

What is the thin sheet-like muscle lying beneath the skin in the anterolateral neck?   Platysma muscle

What muscle divides the neck into anterior and posterior triangles?   Sternocleidomastoid (SCM) muscle

What muscle defines the posterior extent of the neck dissection?   Trapezius muscle

What group of muscles in the anterior neck acts to elevate and depress the larynx?   Strap muscles

What group of muscles defines the deep limit of the neck dissection?   Scalene muscles

What muscle serves to stabilize the scapula and allows abduction beyond 90°?   Trapezius muscle

In what plane are skin flaps raised for neck surgery?   Subplatysmal plane

Major Vascular Structures

What landmark roughly approximates the site of the bifurcation of the common carotid artery?   Upper border of the thyroid cartilage

What are the branches of the internal carotid artery in the neck?   There are none.

**What are the branches of
the external carotid artery
in the neck?**

1. Superior thyroid artery
2. Ascending pharyngeal artery
3. Lingual artery
4. Facial artery
5. Occipital artery
6. Posterior auricular artery
7. Superficial temporal artery
8. Maxillary artery

Fascial Compartments

**What are the layers of the
deep cervical fascia?**

1. Superficial layer—Surrounds entire
   neck enclosing the trapezius, SCM,
   and omohyoid muscles
2. Middle (visceral) layer–Surrounds the
   visceral structures of the anterior neck
3. Deep (prevertebral) layer—Surrounds
   the paraspinous muscles and vertebral
   column

**Which layers contribute to
the formation of the
carotid sheath?**

All of the above

Other Anatomic Topics

**What three structures are
within the carotid sheath?**

Carotid artery, jugular vein, and vagus
nerve

**What are the lymphatic
zones in the neck?**

Zone 1—Submental and submandibular
Zones 2, 3, and 4—Equal thirds of the
    internal jugular chain, with Zone 2
    being the most superior
Zone 5—Posterior cervical triangle

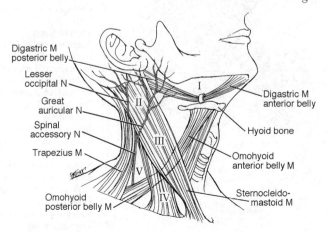

Digastric M
posterior belly

Lesser
occipital N

Great
auricular N

Spinal
accessory N

Trapezius M

Omohyoid
posterior belly M

Digastric M
anterior belly

Hyoid bone

Omohyoid
anterior belly M

Sternocleido-
mastoid M

Describe the location of:

Jugular vein — Lies lateral to carotid artery, deep to SCM

Thoracic duct — Joins the venous system at the junction of the left internal jugular and subclavian veins

Vagus nerve (CN X) — Exits skull at jugular foramen; travels within the carotid sheath

Spinal accessory nerve (CN XI) — Exits skull at jugular foramen, passes deep to the posterior belly of digastric muscle, enters SCM about 4 cm below mastoid process, exits SCM 1 cm superior to Erb's point (greater auricular nerve meets SCM), and enters trapezius two finger breadths above clavicle

Hypoglossal nerve (CN XII) — Exits skull through hypoglossal canal, deep to digastric muscle in the submandibular triangle

Phrenic nerve — Runs lateral to medial on the surface of the anterior scalene muscle

Brachial plexus — Passing between the anterior and middle scalene muscles on the way to axilla

What spinal levels contribute to the:

Phrenic nerve? — C2, 3, and 4

Brachial plexus? — C4–8 and T1

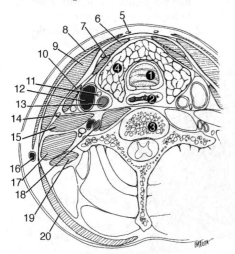

1. Trachea
2. Esophagus
3. Cervical (C7) vertebral body
4. Thyroid gland
5. Anterior jugular vein
6. Sternohyoid muscle
7. Sternothyroid muscle
8. Platysma muscle
9. Sternocleidomastoid muscle
10. Omohyoid muscle
11. Vagus nerve
12. Internal jugular vein
13. Common carotid artery
14. Phrenic nerve
15. Scalenus anterior muscle
16. External jugular vein
17. Scalenus medius muscle
18. Vertebral artery
19. Scalenus posterior muscle
20. Trapezius muscle

CONGENITAL LESIONS OF THE NECK

Branchial Cleft Cyst

What is the most common type?

Second(> 90%)

Which type may communicate with external auditory canal?

First

Which type is theoretical, with few case reports?

Fourth

What is the general location of:
First branchial cleft cysts?

Type I→Usually in close proximity to the auricle and lateral to CN VII
Type II→Typically present below the angle of the mandible as an abscess passing through parotid gland and may be medial, lateral, or between CN VII branches

Second branchial cleft cysts?

Present as a mass at the anterior border of the SCM, and passes between the external and internal carotid artery and ends in the tonsillar fossa

Third branchial cleft cysts (rare)?

Appear anterior to the SCM and pass posterior to the common and internal carotid artery; pierce the thyrohyoid membrane to enter the piriform sinus

What is the usual presentation?

Present as cysts, sinuses, or fistulas usually in children; often become infected

What diagnostic studies are used?

Fistulogram, ultrasound, CT, or MRI

What is the treatment?

Complete surgical excision

Thyroglossal Duct Cyst

What is the usual presentation?

Midline cervical mass that elevates with tongue protrusion

What diagnostic study is used?	Ultrasound to differentiate from thyroid tissue
What is the treatment?	Sistrunk procedure involves resection of cyst, tract, and central hyoid bone.

PENETRATING NECK TRAUMA

What are the two triangles that divide the neck for evaluation of trauma?	Anterior triangle:
	  1. Superiorly: Inferior border of mandible
	  2. Anteriorly: Midline neck
	  3. Posterolateral: SCM
	Posterior triangle:
	  1. Anteriorly: SCM
	  2. Posteriorly: Trapezius
	  3. Inferiorly: Clavicle

What are the three zones of the neck?	Zone I (Sternal notch to cricoid) Zone II (Cricoid to inferior border of mandible) Zone III (Above inferior border of mandible)
What is the first priority of managing neck trauma?	Assuring or establishing a stable airway
With trauma, which triangle is more likely to result in serious injury to vital neck structures?	Anterior triangle
Penetrating trauma to what zones requires arteriogram?	Zones I and III. (Some surgeons believe that arteriograms are also indicated in zone II injuries)
Which vessels should be studied on arteriogram?	All four vessels of the extracranial cerebrovasculature (both carotids and vertebral arteries) and in the case of zone I, aorta, and arch vessels.
What other studies are performed in the evaluation of neck injury?	1. Fiberoptic esophagoscopy or barium cine-esophagogram (Note: Esophagoscopy inadequately evaluates the proximal esophagus.) 2. Bronchoscopy

Traditionally, what structure, when penetrated, requires surgical evaluation for possible injury to vital neck structures?	Platysma muscle. This surgical evaluation is currently controversial, and many surgeons now choose to observe select cases of platysmal penetration.

ONCOLOGIC LESIONS OF THE NECK

Neck Dissection

What are the indications for neck dissection in head and neck cancer?	1. Clinically positive disease (i.e., palpable lymphadenopathy) **and/or** 2. Greater than 25% risk of occult cervical metastases

How are neck nodes staged with regionally metastatic disease?	N0: No detectable nodal disease
	 N1: Single ipsilateral node ≤ 3 cm
	 N2
	     a: Single ipsilateral node > 3–≤ 6 cm
	     b: Multiple ipsilateral nodes ≤ 6 cm
	     c: Bilateral or contralateral nodes ≤ 6 cm
	 N3: Nodes > 6 cm

What is removed in the CLASSIC RADICAL neck dissection?	1. Lymph nodes (and deep cervical lymphatics) from mandible to clavicle, from anterior midline to trapezius 2. Spinal accessory nerve (CN XI) 3. Internal jugular vein 4. SCM 5. Submaxillary gland 6. Omohyoid and digastric muscles
What structures are commonly SPARED in modified (functional) neck dissections?	1. Spinal accessory nerve (CN XI) 2. Internal jugular vein 3. SCM (Note: Each may be spared singly or in combination.)
What are the common complications of neck dissection?	1. Bleeding 2. Facial edema 3. Cerebrovascular accident 4. Chylous fistula 5. Carotid artery rupture 6. Cranial nerve injuries

What complication is associated with bilateral internal jugular vein ligation?	Marked head and neck edema
What additional procedure should be performed on patients requiring bilateral jugular ligation?	Tracheotomy to protect airway
What is the role of radiation therapy in treating metastatic squamous cell carcinoma to the neck?	1. Adjunct to neck dissection for advanced disease 2. May be useful as primary therapy for N0 necks 3. May be useful for recurrent disease following neck dissection

Thyroid Tumors

What is the basic diagnostic and therapeutic approach for the thyroid nodule?	Controversial. One useful algorithm is as follows: 1. The initial step is fine-needle aspiration (FNA), with surgery for malignant cytology, observation for benign cytology, and radionuclide scanning for indeterminate cytology. 2. For nodules noted on radionuclide scanning to be cold or warm, therapy is surgical; for hot nodules, observation is appropriate.
What is the most common histology of benign neoplasms of the thyroid?	Adenomas
What signs and symptoms are suggestive of thyroid malignancy?	1. Rapid growth 2. Firm consistency to nodule 3. Fixation to surrounding tissues 4. Cervical lymphadenopathy 5. Vocal cord paralysis
Approximately what percentage of thyroid nodules are malignant?	Only 5%
What are the malignant neoplasms of the thyroid and their relative frequencies?	1. Papillary adenocarcinoma (70%) 2. Follicular carcinoma (15%) 3. Medullary carcinoma (10%) 4. Anaplastic carcinoma (< 5%) (Other malignancies include lymphoma, sarcoma, metastatic tumors, squamous

cell carcinoma, and mucoepidermoid carcinoma.)

Which thyroid neoplasm is:
Most common? Papillary (> 70%)

Most malignant? Anaplastic carcinoma

Least malignant? Papillary

Associated with psammoma bodies on histology? Papillary

Associated with familial endocrine syndromes? Medullary

Arise from parafollicular cells (C cells)? Medullary

A Hürthle cell tumor (onocytes)? Follicular

Associated with a high incidence of cervical metastases but rarely distant (hematogenous) spread? Papillary

Associated with Hashimoto's thyroiditis? Papillary

What are the most common sites of thyroid metastases? Lungs, brain, and bone

What is the 10-year survival rate for the four types of thyroid carcinoma?
1. Papillary carcinoma→70% to 90%
2. Follicular carcinoma→35% to 50%
3. Medullary carcinoma→approximately 40%
4. Anaplastic carcinoma→ < 10% (5-year survival)

What is the surgical treatment for each type of thyroid carcinoma?
1. Papillary: Most authors suggest total thyroidectomy and regional node dissection for clinically positive nodes. However, patients less than 40 years of age with masses less than 1 cm may be treated with hemithyroidectomy and isthmusectomy.

2. Follicular: Same as papillary
3. Medullary: All patients should undergo total thyroidectomy with paratracheal node dissection and formal neck dissections if clinically positive disease is present.
4. Anaplastic: Many consider surgical therapy to be heroic.

INFECTIOUS LESIONS OF THE NECK

What are the etiologies of deep neck infections?

1. Odontogenic infections
2. Upper respiratory infection
3. Trauma
4. Foreign body
5. Instrumentation (especially IV drug users)

What is the bacteriology?

Usually mixed bacterial infection
  Staphylococcus and *Streptococcus* are the most common aerobes.
  Odontogenic pathogens are the most common anaerobes.

What is the presentation?

Pain, swelling, fever, trismus, dysphagia, respiratory difficulties, fluctuance, and dental complaints

What is the diagnostic study of choice?

CT scan with IV contrast

What is the treatment?

1. Assure or establish adequate airway
2. IV antibiotics
3. Needle aspiration (or surgical drainage if abscess)

URGENT AIRWAY MANAGEMENT

What is the procedure of choice for most emergent airway situations?

Cricothyroidotomy

What are the contraindications for cricothyroidotomy?

1. Children less than 12 years of age
2. Laryngeal trauma
3. Patients with laryngeal or subglottic tumor

How is a cricothyroidotomy performed?

A transverse skin incision is made over the cricothyroid membrane, followed by a stabbing incision directly into the cricothyroid membrane to enter the airway. The back end of the knife handle is inserted into the airway and twisted to further open the incision; then an endotracheal tube is inserted for ventilation (taking care to stay as close to the cricoid cartilage as possible to avoid injuring the glottis).

What is the major advantage of emergent cricothyroidotomy over emergent tracheotomy?

The cricothyroid membrane is the most superficial portion of the trachea and thus requires less dissection to enter the airway.

What other procedure may be used to oxygenate patients emergently?

Transcricothyroid puncture with a 14-gauge catheter

For which patient population is this technique indicated?

Children

What is the limiting factor of this technique?

The patient can be oxygenated but not ventilated.

What gas can be used as a temporizing measure?

Heliox. A helium/oxygen mixture that diffuses into the airway more easily because of its lower molecular weight

May cricothyroidotomies be used for long-term airway support?

Controversial; most support the notion that if tracheotomy is required for more than 3 to 5 days, cricothyroidotomies should be converted to formal tracheostomy to prevent subglottic stenosis.

HEAD AND NECK RECONSTRUCTION

What are the PEDICLED MYOCUTANEOUS flaps used in head and neck reconstruction?

1. Latissimus dorsi
2. Pectoralis major
3. Trapezius

Which flap is most commonly used?	Pectoralis major
What pedicled fasciocutaneous flap is used?	Deltopectoral flap
What is the vascular pedicle for each of the previously described flaps?	1. Pectoralis major→Thoracoacromial artery 2. Latissimus dorsi→Thoracodorsal artery 3. Trapezius→Descending branch of the transverse cervical artery and dorsal scapular artery 4. Deltopectoral flap→Anterior thoracic perforators of thoracoacromial artery
What are the FREE flaps commonly used for head and neck reconstruction?	Radial forearm, fibula, jejunum, scapula, iliac crest, and rectus abdominis
What tissue source may be used in cases of significant injury to the pharynx and esophagus?	Gastric pull-up
Where is the blood supply for this "pedicle"?	Right gastric and gastroepiploic vessels

MISCELLANEOUS TOPICS

Where is the most common neck mass?	Reactive lymph node
What is "quincy"?	Paratonsillar abscess secondary to acute tonsillitis
What is the most common type of teratoma in the head and neck?	Epidermoid cyst
What is leukoplakia?	White patch in oropharynx
When is biopsy indicated in leukoplakia?	For smokers or alcoholics (high risk of head and neck carcinoma)

What is the most common type of branchial cleft anomaly?	Second cleft
What type of schwannoma arises from CN VIII?	Acoustic neuroma
What is the most common benign laryngeal lesion in both children and adults?	Laryngeal papilloma
What tumors of skeletal muscle have a predilection for the head and neck?	Rhabdomyomas
What is Bezold's abscess?	Cervical abscesses secondary to ear infection
What is the most common cause of facial paralysis?	Bell's palsy (etiology uncertain)
What is a maxillary torus?	Benign bony growth found midline in the palate
What is the most common bone tumor in the head and neck?	Osteogenic sarcoma (however, rarely seen in the head and neck)
Which parotid tumor accounts for 70% of all bilateral salivary tumors?	Warthin's tumor
What is an esthesioneuroblastoma?	Rare tumor that develops in the olfactory epithelium
Which facial fracture is characterized by complete craniofacial separation?	Le Fort III
What is odynophagia?	Painful swallowing
What is dysphagia?	Difficulty swallowing
What is Meniere disease and the classic triad of presentation?	Disorder of membranous labyrinth. The triad is tinnitus, hearing loss, and vertigo.

What is a glomus jugulare?   Neoplasm arising from jugular bulb and often extending into the middle ear

What is median rhomboid glossitis?   A congenital defect caused by improper fusion of posterior third of tongue to anterior two-thirds; resembles neoplasm.

What is the most common infection of the neck in children?   Acute cervical lymphadenitis

What is the most common infection of the neck in adults?   Acute cervical lymphadenitis

What is the most common head and neck tumor in children?   Hemangioma

What is vestibular neuritis?   Severe attacks of vertigo thought to be secondary to viral infection

What is ankyloglossia?   Limited movement of tongue because of shortened frenulum

50

Plastic Surgery

Jonathan Winograd, MD

WOUND HEALING

What are the three components of wound healing?	1. Epithelialization (provides a watertight seal) 2. Fibrous tissue synthesis (provides strength) 3. Contraction (moves edges into proximity)

EPITHELIALIZATION

How much time is needed for epithelialization to form a watertight seal?	Twenty-four hours in a wound that is closed primarily
What regulates the proliferation of epithelial cells?	As the layer of epithelial cells progresses across the wound, it thins to the level of single cells, slowing its advance. When this layer comes in contact with other epidermal cells, further lateral growth is halted. The layer then begins to thicken and obtain dimensions similar to those of normal epidermis.
How does the "neoepithelium" of wound healing differ from native epithelium?	It is thinner, has less pigment, and lacks rete pegs (the normal interdigitation of dermal and epidermal layers).
Under what circumstances can proliferative signals trigger epidermoid malignancy?	In wounds in which the cells have altered DNA, i.e., chemical injury or ionizing radiation, or in which the healing process has been subject to repeated breakdown, i.e., burn wounds
What epithet is ascribed for squamous cell carcinoma of chronic wounds?	Marjolin's ulcer

FIBROUS TISSUE SYNTHESIS

What is granulation tissue?

Ingrowing capillary buds and fibroblasts as well as their extracellular matrix. It is the initial tissue deposited within the forming scar.

What is the time course for the scar to form?

Biochemical synthesis by fibroblasts may be evident within 2 days. Visible evidence is present within 4 to 6 days.

When does the collagen content of the wound reach its peak?

The collagen content undergoes a rapid increase from day 5 to day 17, after which it plateaus. Collagen breakdown and synthesis reach an equilibrium; therefore, the amount does not change.

When does the wound achieve its maximum strength?

The wound continues to grow stronger for up to 2 years.

When does the wound achieve 80% to 90% of its final strength?

Within 30 days

Why does the wound continue to grow stronger even though the collagen content has stabilized?

Strength is improved through remodeling of collagen cross-linking, not additional synthesis.

What is secondary healing?

If a wound is reopened after the fifth day of healing, the return of tensile strength is extremely rapid because the collagen already present can be used almost immediately. If tissue > 1 cm away from the edge of the original wound is excised, the effect is abolished.

HEALING BY SECONDARY INTENTION

What is healing by secondary intention?

A prolonged repair process characterized by a larger tissue defect in which **contraction** is the dominant mechanism of decreasing wound size and closing the defect.

How does contraction occur?	Myofibroblasts (specialized fibroblasts with the ability to contract like smooth muscle cells) form within the granulation tissue and begin to contract.
When does this contraction begin?	Four to five days after injury
What are the advantages of healing by secondary intention?	Through this process, large defects can be closed or significantly reduced over a period of weeks to months. The incidence of wound infection decreases in the setting of a contaminated operative field.
What are the disadvantages?	Granulation tissue that is allowed to epithelialize usually results in a substantial scar. Furthermore, contraction can severely limit function, particularly in areas requiring mobility, such as joints.

ABNORMALITIES OF WOUND HEALING

What is a hypertrophic scar?	A cicatrix that shows excessive deposition of collagen within the margins of the healing wound. The scar usually diminishes over time.
What is a keloid?	A scar with excessive deposition of collagen outside the margin of the healing wound. This scar often invades surrounding tissue and recurs after surgical excision. It is more common in African-Americans than in Caucasians.
What is the treatment of hypertrophic scars and keloids?	Excision can be attempted but often results in recurrence. Corticosteroid injections and direct compression, sometimes in combination with keloid excision, have had success in some patients.
What is crucial for success of excision?	Reapproximation of skin edges without tension

What is "proud flesh"?	The production of excessive granulation tissue at the site of expected wound repair
What is the treatment of "proud flesh"?	Excision, chemical cautery, and electrocautery are all effective in abolishing the response.

PRINCIPLES OF WOUND MANAGEMENT

What is the zone of injury?	That region of tissues affected by the energy imparted in a traumatic insult
How can it be assessed?	Appearances are deceiving, and an understanding of the mechanism of trauma, with particular attention to the amount and distribution of the energy imparted, is crucial. (Note: Even in experienced hands, the zone of injury can be incorrectly identified or difficult to ascertain because of microscopic changes that extend beyond the visible boundaries. Final determination may be as late as **72 hours** post trauma.)
What bacterial load poses a threat to otherwise viable tissue in a wound?	A load greater than or equal to 10^5 organisms/g of tissue
When does warm ischemia result in significant injury to muscle versus skin?	Muscle → 6 hours, skin → 12 hours (*Note:* Times are improved by cooling of tissue.)
What are the basic objectives of therapy designed to limit the zone of injury?	1. Maximize blood flow 2. Prevent infection 3. Stabilize the injured area (splinting of tissues)
What initial steps can be taken to limit the zone of injury?	1. Gentle handling of tissue 2. Adequate hemostasis 3. Removal of devitalized tissue 4. Obliteration of dead space 5. Removal of foreign bodies
How is the complex wound prepared for reconstruction?	Serial débridement, irrigation, application of topical antibiotics, physiologic dressing, and systemic antibiotics

What is the quantitative effect of irrigation with jet lavage?

Ninety percent of the bacterial load (or one log value) on average is removed.

What topical antibiotics are effective against the usual pathogens?

Polymyxin B, bacitracin, neomycin, Silvadene, Sulfamylon cream, and silver nitrate are all effective **without** fibroblast toxicity.

What disinfectants can be applied without harm to tissues?

Betadine at a dilution of **1:1000** and sodium hypochlorite at a dilution of 1:100 are both effective antibacterials without significant fibroblast toxicity. Higher levels inhibit epithelialization.

What is the appropriate role for systemic antibiotics in wound management?

Before tissue invasion, antibiotics can be effective as prophylaxis against colonization of susceptible tissue. In chronic wounds, antibiotics are ineffective in lowering tissue contamination levels and encourage colonization by resistant organisms. They should be used only if the wound is a suspected source of sepsis.

Early reconstruction usually helps to prevent hypertrophic scarring and contracture. What areas are exceptions to this rule?

Some limited facial and fingertip soft tissue defects are areas in which contracture alone can close a defect with minimal deformity and good preservation of function.

What is the usual reconstructive sequence from simplest to most complex in wound management?

Primary closure→secondary closure→skin grafts→random flaps→tissue expansion→muscle flaps→free tissue transfer

SKIN GRAFTING

What is a skin graft?

Transfer of a layer of skin (epidermis with a variable thickness of attached dermis) to a recipient bed without an attached blood supply

How does full thickness differ from partial thickness?

Full thickness is the entire dermis; partial thickness is any amount less than full.

How does a graft survive the first 24 to 48 hours?

Plasmatic imbibition or "cell drinking" of nutrients, similar to that of cells in culture. Fibrin is responsible for adherence.

After imbibition, what processes maintain the viability of the graft?

1. Inosculation (vessels of the graft align and anastomose with vessels of the recipient bed)
2. Neovascularization (new vessels grow from the bed into the graft)

Which tissue bed can support a skin graft?

New granulation tissue, peritenon, perineurium, perichondrium, periosteum, and vascularized fat

Which tissue beds cannot support a skin graft?

Poorly vascularized or desiccated tissue, tendon, nerve, cartilage, cortical bone, and irradiated tissue

What bacterial count cannot support graft survival?

$>10^5$ organisms/g tissue

Which organism prevents graft survival at a lower bacterial count, and why?

β-hemolytic strep, because it produces streptokinase, which lyses fibrin and interrupts graft adherence

What other factors affect graft survival?

Any process that disrupts contact with the recipient bed, e.g., hematoma, pus, or shear stress

What is done intraoperatively to reduce the risk of disrupting contact?

Meshing of skin grafts

Do wounds continue to contract after skin grafting?

Yes, but to a variable degree depending on the type of graft used. For split-thickness grafts, some contraction continues, consuming up to 35% of the total area grafted. For full-thickness grafts, significant continued contraction is rare.

Can the skin of the graft itself contract?	Yes, in partial-thickness grafts, although this contraction is improved by providing an adequate amount of graft for coverage
What changes in pigmentation are expected in a skin graft?	Hypopigmentation, initially due to the death of pigmented cells, is followed by hyperpigmentation on their return, with gradual return to baseline.

FLAPS

What are the indications for the use of flaps?	1. Poor recipient bed vascularity 2. Full-thickness defects of eyelid, ear, nose, and lip 3. Exposed tendons 4. Tissue bulk needed for function or filling of dead space
What is a random pattern flap?	A flap that bases its blood supply on the dermal and subdermal plexuses. Its orientation is random because its blood supply does not rely on a particular anatomically defined vascular bundle.
Example?	A V–Y advancement flap (often used in the coverage of fingertip soft tissue loss)
What is an axial or arterial flap?	A flap based on direct cutaneous arteries perforating from an underlying artery
Give an example of an axial or arterial flap.	Flaps for the head and neck where a deltopectoral flap or a nasolabial flap is commonly used for reconstruction.
What is a fasciocutaneous flap and where does it derive its blood supply?	A flap based on intermuscular septae. Its blood supply is derived from vessels that arborize within the septae to form plexuses.
What are the advantages of a fasciocutaneous flap?	It occupies a minimal amount of space, supplies excellent strength, and can be used as a sheath to tendon, bone, or exposed vessels.
Give an example.	Tensor fascia lata flap (often used for its strength in abdominal wall reconstruction)

What is a muscle flap?

A flap consisting of vascularized muscle. If it includes overlying subcutaneous tissue and skin, it is termed a **musculocutaneous** flap.

What are the advantages of a muscle flap?

The bulk supplied by the muscle and subcutaneous tissue aids in the reconstruction of large defects while offering durability in mechanically active areas. The rich blood supply also aids in immunologic defense in infected wounds and provides a means of introducing antibiotics directly into the affected area.

Give an example of a muscle flap.

The pectoralis flap, used for coverage in sternal dehiscence, allows for obliteration of the large dead space and eradication of mediastinal infection.

Example of a musculocutaneous flap?

The TRAM flap, used in breast reconstruction, provides the proper amount and type of tissue for replacement of breast tissue.

What is a free flap?

A flap in which native blood supply is divided and the reconstructed supply is derived from microsurgical anastomoses to local vessels

What are the indications for a free flap?

Tissue requirements greater than can be supplied from available pedicle flaps or unique tissue requirements, e.g., bone

What are the advantages of a free flap?

Limitless reconstructive sources, functional muscle transfer, cutaneous sensation, and expansion of reconstructive tissue types to bone, for example

Give examples of a free flap.

Free TRAM for breast reconstruction and fibular transfer for mandibular reconstruction

Tissue Expansion

How is tissue expansion accomplished?

Silastic prostheses are implanted beneath the tissue to be expanded; then saline is incrementally infused until tissue expansion is complete.

Can expansion damage tissue?

Gradual expansion preserves function and viability of all overlying structures. Damage is almost always the result of too rapid an expansion.

What are the signs of tissue damage?

Neurapraxia, loss of dermal appendages, necrosis of overlying skin, and ultimately exposure of the implant

What are common complications and their management?

1. Seroma—percutaneous aspiration. Use of suction drainage usually avoids seroma formation.
2. Hematoma—percutaneous drainage (rarely successful) followed by exploration for continued hemorrhage; prevention through adequate hemostasis is crucial
3. Infection—early infections mandating removal and replacement in 4 to 6 months. Late infections combined with or resulting from extrusion can be managed with low-volume frequent expansions until expansion is complete.

Why can infected expanders be left in tissue?

Expanded tissue, including the capsule of the implant, has an extensive blood supply, giving it remarkable antimicrobial capabilities.

BURNS

INITIAL ASSESSMENT AND RESUSCITATION

What are the different levels of burn injury?

1. Superficial (first degree)—injury to epidermis, minimal dermal injury
2. Superficial partial thickness (second degree)—involvement of epidermis, moderate amount of dermis
3. Deep partial thickness (second degree)—involvement of epidermis, significant portion of dermis
4. Full thickness (third degree)—complete loss of dermis
5. Fourth degree—injury through dermis, for example, subcutaneous tissue, muscle, bone

Compare the healing and management for each type of burn injury.

1. Superficial—usually progresses to exfoliation and complete healing (e.g., sunburn)
2. Superficial partial—deep dermis viable, which allows healing with reepithelialization within 14 to 21 days. Grafting is rarely required; hypertrophic scarring less common.
3. Deep partial—usually heals within 3 to 4 weeks, with grafting recommended to expedite healing, lessen degree of hypertrophic scarring
4. Full thickness: epithelialization over granulation tissue only, grafting necessary to limit hypertrophic scarring, replace dermal integrity
5. Fourth degree: requires débridement of all necrotic tissue, often complex reconstructive schemes

How are second-degree burns distinguished from third-degree burns on physical exam?

Second-degree burns are usually painful, weeping, and erythematous. Third-degree are painless, tough, dry, and white, gray, or charred in color. (**Note:** Early evaluations are likely to change as the thermal injury evolves.)

What is a simple rule for assessing the percentage of total body surface area (TBSA) involved?

The rule of nines: Head and neck 9%, upper extremities 9% each, anterior chest and abdomen 18%, posterior chest and lower back 18%, lower extremities 18% each.
The rule of palms: patient's palm is roughly equal to 1% of their TBSA.

What is the triage scheme for burn patients?

The scheme depends largely on the particular institution. A general outline follows.
1. Mild (up to 15% TBSA, up to 3% third degree)—can be followed as outpatient
2. Moderate (up to 25% TBSA, up to 10% third degree)—can be followed in community hospital
3. Major (greater than 25% TBSA, greater than 10% third degree, **or** burns of the hands, face, feet, ears, perineum, associated inhalational or

nonburn trauma)—requires management in specialized burn unit

What is the initial treatment of the burn itself?

For minor burns, bullae can be left intact or ruptured. For large burns, bullae are gently débrided. Antibiotic cream (e.g., Silvadene) is applied, with sterile gauze bulk dressing for protection. This dressing is subsequently changed twice daily until healing.

What is the Parkland formula for fluid resuscitation?

1. First 24 hours—Ringer's lactate at 4 cc/kg weight x % TBSA of burn. Half of the calculated volume is administered in first 8 hours, then half over next 16 hours
2. Second 24 hours—5% albumin at 0.5 cc/kg weight x % TBSA of burn plus 2000 cc D5W

(Note: Both calculations do **not** include maintenance fluids!)

What is the rationale for reserving colloid until the second day of fluid resuscitation?

Capillary permeability is increased in the first 24 hours; therefore, colloid would extravasate and worsen edema.

Is it advisable to exceed the Parkland formula if urine output falls?

Maybe. The Parkland formula is a general guideline and should by no means be considered absolute. However, falling urine output in the face of continued aggressive fluid resuscitation may also be an early sign of cardiac or renal abnormalities, and diagnostic measures should be undertaken to exclude etiologies other than intravascular volume depletion for oliguria.

INHALATIONAL INJURY

What is the offending agent in inhalational injury?

Carbon monoxide. The airway also suffers chemical burns from incomplete products of combustion. (Note: The injury is not a thermal injury.)

What are the different components of airway injury?

1. Upper airway obstruction from soft tissue swelling
2. Carbon monoxide poisoning
3. Lower airway or parenchymal lung damage, leading to pneumonia and atelectasis

What are the telltale signs of likely inhalational injury in the history?

1. Closed-space fire
2. Prolonged exposure to smoke

What are the signs and symptoms?

Facial burns, singed facial hair, soot in mouth, hoarseness, wheezing, and bronchorrhea

Can inhalation injury be excluded by a normal CXR and normal ABG?

No. Neither CXR nor ABG need be abnormal in the early stages of even severe airway damage.

Which diagnostic tests are used to assess airway damage?

Flow volume loops to demonstrate an obstructive picture; xenon lung scan to demonstrate adequacy of ventilation; nasopharyngoscopy to directly visualize airways and assess for injury

Do the preceding tests rule out the danger of later obstruction or respiratory collapse?

No! If there is a high clinical suspicion of potential obstruction or a progressive deterioration in oxygen delivery, intubation is mandated regardless of negative test results or early stable appearance.

What measures short of intubation can be taken to support adequate ventilation?

Humidified air to encourage clearance of secretions, aggressive pulmonary toilet, bronchodilators, and supplemental oxygen

What are the common indications for intubation in the burn patient?

1. Upper airway obstruction
2. Large fluid requirements (leading later to soft tissue swelling and pulmonary edema)
3. Worsening hypoxia despite supportive therapy

What are the signs of carbon monoxide poisoning?

Headache, confusion, coma, and arrhythmias

What is the normal level of carboxyhemoglobin?

0% to 5% (versus 5%–10% in smokers)

What is the treatment for CO poisoning and how does it work?

100% oxygen; competes for binding sites on the hemoglobin molecules and helps to reverse cerebral and myocardial hypoxia

What other cause of respiratory collapse is common in major burns even without inhalational component?

Eschar of the thorax may restrict the normal excursion of the chest in respiration; emergency escharotomy of the chest is indicated (see below for illustration).

MANAGEMENT OF THE BURN PATIENT

What are the indications for escharotomy in the burn patient?

Circumferential deep second- or third-degree burns that threaten limb perfusion **or** prevent adequate ventilation.

What is the technique of escharotomy for the limb, thorax, and hand?

Limb—medial and lateral aspects of the limb incised to release eschar and prevent the development of a compartment syndrome
Thorax—incisions over both anterior axillary lines and the costal margin anteriorly, forming a shield that allows adequate respiratory excursion
Dorsum of the hand—longitudinal incisions between the second, third, fourth, and fifth rays

What is the goal of burn wound management?

Conversion of the open, contaminated wound to a closed, healed wound with the lowest possible morbidity

What are the general components of burn wound management?

1. Antibiotic creams and dressing changes—Silvadene, Sulfamylon, or silver nitrate is applied twice daily to keep wound contamination at lower levels and help lower the incidence of sepsis. Eschar is gently débrided as its separation from the wound progresses.
2. Serial excision of eschar and grafting—autografting is performed if donor sites meet demands. Allografting with

cadaveric skin or xenografting with porcine skin is added to cover additional areas.

3. Replacement of allograft with autograft—Allograft must be removed every 3 to 5 days to prevent excessive ingrowth of blood vessels. This cycle must be repeated until autograft is available.

What are the advantages and disadvantages of the different topical antibiotics?

Silvadene—good antibacterial spectrum, little systemic absorption, 8% incidence of sulfa allergy, transient leukopenia not uncommon

Sulfamylon—excellent penetration of eschar and deep burns (e.g., electric burns), broadest antibacterial action (good on heavily infected burns); carbonic anhydrase inhibitor, painful application

Silver nitrate—good for sulfa allergy, useful in TENS, wound discoloration, electrolyte leeching, no penetration of eschar

Bacitracin—suitable for superficial partial-thickness burns of the face or residual small open areas

Betadine Ointment—potent antibacterial action useful against multiresistant organisms; painful application, organic iodine absorption a hazard; fibroblast inhibition

What are the signs of burn wound sepsis?

1. Hemorrhagic or gangrenous discoloration of previously viable tissue
2. Accelerated rapid eschar separation
3. Subcutaneous bleeding
4. Systemic sepsis

How can bacterial invasion of viable tissue be confirmed?

Excisional biopsy of eschar and underlying viable tissue for quantitative culture and sectioning to look for evidence of bacterial invasion

What quantity of bacteria is considered consistent with burn wound sepsis?

$> 10^5$ organisms / g tissue

Why should the use of a Swan-Ganz catheter be avoided unless absolutely necessary in the setting of a major burn?

In addition to the usual risks is an increased risk of seeding the endocardium, pulmonary and tricuspid valves in the face of wound sepsis.

Is antibiotic prophylaxis recommended for major burns and why?

No! As wound colonization is a process of several weeks' duration, antibiotic prophylaxis serves only to encourage resistant organisms earlier in the course of treatment. Only clinically septic patients should be treated with broad coverage until culture data direct more specific therapy.

In large TBSA burns (greater than 60%), what other measures can be used to achieve long-term coverage of wounds?

Epithelial cells of the patient can be cultured in sheets and placed over previous allografts after all epidermal remnants have been removed.

How do major burns affect metabolism and what are the associated risks?

Burn patients enter a hypermetabolic state in which they quickly undergo conversion of muscle protein into glucose unless their significant nutritional requirements are met.

What are the common gastrointestinal sequelae of major burns?

Duodenal and peptic ulceration, gastritis, and acalculous cholecystitis

What is the proper prophylaxis against these conditions?

Tube feeding and the use of antacids have been shown to reduce the incidence of ulceration and bleeding. Tube feedings may prevent biliary stasis and the associated cholecystitis.

Do tube feedings have any advantage over H$_2$ blockade?

Yes. Tube feedings, if begun in the **immediate** post-burn period, prevent bacterial transmigration. Although controversial, H$_2$ blockade **may** also be associated with higher levels of bacteria in the stomach and a higher incidence of pneumonia.

ELECTRICAL BURNS

What are the different patterns of low-tension and high-tension electrical injury?

Low-tension injury—of limited size and usually confined to the hands or mouth, but often of considerable depth because (1) the victim's muscles contract to prolong contact and (2) the current is relatively small and unable to travel long distances

High-tension injury—travels a long path due to the large amount of energy in the current, but the contact is brief because most of these currents connect with the body through an arc traveling through air (1 inch per 10,000 volts)

What are the usual EKG abnormalities of high-tension injury?

Sinus tachycardia and ST segment–T wave changes (can persist for several weeks). Myocardial infarction is rare.

In electric burns of the extremity, what complications commonly arise in the first 24 hours?

Compartment syndromes and rhabdomyolysis (with subsequent acidosis, hyperphosphatemia, hypocalcemia, and myoglobinuria)

What is the topical antibiotic of choice in electrical burns, and why?

Sulfamylon, because of its deep penetration into tissue

In children sustaining electrical burns to the oral commissure, what life-threatening complication occurs in 20% 2 to 3 weeks later?

Necrotic erosion into the labial artery, with significant subsequent hemorrhage

CHEMICAL BURNS

What is the main principle of initial therapy in chemical burns?

Removal of all contaminated clothing and copious irrigation to remove all offending agents

How are the common acids and alkalis neutralized?

Acids—Most are neutralized with the initial tissue reaction. H_2O for additional dilution is sufficient.

Alkalis—Hydroxyl ion penetration is progressive. Copious, prolonged water irrigation and neutralization with Sulfamylon are the treatments of choice.

What are the late complications specific to alkali burns?	Tympanic membrane perforation, parotid fistulas, severe keloids, and early Marjolin's ulcer formation

Hydrofluoric Acid (HF) Burns

How do HF burns differ from other acid burns?	The flouride ion penetrates deeply into tissues, causing liquefaction necrosis and decalcification/erosion of bone.
What is the treatment of HF burn?	Calcium or magnesium solutions (by topical application or direct injection) are used to neutralize the HF by creating insoluble precipitates in tissue. Topical cooling of affected areas slows the progression of the chemical reaction.
How is the vehicle of calcium or magnesium salts determined?	If the concentration of HF exceeds 20%, injection is indicated.
How is the adequacy of neutralization assessed?	Resolution of pain is a reliable gauge of adequate neutralization.

MAXILLOFACIAL TRAUMA

EMERGENCIES

What are the three commonly encountered emergencies of maxillofacial injuries?	1. Airway obstruction 2. Life-threatening hemorrhage 3. Aspiration
What are mechanisms of airway obstruction in maxillofacial trauma?	Soft tissue swelling, fractured teeth or denture fragments, blood, or gross anatomical disruption can all produce obstruction to airflow.
Treatment?	Endotracheal or nasotracheal intubation; in some cases, emergency cricothyroidotomy
Which maxillofacial injuries are commonly associated with serious hemorrhage?	Deep facial lacerations and closed maxillofacial injuries with associated fractures

What is the preferred treatment of hemorrhage in facial lacerations?	Direct pressure and circumferential pressure bandage
What is the danger in blind clamping of vessels through a facial laceration?	Damage to the facial nerve
What is the common source of bleeding in closed maxillofacial injuries?	Arteries and veins adjacent to the walls of fractured sinuses
What are the four common methods of controlling hemorrhage from these injuries?	1. Anterior–posterior nasal packing 2. External compression dressing 3. Selective arterial ligation 4. Maxillary fracture reduction
How is nasal packing frequently accomplished?	Two 30- to 50-cc Foley balloon catheters are inserted through the nares, inflated in the posterior pharynx, and pulled to occlude the posterior choanae. Antibiotic-soaked Vaseline gauze is then packed anteriorly through the nostrils.
Which arteries can be safely ligated to control life-threatening facial hemorrhage?	1. Internal maxillary artery 2. External carotid artery 3. Superficial temporal artery
What are the signs of pulmonary aspiration?	Noisy respiration, hypoxia, decreased lung compliance, and infiltrate on CXR
What is the treatment of pulmonary aspiration?	Supportive therapy (supplemental oxygen ± intubation). Bronchoscopic lavage can help to improve oxygenation.

SOFT TISSUE WOUNDS

What is the optimal time for facial wound closure?	Due to the excellent blood supply, closure can be performed up to 24 hours after this wound occurs. Closure after fracture reduction also avoids manipulation of the repair.

What are the standard methods of wound cleansing?	Pressure irrigation via 20-gauge angiocatheter, scrubbing or mechanical removal of debris, and sharp débridement
What are the long-term sequelae of retained debris?	Nidus for infection and "tattooing" of skin (foreign material can be incorporated into the forming scar). Later revision is usually unsatisfactory.
What are the common guidelines for extent of débridement?	Conservative resection (1–2 mm) is the rule. "Devitalized" tissue often survives in the facial region.
Are there any exceptions to débridement?	Resection should be avoided in the area of the vermilion, oral commissures, eyelid margin, nostrils, and distal nose.
What are the indications for prophylactic antibiotics?	1. Lacerations of the oral cavity, including compound fractures 2. Fractures involving teeth 3. Sinus fractures 4. Animal bites (Note: Antibiotics are not indicated in uncomplicated facial lacerations.)
What is the postoperative wound care?	Suture lines are cleansed with 1:1 peroxide/saline on cotton tip applicators followed by bacitracin (facial) or bacitracin ophthalmic ointment t.i.d. (periorbital).
What is the postoperative care for intraoral wounds?	Irrigation every 4 hours with bactericidal mouthwash or 1:1 peroxide/saline.
Is early scar revision commonly indicated?	No. Despite the appearance of initial scarring, revision is indicated only for functional problems (i.e., ectropion or obvious malalignment). Maturation with cosmetic improvement occurs for up to 1 to 2 years.

FACIAL NERVE

What are the terminal branches of the facial nerve *and* what muscles do they innervate?	The arborization of the terminal branches of the facial nerve is variable. The following general divisions are described:

1. Frontal–temporal—muscles of forehead and superficial temporal region, including orbicularis oculi and frontalis and excluding temporalis (trigeminal)
2. Zygomatic—muscles of lower orbit, midface, including orbicularis oculi, excluding masseter (trigeminal)
3. Buccal—muscles of cheek and mouth, including orbicularis oris
4. Mandibular—muscles of lower lip and chin, including orbicularis oris
5. Cervical—platysma, distal anastomosis to mandibular branch
6. Posterior auricular—occipitalis, auricularis posterior

Which facial nerve lacerations require repair?

Proximal to a line drawn from the lateral canthus to the nasolabial sulcus, all lacerations of facial nerve branches should be repaired, under magnification, with fine sutures. Distal to the line, the branches are too small. The cervical branch requires no repair.

What components of the facial nerve contribute to lacrimation, salivary secretion, and taste?

1. The **chorda tympani** passes through the petrotympanic fissure, supplies taste to the anterior two-thirds of the tongue and innervates the submandibular and sublingual glands.
2. The **greater petrosal nerve** passes through the pterygopalatine fossa to innervate the lacrimal glands.

If facial paralysis is accompanied by loss of taste, lacrimation, or salivary secretion, how does this combination add to the diagnostic impression?

Because only the branchial motor branches and a sensory nerve to the posterior auricle exit the stylomastoid foramen, this would imply a more proximal lesion of the facial nerve.

TRIGEMINAL NERVE

Is the trigeminal ganglion intracranial or extracranial?

Intracranial

Where do the three branches of the trigeminal nerve exit the skull?

The superior orbital fissure (V_1), the foramen rotundum (V_2), and the foramen ovale (V_3)

What muscles does the trigeminal nerve innervate?

Muscles of mastication (temporalis, masseter, and pterygoids); tensor tympani, tensor veli palatini, mylohyoid, and the anterior belly of the digastrics

What is the distribution of sensory innervation among the three branches?

The distribution corresponds to the three embryologic divisions of the face:
Frontonasal process is V_1—forehead, nasal dorsum, innervation of frontal anterior dura
Maxillary process is V_2—cheek, palate, and maxillary half of oral cavity
Mandibular process is V_3—lower third of face, mandibular half of oral cavity, tongue

Are lacerations of the trigeminal nerve routinely repaired, and why?

Yes. Because the motor function of the trigeminal is essential, repair of motor branches is usually undertaken.

Is sensory nerve repair necessary for protective sensation?

The majority of sensory innervation in the face has a high degree of overlap and does not mandate sensory nerve repair.

PAROTID GLAND

Which duct drains the parotid gland?

Stensen's duct

Where is the duct located?

The duct extends anteriorly from a point just anterior to the masseter and a finger's breadth below the zygomatic arch to the region of the second maxillary bicuspid.

Is it imperative to repair lacerations of the parotid gland?

No. Salivary drainage from parotid trauma stops spontaneously **unless** Stensen's duct is involved.

How is the duct repaired?

Ductal lacerations are repaired with fine sutures under magnification over a stent.

What injury is commonly associated with ductal laceration?	Lacerations and blunt trauma to the buccal branch of the facial nerve, whose course parallels that of the duct

FACIAL FRACTURES

What are the common signs of facial fractures?	Contusions, bruises, or lacerations; pain or localized tenderness; anesthesia or paresthesia; paralysis; malocclusion; visual disturbances; facial deformity, often palpable, or asymmetry; crepitus
What radiographic evaluation should be performed?	CT scans with coronal reconstructions are the definitive diagnostic modality for facial trauma; however, plain film evaluation may be indicated or sufficient in certain cases, as will be discussed next.
What are the structures viewed on the following films: Waters', Towne, lateral and AP skull, AP and lateral oblique mandible, Panorex?	1. Waters'—frontal, supraorbital, orbital, zygomaticomaxillary, and nasal areas. 2. Towne's—condylar and subcondylar region of the mandible and floor of the orbit 3. Skull—sinuses, frontobasilar, and nasoethmoid areas 4. Mandible—body, symphysis, condylar, and coronoid mandible areas 5. Panorex—entire mandible and lower maxilla
What additional study should be obtained before the reconstruction of fractures involving the occlusion?	Maxillary and mandibular dental impressions
What are the specific signs of a nasal fracture?	Lateral nasal deviation, retrusion, or flattening; dislocation of the septum; difficulty breathing; nasal or periorbital hematomas; lacerations over the bridge; bleeding
What treatment is indicated for an isolated nasal fracture?	Closed reduction and manipulation

What are the five anatomic attachments of the zygoma?

1. Posterior—temporal bone
2. Anterior/superior—frontal bone
3. Medial—sphenoid bone
4. Anterior—maxillary bone
5. Anterior/inferior—maxillary alveolus

What are the 10 common signs of zygoma fractures?

Periorbital and subconjunctival hematoma; depression of lateral canthus; recession of malar prominence; step-off or tenderness of inferior orbital rim, anterior maxillary wall; unilateral epistaxis (through maxillary antrum); orbital entrapment inferiorly; infraorbital nerve numbness; globe dystopia or enophthalmos; intraoral hematoma of superior buccal sulcus; difficulty chewing due to impingement of the arch on the coronoid process

What is a nasoethmoidal orbital (NOE) fracture?

A fracture that includes the nose and medial orbital rim

What percentage of NOE fractures are bilateral?

Sixty-six percent

What are the common signs of an NOE fracture?

Depressed nasal dorsum; tenderness over medial canthal ligament; telecanthus (increased distance between eyes); eyelid "spectacle" hematomas; epistaxis; nasal laceration; mobility of the medial orbital rim with direct pressure or intranasal traction

What is the Furnas traction test and what does it test for?

The test is accomplished by palpating the medial canthal region while applying lateral traction on the eyelid. If the medial canthal ligament is intact, it should be palpable during this maneuver as a "bowstring."

What are the signs of a frontal sinus fracture?

Soft tissue trauma to the forehead; epistaxis; depression of the frontal bone

Which frontal sinus fractures require surgery?

Only displaced fractures require open reduction and fixation (wire or plates).

What is the treatment for comminuted frontal sinus fractures in which depressed fragments cannot easily be reduced and fixed?

Sinus obliteration or cranialization

What determines whether frontal sinus obliteration or cranialization is performed?

An intact posterior wall mandates sinus obliteration whereas a severely disrupted wall dictates cranialization. (Note: Mucosa must be removed from all fracture fragments and from remaining sinus walls in either case to isolate the cranial cavity from the nasal cavity.)

What is a common complication of frontal sinus fractures?

Mucocele (due to incomplete removal of sinus mucosa)

What are the common signs of supraorbital fractures?

Soft tissue trauma; depression or irregularity of superior orbital rim; numbness in supraorbital nerve distribution; eyelid ptosis; downward and outward protrusion of globe; superior orbital fissure or orbital apex syndrome

What are the common signs of an orbital floor fracture?

Periorbital and subconjunctival hematoma; anesthesia of the infraorbital nerve; diplopia on upward or downward gaze (entrapment of the inferior rectus and/or inferior oblique); enophthalmos; globe dystopia; orbital emphysema; ipsilateral epistaxis from maxillary sinus; positive forced duction

What is a forced duction exam and what does it demonstrate?

Forced duction is performed by applying topical anesthetic to the globe, grasping the inferior conjunctiva, and testing whether upward movement of the globe is possible. If movement is restricted, it is likely due to entrapment of the inferior rectus within an orbital floor fracture.

What is the Le Fort classification system for maxillary fractures?

Le Fort I—transverse fracture separating the maxillary alveolus from the upper midfacial skeleton
Le Fort II—fracture separating a pyramidal nasomaxillary segment from

the zygomatic and orbital facial
skeleton
Le Fort III—fracture separating the
facial bones from the cranial skeleton
through the upper orbits and nose

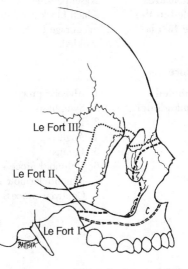

Le Fort III

Le Fort II

Le Fort I

BATTISTA

**What are the diagnostic
signs of Le Fort fractures?**

Malocclusion; mobility of maxillary
alveolus in reference to the upper
portion of the facial or cranial skeleton
from which it is severed; signs of
zygomatic, orbital, nasal or NOE
fractures detailed previously; elongated
and depressed midface; profuse
nasopharyngeal bleeding

CSF Rhinorrhea

**What fractures are
commonly associated with
CSF rhinorrhea?**

Fifty percent to seventy-five percent of
frontal basilar and NOE fractures;
twenty-five percent of Le Fort II and
III fractures.

**What is the bedside test
for CSF rhinorrhea?**

If bloody nasal drainage representing
CSF is blotted onto a white paper towel, a
clear ring extends out from a central spot
of blood (called the double-ring sign).

**What is the management
of CSF rhinorrhea?**

Fistulas associated with displaced
fractures usually undergo direct repair.
Those not associated with displaced
fractures often resolve over a 2-week
period.

Is antibiotic prophylaxis warranted?

Yes, but only for 2 or 3 days after fracture reduction. Long-term prophylaxis leads to the development of resistant organisms.

What routine measures should be avoided in the setting of a CSF fistula?

Nasal packing and nasogastric tubes, which block nasal drainage and encourage bacterial growth, should be avoided.

Mandible Fracture

What are the labeled regions of the mandible?

1. Alveolar process
2. Symphysis
3. Body
4. Angle
5. Ramus
6. Coronoid process
7. Mandibular notch
8. Condylar process

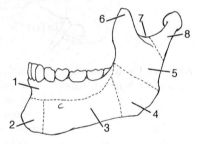

What is the anatomic distribution of fractures of the mandible?

A third in the condylar–subcondylar area, a third at the angle, a third in the body–symphysis.

What percentage of mandible fractures are bilateral?

> 50%

Do mandible fractures more commonly compound externally or intraorally?

Most compound intraorally; thus, a thorough exam of the oral cavity is essential.

What are the common signs of a mandible fracture?

Intraoral or external soft tissue trauma; occlusal abnormality; numbness in distribution of mental nerve; bleeding from a tooth socket; fractured or missing teeth; trismus; open bite, abnormality of

arch, or intercuspation of teeth;
bleeding from the ear (laceration of
anterior wall of ear canal from condylar
fracture); intraoral odor

RECONSTRUCTIVE PRINCIPLES

**What are the indications
for exploration of orbital
floor or medial wall
fractures?**

Diplopia of primary gaze or downward
gaze persistent for 2 weeks,
enophthalmos greater than 3 mm, and
other upper facial fractures requiring
surgery

**What is the primary goal
of orbital wall
reconstruction?**

Restoration of globe support and
reestablishment of normal proportions of
bony volume to orbital content. This
combination almost always requires an
implant of the orbital floor, using
alloplastic or autogenous materials.

**Which complicating factors
make nasoethmoidal
fractures particularly
challenging?**

1. Fragility of the bones makes
   comminution and bone loss common.
2. Associated injuries to the lacrimal
   system, medial canthal tendon, and
   cranial cavity

**What is the basic approach
to reconstruction of the
NOE fracture?**

Interosseous plating or wiring with bone
grafting as needed. Telecanthus is
corrected by transnasal canthopexy.

**Do nondisplaced fractures
of the zygomatic arch or
zygoma require treatment?**

No, neither require treatment unless
subsequent displacement is noted.

**What is the basic approach
to displaced zygoma
fractures?**

Depressed arch fractures require
elevation alone. The remainder require
reduction and fixation to the maxillary
and frontal articulations.

**What is intermaxillary
fixation (IMF)?**

Two arch bars are conformed to fit the
maxillary and mandibular teeth and then
fastened with circumdental wires. The
arch bars are then wired to each other
to restore the proper occlusal
relationship.

If used alone, how long is IMF left in place?	Between 6 and 8 weeks
What is the general goal of MAXILLARY fracture treatment?	Restoration of the articulations with the three maxillary buttresses, the zygomatic, nasofrontal, and the pterygomaxillary, in order to reestablish the normal occlusal relation.
How is this accomplished?	IMF is used to reestablish the occlusion. Plate and screw fixation of fracture fragments with and without bone grafting restores the maxillary buttresses.
What is the general goal for MANDIBULAR fracture treatment?	Restoration of normal occlusion
How is this accomplished?	With IMF. However, because the incidence of multiple mandible fractures is high and the muscles of mastication exert considerable force on fracture fragments, open reduction and fixation with heavy plates and screws may be needed to achieve stability of the arch.
Which mandibular fractures are rarely treated with open reduction–fixation, and how are they managed?	1. Ramus and coronoid fractures (rarely displaced due to muscle protection)— brief IMF or soft diet is the rule 2. Condylar fractures—if isolated, IMF for 3 weeks only, followed by physiotherapy to restore TMJ function 3. Alveolar fractures—often treated with a single arch bar, with IMF added if unstable

HAND SURGERY

ANATOMY

How does the skin of the hand differ on dorsal and ventral sides, and what are the functional implications?	Palmar skin is thick, tethered, irregularly surfaced and moist, with subcutaneous fat beneath, providing padding, stability and friction, for a strong grip. Dorsal skin is thin and mobile, with little fat, providing freedom for the motion of the various joints.

What is the function of the tendon synovial sheaths?

The sheaths (consisting of tenosynovium) act as a mesentery, providing nutrient blood flow and lubrication for gliding of the tendons.

Extrinsic flexors of the hand

What are the extrinsic flexors of the hand?

Digital—flexor pollicis longus (FPL), flexor digitorum profundus (FDP), flexor digitorum superficialis (FDS)
Wrist—palmaris longus (PL), flexor carpi radialis (FCR), flexor carpi ulnaris (FCU)

Where do the extrinsic flexors have their insertions?

FPL and FDP—volar base of distal phalanx
FDS—volar middle phalanx
FCU—pisiform and hamate bones
FCR—volar base of second and third metacarpal
PL—superficial palmar fascia

How is each extrinsic flexor tested?

FPL—flexion of thumb interphalangeal joint with metacarpophalangeal joint extended
FDP—flexion of distal interphalangeal joint with proximal interphalangeal (PIP) joint held in extension
FDS—flexion of PIP with other fingers held in extension. Ulnar three FDP tendons share muscle belly and must be eliminated through extension of other digits during FDS testing.
FCU, FCR, PL—wrist flexed while tendons palpated

Where are the tendon sheaths of the flexors located?

The proximal sheaths start one finger breadth proximal to the flexor retinaculum and reach to the proximal transverse palmar crease. The separate sheaths unite during development to form a common sheath, except for the sheath of the thumb. Distal sheaths begin at the palmar (volar) plate of the MCPs and extend to the distal insertion of the flexor tendons. For the thumb and small fingers, the distal and proximal sheaths are continuous.

Does the sheath of the thumb communicate with the other flexor sheaths?

Yes, in 50% of individuals

What are the structure and function of the fibro-osseous tunnels of the flexor tendons?

The tunnel is a fibrous sheath in each digit which runs from the metacarpal head to the insertion of the tendon on the distal phalanx. Thickenings known as pulleys guide the tendon during excursion. There are five annular (A–A5) and three cruciate (C–C3) pulleys.

Which pulleys are considered the most functionally important?

The A2 and A4 pulleys, over the proximal and middle phalanges, respectively

Extrinsic Extensors of the Hand

How many dorsal compartments and extensors are present in the hand?

Six dorsal compartments which contain the nine separate extensors

What are the extrinsic extensors of the hand?

Compartment: Extensors (radial to ulnar)

First: Abductor pollicis longus (APL), extensor pollicis brevis (EPB)

Second: Extensor carpi radialis longus (ECRL), extensor carpi radialis brevis (ECRB)

Third: Extensor pollicis longus (EPL)

Fourth: Extensor digitorum communis (EDC), extensor indicis proprius (EIP)

Fifth: Extensor digiti minimi (EDM)

Sixth: Extensor carpi ulnaris (ECU)

What are the insertions of the extensors?

APL—base of thumb metacarpal

EPB—base of proximal phalanx

ECRL—base of index metacarpal

ECRB—base of middle metacarpal

EPL—base of distal phalanx thumb

EDC—base of both middle and distal phalanges

EIP—dorsal expansion of index finger, which inserts as above

EDM—dorsal expansion of small finger, which inserts as above

ECU—base of small finger metacarpal

How is each of these muscles tested?

APL or EPB—Abduct or extend, respectively, the thumb while palpating radial side of anatomic snuff-box.

ECRL and ECRB—Extend closed fist and palpate the two adjacent tendons.

EPL—Extend thumb while palpating ulnar side of snuff-box; lift thumb off table with hand flat on palm.

EDC—Straighten fingers watching for MCP extension.

EIP—Extend index finger only, with hand closed in a fist.

EDM—Extend small finger only, with hand closed in a fist.

ECU—Extend and ulnar-deviate wrist with closed fist; palpate tendon just distal to ulnar head.

Where are the synovial sheaths of the extensors?

They extend proximally one finger breadth from underneath the extensor retinaculum and distally one finger breadth onto the dorsum of the hand. There are six, one corresponding to each of the six compartments.

What is extrinsic extensor tightness?

If extensors limit the range of passive flexion of MCP and PIP joints combined, extrinsic tightness exists.

How is extrinic extensor tightness tested?

By passively flexing the PIP joints with MCP joints first in extension and then in flexion. If flexion of PIP joints is decreased by MCP flexion, tightness has been demonstrated.

What are the intrinsic muscles of the hand?

The muscles of the thenar and hypothenar eminences, the lumbricals, interossei, and adductor pollicus

What are the thenar muscles and their functions?

Abductor pollicis brevis—abducts the thumb with APL

Flexor pollicis brevis—flexes thumb MCP

Opponens pollicis—pulls thumb medially and forward across palm

How is thenar function evaluated?	Thumb and small fingertips are brought together with nails parallel (opposition); the thumb is raised 90° above the plain of the palm (abduction). The thenar eminence is observed for contraction and symmetry with the opposite side.
What is the function of the *ad*ductor pollicis and how is it tested?	Thumb adduction. Tested by holding a piece of paper between the thumb and radial index proximal phalanx—if weak, the IP of the thumb flexes, known as "Froment's sign."
What is the function of the lumbricals?	Flexion of MCP's and extension of IP's
How are the lumbricals tested?	By simultaneously accomplishing both MCP flexion and IP extension
What are the functions of the interossei (dorsal and palmar)?	Palmar interossei adduct (PIO) digits, whereas dorsal interossei (DIO) abduct digits.
How are the interossei tested?	The most stringent test is to place the palm flat on the table, hyperextend the digits, and then abduct and adduct them. The first DIO can be palpated during the abduction of the index finger.
What are the muscles of the hypothenar eminence?	Abductor digiti minimi, flexor digiti minimi, and opponens digiti minimi (like the thenar eminence)
How are the hypothenar muscles tested?	To test abduction, abduct the small finger while observing for dimpling of the eminence. Opposition can be tested as described above for the thenar eminence.
What is intrinsic muscle tightness?	Tightness is defined as limited PIP passive flexion during MCP flexion, which puts tension on the intrinsics. It is relieved by MCP extension, which relaxes the intrinsics.

Nerves of the Upper Extremity

What are the three primary nerves innervating the upper extremity?	Median, ulnar, and radial nerves

What is the anatomic course of the median nerve in the forearm?

The median nerve enters the forearm through the pronator teres and gives off the anterior interosseous branch in the proximal forearm. It then runs between the flexor digitorum profundus and sublimis, entering the radial side of the carpal tunnel at the wrist.

What is the anatomic course of the ulnar nerve in the forearm?

The ulnar nerve runs behind the medial epicondyle of the humerus, between the two heads of flexor carpi ulnaris, and lies between the flexor digitorum profundus and flexor carpi ulnaris. It branches from the dorsal cutaneous branch in the distal forearm and then enters Guyon's canal at the wrist ulnar to the ulnar artery.

What is the anatomic course of the radial nerve in the forearm?

The radial nerve enters the cubital fossa between the brachialis medially and the brachioradialis and the extensor carpi radialis longus laterally, and divides into superficial and deep branches at the lateral epicondyle of the humerus. The deep branch runs between superficial and deep layers of the supinator, entering the posterior compartment of the forearm. The superficial branch runs under the brachioradialis and above the supinator and pronator teres muscles, eventually coursing dorsally at the wrist.

What muscles are innervated by the median nerve in the forearm?

Pronator teres, flexor carpi radialis, palmaris longus, flexor digitorum superficialis, flexor digitorum profundus (radial), flexor pollicis longus, and pronator quadratus

What muscles are innervated by the ulnar nerve in the forearm?

Flexor carpi ulnaris, flexor digitorum profundus (ulnar)

What muscles are innervated by the radial nerve in the forearm?

Extensor carpi radialis brevis, supinator, extensor digitorum communis, extensor digiti minimi, extensor carpi ulnaris, abductor pollicis longus, extensor pollicis longus, extensor pollicis brevis, extensor indici proprius, °anconeus, °brachioradialis, °extensor carpi radialis longus, and °triceps (° innervated above the elbow)

What are the sensory territories of the hand?

(Note: Variability in the sensory innervation is common, and may even consist of contribution from the lateral cutaneous nerve of the forearm [musculocutaneous nerve] or the posterior cutaneous nerve of the forearm [radial nerve]).

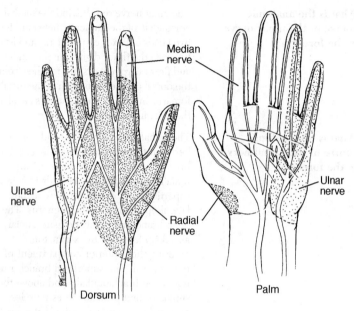

Median nerve

Ulnar nerve

Radial nerve

Ulnar nerve

Dorsum

Palm

How is sensory testing of the fingers best accomplished?

Tactile gnosis (tested by two-point discrimination) is the best indicator of nerve function. Two prongs (for example, from a paper clip) are pressed against the skin while the patient identifies the sensation as a single or double point. This test is done with the probes both stationary and moving, and the minimal distance at which two points can be distinguished is determined. Abnormal is defined as > 6 mm static or > 3 mm moving required for detection of two points.

What is the best substitute in the uncooperative or unresponsive patient, or the child?

The immersion test (where the hand is placed in water for 5–10 minutes and then observed for wrinkling of the glabrous skin) is a good substitute. Denervation of the skin prevents wrinkling.

What is the course of the median nerve in the hand, and what are the structures that it innervates?

The median nerve exits the carpal tunnel, branching into the thenar motor branch, common digital nerves (to the thumb, index finger, middle finger, and radial half of ring finger), the first and second lumbricals, and the sensory branches to the radial palm.

What is the course of the ulnar nerve in the hand, and what are the structures that it innervates?

The ulnar nerve exits Guyon's canal and divides into deep and superficial branches. The deep branch supplies the hypothenar muscles, the interossei, the third and fourth lumbricals, adductor pollicis, and deep flexor pollicis brevis. The superficial branch supplies the palmaris brevis, the common digitial nerves (to small and ulnar half of ring finger), and sensation to the ulnar palm.

What is the course of the radial nerve in the hand, and what are the structures that it innervates?

After traveling beneath the brachioradialis tendon, the superficial branch of the radial nerve provides sensation to the radial half of the dorsum of the hand, to the entire dorsum of the thumb, and to the index and radial half of the middle finger dorsum proximal to the PIP joints.

Arteries of the Upper Extremity

What is the course of the arteries supplying the forearm?

At the elbow, the **brachial artery,** lying between the median nerve medially and the biceps tendon laterally, divides into ulnar and radial arteries. The **radial artery** runs under the belly of the brachioradialis proximally and then courses superficially to the wrist, just radial to the flexor carpi radialis. The **ulnar artery** gives off the common interosseous artery, which follows the interosseous membrane after dividing into anterior and posterior branches.

The ulnar artery crosses under the flexor digitorum superficialis and runs along its ulnar border, entering Guyon's canal at the wrist, with the ulnar nerve.

What is the arterial supply to the hand?

There are four major arterial arches of the hand and wrist. The **palmar carpal arch** and **dorsal carpal rete** receive contributions from the interosseous, radial, and ulnar arteries. The **deep palmar arch** also receives contributions from all four forearm vessels. The **superficial palmar arch** receives input primarily from the radial and ulnar arteries.

What is the arterial supply to the digits?

Each digit is supplied with two **dorsal digital arteries,** which extend distally to the PIP joint level, receiving the same tributaries as the dorsal carpal rete. Two **palmar digital arteries,** which course with the digital nerves to the tips of the digits, are supplied by both the deep and superficial palmar arches.

What test assesses the contributions of ulnar and radial arteries to the blood supply to the hand?

The Allen test. The radial and ulnar arteries are compressed manually and the hand exsanguinated by making a fist. One artery is released and the filling time observed. Normal time for this test is 5 seconds.

How is the arterial supply to the finger assessed for bilateral contribution?

An Allen test can also be done on the digits by compressing both of the palmar digital arteries and assessing refilling time after release of a single artery.

What are the eight bones of the wrist?

From Radial To Ulnar
Proximal: Scaphoid, Lunate, Triquetrum, Pisiform
Distal: Trapezium, Trapezoid, Capitate, Hamate

Which motions of the hand are accomplished by the intercarpal and radiocarpal joints and which by the radioulnar joints?

Flexion, extension, radial and ulnar deviation are accomplished by the wrist and radiocarpal joints alone. Supination and pronation are accomplished by the proximal and distal radioulnar joints.

What are the fixed and mobile units of the hand?

Fixed unit—metacarpals of the index and middle fingers are rigidly attached to the distal carpal row
Mobile unit—the other metacarpals and phalanges are suspended from this unit

In what position is the hand usually splinted?

Intrinsic plus position (or position of safety): Wrist—35 degrees of extension; MCPs—45 to 70 degrees of flexion in a cascade from index to small; IP's—10 degrees of flexion each; thumb—abduction of metacarpal, MCP and IP in neutral

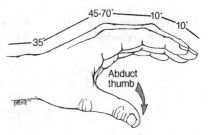

When is the intrinsic plus position used and why?

For most hand injuries requiring immobilization; it prevents permanent contractures of collateral ligaments and decreases the loss of mobility during splinting.

When is this position contraindicated?

With flexor tendon injuries

HAND EMERGENCIES

Traumatic Amputations

What is the general cause of life-threatening hemorrhage in the forearm and hand?

Usually a **partially** transected artery (versus completely transected arteries, which can retract into the surrounding tissue as well as initiate vasospasm effectively, thus reducing the risk of life-threatening hemorrhage)

Treatment?

1. Direct pressure and elevation stop the majority of severe bleeding.
2. A tourniquet 100 to 150 mm Hg above systolic blood pressure can be

applied as a temporizing measure for 30 minutes at a time, with 5-minute rests in between to assess for control of bleeding and for patient comfort.

What are the indications for replantation of amputated digit?

1. Multiple injured digits (even with only a single amputation if other digits are severely injured)
2. Thumb amputations (especially if proximal to the IP joint)
3. All amputations in children
4. Clean amputations (sharp division) at the hand, wrist, or distal forearm

Is replantation commonly limited by technical considerations?

No; although restoration of blood supply is not always possible in a severely injured amputated part, more often reattachment and viability are possible. (Note: If the reattached part will offer no significant functional advantage over amputation, replantation should be avoided.)

What are the relative contraindications to replantation?

1. Severe crush or avulsion
2. Amputation between the MCP and PIP joints of a single digit
3. Heavily contaminated wound
4. Smoking history

What are the absolute contraindications to replantation?

1. Severe medical problems or associated injuries increasing the risk of surgery
2. Multilevel injury to the amputated part
3. Inability to stop smoking for 3 months post replant
4. Psychiatric illness that precipitated self-amputation

Preoperative preparation in patient with amputated digit?

Débridement of stump with irrigation and dressing with nonadherent gauze, tetanus prophylaxis, IV antibiotics, and IV hydration

What is the preparation of the amputated part?

Débridement with irrigation, wrapping in gauze moistened with lactated Ringer's or normal saline, and placement of wrapped part in sealed container that is immersed in an ice bath

How is an incompletely amputated part prepared?

The treatment is identical with the additional step of detorquing intact vessels to restore blood supply. The attached part is cooled in insulated ice packs instead of in the previously mentioned ice bath.

Mangling Injury

What are the guiding principles in the initial treatment of a severe mangling injury?

1. Adequate débridement of devitalized tissue and debris with loose closure, delayed primary closure, or skin grafting to avoid tension caused by swelling
2. Opening of investing fascia prophylactically to prevent a potential compartment syndrome
3. Serial débridements every 2 to 3 days as needed

What is the initial treatment of mangled parts that are unlikely to regain function but maintain an adequate blood supply? Why?

Mangled parts, such as a severely injured finger, are often left intact because they are an excellent source for autologous grafting of skin, bone, articular surface, nerve, artery, and tendon.

Compartment Syndrome

What is the mechanism of compartment syndrome?

Accumulation of fluid (either blood or exudate) within a fascial compartment builds pressure that obstructs venous outflow. As arterial inflow continues, the pressure continues to increase until arterial inflow is decreased, causing ischemia and further progression of the fluid accumulation as tissue injury worsens.

What compartments can be affected in the forearm and hand?

Volar or dorsal compartments in the forearm and intrinsic muscle compartments in the hand

What are the cardinal signs of a compartment syndrome?

1. Gross appearance—swollen, tense, tender hand or forearm
2. Muscles—tender and increased pain on passive extension
3. Nerves—pain (early), followed by paresthesias (later), followed by anesthesia (late)
4. Pulselessness (late!)

How can compartment syndrome be distinguished from simple swelling?

Compartment pressures can be measured. Pressure greater than 30 mm Hg is considered a true compartment syndrome. However, since pressures can evolve rapidly (and may be incorrect due to technical considerations), a high clinical suspicion should lead to repeat measurements or prophylactic fasciotomies even in the face of "normal" pressures.

HAND INJURIES REQUIRING URGENT TREATMENT

Burns

Which hand burns are usually more severe: scald or flame?

Flame burns more often involve full-thickness dermal injury, whereas scalds are usually only partial-thickness burns.

What region of the hand is least susceptible to injury?

The palm, because of its relatively thick dermis, can often resist full-thickness loss better than the dorsum can.

What is the management of partial-thickness burns of the hand?

1. Splinting in the position of safety
2. Application of Silvadene twice a day
3. Frequent range-of-motion physical therapy
4. If not healed in 2 weeks, skin grafting to avoid scarring, particularly on the dorsum
5. Wound checks to ensure rapid progression of healing
6. Pressure garments to reduce hypertrophic scarring after wounds are covered

What is the management of full-thickness burns?

1. Early excision and grafting
2. Emergency escharotomy and carpal tunnel release (if compartment syndrome is a concern)

How are deeper burns (e.g., fourth degree) managed?

1. Adequate and frequent serial débridements
2. Similar to mangling, nonfunctioning viable parts may be used as a source of tissue for reconstruction.

How is the management of tar burns different from the management of other thermal burns?

Tar can act initially as a protective dressing. If antibiotic-impregnated Vaseline is applied every 6 to 12 hours, the tar slowly dissolves out of the wound.

What is the voltage threshold for significant travel through tissue?

500 volts is required for current to pass through tissues of least resistance, which include both blood vessels and nerves.

What precaution must always be considered in electrical injuries of > 500 volts?

Because of tissue penetration, deep tissue necrosis may ensue, mandating:
1. A more extensive débridement than might be anticipated by examination
2. Careful observation for a compartment syndrome

For details of chemical burn treatment, see the burn section of this chapter.

Cold Injury

What determines the extent of cold injuries?

Duration of exposure and temperature

What can increase the extent of such injuries?

Wetness, dependency of the affected part, vasospasm, open wounds, constrictive wrappings, and immobile body positions

What is the progression of signs and symptoms as injury progresses?

Early injury—burning and itching, erythema
Late injury—pallor, coldness, and numbness

What are the signs and symptoms as the tissues are rewarmed?

Burning, paresthesias, aching. Erythema and vesicles (clear or hemorrhagic) that may progress to ulcers

How is therapeutic rewarming accomplished?

Rewarming takes place in **lukewarm** water (40°–42°C) until normal color and warmth return. Analgesia is often required during this process.

What is the next step in therapy?

As with thermal injuries, the hand is splinted and dressed. Vesicles are left intact and débrided after rupture or hardening.

How are ruptured vesicles managed?

Once the depth of the injury has been determined, the wounds are treated in the same manner as burns of similar extent.

What more aggressive modes of therapy are occasionally instituted in the management of cold injury?	1. Core rewarming for systemic hypothermia (if present) initiated along with rewarming of the frostbitten part. 2. Antithrombotics to prevent thrombosis of affected vessels 3. Temporary sympathectomy with nerve block to improve blood flow (Note: Neither antithrombotics nor temporary sympathectomy is proved conclusively to decrease tissue necrosis in the affected parts.)

SIMPLE INFECTIONS OF THE HAND

Paronychia

What is a paronychia?	An infection of the periungual tissue which can extend under the nail or onto the finger pad
What is the most common causative organism?	*Staphylococcus aureus*
What is the treatment?	1. Elevation of the nail margin and removal of the affected portion of the nail plate 2. Soaks and antibiotic therapy (usually a penicillin effective against *Staphylococcus aureus*) 3. Drainage of abscess (if present) and protection of the nail matrix with nonadherent gauze
What additional cause must be considered for chronic paronychiae, especially with occupational risks such as dishwashing?	Chronic fungal infections are common in these cases; consider antifungal therapy.

Felon

What is a felon?	Infection of the finger-pad soft tissue. Presents as a swollen, painful, tense finger pad.

How may it progress if untreated?	Osteomyelitis of the distal phalanx
What is the treatment?	A longitudinal incision at the nail–skin margin is carried down to just before the anterolateral border of the distal phalanx. The longitudinal fibrous septae of the finger pad are incised to reach the abscess cavity and allow evacuation. A wick is placed to provide continued drainage. Soaks and an antibiotic active against *Staphylococcus aureus* are also indicated.
If the felon has progressed to osteomyelitis, what additional therapy is needed?	Débridement of devitalized bone, then prolonged antibiotic therapy for 4 to 8 weeks

Herpetic Whitlow

What is a herpetic whitlow?	A herpes simplex vesicle or ulcer on the finger (often seen in dental or medical personnel who do not use adequate precautions)
What tests may be used for diagnosis?	A Tsanck smear of lesional fluid, scrapings for giant cells, fluorescent antibody testing of lesion fluid, or culture of the lesion for virus
What is the treatment?	Topical acyclovir ointment should be applied every 3 hours for 48 hours with 5 days of oral acyclovir to start simultaneously. Incision and débridement should be avoided. Antibacterial antibiotics are indicated only in cases of suspected superinfection.

COMPLEX INFECTIONS OF THE HAND

Suppurative Tenosynovitis

What is suppurative tenosynovitis?	A bacterial infection of the tendon sheath usually following penetrating trauma

Is it more common in extensor or flexor tendon sheaths?

Flexor

What are Kanavel's four signs of flexor tenosynovitis?

1. Flexed posture of the affected digit
2. Tenderness along the sheath with erythema
3. Pain on passive extension of DIP joint
4. Fusiform swelling (sausage-like finger)

Which sign is the strongest indicator of tenosynovitis?

Pain on passive extension of the DIP joint

What is a horseshoe infection?

Suppurative tenosynovitis that has spread in a horseshoe pattern from either ring or small finger through palm to affect the other digit. May develop because the small finger and thumb tendon sheaths both extend from the palm and often communicate.

What is the immediate treatment of suppurative flexor tenosynovitis?

Incisions are made over the proximal sheath and at the level of the middle phalanx. A No. 5 French catheter is inserted between the A4 and A5 pulleys, and the sheath is irrigated with a bacitracin solution.

What additional treatment accompanies the operative drainage?

IV antibiotics, splinting in the intrinsic plus position with elevation, and irrigation of the sheath every 4 to 6 hours with bacitracin solution through an indwelling catheter until the infection resolves

Deep-Space Infections

What are the two areas for deep-space infections of the hand?

1. Midpalmar (between the flexor tendons and the metacarpals of the ulnar three digits)
2. Thenar (between the flexor tendon of the index finger and the adductor pollicis)

What is the treatment?

1. Incision and débridement with drain placement. The midpalmar space is drained with a palmar incision between the third and fourth rays, the thenar space through a dorsal incision of the thumb web space
2. IV antibiotics

What are the common sources of septic arthritis?

1. Direct inoculation from penetrating trauma
2. Hematogenous spread

What are the common pathogens for penetrating trauma?

For trauma, especially of the MCP joint, the infection is often the product of human tooth penetration and inoculation. *Staphylococcus aureus* is the most commmon, but mixed gram-positive and gram-negative cultures are frequent.

Which organsim is classically associated with human bites?

Eikenella corrodens, a gram-negative bacillus

What are the common pathogens for hematogenous spread?

Although any pathogen can cause septic arthritis in this manner, *Neisseria gonorrhoeae* must always be considered.

Treatment of septic arthritis?

Incision and débridement with drain placement. Antibiotic coverage includes a penicillin with activity against *Staphylococcus aureus* and an aminoglycoside.

How is mycobacterial infection usually contracted?

From a puncture wound in the setting of soil or water

What is the usual presentation of mycobacterial arthritis?

A synovitis of a tendon sheath or joint develops approximately 6 weeks post-trauma.

How is mycobacterial arthritis diagnosed and treated?

Culture or the finding of multinucleated giant cells confirms the diagnosis. Long-term antibiotic therapy is required.

TENDON LACERATIONS

What flexor tendon injuries can be treated in the emergency room setting?

None! Although careful inspection is acceptable in the emergency room, virtually ALL flexor tendon injuries require operative exploration, therapy, or both.

What extensor tendon injuries can be treated in the emergency room?

Any laceration in which both ends can be easily visualized for repair can be treated in the emergency room. Multiple tendon injuries or those with difficult exposure (i.e., more proximal) should be attempted only in the operating room.

What are the zones used to describe flexor tendon lacerations?

Zone I—mid finger pad to distal half of middle phalanx
Zone II—proximal half of middle phalanx to MCP joint, inclusive of the MCP
Zone III—distal palmar crease to midpalm
Zone IV—midpalm to wrist crease, carpus included
Zone V—wrist crease and proximal

Which zone is also called "no man's land"?

Zone II

What is the usual mechanism of a Zone I flexor injury?

Avulsion of the tendon insertion during grasping

Why is flexion often intact in a Zone I flexor injury?

The vinculum, a mesentery for the tendon, often stays connected to the distal phalanx.

Why are functional results of flexor tendon repair notoriously poor in Zone II?

Zone II requires smooth gliding of the FDS and FDP tendons within the narrow confines of the fibro-osseous tunnel of the tendon sheath. Repair without significant adhesion formation is difficult and often requires revision.

Injury to what structures often accompanies Zone III flexor injuries?

The superficial transverse vascular arch, the median nerve at its division into terminal branches, and the thenar motor branch of the median nerve

Why is operative exploration mandatory for Zone IV flexor injuries?

Exposure is technically demanding because it is located within the carpal tunnel.

Why are Zone V flexor lacerations, which are easily repaired, usually devastating injuries?

Tendon healing (which is generally good) often is overshadowed by a severe accompanying nerve injury (which generally recovers only partially).

What are the initial steps taken before operative repair of flexor tendons?

Débridement, loose closure, splinting in the intrinsic plus position except with the wrist in slight flexion

How long can surgical repair be delayed?

Although some controversy exists on the exact timing, repair within 6 days prevents significant contraction.

What is the usual method of tendon reapproximation?

A modified Kessler suture is widely used because of its good tensile strength, placement of the knot within the repair, and relatively small amount of ischemia induced.

What are the three major complications of partial tendon lacerations?

1. Delayed rupture
2. Trigger phenomenon
3. Decreased range of motion

Which partial tendon lacerations should be repaired?

Any laceration > 50% of the diameter **or** near the proximal pulley should be repaired. (*Note:* Controversy exists over the indications for repair, because rates of rupture may be higher in repaired tendons and tensile strength may be decreased.)

How is the tendon repaired?	Approximation of the epitenon with fine sutures
What are the zones used to describe extensor tendon lacerations?	Zones I and II—distal phalanx, DIP joint Zones III and IV—central slip or lateral slips of the long extensor tendon, fibers of the intrinsic expansion, and the oblique and transverse fibers of the extensor aponeurosis Zone V—the MCP region Zone VI—digits proximal to MCP and area of extensor retinaculum
What is the usual mechanism for Zone I and II extensor injuries?	A blow to the extended digit, forcing flexion of the DIP joint and avulsion of the tendon with or without a fragment of bone
What is the resultant deformity?	Mallet finger (DIP joint flexion). Eventually the PIP joint becomes hyperextended through a proximal shift in the action of the extensors after distal rupture and a swan-neck deformity result.
What is the most common resultant deformity of a Zone III or IV injury?	Boutonnière deformity (PIP joint flexion and DIP joint hyperextension)
What is the general treatment of extensor tendon injuries?	Open lacerations—direct repair of the tendon with subsequent splinting for 6 to 8 weeks (K wire for fixation of joint(s); closed rupture—splinting in neutral or hyperextension for 6 to 8 weeks ($\pm$ K-wire fixation)
How are lacerations to the extensor aponeurosis treated?	Splinting as previously described, with or without suture closure of the defect

NERVE INJURIES

What happens to peripheral nerves proximal to the site of injury?	Retrograde degeneration of axons (1–2 cm) with Schwann cell proliferation; degenerative changes of the neuronal cell body (may reverse within 40 to 120 days); axonal sprouting within 1 week that grows centrifugally from the site of transection

What happens to peripheral nerves DISTAL to the site of injury?

Wallerian degeneration (axonal disintegration progressive to the entire length of the distal segment); removal of debris by macrophages; Schwann cell proliferation within the neural tube and outside of the distal stump

Which types of nerve injuries mechanistically have the best prognosis?

From best to worst, laceration > crush > stretch (corresponds to the size of the zone of injury)

What other factors worsen prognosis?

More proximal injuries (due to increased length of wallerian degeneration) and older age of the patient

What is the initial treatment of nerve injuries?

Thorough débridement and closure (if possible) to best preserve the integrity of divided nerve stumps

What is the best timing of repair for nerve lacerations?

Either primary repair **or** delayed primary repair, within 7 to 10 days

What is the indication for delayed repair, and how long can the patient wait without significant worsening of functional recovery?

Delayed in cases where nerve function may return, i.e., closed injury such as a crush or stretch injury. Delays of 5 to 6 months are possible.

What are the principles of nerve repair?

Tensionless reapproximation with minimal suturing, the least undermining possible, accurate fascicular alignment

What is the indication for nerve grafting?

When tensionless reapproximation is not possible

What nerves are usually used for grafting?

Sural and superficial radial nerves

FRACTURES OF THE HAND

Extra-articular Fractures of the Hand

What is the standard treatment for nondisplaced extra-articular fractures of the metacarpals and phalanges?

Splinting in the intrinsic plus position with guarded motion to commence in 10 to 14 days. Stable phalangeal fractures may then be placed in a digital splint or "buddy taped" for 2 to 3 weeks. Metacarpal fractures remain splinted for 2 to 3 weeks.

When can displaced metacarpal and phalangeal fractures be treated with closed reduction?

Whenever closed reduction is able to correct for angulation or rotational deformity

What is boxer's fracture?

A fracture of the fifth metacarpal neck

How is this metacarpal fracture unique?

Usually volar angulation is not well tolerated in the metacarpals; however, because of the mobility of the fifth metacarpal, up to 40 degrees of volar angulation can still give acceptable function.

Intra-articular Fractures of the Hand

What features of intra-articular fractures must be considered in deciding the most appropriate treatment?

1. Ligamentous injury and the consequent joint instability
2. The integrity of the articular surface, which will greatly influence long-term functional recovery

What is the significance of small bone fragments seen on radiographs of intra-articular fractures?

Frequently these fragments point to an avulsion of a ligamentous attachment, which may have important consequences for joint stability.

What are the similarities and differences between a Bennett's fracture and a Rolando's fracture?

Both are intra-articular fractures of the base of the thumb metacarpal. A Bennett's fracture is by definition unstable because the APL displaces the shaft proximally and radially away from the other intra-articular fracture fragment. A Rolando's fracture is a Y- or T-shaped fracture of the base.

What is the treatment of these fractures?

Open reduction and internal fixation are frequently required of both.

What is the treatment of PIP intra-articular fractures?

Splint if < 25% of articular surface; ORIF if > 25% and unstable

What are the indications for ORIF in DIP intra-articular fractures?

1. > 30% of articular surface involved
2. Palmar subluxation of the distal phalanx
3. Proximal displacement of the fracture fragment (may result in extensor lag)

Nonoperative treatment of an intra-articular fracture of the DIP?	Splinting of the digit in the intrinsic plus position with progression to a digit splint or "buddy taping" within 2 or 3 weeks

DISLOCATIONS OF THE HAND

Which are the most typical dislocations of the DIP, PIP, and MCP joints?	For DIP and PIP, dorsal and lateral. For the MCP (including thumb), usually dorsal.
What is the treatment of these dislocations?	Closed reduction and splinting (degrees of flexion depend on joint)
What is the next step if instability of the joint persists?	Closed reduction and percutaneous fixation, followed by ORIF if this is unsuccessful
What is gamekeeper's thumb?	Disruption of the thumb's ulnar collateral ligament; usually incurred by lateral stress while grasping an object
How is degree of instability assessed?	Radiographic stress views under digital block for analgesia (Note: A fracture **must** first be ruled out with x-ray before stressing is allowed.)
What is the treatment of gamekeeper's thumb?	Thumb spica cast if there are < 40 degrees of instability or a nondisplaced fracture; for > 40 degrees of instability or a displaced fracture, ORIF is required.
Treatment of carpal–metacarpal (CM) dislocation?	Usually the ligamentous disruption is significant and requires at least percutaneous fixation after reduction.
Which CM dislocations are frequently associated with fracture?	Thumb dislocations (Bennett's fracture)

FRACTURES AND DISLOCATIONS OF THE WRIST

How is a scaphoid fracture diagnosed?	Snuff-box tenderness. Multiple radiographic views of the wrist, especially an oblique, are often needed for diagnosis.

What should be done if fracture is suspected, but x-ray examination is negative?

Potential scaphoid fractures should be treated expectantly and followed up with repeat imaging and exams.

How is a nondisplaced scaphoid fracture treated?

Cast with wrist in neutral and thumb in abduction for 4 to 6 weeks. Continue close radiographic follow-up.

What is a classic complication of proximal scaphoid fractures?

Avascular necrosis of the proximal fragment. This condition can be prevented in that union can often be obtained with conservative management.

What is the usual mechanism for a hook, or hamate, fracture?

Striking a solid object while grasping a solid object

What is the treatment of hook, or hamate, fracture?

Four to six weeks of cast immobilization. Excision of the hook is indicated for nonunion.

What is Kienböck disease?

Traumatic malacia of the lunate. Susceptible individuals undergo avascular necrosis in response to single or multiple traumas.

What is the treatment of Kienböck disease?

Complex reconstructive techniques including bone grafting and fusions

How is a lunate dislocation diagnosed?

Lateral wrist radiograph demonstrates volar displacement of the lunate. (Note: Dorsal lunate dislocations are rare.)

How is a perilunate dislocation diagnosed?

Lateral wrist radiograph demonstrates alignment of the lunate and dorsal displacement of the capitate and digits. (Note: Volar perilunate displacement is rare.)

How are lunate and perilunate dislocations treated?

Successful closed reduction followed by casting in thumb spica cast with 20 degrees of wrist flexion. ORIF is often necessary.

What is scapholunate dissociation and how is it diagnosed?	Disruption of the volar radioscapholunate ligament and the interosseous scapholunate ligament. Diagnosed by AP wrist radiograph showing a gap between scaphoid and lunate and an axially oriented scaphoid.
Treatment of scapholunate dissociation?	Closed reduction with K-wire fixation or ORIF followed by immobilization in volar flexion

NERVE COMPRESSION SYNDROMES

Carpal Tunnel Syndrome

Risk factors for carpal tunnel syndrome?	Rheumatoid arthritis, Colles' fracture, pregnancy, diabetes mellitus, thyroid disease, and occupations requiring leaning or banging on the base of the palm (Note: The largest proportion of affected individuals has no known risk factors.)
What are the signs and symptoms?	1. Pain, paresthesias, numbness in the median nerve distribution. Pain may also be referred to the shoulder or elbow 2. Thenar atrophy secondary to motor branch disease 3. Decreased thumb pronation from APB weakness
What simple clinical tests can aid in diagnosis?	1. Phalen's test—elbows are placed on the table, wrists resting in flexion. Symptoms will be induced in 60 seconds. 2. Tinel's sign—paresthesias are elicited by tapping over the carpal tunnel.
What is the differential diagnosis?	Thoracic outlet syndrome, cervical radiculopathy, and other peripheral neuropathies
How can compression be distinguished from other peripheral nerve syndromes?	Nerve conduction studies and electromyography can be used to accurately diagnose the presence of compression and to pinpoint its location.

How does carpal tunnel differ clinically from high median compression in the forearm?

High median compression causes flexor weakness in FDP and FPL as well as a less well-defined sensory loss.

What is the nonoperative treatment of carpal tunnel syndrome?

Splinting of the wrist at night in a neutral or slightly extended position, corticosteroid injections into the carpal tunnel

What is the operative treatment of carpal tunnel syndrome?

Decompression of the carpal tunnel by release of palmar fascia and transverse carpal ligament, neurolysis, and relaxed closure of the tunnel

Ulnar Nerve Compression

Most common site of ulnar nerve compression?

At the elbow as the nerve passes through the cubital tunnel

Signs and symptoms?

Pain, paresthesias, numbness in the ulnar distribution; weakness of the interossei, adductor pollicis, FCU, and FDP to ring and small fingers

What is the nonoperative treatment of ulnar nerve compression?

Padding at the elbow

What is the operative treatment of ulnar nerve compression?

Release of the nerve from the cubital tunnel with rerouting anterior to the medial humeral epicondyle

As it is uncommon on its own, what other conditions often precipitate ulnar nerve compression at the wrist?

1. Ulnar artery aneurysm or compressing thrombosis
2. Repetitive trauma
3. Anterior dislocation of the ulnar head
4. Ganglion of the pisohamate joint
(Note: The location of nerve compression, as with carpal tunnel, can be determined by nerve conduction studies and electromyography.)

Where is the radial nerve most susceptible to compression?

The mid-humerus posteriorly as it runs along the bone

Common mechanisms of injury?

Prolonged pressure (e.g., "Saturday night palsy," trauma, heavy triceps use)

What are the symptoms?	Pain, paresthesias, numbness in radial distribution; weakness of wrist extension, digit extension at the MCP's, and thumb extension
What is the treatment?	Most of these compressions are self-limited (e.g., neurapraxia) and not an ongoing compression. They respond to conservative therapy of a "cock-up" wrist splint, which allows the fingers to function through muscles until recovery of the nerve.

FINGER-PAD DEFECTS

What is the treatment of tissue defects of the finger-pad with bone and soft tissue mostly intact?	The amputated pad can be used to fashion a full-thickness graft. Exposed bone may be rongeured smooth, and soft tissue closed over it for padding. Grafts can often be secured with only a nonadherent compression dressing.
What are the options for larger defects?	Local V–Y advancement flaps or pedicle flaps derived from the thenar eminence or adjacent finger (cross finger flap).
When are the pedicle flaps divided postoperatively?	Two weeks

NAIL AND NAIL-BED INJURIES

What is the treatment of subungual hematoma WITHOUT severe disruption of the nail plate from the matrix?	Trephination—holes are punched or burned through the nail plate to allow drainage
Which injury commonly accompanies subungual hematomas?	Distal phalanx fractures
How does the risk of this concurrent injury alter management?	Radiographs should always be obtained, and sterile technique should be used for trephination (can convert a closed fracture into an open one).

Treatment of lacerations of the nail bed?	Repair with fine absorbable sutures. Exposed matrix may be covered with nonadherent gauze or the nail may be used as a splint.
What is the treatment of avulsions of the germinal matrix?	The germinal matrix should be replaced in the eponychial fold and either sutured in place or held with nonadherent gauze.

ARTHRITIS

Rheumatoid Arthritis

What are the common manifestations of rheumatoid arthritis in the hands?	1. Trigger fingers 2. Wrist tenosynovitis 3. Extensor tendon rupture 4. Carpal tunnel syndrome 5. Fibrosis and shortening of the intrinsics
What are the expected deformities as disease progresses?	1. Ulnar drift of the digits 2. Extensor lag at the MCP's 3. Swan-neck and boutonnière deformities 4. Degeneration of articular surfaces and bone mass
Treatment of arthritis?	In addition to the systemic treatment with anti-inflammatory medication, attempts may be made to salvage function through reconstruction, replacement, and removal of diseased structures in selected patients.
In osteoarthritis, what are the most commonly involved joints of the hand?	IP joints of the digits and the basal joint of the thumb
What are Heberden's and Bouchard's nodes?	Osteophytes of the DIP and PIP joints, respectively
Treatment of osteoarthritis?	NSAIDs are the mainstay of early therapy. For advanced degenerative changes, reconstructive decisions similar to those for rheumatoid arthritis are sometimes indicated.

MISCELLANEOUS HAND CONDITIONS

Trigger Finger

What is the pathophysiologic mechanism of a trigger finger?

Triggering is caused by a discrepancy between the flexor tendons and the proximal sheath, specifically the **A1 pulley.**

What are the etiologies?

Idiopathic, tenosynovitis, post-traumatic, and rheumatoid arthritis

What is the treatment?

Steroid injections into the sheath with or without splinting of the IP joints in extension. If this fails, operative opening of the proximal sheath is performed.

de Quervain's Stenosing Tenosynovitis

What is de Quervain's stenosing tenosynovitis?

A tenosynovitis of the first dorsal compartment (APL and EPB), with or without triggering, secondary to the inflammation

What are the signs and symptoms?

Pain over the tendon sheaths with motion of the thumb; thickness and tenderness over the first compartment

Clinical tests used to make the diagnosis?

1. Finkelstein's test—thumb is flexed and grasped by digits; then fist is ulnar deviated, which elicits pain over the radial styloid
2. Forceful abduction or extension of the thumb, which elicits pain

What other pathologic process can mimic the symptoms of de Quervain's; how can the two be distinguished?

Arthritis of the thumb carpometacarpal joint. This condition can be diagnosed by forcefully grinding the metacarpal on the trapezium, which elicits pain and crepitus in the case of arthritis.

What is the treatment?

Steroid injections within the first dorsal compartment with or without splinting. If unsuccessful, operative release of the fibro-osseous sheaths of the first compartment is performed.

Dupuytren's Fasciitis and Contracture

What is Dupuytren's fasciitis and contracture?
Painless thickening of the palmar fascia due to fibrous proliferation, which frequently begins as a nodule and may progress to a contracture of the MCP, PIP, or DIP joint with functional loss of the digit

Whom does it typically affect?
Middle-aged patients, 7:1 ratio of men to women. Alcoholics, chronic invalids, epileptics, and patients with liver disease, diabetes mellitus, or pulmonary tuberculosis are at increased risk.

What are the most frequently affected regions of the hand?
1. Digits in order of decreasing frequency: ring > small > middle > thumb > index
2. Joints, in decreasing order: MCP > PIP > DIP

What is the treatment?
Lysis of constricting fascial bands provides temporary relief. To prevent recurrence, removal of the palmar fascia must be complete. Local corticosteroid injections are ineffective.

Ganglion Cyst

What is a ganglion cyst?
An outpouching of synovium from an underlying joint or tendon sheath. Because it continues to produce synovial fluid, it may be firm to palpation.

What are the most common locations?
Dorsoradial wrist, volar radial wrist, flexor tendon sheath between the A1 and A2 pulleys, and DIP dorsally (referred to as a mucous cyst)

What is the treatment?
Aspiration may be attempted. If not successful, operative removal of the cyst and a small cuff of joint capsule or tendon sheath from which it emanates is performed.

Ligament Sprain

What is the treatment of a stable ligament sprain, once fractures or unstable tears are excluded?
Splinting in the intrinsic plus position, elevation, ice for 24 to 48 hours, analgesics for pain control

51

Thoracic Surgery

Kirk J. Fleischer, MD

THORACIC WALL

CONGENITAL LESIONS

What are the two most common types?	1. Pectus excavatum—funnel-shaped posterior displacement of the sternum (most common type) 2. Pectus carinatum—anterior sternal displacement ("pigeon breast")
What is the etiology?	Congenital abnormality in the development of the costal cartilages resulting in secondary sternal displacement
What is the most common complication?	Poor self-esteem and psychological complications. Significant cardiorespiratory compromise is rare, although it has been described in patients with more severe pectus excavatum (especially with exercise).
What are the indications for treatment?	Almost all patients should have surgical repair before age 5 to avoid the aforementioned complication, because the defect progresses with time.
What is the surgical procedure?	Resection of involved costal cartilages with preservation of the perichondrium (for regeneration of new cartilage), followed by fixation of sternum in proper position with segments of resected cartilage (or temporary metal bar in patients > age 12)
Which alternative technique corrects pectus excavatum?	Sternal turnover—Anterior chest wall removed as free graft, flipped over, and secured to rib cage

ACQUIRED LESIONS

Chest Wall Tumors

What are the most common benign chest wall tumors?	Chondroma, fibrous dysplasia, and lipoma
What are the most common malignant chest wall tumors?	Locally invasive malignancies (breast, lung) and metastases (kidney, colon, etc.), versus most common primary chest wall tumors, which are fibrosarcoma and chondrosarcoma
What percentage of benign versus malignant tumors present as painful, palpable mass?	Benign—66% (versus malignant—95%)
What is next on differential diagnosis of a painful chest mass?	Pulmonary infection with invasion into chest wall (i.e., Actinomyces, Nocardiosis)
Which features suggests an infectious etiology?	Fluctuation in size of mass over time and constitutional symptoms (lethargy, low-grade fever, weight loss)
Which type demonstrates a classic "onion-peel" appearance on X-ray?	Ewing's sarcoma
Which type demonstrates a classic "sunburst" appearance on X-ray?	Osteogenic sarcoma (osteosarcoma)
What is the treatment of benign tumors?	Wide excision, because of difficulty determining malignant potential by histologic evaluation (Note: The "classic" 4-cm margin of the excision is controversial and evolving.)
What is the treatment of malignant tumors?	Wide excision and occasionally resection of the entire involved bone (especially if high-grade tumor involving the sternum)

How is resultant defect reconstructed?

Goretex patch, methylmethacrylate plate and mesh "sandwich," or Prolene mesh. A muscle or musculocutaneous flap should also be rotated over the defect.

What is a pneumatocele?

Herniation of lung through defect in chest wall (due to trauma, surgery, or congenital defect)

Tietze Syndrome

What is Tietze syndrome?

Nonsuppurative inflammation involving costochondral cartilages (idiopathic)

Presentation and usual course?

Local pain and swelling; often resolves spontaneously

PLEURA

PNEUMOTHORAX (PTX)

What is pneumothorax?

Air or gas in the pleural space

What are the symptoms?

Small PTX (< 20% or 25%)—Usually asymptomatic; large PTX—ipsilateral chest pain, shortness of breath, and cough

What is the basic significance of a PTX?

Potential for tension PTX, a rapidly life-threatening complication (intrathoracic pressure, venous return, cardiac output and cardiogenic shock)

How can visualization of PTX on CXR be facilitated?

Perform CXR at end-expiration.

What is the conservative management for pneumothorax?

Observation for 24 hours, nasal cannula or face-mask oxygen (to expedite rate of resorption of PTX), serial CXRs (every 8–12 hours to follow size of PTX). If same size or smaller at 24 hours, discharge to home with weekly follow-up CXRs until PTX resolved.

What is the average rate of resorption of air from the pleural space per day?

Between 50 and 75 ml per day

What patients are candidates for observation?

Stable (no change in size over time), small PTX in a reliable, alert, nonintubated patient

What is the acute management of unstable patients?

Emergency needle aspiration with 14-gauge needle into intercostal space (ICS) 2 at midclavicular line followed by chest tube (thoracostomy) placement

What are the indications for tube thoracostomy?

Large PTX, PTX increasing in size during observation, unstable patient, patient on mechanical ventilation (regardless of size of PTX), bilateral PTX, tension pneumothorax

What are the classic sites for insertion?

Midaxillary or posterior axillary ICS 5 or 6

What size tube should be used for pure PTX (i.e., no concurrent hemothorax)?

20 or 24 French (36 or 40 French if hemothorax present)

What is the technique for tube thoracostomy placement?

Incise skin over rib, use Kelly clamp to bluntly form subcutaneous tunnel (directed posteriorly) and enter pleural cavity immediately over rib (to avoid neurovascular bundle); insert tube and secure to skin.

What is the management after insertion of the tube thoracostomy?

Connect with underwater seal drainage system (Pleuravac) at 20 cm H_2O of suction; when the air leak has sealed and all the air has been evacuated (no "air" leak in Pleuravac), the suction can be turned off (now the tube is to "water" seal); if PTX remains resolved by CXR at 24 hours, tube may be removed.

Surgery for Pneumothorax

What are the most common indications for surgery?

Recurrent spontaneous PTX, persistent air leak (> 3–10 days, "complicated" PTX), underlying lung disease (e.g., blebs)

What is the standard surgical approach?

Transaxillary thoracotomy (Note: Thoracoscopic techniques are rapidly gaining in popularity.)

What nerves may be injured with this incision?

Long thoracic or thoracodorsal nerves

What is the procedure of choice?

Pleurodesis (formation of adhesions between visceral and parietal pleura to obliterate potential space) [vs. pleurectomy now rarely performed]. Resection of bullae or blebs with stapler may also be indicated.

How is this procedure performed?

Direct parietal pleural abrasion with sponge or application of a sclerosing agent (talc, bleomycin, or tetracycline) [Note: Variable success can also be achieved by instilling these agents via chest tube to avoid surgery in high-risk patients.]

Spontaneous Pneumothorax

What is the most common general etiology?

Rupture of apical emphysematous bulla (Note: Only 15% of these bullae are visualized on CXR.)

What patient population is at highest risk?

Tall, thin males (M:F ratio 10:1), age 20 to 35 years old, often cigarette smoker but no COPD (Primary or idiopathic spontaneous PTX)

What percentage of patients have underlying lung disease?

Only 30% (Secondary spontaneous PTX)

What are the most common conditions associated with spontaneous PTX?

COPD, metastatic disease, and *Pneumocystis carinii*

What is the most important factor in prediction of recurrence rate?

Number of previous episodes (e.g., recurrence rate increases with each episode; after first, risk = 30%–50%, second = 50%–65%, third = 80%)

What is the recurrence rate after surgery?

Only 10%

Traumatic Pneumothorax

See the *Thoracic Trauma* section.

PLEURAL EFFUSION

What are the two types of effusions and their etiologies?	1. Transudative—Congestive heart failure, nephrotic syndrome, and cirrhosis 2. Exudative—malignancy, trauma, infection, pancreatitis, and infarction
What are the most common causes of the following biochemical findings of an effusion: **Glucose < 60 mg / 100 ml?**	Malignancy, TB, pneumonia, or rheumatoid
Elevated amylase?	Pancreatitis, esophageal rupture, or malignancy
pH < 7.2?	Pneumonia, esophageal rupture (especially if < 6.5), malignancy, tuberculosis, systemic acidosis, rheumatoid, or hemothorax
Treatment of effusion varies depending on the etiology. If thoracentesis is performed, why should a massive effusion be evacuated in stages?	Flash pulmonary edema or circulatory collapse may occur if too large a volume is initially drained. Although this is rare, a safe limit to remove at one time is about 1500 ml.

EMPYEMA

What is empyema?	Pleural effusion due to infection (Note: Does not have to be frank pus; a positive Gram stain or culture is sufficient)
What are the three empyema phases?	Exudative, fibropurulent, and chronic (or organized)

What is the time course of these phases?

Exudative—0 to 24 hrs
Fibropurulent—24 to 72 hrs
Organized— > 72 hrs

What are the fluid characteristics of each of these phases?

Exudative—Thin, serous; pH >7.3,
    normal glucose, protein < 2.5, WBC
    < 15,000
Fibropurulent and organized—
    progressively more thick and purulent;
    pH < 7.3, low glucose, increased
    protein, and WBC > 15,000

Which characteristic gross feature develops as the untreated empyema matures?

Fibrous peel or rind around lung
(resulting in the classic "trapped lung
preventing lung reexpansion)

What is the most common etiology of empyema?

Pneumonia (develops in 1% of cases)

What are the most common associated organisms?

Staphylococcus aureus (most common),
Streptococcus, and gram negative
organisms (e.g., Pseudomonas,
Klebsiella, *E. coli*)

Which infection classically develops into empyema early in the course of the pneumonia and rapidly progresses to the fibropurulent phase?

Streptococcus pneumoniae

Which infection is characterized by extreme clinical toxicity?

Klebsiella

What is the classic CXR finding of empyema?

Multiple air–fluid levels due to
loculation of empyema by fibrous septae
(these loculations frequently complicate
drainage by tube thoracostomy)

What is the treatment of empyema in the exudative phase?

IV antibiotics and complete drainage via
thoracentesis

What should be done if fluid reaccumulates after drainage of exudative-phase empyema?

Place tube thoracostomy for drainage.

What is the treatment of empyema in the fibropurulent phase?

Controversial. Many surgeons advocate initial attempt at chest tube drainage before surgical intervention, whereas others favor surgery first.

What are the surgical options for drainage of fibropurulent empyema?

Thoracoscopic drainage; limited thoracotomy ± subperiosteal resection of short (5 cm) section of rib

What is the treatment of empyema in the organized phase?

Decortication—-Removal of fibrous peel, empyema, and pleura in affected regions via thoracotomy (Note: Decortication may be necessary in the fibropurulent phase if trapped lung is discovered at surgery.)

What is the surgical management of organized empyema in high-risk patients?

Eloesser flap (open pleurocutaneous fistula)—Remove rib, unroof empyemic cavity, and sew flap of skin to parietal pleura

What is the current management of empyema following pneumonectomy?

Drain pleural space, IV antibiotics, and status of bronchial stump (leak versus intact) by bronchoscopy to determine if surgical repair is necessary

CHYLOTHORAX

What is chylothorax?

Pleural effusion composed of lymphatic fluid or chyle due to disruption of thoracic duct

What is the course of the thoracic duct?

Cisterna chyli in the abdomen; aortic hiatus right side of vertebral column crosses to left side at T5 to T7; empties into left subclavian vein

What is the normal volume of flow per day through the duct?

Two liters! (accounts for frequency of massive effusions in chylothorax)

What are the etiologies of chylothorax?

Iatrogenic injury at the time of operative dissection along anterior vertebral surface (esophageal, aortic, or orthopedic surgery) or in left neck, blunt trauma, malignancy, and central venous catheter placement

How is the diagnosis made?

Biochemical and microscopic evaluation of pleural fluid (lipid/lymphocytes in chylothorax); lipid load test (high lipid meal results in increased volume and milky appearance of pleural fluid); lymphangiogram (visualize leak)

What is the conservative treatment of chylothorax?

NPO with parenteral hyperalimentation or PO medium-chain triglycerides (absorbed directly into blood rather than lymphatics)

Reexpansion of lung and drainage of fluid with chest tube (or repeated thoracentesis)

What complications may arise during course of conservative therapy?

Dehydration, malnutrition (chyle contains lipid absorbed from bowel), and immunocompromise (due to loss of lymphocytes)

When should surgical intervention be considered?

After 3 to 4 weeks of unsuccessful conservative treatment

Chest tube output > 1000 ml/24 hr for > 1 week

What are the surgical options?

Pleurodesis (with talc, etc.)

Open or thoracoscopic ligation of thoracic duct (extensive collaterals permit chylous return from gut)

Pleuroperitoneal shunt (i.e., Denver)

Where should the ligation be performed?

Low in the mediastinum. Ligate the bundle of tissue between the aorta and azygous vein on the right side of the vertebral column near the diaphragm.

PLEURAL TUMORS

Primary Pleural Tumors

What is the most common type of primary pleural tumor?

Mesothelioma

What are the risk factors?	Asbestos exposure and tobacco abuse
Compare benign versus malignant pleural tumors to answer the following questions.	
Which type is more common?	Malignant
Which type is more closely linked to asbestos exposure?	Malignant
Which type is associated with a paraneoplastic syndrome?	Benign (Hypertrophic pulmonary osteoarthropathy—clubbing, arthralgia, etc.)
How do the treatments of benign versus malignant tumors compare?	Benign—Resection Malignant—Palliative radio-/ chemotherapy ± resection
Compare the prognosis of benign versus malignant tumors.	Benign—90% cure with resection Malignant—death (no cure; mean survival 15–18 months)
What is the characteristic gross feature of the malignant type?	Encasement of lung with tumor
What is the main route of spread?	Relentless local invasion (Note: Metastases are an uncommon and late occurrence.)

Metastatic Pleural Tumors

Metastatic pleural tumors account for what percentage of pleural tumors?	Ninety percent!
What are the most common sources (primary tumors)?	Lung, breast, stomach, and pancreas

TRACHEA

ANATOMY

Which nerves are most likely to be injured during tracheal surgery?	Recurrent laryngeal nerves
What is the blood supply to the trachea?	Inferior thyroid artery (upper trachea) and bronchial arteries (lower trachea)
Why is the safest surgical approach in the AP plane?	Blood supply enters via lateral walls, and recurrent laryngeal nerves run along the lateral walls.
What percentage of the tracheal length may be safely resected in children vs. adults?	Children—33%; adults—50% to 60%

TRACHEAL STENOSIS

What are the etiologies?	Intubation injury, tracheal tumors, and trauma
What is the criterion for a "critical stenosis" in an adult?	Intraluminal diameter < 4 mm
What is the usual presentation?	Cough, stridor, dyspnea, wheezing
Why are many patients with tracheal stenosis on steroids preoperatively?	Because the wheezing that frequently accompanies the stenosis is misdiagnosed as "asthma" (Note: Wean steroids before tracheal resection!)
Should a flexible or rigid bronchoscope be used for preoperative evaluation in most cases and why?	Rigid bronchoscope because it can provide immediate airway (in addition to allowing better suctioning, larger biopsies, and coring out/sequential dilating technique for tumors).
What is the primary cause of technical problems with the tracheal anastomosis?	Excessive tension on the anastomosis

What maneuvers can be performed to reduce this problem?	Cervical flexion (secure chin to chest with heavy suture), suprahyoid laryngeal release, and mobilization of bilateral lung hila
What should be done to reduce the risk of tracheoesophageal fistula?	Interpose muscle flap between tracheal suture line and esophagus
What is the most common acute complication of tracheal surgery?	Laryngeal edema
What is the appropriate management?	Restrict fluids, administer racemic epinephrine and brief course of steroids
What is the most common late complication of tracheal surgery?	Granulations at suture line
What is the appropriate management?	Bronchoscopic removal of granulations ± exposed suture; ± short course of steroids
Where are postintubation tracheal stenoses most commonly found?	1. At the level of the endotracheal tube or tracheostomy cuff 2. At the level of the tracheostomy stoma
What tracheal lesion is often seen between these stenoses?	Segment of tracheomalacia
What is the consequence of this lesion?	With inspiration, the malacic segment collapses (exacerbates the airway obstruction).
What is the etiology of the cuff stenosis?	Circumferential mucosal ischemia with resultant fibrosis
What is the standard treatment of postintubation tracheal stenosis?	Resection with end-to-end anastomosis
What are the treatment options for high-risk patients?	Repeated dilations, laser ablation, or stent placement (i.e., trach tube or Silastic T-tube)

Tracheal Tumors

What is the incidence of malignant tracheal tumors in children versus adults?	Children— < 10%; adults— > 80%!
What are the most common malignant types in adults?	1. Squamous cell carcinoma 2. Adenoid cystic carcinoma
What is the most common benign type in adults?	Squamous papillomas
What is the most common type in children?	Hemangioma
Which tumor classically presents with extensive proximal and distal submucosal spread?	Adenoid cystic carcinoma
What is the usual presentation of tracheal tumors?	Cough, dyspnea, stridor, hemoptysis, hoarseness, and wheezing
Why are distant metastases infrequent?	Patients often die early because of asphyxia from tracheal obstruction
How is the diagnosis usually confirmed?	Bronchscopic biopsy
When is this diagnostic technique contraindicated?	1. Highly vascular tumors (e.g., hemangiomas, carcinoids) 2. Critical tracheal stenosis
How can the bronchoscope be used to temporarily stablize the critically stenosed airway?	Core out intraluminal tumor with bronchoscope tip or endoscopic dilation.
What is the treatment of benign tumors?	Local resection (usually)
What is the treatment of malignant tumors?	Resection ± radiation therapy (pre- or post-op)

What is the best treatment for high-risk patients?	Placement of Silastic (Montgomery) T-tube stent
Compare incision used for upper versus lower tumors.	Upper—Collar incision ± vertical sternal extension Lower—Posterolateral thoracotomy

ACQUIRED ESOPHAGORESPIRATORY FISTULA

What is the usual presentation of small fistula?	Chronic cough, weight loss, and recurrent lung infections
What is the usual presentation of large fistula?	Paroxysmal coughing after eating or drinking (Ono's sign)

Nonmalignant Fistulae

What are the most common etiologies of nonmalignant fistulae?	Erosion by the tracheal tube cuff and blunt chest trauma
What are the usual infectious etiologies?	Tuberculosis and histoplasmosis
What is the surgical treatment for nonmalignant fistulae?	Divide fistula, repair esophageal and tracheobronchial defects, and separate the repairs with muscle, pleural, or pericardial flap (occasionally tracheal resection is also indicated if segment is severely diseased).
What steps should be taken if the patient is still being mechanically ventilated?	The incidence of anastomotic breakdown is high if attempt to repair before extubation. Thus, staged approach is recommended: First, position the cuff of the endotracheal tube below the fistula, remove nasogastric tube, and place gastrostomy/feeding jejunostomy until patient can be extubated. Then after extubation, repair as described previously.

Malignant Fistulae

What are the most common etiologies of malignant fistulae?	Esophageal (85%) and lung (10%) carcinoma

What are the surgical treatment options in the setting of esophageal carcinoma?

1. Esophageal exclusion (suture or staple proximal and distal ends) and bypass (usually with stomach or colon anastomosed to cervical esophagus)
2. Esophageal intubation with endoprosthesis (for the high-risk patient)

(Note: Resection of the fistula is contraindicated in the setting of carcinoma.)

What is the prognosis in the setting of malignancy?

Eighty percent mortality in 3 months (i.e., the fistulae develop late in the course of the disease)

TRACHEOINNOMINATE ARTERY (TA) FISTULA

What is the etiology?

Erosion into innominate artery by tracheostomy tube

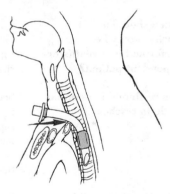

How can the potential for the future development of TA fistula be dramatically reduced at the time of tracheostomy?

Place tracheostomy no lower than the third tracheal ring.

How can the risk in patients with chronic tracheostomy be reduced?

Avoid cuff overinflation (to avoid mucosal ischemia,etc.)

What sign occurs in 50% of patients before massive hemorrhage?

Transient sentinel bleed (especially significant if between 1–2 weeks after tracheostomy)

What is the emergency (bedside) treatment?	Hyperinflate cuff and apply suprasternal pressure. If still massively bleeding, bluntly dissect innominate artery off trachea via the cutaneous stoma, and compress the artery anteriorly against sternum.
What is the definitive surgical treatment?	Median sternotomy, resect innominate artery segment in contact with trachea, oversew the arterial stumps (bypass rarely indicated due to the extensive collateral flow), and secure muscle flap over stumps. (Note: Tracheal defect allowed to granulate closed.)

TRACHEOSTOMY

What are the indications?	1. Chronic respiratory failure 2. Copious tracheobronchial secretions 3. Upper airway obstruction or injury
When should a tracheostomy be performed in a ventilator-dependent patient?	Controversial; however, most experts now agree that if longer term ventilatory support is necessary, tracheostomy should be performed within 7 days.
Where should incision be made in trachea?	Second and third cartilages (Note: There is no definitive evidence concerning the superiority of vertical versus horizontal incision, the removal of segment of cartilage, or formation of a tracheocutaneous flap.)
What are the possible long-term complications?	Sepsis, hemorrhage, and tracheal stenosis

LUNG

ANATOMY

What is the blood supply to the lung?	Pulmonary arteries (primarily for gas exchange) and bronchial arteries from aorta and intercostal aorta (supply lung parenchyma)
What is the most common accessory lobe?	Azygous lobe (due to the developing lung forming a pleural mesentery-like structure around the azygous)

What is the location of this accessory lobe?	Right upper lobe region
Which is the "eparterial bronchus" and why is it so named?	Right upper bronchus. It is the only bronchus that lies superior to the pulmonary artery.
Which nerve runs anterior to the hilum?	Phrenic nerve
Which nerve runs posterior to hilum?	Vagus nerve
Which vessel must be divided for adequate exposure of right bronchus or carina from right thoracotomy?	Azygous vein

Refer to end of this section for illustration of the segmental anatomy of the lung.

CONGENITAL LUNG LESIONS

What is the most common etiology of lung hypoplasia?	Diaphragmatic hernia (herniated bowel preventing normal growth of lung)
What are the two classic lesions of congenital cystic lesions of the lung?	1. Bronchogenic cysts 2. Lung sequestration

Bronchogenic Cysts

What is a bronchogenic cyst?	Congenital cyst in lung (or mediastinum) likely secondary to failure of canalization of bronchial system with associated dilation of more proximal bronchi
What is the usual presentation in an infant or child?	Respiratory insufficiency, compression atelectasis, and pneumothorax
What is the usual presentation in an adult?	Recurrent pneumonia and sepsis
What is the classic CXR finding?	Smooth density extending from mediastinal border at the level of carina (fluid- and/or air-filled)

Sequestration

What is a lung sequestration?	Lung tissue not connected with tracheobronchial tree
What other anatomic feature characterizes this lung tissue?	Receives blood supply from anomalous systemic arteries (instead of pulmonary arteries)
What are the most common origins of these vessels?	Thoracic aorta (70%); assorted infradiaphragmatic sources (30%) (usually via the inferior pulmonary ligament)
What percentage also have abnormal pulmonary venous anatomy?	Only 10%
What are the two types of sequestration?	Intralobular and extralobular
What feature distinguishes them?	Intralobular—surrounded by normal lung parenchyma Extralobular—surrounded by its own pleura (outside normal lung parenchyma)
Which type usually presents in children versus adults?	Extralobular—children; intralobular—adults
What is the most common location in the lung?	Posterior basal regions of lower lobes
How does sequestration usually present in the adult?	Recurrent pneumonia or lower lobe abscess refractory to antibiotic therapy
How is the diagnosis made?	Chest and abdominal CT scan with contrast or arteriogram(anomalous **systemic** arterial supply)
What is the treatment?	Antibiotic therapy and surgical resection (**Beware:** If blood is supply infradiaphragmatic, the vessel may quickly retract below the diaphragm when transected.)

LUNG INFECTIONS

Lung Abscess

What are the etiologies of lung abscess?

Aspiration pneumonia (50%), primary necrotizing pneumonia (20%), bronchial obstruction secondary to neoplasm (10%–20%), septic emboli, and infection of pulmonary infarction

What are the primary risk factors for aspiration pneumonia?

Altered mental status (alcoholism, epilepsy), poor dentition, periodontal infections, and vocal cord dysfunction

What is the most common group of organisms causing aspiration pneumonia and abscess?

Anaerobic bacteria (e.g., *Bacterioides, Peptostreptococcus, Fusobacterium*)

What are the classic sites of aspiration pneumonia in the lung?

1. Posterior segment of right upper lobe
2. Superior segment of left lower lobe

Why these segments?

They are the most dependent lobes in the supine patient.

What are the most common causes of primary necrotizing pneumonia?

Staphylococcus aureus, gram-negative organisms (especially *Klebsiella*), and mycobacteria

What findings on CXR or CT scan would suggest presence of an associated carcinoma?

Thick-walled or large (> 6 cm) abscess

What is the usual presentation?

Fever and malaise followed by cough with copious, fetid sputum production

What does this latter sign indicate?

Abscess has eroded into airway (and drainage of abscess contents into tracheobronchial tree).

What CXR finding is present at this stage?

Cavitary lesion with air–fluid level(s)

With this presentation, what other lesions are in the differential diagnosis?

Bronchiectasis and cavitary carcinoma

In addition to the routine CXR and CT scan, what diagnostic procedure should be performed on all patients, and why?

Bronchoscopy. **Must** rule out carcinoma!

What complications are associated with aspiration pneumonia?

Bronchopleural fistula and pneumothorax, massive hemoptysis, and metastastic abscess (most commonly to the brain)

What is the conservative treatment of lung abscess?

High-dose IV antibiotics (penicillin, clindamycin) and "internal drainage" (via coughing and repeated bronchoscopy)

How effective is this treatment?

Successful in 95%

What is the surgical treatment?

Percutaneous or open drainage of abscess; in some cases, lung resection

What are the indications for surgery?

1. Unresponsive to 3 to 8 weeks of conservative therapy
2. Massive hemoptysis
3. Suspicion of carcinoma
4. Pyopneumothorax and empyema (suggesting bronchopleural fistula)

Bronchiectasis

What is bronchiectasis?

Chronic dilation of distal bronchial tree (usually the second–fourth-order segmental bronchi)

What is the most common etiology?

Destructive pneumonia (bacterial or viral)

What rare congenital syndrome includes bronchiectasis in its triad of lesions?

Kartagener syndrome (triad also includes situs inversus and sinusitis)

What is the usual presentation?

Chronic cough productive for characteristic copious, purulent, fetid sputum (especially in morning)

What is the gold standard for diagnosis?

Bronchogram (using contrast solution Lipiodol) [Note: Although thin-cut CT is gaining in popularity, a bronchogram still defines the anatomy best and should be done in any potential candidate for surgery.]

What are the indications for surgery for bronchiectasis?

1. Recurrent pulmonary infections
2. Significant hemoptysis
3. Brain abscess due to bacterial emboli
4. Continuous copious sputum

What is the procedure of choice for bronchiectasis?

Resection of affected regions (Note: the diffuse nature of the disease prevents most patients from undergoing surgery)

Tuberculosis (TB)

What is the responsible organism and route of transmission?

Mycobacterium tuberculosis by aerosolized droplets

What percentage of infected individuals have clinically significant tuberculosis?

Only 5% to 15%

What is the most common region of lung to be affected?

Apices of lung

What is the evolution of the parenchymal lesion?

Pulmonary infiltrate—caseous necrosis—fibrosis and calcification (granulomas)

What is a Gohn complex?

Parenchymal lesion plus enlarged hilar lymph nodes

What is a Rasmussen aneurysm?

Dilated branch of pulmonary artery within or near a TB cavity

What is the usual presentation of these aneurysms?

Hemoptysis

What are the indications for surgical resection for tuberculosis?

Failure of anti-TB medical therapy (e.g., isoniazid, rifampin, pyrazinamide) as manifested by persistently positive sputum, massive or recurrent hemoptysis, bronchopleural fistula, or mass lesion in a region of TB (to exclude malignancy)

Mycotic Infections

What are the most common mycotic infections in the United States?

Histoplasmosis (most common), coccidioidomycosis, *Aspergillus,* and blastomycosis

What organism has traditionally been grouped with fungal infections but is bacterial in origin?

Actinomycosis

Which of these infections is associated with:
    Dental abscesses?

Actinomycosis

    Thin-walled cavity with air–fluid level?

Coccidioidomycosis

    Chronic papulopustular skin ulcers?

Blastomycosis

    Abscesses containing "sulfur granules"?

Actinomycosis

What is a mycetoma?

Classic "fungus ball" composed of *Aspergillus*

What is the usual predisposing lesion of a mycetoma?

Cavity secondary to *Mycobacterium tuberculosis*

What is the classic finding on upright CXR?

Radiolucent crescent (small ball in larger round cavity)

What is the medical treatment of pulmonary fungal infection?

Amphotericin B for all infections **except** Actinomycosis, which requires penicillin

What are the indications for surgical intervention for mycotic pulmonary infections?

Often controversial especially with noncavitary lesions (nodules); however, most agree that excision is indicated for cavitary lesions refractory to medical treatment and recurrent hemoptysis.

MASSIVE HEMOPTYSIS

What are the etiologies?

Lung abscess, bronchiectasis, trauma, and, much less frequently, tumor

What is the most common etiology?

Mycetoma (see *Mycotic Infections* section)

What is the usual cause of death?

Asphyxia (not hemorrhagic shock)

What is the acute management of massive hemoptysis?

Protect the nonbleeding lung! Place patient on side (with bleeding side down if known pathology on one side); use rigid bronchoscopy to determine side of bleeding (right vs. left); insert Fogarty venous occlusion catheter into bleeding bronchus and endotracheal tube into trachea or nonbleeding bronchus (the latter may require flexible bronchoscope).

What is the definitive treatment of massive hemoptysis?

Lobectomy or pneumonectomy

What is an option for high-risk patients?

Selective bronchial artery embolization (Note: Rebleeding rate is significant and many surgeons believe that elective resection is prudent if patient's condition improves.)

BENIGN LUNG TUMORS

Account for what percentage of primary lung tumors?

Less than 1%

What are the different types?

1. Hamartoma
2. Carcinoid
3. Adenoid cystic
4. Mucoepidermoid

Which are actually low-grade malignant tumors?	Carcinoid, adenoid cystic, and mucoepidermoid (Note: These types of tumors were traditionally called "bronchial adenomas.")
Why?	Ten percent to fifteen percent metastasize
Which type is most common?	Carcinoid (accounts for 85% of these low-grade malignant tumors)
Carcinoids arise from what origin cell?	Kulchitsky's cell (neuroendocrine argentaffin cells)
What are the features of the carcinoid syndrome?	Cutaneous flushing, diarrhea, bronchoconstriction, and right-sided valvular disease (tricuspid, pulmonary)
What percentage of patients develop this syndrome?	Only 3%
What is the appearance of carcinoid on bronchoscopy?	Red (very vascular tumors)
What is the usual presentation of benign lung tumors?	Central tumors—cough, pneumonia, dyspnea, or hemoptysis Peripheral tumors—characteristically asymptomatic (found incidentally on CXR as a well-defined, slightly lobulated mass)
What is the treatment?	Central tumors—Sleeve resection Peripheral tumors—wedge resection or enucleation

PRIMARY MALIGNANT LUNG TUMORS

What percentage of male versus female cancer deaths are due to lung cancer in the United States?	Male—35%; female—20% (now the leading cancer killer in **both** men and women after it surpassed breast cancer in 1986)

What are the risk factors?

Tobacco abuse (benzopyrene), toxic exposure (e.g., asbestos, radon), and preexisting lung disease (Note: Considering that the majority of smokers do not develop lung cancer, there is likely an inherited predisposition to the development of carcinoma.)

What are the four types of lung carcinoma?

Squamous cell (most common), adenocarcinoma, small cell (oat cell), and large cell

Which of these types is (are):

Usually found centrally?

Squamous cell (70%), small cell (80%), and large cell (60%) [versus adenocarcinoma, which is peripheral in 75% of cases]

Highly malignant?

Small cell (considered by many to be a systemic disease at time of diagnosis)

Usually associated with heavy smoking history?

Squamous cell and small cell

Often arise in tuberculosis scar?

Adenocarcinoma

Which oncogene frequently:

Has point mutations in adenocarcinoma?

K-*ras*

Is amplified in small cell carcinoma?

myc family (especially c-*myc*)

What is the most consistent chromosome deletion?

p14 to p23 on chromosome 3 (small cell carcinoma)

Presentation of Primary Malignant Lung Tumors

What percentage are asymptomatic?

Only 10% to 20%

What are the symptoms?

Cough (most common symptom), hemoptysis (usually blood-streaked sputum), chest pain, dyspnea, anorexia, and weight loss

What is the etiology of hoarseness that may accompany lung carcinoma?	Invasion of recurrent laryngeal nerve (direct or metastatic lymph node)
What side will usually be involved, and why?	Left. Left laryngeal nerve loops low around the aortic arch (versus right nerve loops around the more cephalad subclavian artery)
What are the mechanisms by which lung carcinoma can cause dyspnea?	Bronchial obstruction, pleural effusion, and invasion of phrenic nerve with resultant paralysis of hemidiaphragm

Pancoast's tumor

Where in the lung is Pancoast's tumor located?	Superior pulmonary sulcus in apical part of lung
What is the most common type of carcinoma associated with the syndrome?	Squamous cell carcinoma
Are these tumors slow- or fast-growing?	Usually slow growing with late dissemination
What are the classic signs and symptoms?	Horner syndrome (ptosis, anhidrosis, miosis), pain in shoulder, and motor/sensory deficits in arm (especially in distribution of C8, T1, and T2)
What is the etiology of these findings?	Invasion of the cervical sympathetic chain and brachial plexus

Nonmetastatic systemic syndromes

What are the hormone-related nonmetastatic systemic syndromes associated with lung carcinoma?	Cushing syndrome (most common), SIADH, and hypercalcemia
What is the most common type of lung carcinoma associated with each syndrome and the hormone associated with it?	Cushing—Small cell, ACTH SIADH—small cell, ADH Hypercalcemia—squamous cell (PTH-like peptide)

What are two additional paraneoplastic syndromes?	Neuromyopathies (e.g., Eaton-Lambert syndrome) and pulmonary hypertrophic osteoarthropathy (PHO)
What are the characteristics of PHO?	Clubbing of fingers; swollen tender joints; symmetrical subperiosteal osteitis and new bone formation in extremities

Diagnosis and Staging of Primary Malignant Lung Tumors

Screening studies

What are the most commonly used screening studies in the diagnosis and staging of primary malignant lung tumors?	Sputum cytology and CXR
Which types of tumors are generally better detected by each?	Sputum cytology is better for central tumors (especially squamous cell); CXR is better for peripheral tumors
What percentage of patients with a positive sputum cytology have lung carcinoma?	Between 65% and 75% (the remainder have head/neck or esophageal carcinoma)

Diagnostic studies

What techniques are used to obtain a tissue biopsy for preoperative diagnosis?	1. Bronchial or transbronchial biopsy 2. Percutaneous transthoracic fine-needle aspiration (FNA) 3. Open lung biopsy or mediastinoscopy
What bronchoscopic findings in the laryngeotracheal region suggest incurability?	1. Vocal cord paralysis (recurrent laryngeal nerve invasion) 2. "Blunting" of the tracheal carina (adjacent lymph node enlargement or direct invasion of carcinoma)
What is the most common complication of bronchial biopsy and FNA?	Pneumothorax (up to 30% of patients develop PTX with FNA; 10% require tube thoracostomy)
How reliable are the results of FNA?	If positive, it is diagnostic; if negative, unreliable.

Staging of Lung Carcinoma

What are the steps in staging carcinoma?

TMN system:
1. Stage primary tumor (T0–T4)
2. Assess lymph node involvement (N0–N3)
3. Clinically and radiographically evaluate for distant metastases (M0–M1)

What are the criteria for stage I tumor?

No positive lymph nodes, no direct invasion of adjacent structures, and > 2 cm from the carina (if closer, resectability is very difficult)

What are the basic distinguishing features of stages II through IV tumors?

Stage II—Positive lymph nodes (ipsilateral lung only)
Stage III—Direct invasion of adjacent structures **or mediastinal** nodal metastases
Stage IV—Distant metastases

What features of tumor determine its T stage?

Size, distance from carina, ± atelectasis in involved lung, ± pleural effusion, and ± invasion into neighboring structures (e.g., pleura, chest wall, esophagus)

How is lymph node involvement assessed?

CT scan, mediastinoscopy, mediastinotomy, and/or thoracoscopy

What size lymph nodes are considered suspicious for carcinoma?

> 1 cm

How is mediastinoscopy usually performed?

3-cm incision in suprasternal fossa, dissect to pretracheal fascia; fascia is divided; plane anterior to trachea is bluntly developed with finger to carina, and scope inserted and advanced along trachea.

Which important region cannot be evaluated by mediastinoscopy?

Aortopulmonary window (lymphatic drainage of the left lung). Thus, if biopsy is wanted from this region, mediastinotomy must be used.

How is mediastinotomy performed?	Anterior parasternal incision, then short segment of costocartilage is removed (Chamberlain procedure) and scope inserted.
Which symptom would encourage going directly to mediastinotomy, and why?	Hoarseness. Left recurrent laryngeal nerve passes through aortopulmonary window.
What percentage of patients have distant metastases at time of diagnosis?	Between 50% and 60%
What are the most common sites of blood-borne metastases?	Brain, bone, adrenals, liver, and kidneys
For what stages should metastatic workup be performed?	Stages II and III (in stage IV, already have evidence of distant spread)
What is the standard metastatic workup?	1. Brain CT (or MRI) 2. Abdominal CT (or good-quality ultrasound) 3. Bone scan (optional)

Management of Primary Malignant Lung Tumors

Preoperative evaluation

What study must be performed to determine if patient with Primary Malignant Lung Tumor can tolerate lung resection?	Pulmonary function tests (PFTs)
What is essential to reduce risk of ventilator dependence postoperatively?	Postoperative FEV1 must be ≥ 0.8 or 1.0 L
How may a preoperative FEV1 of 1.2 L be satisfactory for safe pneumonectomy?	Must consider the contribution of **each lung** to FEV1. Split lung function (Xenon) test may show that the diseased lung contributes only a small amount to the preoperative FEV1.

What room air PaO2 and PaCO2 would be considered too high a risk for surgery?	PaO2 < 50 mm Hg , PaCO2 > 50 mm Hg
What are accepted signs of inoperability?	1. Positive supraclavicular, scalene, contralateral mediastinal or hilar lymph nodes 2. Malignant pleural effusion 3. Involvement of tracheal carina 4. SVC syndrome 5. Recurrent laryngeal or phrenic nerve paralysis 6. Involvement of main pulmonary artery 7. Distant metastases 8. Horner syndrome (Note: Not all surgeons would agree that some of these signs are contraindications for surgery.)
By these criteria, what percentage are incurable on presentation?	Sixty-six percent (and almost half the remainder are medically poor candidates for surgery)

Radiotherapy (XRT)

What are the indications for XRT?	1. Inoperable patients due to extent of disease or medical condition 2. Recurrence of carcinoma after surgery
What is the standard dosing regimen?	From 5000 to 6000 rads, 5 times per week, 5 to 6 weeks
What are the early thoracic complications of XRT?	Radiation pneumonitis and esophagitis (usually mild)
Which complication of an inoperable lesion often dramatically responds to XRT?	SVC syndrome

Chemotherapy

What are currently the most effective chemotherapeutic agents?	For small cell: Cyclophosphamide, vincristine, and doxorubicin For non–small cell: cisplatin, VP16, Taxol (Note: Unfortunately, overall results with chemotherapy have not been impressive.)

Chemotherapy is most commonly used in the treatment of what type of lung carcinoma?

Small cell carcinoma (80% disseminated at diagnosis)

Surgical treatment

What percentage of patients are surgical candidates?

Only 25%

What is the most commonly used surgical approach?

Posterolateral thoracotomy through ICS 5 or 6

What are the indications for median sternotomy?

1. Patients with marginal pulmonary function
2. Multiple bilateral wedge resections

What are the surgical options (from least to most extensive resection)?

Wedge resection—Segmentectomy—Lobectomy—Sleeve resection of bronchus with lobectomy—Pneumonectomy

Which is most commonly performed?

Lobectomy

What is a sleeve resection?

Removal of segment of bronchus (and accompanying lobe) followed by end-to-end anastomosis of remaining proximal and distal bronchial ends

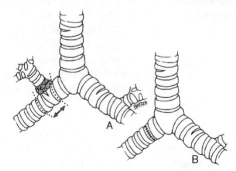

What is the benefit of a sleeve resection?

Preservation of uninvolved distal lung

What should be done to reduce risk of bronchopleural fistula?	Wrap bronchial stump or anastomosis with a pleural, intercostal muscle, or pericardial flap
Is suture or staple closure preferred for bronchial transection?	Staple (more secure; reduced risk of bronchopleural fistula)
What is the most common postoperative complication following lung resection?	Supraventricular tachycardia
What is the mortality rate of right versus left pneumonectomy?	Right—10%; Left—only 1% to 6%
What is the mortality rate of lobectomy?	2% to 5 %

METASTATIC LUNG TUMORS

What percentage of patients with carcinoma develop metastases to the lung?	Thirty percent
What are the most common sources?	Colon (30%), breast (15%), and kidney (7%)
What are the primary criteria in consideration for potential resection?	1. Metastatic disease isolated to the lung 2. Primary carcinoma controlled 3. Metastases potentially resectable (technically and in terms of patient's predicted reserve after resection of lung parenchyma) (Note: Number of metastases is not an exclusion criterion if these other criteria are met.)
Which groups of carcinomas preferentially metastasize to the lung?	1. Soft tissue sarcomas 2. Osteogenic sarcomas 3. Renal carcinomas (Note: Patients with one of these tumors have the most improved survival, e.g., > 50% survival at 5 years with osteogenic sarcoma.)

Some metastases may be so small that they are undetectable at time of surgery. What is the reported increased risk associated with a later, second resection?

No increased risk; postoperative survival same.

SOLITARY PULMONARY NODULES (SPN)

What are SPN?

Peripheral, fairly smooth, well-circumscribed lesion ("coin lesion") noted on CXR of asymptomatic patient

What is the differential diagnosis?

1. Primary lung carcinoma
2. Metastasis to the lung
3. Granulomatous disease (e.g., histoplasmoma, tuberculoma)
4. Benign lung tumors (e.g., hamartoma)
5. Arteriovenous fistulae

What percentage are malignant?

Only 5% to 10%

What patient variable dramatically increases the risk of malignancy?

Age (e.g., in patients > 50 years, more than 80% are malignant!)

What features on CXR suggest malignant etiology?

1. Large size (almost all > 4 cm are carcinoma)
2. Indistinct or highly lobulated margins
3. Growth in size since last CXR
4. Doubling time (DT) between 35 and 280 days

What features on CXR would suggest benign etiology?

1. Small size (almost all < 1 cm are benign)
2. Distinct margins
3. Calcifications (especially if concentric or heavily calcified)
4. Satellite lesions
5. No growth in > 1 year (DT > 465 days) **or** very rapid growth (DT < 35 days)

What finding suggests metastastic disease?

Multiple nodules

SPN in the setting of what syndrome is malignant in 80% of cases?

Pulmonary hypertrophic osteoarthropathy (PHO)

What is the surgical algorithm if uncertain of diagnosis?

1. Determine if patient is operative candidate for lung resection.
2. If candidate, perform wedge resection for frozen sections: If benign—end of procedure; if malignant—perform definitive therapy (e.g., lobectomy)

SEGMENTAL ANATOMY OF THE LUNG (Jackson and Huber Nomenclature)

Right

Upper lobe:
1. Apical segment
2. Posterior
3. Anterior

Middle lobe:
4. Lateral
5. Medial

Lower lobe:
6. Superior
7. Medial basal
8. Anterior basal
9. Lateral basal
10. Posterior basal

Left

Upper lobe:
1.& 2. Apical segments
3. Anterior
4.& 5. Superior and inferior (lingular)

Lower lobe:
6. Superior
7.& 8. Anteromedial basal
9. Lateral basal
10. Posterior basal

MEDIASTINUM

ANATOMY

What are the anatomic compartments of the mediastinum?	Anterior (and superior), middle, and posterior
What are the major landmarks between these compartments as noted on lateral CXR?	A = plane between sternal angle and disc between T4 and T5; B = plane just anterior to pericardium; C = plane posterior to heart and between trachea and esophagus.

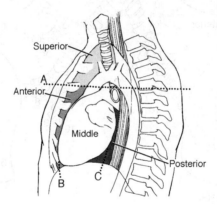

MEDIASTINAL MASSES

What are the four most common classes of mediastinal masses?	1. Neurogenic tumors (20%) 2. Thymoma (20%) 3. Cysts (20%) 4. Lymphoma (15%)
What are the other major classes of masses?	Germ cell, mesenchymal, endocrine, and primary carcinoma
What is the incidence of masses in each mediastinal compartment?	Anterior—55% Middle—25% Posterior—20%
What are the three most common masses and their relative frequencies in each compartment?	Anterior—Thymoma (30%), lymphoma (25%), and germ cell tumors (15%) Middle—pericardial cyst (35%), lymphoma (20%), and bronchogenic cyst (15%)

Posterior—neurogenic tumor (50%), bronchogenic cyst (20%), and mesenchymal tumor (10%)

What percentage of mediastinal masses are benign versus malignant?

Benign—60%; malignant—40%

What percentage of masses in each compartment are malignant?

Anterior—60% Middle—30% Posterior—15%

Which age-group has the highest incidence of malignancy, and why?

Age 30 to 40 (55% of masses are malignant); corresponds to peak incidence of germ cell tumors and lymphoma

What are the most common malignant types in adults?

1. Lymphoma
2. Thymoma
3. Mesenchymal tumors

What are the most common malignant types in children?

1. Neurogenic tumors
2. Lymphoma

What are the symptoms?

Most patients are asymptomatic. Symptoms include chest pain, dyspnea, fever, and cough.

Why is presence/absence of symptoms diagnostically important?

Presence correlates with malignancy. Asymptomatic—only 5% malignant versus symptomatic—50%.

Why is this correlation less applicable with children?

Airway is more compliant and has smaller diameter; thus, more susceptible to compression by mass.

How is the diagnosis made?

Chest x-ray and CT scan to establish working diagnosis (via mass location, size, density, and relationship to other mediastinal structures); followed by tissue biopsy via mediastinoscopy, mediastinotomy, or occasionally fine-needle aspiration for definitive diagnosis (see *Primary Malignant Lung Tumor* section for discussion of mediastinoscopy/otomy)

What is the treatment of the majority of mediastinal masses?	Surgical resection
What are the exceptions?	1. Lymphoma, malignant germ-cell tumors, and tumors that are widely metastatic receive medical treatment (chemo-/radiotherapy). 2. Pericardial cysts are now usually observed.

Neurogenic Tumors

What percentage of neurogenic tumors are malignant?	Adults—10% to 20%; children—20% to 40%
What is the most common location?	Paravertebral gutters (posterior compartment)
Arise from what three neural structures?	Intercostal nerve sheaths, autonomic (sympathetic) ganglion, and paraganglia cells
What are the main neurogenic mediastinal tumors arising from each structure?	Nerve sheath tumors—neurilemmoma (or schwannoma), neurofibroma, neurosarcoma Autonomic ganglion tumors—ganglioneuroma, ganglioneuroblastoma, neuroblastoma Paraganglionic tumors—pheochromocytoma, chemodectoma
Which type(s) of neurogenic tumor:	
Is most common?	Neurilemmoma (40%–60%)
Produce catecholamines?	Paraganglionic tumors
Are hormonally active?	Autonomic ganglion and paraganglionic tumors
Arise from aortic arch or vagus nerve?	Chemodectomas (from chemoreceptor cells)

Are associated with a classic-named neurologic disorder?	Nerve sheath tumors (von Recklinghausen disease)
Presentation?	Chest wall pain (from compression of nerve by mass or bony erosion); neurologic deficit (from direct compression of spinal cord or pathologic vertebral fracture); syndromes associated with the hormonally active tumors (hypertension, flushing, and sweating; diarrhea, abdominal distension, and anorexia)
What percentage of neurogenic mediastinal masses have intraspinal extension?	Ten percent
Results in what classic tumor shape?	Dumbbell (intraspinal and paraspinal masses connected by isthmus of tissue as it passes through the intervertebral foramen)
What is the treatment of neurogenic tumors?	Surgical excision
What special precaution should be taken with dumbbell tumors during surgery?	Avoid excessive traction on intrathoracic portion of tumor during excision (can cause intraspinal hemorrhage and paraplegia); intraspinal portion should be removed by neurosurgical team after intrathoracic excision complete.
What percentage of thymomas are malignant?	Fifty percent
How is malignancy diagnosed?	1. Identification of tumor invasion (Note: Until recently, it has been taught that the diagnosis of invasion could only be made intraoperatively by the surgeon; however, it is now accepted that the pathologist can make the diagnosis of microscopic capsular invasion from a surgical specimen.) 2. Identification of metastases (usually to pleura, rarely to lymph nodes)

Classically associated with what systemic syndrome?

Myasthenia gravis

Seen in what percentage of patients with thymoma?

From 30% to 50% (Note: Only 10% of patients with myasthenia gravis have thymoma.)

What is the primary clinical feature of this syndrome?

Easy fatigability and symmetrical weakness of skeletal muscle (especially extraocular muscles)

What is the medical treatment of this syndrome?

Anticholinesterase agents (neostigmine, pyridostigmine bromide) and steroids

What is the treatment of thymoma?

Total thymectomy often via median sternotomy (Note: Important to resect all adjacent mediastinal fat tissue)

What nerves are at risk of injury because of proximity to thymus?

Phrenic nerves

Which patients with myasthenia gravis should have thymectomy?

Essentially all should undergo thymectomy eventually **even** if no thymoma is present. (May delay surgery if symptoms are mild and well controlled with anticholinesterases)

What is the preoperative preparation?

Discontinue anticholinesterases, plasmapheresis; if patient on steroids, continue until after surgery (to avoid adrenal insufficiency), then rapidly wean.

What is the key postoperative complication in patients with myasthenia gravis?

Respiratory failure (Note: Monitor closely after extubation!)

What percentage of patients demonstrate symptomatic improvement versus complete remission after thymectomy?

Symptomatic improvement—60% to 85%; complete remission—20% to 35% (Note: Maximal improvement may take between 3 months to 3 years postoperatively.)

What is the adjunctive therapy for malignant thymoma?

Postoperative radiation therapy (XRT)

Mediastinal cysts

What are the types of mediastinal cysts?

Bronchogenic, enteric, and pericardial

Which is the most common type?

Bronchogenic (35%)

What is the usual appearance on CT scan?

Mass with near-water density

What is the most common site of each type of cyst?

Bronchogenic—posterior to carina (or main stem bronchus)
Enteric—no dominant site
Pericardial—right costophrenic angle

What is the treatment?

Bronchogenic and enteric cysts—surgical excision (for definitive diagnosis and to avoid possible future malignant degeneration)
Pericardial cysts—usually observed (although some surgeons will percutaneously aspirate them)

Lymphoma

What are the types of lymphoma?

Hodgkin and non-Hodgkin

Specifically which subtype of each is most common in the mediastinum?

Hodgkin—nodular sclerosing; non-Hodgkin—lymphoblastic

Which general type is more locally aggressive?

Non-Hodgkin

How is the diagnosis made?

Biopsy via mediastinoscope (fine-needle aspirate does not provide sufficient tissue); occasionally, anterolateral thoracotomy necessary for isolated hilar lymph node involvement

What is the treatment?

Chemotherapy (MOPP, CHOP, or APO protocols); radiotherapy

What is the overall 5-year survival rate?

Hodgkin—75%; non-Hodgkin—50%

Germ-cell tumors

What are the types of germ-cell tumors?	Teratodermoid, seminomatous, and nonseminomatous
Which types are always malignant?	Seminomatous and nonseminomatous
What are examples of teratodermoid type?	Dermoid cyst and teratoma
What are examples of nonseminomatous type?	Embryonal cell, choriocarcinoma, endodermal cell (or yolk sac), and malignant teratoma
What is the overall most common germ-cell tumor?	Teratoma
What is the most common malignant germ-cell tumor?	Seminoma
What are the nonspecific serum tumor markers frequently elevated in germ-cell tumors?	Alpha-fetoprotein (AFP) and human chorionic gonadotropin (β-hCG)
What is the incidence of elevated levels of these markers in seminomatous versus nonseminomatous tumors?	Seminomatous—none have increased AFP, only 10% have increased β-hCG Nonseminomatous—90% have elevated AFP and/or β-hCG (Note: Regardless of biopsy results, if AFP is elevated, tumor is **non**seminomatous.)
Which type has best prognosis, and why?	Seminoma. Very radiosensitive.
What is the treatment of teratodermoid?	Surgical excision for both benign and malignant types
What is the treatment of seminoma?	Radiotherapy (4500–5000 rads over 6 weeks); ± chemotherapy
What is the treatment of nonseminoma?	Cisplatin-based chemotherapy

How are response to therapy and relapses monitored?	Serial levels of aforementioned tumor markers and CT scans
What are the most common types of mesenchymal tumors?	Lipoma and fibroma
What are the most common types of endocrine tumors?	Ectopic thyroid and parathyroid neoplasms; carcinoids

Miscellaneous Facts about Mediastinal Masses

Which mediastinal mass(es) is(are) associated with:

Vertebral anomalies?	Enteric cyst
Radiologic evidence of tooth within mass?	Teratoma
Hypoglycemia? Why?	Neurosarcoma; secretes an insulin-like substance; called the Doege-Potter syndrome.
Gynecomastia?	Nonseminomatous germ-cell tumors
Characteristic fever pattern?	Hodgkin lymphoma (Pel-Ebstein fever)
Hypertension?	Pheochromocytoma and chemodectoma
Red-cell aplasia?	Thymoma
Cushing syndrome?	Thymoma, primary carcinoma, and carcinoid (mediastinal)
Ulceration into bronchus, esophagus, or lung?	Enteric cyst (gastric mucosa subtype)
Large size? Why?	Mesenchymal tumors. These tumors characteristically do not fix to or invade adjacent structures so they remain asymptomatic until late.

Identified chromosomal abnormalities (Klinefelter syndrome, 5q deletion, trisomy 8)?	Nonseminomatous germ-cell tumors
Ptosis and diplopia?	Thymoma with associated myasthenia gravis
Increased levels of VMA (vanillylmandelic acid) and HVA (homovanillic acid) in urine?	Pheochromocytoma
Increased uptake with 131I-MIBG (metaiodobenzylguanidine) scan?	Pheochromocytoma
Cerebellar and truncal ataxia with darting eye movements?	Neuroblastoma; called opsomyoclonus.
Nights sweats and pruritis?	Lymphoma
Cells from all three germ layers: endo-, meso-, and ectoderm?	Teratoma
Eaton-Lambert syndrome?	Thymoma (Note: Thymomas are associated with more systemic syndromes than is any other mediastinal mass.)

MEDIASTINITIS

Acute (Suppurative) Mediastinitis

What are the most common etiologies?	1. Postoperative infection after open heart surgery (median sternotomy; leading cause) 2. Esophageal perforation (iatrogenic, spontaneous, or traumatic)
What are the most common bacterial organisms?	*Staphylococcus* (*S. aureus*, *S. epidermidis*) accounts for 75% of cases; remainder due to gram-negative organisms (e.g., *Pseudomonas*, *Enterobacter*)

What is the usual presentation?	Fever, chest pain, tachycardia, leukocytosis; in postop mediastinitis, sternal instability and swollen, erythematous wound with serous drainage; in perforation, subcutaneous emphysema (palpable crepitus) and mediastinal emphysema (auscultated Hamman's crunch)
How is the diagnosis made?	Usually made on **clinical** grounds (aforementioned signs); CT scan may reveal abscess or mediastinal gas
What is the treatment?	Surgical debridement, irrigation and drainage, followed by wound closure; IV antibiotics
What are the goals of wound closure?	Clear residual infection, protect exposed underlying viscera and vessels, and obliterate any mediastinal dead space
What is usually used to achieve these goals?	Muscle flap (pectoralis major or rectus abdominis)

Chronic Mediastinitis

What are the etiologies?	Granulomatous infection (usually histoplasmosis, but also *Mycobacterium tuberculosis*)
What is the mechanism?	Granulomata enlarge until they rupture and release their caseous contents into the mediastinum, resulting in intense fibrotic reaction.
What is the most common indication for surgical intervention?	Superior vena cava syndrome due to obstruction by fibrosis and enlarged calcified lymph nodes

ESOPHAGUS

ANATOMY

What are the anatomic narrowings of the esophagus?	Upper esophageal sphincter (UES), midthorax (due to external compression by left bronchus and aortic arch), and lower esophageal sphincter (LES)

Which is the most narrow?	UES
Which type of muscle makes up the muscularis layer?	Skeletal muscle (upper third), smooth muscle (lower third), mixed smooth and skeletal (middle third)
Which named muscle forms the UES?	Cricopharyngeal muscle
At what tracheal and vertebral level is it located?	Cricoid cartilage and T1 vertebra
Unlike most of the gastrointestinal tract, the esophagus lacks what gross feature?	Serosa
What is the arterial supply of the esophagus?	1. Inferior thyroid artery 2. Bronchial arteries 3. "Esophageal arteries" from aorta 4. Inferior phrenic artery 5. Left gastric artery
Which named nerves travel with the esophagus?	Right and left vagus nerves
Which of these nerves is located on the anterior surface?	Left
Which nerves form the intramural autonomic nervous system of the esophagus?	Auerbach's plexus (in between the longitudinal and circular muscle layers) and Meissner's plexus (within submucosa)

ESOPHAGEAL MOTILITY DISORDERS

What are the types of primary motility disorders?	1. Oropharyngeal dysphagia 2. Achalasia 3. Diffuse esophageal spasm
What is the classic type of secondary motility disorder?	Scleroderma

What is the most common symptom?	Dysphagia (difficulty swallowing), notably to both solids and liquids
Which type is associated with increased risk of carcinoma?	Achalasia
What diagnostic tests should be administered?	1. Barium esophagogram 2. Manometry
Which feature of these disorders often makes diagnosis difficult?	Intermittent nature of symptoms. During asymptomatic intervals, esophagogram and manometry findings are usually normal!

Oropharyngeal Dysphagia

What is the physiologic lesion in oropharyngeal dysphagia?	UES does not relax during swallowing.
What are the general groups of etiologies?	Neurogenic disorders (e.g., stroke, brain tumor, multiple sclerosis); myogenic disorders (e.g., muscular dystrophy, myasthenia gravis); structural causes (Zenker's diverticulum); mechanical causes (e.g., webs, tumors); postoperative scarring; and gastroesophageal reflux
What are the symptoms?	Cervical dysphagia, intermittent hoarseness, weight loss, and excessive saliva expectoration
Finding on barium esophagogram?	Prominent posterior cricopharyngeal bar
What is the treatment?	Varies widely depending on the etiology
What must be confirmed before surgery, and why?	Competence of LES (by manometry and acid reflux test). Myotomy makes the UES incompetent, and in the presence of LES incompetence, tracheobronchial aspiration occurs.
If surgery is undertaken, which procedure is performed?	Cervical esophagomyotomy (longitudinal incision of muscular layers of the esophagus) to reduce resistance to swallowing

What incision is used?

Oblique **left** cervical incision, parallel to the anterior border of sternocleidomastoid muscle

Why is it important to avoid disruption of mucosa during the procedures for treatment of esophageal motility disorders?

1. Perforated mucosa increases incidence of postoperative strictures and infection.
2. Risk of life-threatening mediastinitis

What is the management of intraoperative injury to esophageal mucosa?

Primary repair of mucosa. Esophagogram on postop day 1. If leak present **or** if esophageal emptying unsatisfactory, drains (neck drain or chest tube and nasogastric tubes) should remain in place and parenteral hyperalimentation initiated; then, on postop day 10, perform follow-up esophagogram to confirm closure of leak before removal of drains. If esophagogram is normal, follow routine postoperative management.

Achalasia

What is the suspected anatomic etiology?

Absence or degeneration of esophageal ganglionic (Auerbach's) plexus

Which infection causes a similar lesion?

Trypanosoma cruzi (Chagas' disease)

What are the symptoms?

Dysphagia, effortless **regurgitation** after meal (**not** vomiting and **no** sour taste, unlike gastroesophageal reflux), and weight loss

What are the findings on barium swallow?

1. Distal "beak" (dilated body and narrowed distal segment)
2. Tortuous esophagus (in more severe cases)

What are the associated manometric findings?

1. Absent peristalsis in esophageal body
2. LES failing to relax during swallowing
3. High resting pressure in LES (Note: Not all features may be present.)

What lesions may mimic achalasia?	1. Distal esophageal obstruction due to tumor at cardia 2. Reflux stricture (Note: Esophagoscopy should be performed to exclude these diagnoses.)
What are the complications?	Aspiration pneumonia and lung abscess; esophageal carcinoma (squamous cell); epiphrenic diverticulum
What percentage of patients with achalasia develop esophageal carcinoma?	Only 1% to 10% (after 15–25 years of achalasia)
What are the indications for treatment?	All patients should undergo treatment.
What is the primary goal of treatment?	Relieve obstruction due to the nonrelaxing LES
What is the standard interventional regimen?	Initially, pneumatic (or hydrostatic) dilation of LES should be attempted; if this fails, perform esophagomyotomy.
What is a major drawback of the initial aforementioned intervention?	Associated with the highest risk of esophageal perforation of any procedure (2%–10%)
What is the standard surgical procedure?	Heller's myotomy (or variant thereof)—Muscular layers of distal esophagus **and** esophagogastric junction divided (5–7 cm) and carefully dissected from underlying mucosa for 50% of circumference (to allow mucosa to protrude)
What incision is used?	**Left** posterolateral thoracotomy
What technical features of the procedure evoke controversy?	1. Distal extent of the myotomy 2. The necessity for a concurrent antireflux procedure (preferably a partial fundoplication—Dor or modified Belsey techniques)

Diffuse Esophageal Spasm (DES)

What is the physiologic lesion?	Strong, **non**peristaltic contractions of esophagus
Which symptom distinguishes it from achalasia?	Chest pain
Which feature makes initial evaluation difficult?	Pain is angina-like, associated with stress, **and** relieved by nitrates (thus, very difficult to exclude myocardial etiology).
What feature of the dysphagia distinguishes it from that associated with neoplasm, strictures, or rings?	Just as severe with liquids as with solids
What are the findings on barium esophagogram?	1. "Corkscrew" esophagus 2. Muscular hypertrophy sometimes noted on double-contrast swallow
What percentage of barium swallows are normal in DES?	More than 50%
What are the manometry findings?	Nonperistaltic contractions and spasms (high-amplitude or tertiary contractions), **normal** sphincter tone and function (in 75%)
What are the complications?	Hiatal hernia, epiphrenic diverticulum
What is the medical treatment?	Lifestyle changes to reduce stress, smooth muscles relaxants (nitrates and calcium channel blockers)
What indication for surgery has the most successful outcome?	Persistent dysphagia unresponsive to medical treatment (versus surgery for pain is usually unsuccessful)
What is the procedure?	Long esophagomyotomy (from aortic arch to cardia) **plus** antireflux procedure (preferably a partial fundoplication—modified Belsey technique)

Scleroderma

What percentage of patients with scleroderma have symptoms referable to esophageal involvement?

More than 50%

What characteristic pathologic changes occur in the esophagus?

Atrophy of muscularis and fibrotic replacement of the smooth muscle (distal two-thirds of esophagus)

What is the resultant physiologic lesion?

Weak, nonpropulsive contractions of distal esophagus and loss of LES tone

What are the symptoms?

Heartburn (due to reflux), epigastric fullness, and sensation of slow emptying of esophagus

What is the treatment?

Antireflux procedure (fundoplication); in advanced cases, esophagectomy may be required.

ESOPHAGEAL DIVERTICULA

What are the general mechanisms of esophageal diverticula formation?

Pulsion—Pushing out of segment of esophageal wall by intraluminal force
Traction—Pulling out of segment by external traction

What are the most common primary etiologies of diverticula due to each mechanism?

Pulsion—Abnormal esophageal motility
Traction—Inflamed mediastinal lymph nodes

What are specific examples of each type of diverticula?

Pulsion—Pharyngoesophageal (Zenker's) and epiphrenic diverticulae
Traction—Midesophageal (parabronchial) diverticulae

Which are "true" versus "false" diverticula?

Pulsion types are false diverticula (mucosa and submucosa protrude through a defect in muscular portion of wall).
Traction types are true diverticula (mucosa, submucosa and muscular portion of wall).

What are the symptoms?	Dysphagia, retrosternal chest pain, regurgitation of undigested food, cough, severe halitosis, and gurgling sounds in throat
Which diagnostic study is indicated?	Barium esophagogram (Note: Avoid esophagoscopy because of the increased risk of perforation.)
What other study should also be done as part of workup?	Manometry (to assess the esophageal motility disorder in pulsion types)
What are the indications for treatment?	All **symptomatic** patients should undergo surgical repair
Which type rarely requires treatment?	Midesophageal (because rarely symptomatic)

Pharyngoesophageal (Zenker's) Diverticulum

What is the specific location in the esophagus?	Posterior midline within inferior pharyngeal constrictor between thyropharyngeus and cricopharyngeal muscles (Killian's triangle)
Which anatomic landmark is used to locate the sac intraoperatively?	Cricoid cartilage
What motility disorder is associated with pharyngoesophageal diverticulum?	Oropharyngeal dysphagia
What is the current standard surgical treatment?	Diverticulotomy and cricopharyngeal myotomy
What alternative surgical procedure is gaining popularity, and why?	Diverticulopexy (mobilize, invert, and tack pouch to the anterior spinal fascia). Significantly reduced risk of postoperative leak/fistula.
What occurs if myotomy is not performed?	Diverticulum recurs.

Epiphrenic Diverticulum

What is the location in the esophagus?	Distal esophagus (usually within 10 cm of cardia)
What motility disorder is associated with epiphrenic diverticulum?	Diffuse esophageal spasm and achalasia
What is the treatment?	Diverticulectomy; long esophagomyotomy or modified Heller myotomy; ± antireflux procedure (controversial)
Which incision should be used?	Left posterolateral thoracotomy (best access to distal esophagus)

ESOPHAGEAL PERFORATION

What is the most common etiology?	Iatrogenic (esophageal endoscopy or dilatation procedures, paraesophageal surgical procedures)
What are the other etiologies?	Boerhaave syndrome (most common non-iatrogenic etiology), trauma, swallowed foreign body, and caustic injuries
Why does the esophagus tend to rupture at lower pressures than the remainder of the gastrointestinal tract?	Lacks serosa (Collagen fibers of serosa provide considerable strength to alimentary tract wall.)
What is the usual presentation?	Chest pain, dysphagia, nausea, fever, tachycardia, and (not infrequently) hypotension
What is the classic sign of cervical rupture?	Subcutaneous (SQ) emphysema in neck and anterior thorax (crepitus)
What is the classic sign of intrathoracic rupture?	Hamman's crunch (crackles auscultated as heart beats against emphysematous mediastinum). (Note: The mediastinal air may eventually dissect to skin and also result in SQ emphysema.)

Why may patient with esophageal rupture become acutely unstable?

1. Tension pneumothorax (due to concurrent tear in mediastinal pleura)
2. Hypovolemic shock (rates of fluid accumulation in the mediastinum as high as 1 L/hour have been reported.)

What is the first study performed if perforation is suspected?

CXR

What are the classic findings on this study?

Subcutaneous or mediastinal emphysema, or both; widened mediastinum; ± pleural effusion or pneumothorax (if pleura torn)

What is the diagnostic study of choice?

Contrast esophagogram (first, use water-soluble Gastrografin; if not diagnostic, use barium) (Note: Endoscopy is **rarely** indicated.)

What biochemical test from thoracentesis sample of effusion would suggest perforation?

Elevated amylase (especially if isoenzyme from salivary glands)

What life-threatening condition develops with esophageal perforation?

Mediastinitis (primarily due to the **virulent** oral flora bacteria free in the mediastinum)

What is the key prognostic factor?

Duration between event and corrective surgery

Why?

Infection usually does not establish until 18 to 24 hours after the event (but once it develops, treating resultant empyema and suppurative mediastinitis is very difficult).

What is the treatment of cervical esophageal perforations?

Surgical exploration, drainage of retropharyngeal space and upper mediastinum with Jackson-Pratt drains, repair of perforation (if located), and IV antibiotics (Note: Occasionally in patients with limited extravasation, observation and antibiotics are sufficient)

What is the postoperative management regimen of cervical perforations?

Closely follow for evidence of mediastinitis; on day 5 to 7 perform contrast esophagogram Gastrografin, **then barium**—if no leak, drains removed and PO intake may be initiated.

In the treatment of thoracic (and abdominal) esophageal perforations, what is the most important factor in determining the course of treatment?

Interval between perforation and diagnosis

Why?

With late diagnosis, mediastinitis is well established, and any esophageal repair will likely break down because of inflammation, tissue friability, and infection.

What are the generally accepted intervals for "early" versus "late" diagnosis?

Early—Less than 8 hours; late—more than 24 hours (The interval between 8 and 24 hours is controversial and best left to the surgeon's judgment.)

What is usually recommended for early diagnoses?

Direct repair of esophageal leak **plus** drainage (mediastinal and pleural tubes); ± definitive treatment for any underlying esophageal pathology (e.g., myotomy for achalasia) [Note: Treatment of underlying lesions should be undertaken only **if** it can be done **without** jeopardizing the repair of the esophageal leak. In very select cases (e.g., carcinoma), esophagectomy may be indicated.]

What procedure can reduce the risk of fistula when primary repair is performed?

Reinforce esophageal suture line with flap of pleura, intercostal muscle, or diaphragm.

What procedure is usually recommended for late diagnoses (controversial)?

Drainage plus diversion-exclusion of esophagus (end cervical esophagostomy [spit-fistula], distal cervical esophagus stapled, (cardioesophageal junction ligation, gastrostomy/jejunostomy tubes)

Although this procedure is safe, what is its major drawback?

Patient requires a second major surgical procedure to reestablish the continuity of the gastrointestinal tract (usually left colonic interposition).

What are Cameron's criteria for use of nonoperative treatment for patients with thoracic perforation?

1. **Contained leak** (isolated within mediastinum)
2. Self-draining back into esophagus
3. Minimal symptoms
4. No (or minimal) signs of clinical sepsis

What are the components of nonoperative management?

NPO, parenteral hyperalimentation, and IV antibiotics

Iatrogenic Perforation

What are the most common sites of iatrogenic perforation?

Just proximal to upper esophageal sphincter, gastric cardia, or an esophageal pathology (e.g., stricture)

Are iatrogenic perforations usually diagnosed earlier or later than those in Boerhaave syndrome?

Earlier, because the procedure forces the surgeon to consider perforation early in the symptomatic patient (perforation is often initially missed in Boerhaave syndrome because of the relative infrequency of the disease)

What is the inciting event in Boerhaave's syndrome?

Forced vomiting (against closed glottis)

What is the most common site of perforation?

Less than 5 cm above gastroesophageal (GE) junction on left side

What percentage of patients have preexisting esophageal lesion?

Only 10%

HIATAL HERNIA

What is a hiatal hernia?

Herniation of abdominal viscera (usually stomach) through diaphragm via the esophageal hiatus

What are the types?	Type I—Sliding (or axial) Type II—paraesophageal (or rolling) Type III—combined type I and II

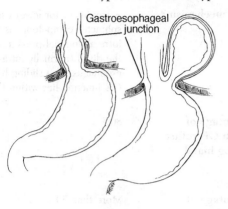

What are the frequencies of each type?	Sliding—More than 90% Paraesophageal—Less than 5% Combined—Less than 1%
What are the basic anatomic differences between type I and II hiatal hernias?	Sliding—cephalad migration of gastroesophageal (GE) junction; no peritoneal hernia sac; phrenoesophageal (PE) membrane intact. Paraesophageal—GE junction in normal position; true hernia sac into which the stomach (± other viscera) herniates; deterioration of PE membrane
What is the usual age of presentation?	Age 60 to 70
What factors contribute to the development of hiatal hernias?	Aging with associated weakening of musculoligamental structures, obesity
What is the classic CXR finding of hiatal hernia?	Retrocardiac shadow, often with air–fluid level (best seen on lateral view)

Sliding Hiatal Hernia (Type I)

What are the symptoms?	Heartburn, regurgitation of sour-tasting fluid, and dysphagia

What is the etiology of symptoms?

GE reflux

What is the mechanism?

A key factor for lower esophageal sphincter competence is the higher intra-abdominal pressures surrounding the distal (normally intra-abdominal) esophagus. In a sliding hiatal hernia, the GE junction lies within the chest.

What percentage of patients with GE reflux have a sliding hiatal hernia?

80%

What percentage of patients require no treatment?

More than 50%

What percentage require surgery?

Only 15%

What are the indications for surgical treatment?

1. Failure of medical therapy for GE reflux (H_2 blockers, omeprazole)
2. Patients who require long-term omeprazole for control of symptoms (currently not FDA approved for long-term use)

What is the surgical procedure?

Antireflux procedure (several types including Nissen and Belsey techniques)

What are the basic objectives of these procedures and how are they achieved?

Anitreflux procedures reduce the hiatal hernia, restore and secure the GE junction (LES) to its original intra-abdominal position. Achieved by:
1. Tightening the dilated esophageal hiatus via reapproximation of the diaphragmatic crura
2. Performing some form of fundoplication (wrap part of fundus partially or completely around the distal esophagus/GE junction). [Note: Remember to protect the vagus nerves.]

What is the procedure of choice for patients with insufficient esophageal length to each abdomen (e.g., due to strictures)?	Collis gastroplasty with formation of "neo-esophagus" by stapling (GIA) along the fundic side of a bougie placed through the esophagus along the lesser curvature of the stomach. Then proceed with fundoplication and the rest of the procedure.

Paraesophageal Hiatal Hernia (Type II)

What are the symptoms?	Mild obstructive symptoms (e.g., dysphagia, postprandial fullness in chest and belching, mild regurgitation); **usually** asymptomatic
What is the mechanism of symptoms?	Intraluminal pressure changes result in enlargement of the gastric sac as ingested food displaces fundic air bubble.
What are the complications?	Gastric incarceration, strangulation, or volvulus-obstruction; gastric hemorrhage or ulceration (due to stasis in gastric sac)
What percentage of patients require surgery?	One hundred percent (although some may not be surgical candidates because of poor medical condition)
Why?	High mortality (20%–25%) associated with severe complications that usually develop acutely in a previously asymptomatic (or only mildly symptomatic) patient with paraesophageal hiatal hernia
What is the basic surgical procedure?	Reduction of the hiatal hernia contents into the abdomen, anchoring of stomach within abdomen, resection of hernia sac, and repair of the dilated esophageal hiatus (by reapproximating diaphragmatic crura)
Which incision is used?	Left posterolateral thoracotomy or midline laparotomy

What are the surgical options for intra-abdominal "anchoring" of stomach?	1. Anterior gastropexy (suture anterior gastric wall to posterior rectus sheath) 2. Hill posterior gastropexy (suture lesser curvature of stomach to preaortic median arcuate ligament) 3. G-tube 4. Antireflux procedure (often performed this primarily to keep stomach in the abdomen)
Why is induction of anesthesia often dangerous in these patients?	Adequate preoperative decompression of gastric contents difficult, and thus patients at high risk of aspiration
What additional procedure is often recommended (controversial)?	Antireflux procedure (fundoplication): controversial because many patients with paraesophageal hernias do **not** have classic symptoms associated with reflux nor do they have positive acid reflux tests

BENIGN ESOPHAGEAL TUMORS

Account for what percentage of esophageal tumors?	Only 1%
What are the most common types?	1. Leiomyoma (66%) 2. Congenital esophageal cyst (also called enteric cyst or esophageal duplication cyst) [See *Mediastinal Masses* section]
How is the diagnosis made?	1. Barium esophagogram 2. Esophagoscopy (to rule out carcinoma)

Leiomyoma

What are the symptoms?	Dysphagia, chest pain. If < 5 cm in size, often asymptomatic
What is the classic finding on barium esophagogram?	Smooth narrowing of lumen with intact mucosa (**intramural** mass)
How is esophagoscopic protocol different with leiomyoma versus carcinoma, and why?	Mass is not biopsied. Scarring from biopsy makes excision more difficult.

What are the indications for treatment?	1. Symptomatic patient (chest pain, dysphagia) 2. Mass > 5 cm in size
What is the procedure?	Surgically enucleate from esophageal wall via extramucosal approach.
What incision should be used?	Posterolateral thoracotomy (right if in upper two-thirds, left if in lower one-third)
Why should endoscopic removal be avoided?	Increased risk of esophageal rupture and late stricture (due to disruption of mucosa)

MALIGNANT ESOPHAGEAL TUMORS

What areas of the world have high incidence?	China, Iran, and South Africa
What are the most common types of esophageal carcinoma?	1. Squamous cell (90%–95%) 2. Adenocarcinoma (2%-8%)
What are the risk factors for each of these types?	Squamous cell—Alcohol, tobacco, some diets (e.g., nitrosamines), achalasia, chronic ingestion of hot beverages or foods, and lye strictures Adenocarcinoma—Barrett's esophagus (transformation of epithelium in distal esophagus from squamous to columnar due to reflux)
What is the most common general esophageal region for each type?	Squamous cell—Upper half Adenocarcinoma—Lower half
What anatomic factors contribute to the high frequency of local tumor invasion and lymphatic spread on presentation?	No serosal layer; extensive lymphatic drainage of the mediastinum with cervical and abdominal collaterals
What is the usual presentation?	Dysphagia (most common symptom), weight loss, chest pain, odynophagia (Note: **Insidious** onset is characteristic of esophageal carcinoma.)

Are solids or liquids more easily swallowed?

Liquids (With achalasia, solids are more easily swallowed.)

What are signs of unresectability?

1. Hoarseness (invasion of recurrent laryngeal nerve)
2. Horner syndrome
3. Paralysis of diaphragm (invasion of phrenic nerve)
4. Malignant pleural effusion
5. Fistula formation
6. Airway invasion
7. Vertebral invasion

Which diagnostic studies are indicated?

Barium esophagogram (± cine technique), esophagoscopy, bronchoscopy, CT scan of chest and abdomen

What are the two gross "types" of esophageal carcinoma noted on barium swallow?

Fungating irregular lesion (upper "shelf" or "apple core" appearance); smooth annular lesion

Why should esophagoscopy be performed?

To biopsy for definitive tissue diagnosis, to confirm location and length of tumor, to determine if Barrett's esophagus is present, and to determine if gastric invasion is present

Why should bronchoscopy be performed?

To rule out fistula with tracheobronchial tree and evaluate for coexistent bronchogenic carcinoma (common risk factor of smoking)

What is the primary goal of staging the esophageal carcinoma?

To determine if the surgical procedure is to be performed for cure vs. palliation (Note: Curative procedure requires resection of tumor and all potentially involved lymph nodes with negative margins.)

What percentage of patients are potentially curable on presentation?

Only 20% to 25%

What are the four stages of esophageal tumors (American Joint Committee on Cancer, AJCC)?

Stage I—localized to submucosa and no lymph node metastasis
Stage II—invasion into muscularis, regional lymph node metastasis, or both
Stage III—extension into adventitia and regional lymph node metastasis; invasion into adjacent structures regardless of status of lymph nodes
Stage IV—distant metastasis

What is the most common stage to present to the surgeon?

Stage III (> 95%) [Note: The exceptions are the patients with Barrett's esophagus, who are frequently diagnosed earlier due to their close follow-up.]

What are the two goals of treatment?

1. Treat the dysphagia by providing unobstructed swallowing for the remainder of the patient's life (90% successful).
2. Attempt to cure the carcinoma (rarely successful).

What are the three major treatment strategies?

1. Localized endoscopic control—insertion of polyvinyl "funnel esophageal tube" (to maintain patency), endoscopic laser debulking of tumor
2. Single mode therapy—Surgical resection or radiation therapy (**rarely** chemotherapy)
3. Combined therapy—neoadjuvant therapy)—chemoradiation therapy (or chemotherapy) followed by surgical resection

What are the indications for non-operative treatment?

1. Poor surgical candidate—advanced age, poor pulmonary reserve (FEV_1 < 1.25 L), other significant comorbid pathology (e.g., ejection fraction < 40%)
2. Inoperable due to local invasion into aorta, tracheobronchial tree, or vertebra

What is the radiation dose for palliation versus for cure?

4000 to 5000 rads for palliation, 5000 to 7000 rads for cure (Note: Radiation therapy alone is of **no** benefit as a preoperative adjunctive therapy.)

What are the most frequently used chemotherapeutic agents?

Cisplatin and 5-FU

What is the surgical procedure for esophageal carcinoma?

Partial esophagogastrectomy—Resection of esophagus (variable lengths depending on surgical approach) plus proximal portion of stomach

What are the two most commonly used approaches?

1. Transhiatal esophagectomy (THE)
2. Transthoracic (Ivor-Lewis) esophagectomy (TTE)

What are the basic differences between the approaches?

THE—laparotomy plus cervical incision (part of thoracic dissection performed blindly), anastomosis done in the neck
TTE—laparotomy plus thoracotomy (permits direct visualization of resection), anastomosis performed in the chest

Which procedure has improved survival?

Same survival rate (despite claims by proponents of TTE that it provides improved chance for cure due to a more complete mediastinal lymph node resection and less risk for life-threatening hemorrhage)

What are the proven benefits of THE?

1. Better tolerated by those with respiratory insufficiency (because no thoracotomy)
2. Cervical anastomotic leak is nonfatal whereas thoracic leak has 50% mortality; thus, overall lower mortality (particularly in high-risk groups) may in fact be lower with THE.

What is the primary indication for TTE?

Tumor unresectable via THE owing to fixation to vital mediastinal structures (e.g., trachea, aorta) as determined **at the time of surgery** by the surgeon palpating the tumor through the esophageal hiatus

How is the continuity of the gastrointestinal tract reestablished?

Gastric pull-up (95%) or colonic interposition (5%) [substernal or posterior mediastinal routes]

What vessels are perserved when mobilizing stomach cranially?	Right gastric and right gastroepiploic vessels
In addition to the esophagectomy, what additional procedures are usually performed?	1. Feeding jejunostomy (Note: Feeds may start in the recovery room.) 2. Pyloroplasty/pyloromyotomy if gastric pull-up used (vagus nerves severed with resection; thus, major control of pylorus lost and may result in gastric outlet obstruction)
What is the mortality rate from esophagectomy?	Five percent
What postoperative adjunctive therapy is recommended?	XRT
What is the 5-year survival rate for each stage after treatment?	Stage I—85%; stage II—35%; stage III—15%; stage IV—0% (AJCC staging)

CORROSIVE ESOPHAGEAL INJURIES

How are these burns classified?	First degree—Only mucosal erythema and edema Second degree—erythema, edema, **and** ulceration (**partial** esophageal circumference) Third degree—**circumferential** esophageal ulceration and mucosal sloughing
Which diagnostic studies should be performed on initial evaluation?	Esophagoscopy followed by barium esophagogram
What contraindicates the first study?	Evidence of laryngeal or pharyngeal burn (stridor, hoarseness, dyspnea). Admit and monitor for airway obstruction (maximal edema sometimes delayed 6–24 hours!) before diagnostic evaluation of esophagus

What is the treatment of each type/degree of burn?

First degree—Brief observation; continue PO intake, and discharge home

Second degree—Antibiotics for 3 weeks; continue PO intake, follow-up with endoscopy after 3 weeks

Third degree—Same as second **plus** large gastrostomy (Note: Some also advocate steroid therapy to reduce incidence of stricture formation.)

What are the late sequelae of corrosive injury?

Stricture formation (most common), malignant degeneration, and hiatal hernia (fibrotic esophagus retracting stomach into chest)

What is the treatment of the most common sequela?

Repeated bougie dilatation of stricture (safest approach being **retrograde** through gastrostomy); alternatively, balloon dilatation

How long is this treatment continued?

Until a permanently patent lumen develops or 6 months of unsuccessful conservative treatment (Then consider esophagectomy.)

OTHER ESOPHAGEAL LESIONS

Esophageal Webs

What is the most common symptom?

Dysphagia

What are the types and general location of each in esophagus?

Plummer-Vinson syndrome (PVS) web— Upper esophagus

Schatzki's ring—Distal esophagus (at squamocolumnar junction)

What is the etiology of each type?

Uncertain, but presumed etiology for PVS is iron deficiency and for Schatzki's is gastroesophageal reflux

What is the target population of PVS?

Middle-aged women

What are the characteristic findings on physical exam of this population?

Edentulous, spoon-shaped fingers with brittle nails, and atrophic oral mucosa

What is the treatment?   Dilation of web plus iron supplements in PVS; antireflux procedure in Schatzki's

Acquired Esophageal Fistula

What is the most common etiology?   Malignancy

See the *Acquired Tracheoesophageal Fistula* section.

BARIUM ESOPHAGOGRAM

What is the most likely diagnosis for each of the following line drawings of various barium studies (several possibilities are present; try to pick the best)?

A. Diffuse spasm
B. Achalasia (moderate)
C. Carcinoma: Annular type
D. Zenker's diverticulum
E. Diffuse spasm with epiphrenic diverticulum
F. Leiomyoma
G. Carcinoma: Fungating type
H. Sliding hiatal hernia (type I) with Barrett's esophagus and esophageal stricture due to reflux
I. Schatzki's ring
J. Achalasia (severe)

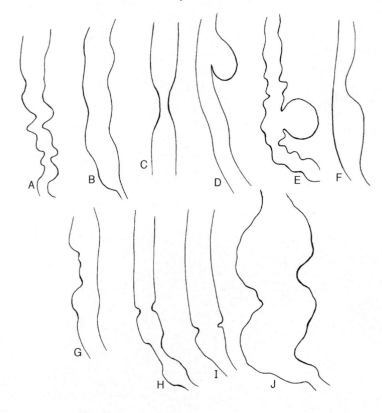

THORACIC TRAUMA

INITIAL MANAGEMENT OF THORACIC TRAUMA

What are the immediate priorities on admission to ER?

ABCs of resuscitation (airway, breathing, circulation; primary survey of ATLS)

What are the IMMEDIATELY life-threatening thoracic injuries identified on PRIMARY survey of ATLS?

1. Airway obstruction
2. Tension pneumothorax (PTX)
3. Open PTX
4. Flail chest
5. Massive hemothorax
6. Cardiac tamponade

What are the POTENTIALLY life-threatening thoracic injuries identified on SECONDARY survey of ATLS?

1. Pulmonary contusion
2. Myocardial contusion
3. Aortic disruption
4. Traumatic diaphragmatic hernia
5. Tracheobronchial disruption
6. Esophageal disruption

What is the standard regimen for establishing venous access in the thoracic trauma patient?

First, insert 14-gauge IV in the antecubital fossa. Then, insert 8.5 French trauma catheter in subclavian or internal jugular vein on the same side as the chest injury. If patient is in shock, insert another 8.5 French catheter into a femoral vein (thus, providing the unstable patient with venous access above and below the diaphragm).

What are the most common causes of persistent, unexplained hypotension despite volume resuscitation and tube thoracostomy?

1. Occult hemorrhage (intra-abdominal, retroperitoneal, femoral/thigh)
2. Pericardial tamponade

What are the indications for emergency room (ER) thoracotomy?

1. Exsanguinating penetrating thoracic trauma
2. Patient who becomes pulseless en route to hospital or during ER resuscitation

(Note: In the vast majority of cases, thoracotomy is **not** indicated if no signs of life were noted before hospital evaluation.)

Which incision is used for ER thoracotomy?	Left anterolateral thoracotomy (± extension across sternum to right chest—partial or complete "clam-shell" incision)
What is the sequence of the basic objectives of an ER thoracotomy?	1. Rule out or treat pericardial tamponade with longitudinal pericardiotomy. 2. Do bimanual compressions if heart is asystolic. 3. Clamp descending aorta. 4. Identify and temporarily control intrathoracic bleeding.
What is the most frequent general mistake resulting in patient demise?	Delay in surgery for diagnostic studies in the labile trauma patient
What regions of the body are included in the prep and draping for surgery?	From the mid-neck to bilateral mid-thighs!
Why include the most inferior region in the prep?	The groins are included to provide access to: 1. Femoral vessels if femoral–femoral cardiopulmonary bypass becomes necessary 2. Saphenous vein if autologous graft is needed for vascular repair

CHEST WALL TRAUMA

Rib Fractures

What is the most frequently fractured region of the ribs?	Posterior angle (especially ribs 5 through 9)
Which fractures are frequently missed on CXR?	Anterior rib fractures (not easily visualized at the costochondral junction)
What is the significance of fractures of ribs 10 through 12?	High incidence of associated injuries to spleen or liver

What is the treatment of rib fracture?

Analgesia. In more severe cases, admission for observation and respiratory therapy (to prevent atelectasis and pneumonia). (Note: External splinting or taping of chest is **contraindicated**.)

What general regimens are used for analgesia?

Most single fractures can be treated with oral analgesics. Multiple rib fractures may require intercostal/epidural nerve blocks or intrapleura analgesia.

What is the significance of first and second rib fractures?

Kinetic energy required to fracture these ribs is great; thus, they are frequently associated with severe intrathoracic injury.

What additional diagnostic studies should be strongly considered in these patients?

Esophageal swallow and aortic arteriogram (due to the increased risk of esophageal and aortic or great vessel injuries)

What is flail chest?

≥ 3 adjacent ribs fractured in > 1 site

What is the classic physical finding in flail chest?

Paradoxic movement of a segment of chest wall with respiratory cycle (segment moves in with inspiration, out with expiration)

Flail chest is frequently associated with what intrathoracic lesion?

Pulmonary contusion

Approximately what percentage of patients with flail chest require mechanical ventilation?

Only 50%! (in the past, **all** patients were intubated; however, a more conservative approach has resulted in reduced morbidity.)

Sternal Fractures

How is the diagnosis of sternal fractures confirmed?

Lateral CXR

What is the significance of sternal fractures?

High incidence of associated intrathoracic injuries (myocardial and pulmonary contusions, disruption of the tracheobronchial tree)

Which sternal fractures should be treated?	Unstable fractures (mobile fragments on anterior compression of chest)
Why?	Reduce risk of pseudarthrosis and resultant chronic pain
Which procedure is used?	Stabilization with vertical wire sutures

PLEURAL TRAUMA

Traumatic Pneumothorax (PTX)

Injury to what structures may cause traumatic pneumothorax (PTX)?	Chest wall, tracheobronchial tree, lung, or esophagus
What is an open PTX?	PTX associated with chest-wall defect ("sucking chest wound," e.g., close-range shotgun blast)
What is a tension PTX?	PTX associated with one-way flap air leak (chest wall or bronchopleural) resulting in trapped **air under pressure** in hemithorax—causes collapse of ipsilateral lung, mediastinal shift, and compression of contralateral lung
What is the usual presentation of simple PTX?	Respiratory distress, chest pain; decreased breath sounds and hypertympany to percussion on affected side, collapsed lung on CXR
What is the usual presentation of tension PTX?	Significant respiratory distress, hypotension, tachycardia, cyanosis, and tracheal shift (away from PTX) [Note: This is a **clinical** diagnosis!]
What is the appearance of PTX on supine CXR?	Diffuse radiolucency in the anterior costophrenic region
What is the treatment of simple PTX?	Tube thoracostomy in midaxillary line ICS 5 or 6 (36–40 French is usually recommended for traumatic PTX because of the frequency of hemopneumothorax); see *Pneumothorax* section for more detailed discussion of technique

What should be done if lung does not completely reexpand?

Initially, a second chest tube should be placed; if the lung still is not reexpanded (or persistent air leak is present), bronchoscopy should be performed to rule out tracheobronchial lesion.)

What is the treatment of open PTX?

Cover wound with occlusive dressing while tube thoracostomy is performed distant from the chest wall defect; then perform operative repair.

What is the treatment of tension PTX?

Convert to simple PTX by emergency needle aspiration with 14-gauge needle in ICS 2 at midclavicular line; then perform tube thoracostomy.

What are the indications for placement of tube thoracostomy if severe lung injury is suspected, but no PTX is evident on CXR and no respiratory distress is present?

1. Patient requiring positive pressure ventilation (general anesthesia) for operative intervention of other injury (e.g., cranial)
2. Patient transferred by air or ground transport to another center

Hemothorax

What are the most common sources of bleeding?

Intercostal artery or internal mammary artery (85%). Other sources include fractured ribs, deep pulmonary laceration, aorta, and occasionally the heart.

How much blood can a hemithorax hold?

From 2 to 2.5 L

What is the usual presentation?

Dyspnea, decreased breath sounds, and dullness to percussion on affected side

What are the associated CXR findings?

Diffuse hazy hemithorax on supine CXR, effusion noted on upright CXR (air–fluid level of concurrent PTX)

What is the treatment?

Large-bore intravenous access for rapid fluid resuscitation—then **(and not before)** tube thoracostomy (36–40 French tube); ± autotransfusion

Why is it important that all of the blood be evacuated from pleural cavity?

Fibrothorax may develop from organized clot.

What is the treatment for this complication?

Decortication via posterolateral thoracotomy (fibrous peel removed relatively easily when performed before 3–4 weeks)

What are the indications for urgent thoracotomy?

1. > 1500 ml of blood on placement of chest tube
2. > 200 to 300 ml/hr for > 3 consecutive hours
3. > 2,500 ml over 24 hours (Note: One might consider thoracotomy at much lower volumes in the elderly patient.)

What percentage of patients require thoracotomy?

Only 10%

What should be done if exsanguinating bleeding from the lung is encountered?

Clamp hilum with atraumatic clamp to provide control of hemorrhage until lesion can be identified and repaired (or resected).

TRACHEOBRONCHIAL TRAUMA

What is the most common mechanism of injury?

Motor vehicle accidents (hyperextended neck striking the dashboard or steering wheel)

What are the classic findings on physical exam?

Subcutaneous emphysema (especially with cervical tracheal injury), auscultation of mediastinal emphysema (Hamman's crunch) (Note: External evidence of neck or chest injury is often minimal even in the setting of airway disruption.)

What are the associated CXR findings?

Pneumomediastinum, PTX, and subcutaneous emphysema

What would significantly increase suspicion of tracheobronchial disruption after placement of tube thoracostomy?

1. Persistent air leak
2. Incomplete reexpansion of lung
3. Worsening respiratory status/ symptoms when tube placed to suction because of resultant increase in flow through tracheobronchial lesion (almost pathognomonic)

How is definitive diagnosis made?

Bronchoscopy

What is the acute management of tracheobronchial trauma?

Establish a secure airway via intubation (use flexible bronchoscope to guide endotracheal tube if tracheal injury present)

What are the indications for surgical repair?

1. Persistent air leak (> 2 weeks)
2. Large air leak with respiratory compromise due to incomplete expansion of lung

What procedure is used?

Primary repair and pleural or muscular flap wrap around the suture line

What procedure can be performed if primary repair of trachea is not feasible at time of injury?

Bronchoscopic placement of a silicone tracheal T-tube (Montgomery)

What is the major chronic sequela of unrecognized tracheobronchial disruption?

Stricture formation with increased risk of necrotizing infection (seen more frequently in partial obstruction than complete)

PULMONARY TRAUMA

Pulmonary Contusion

What is the mechanism?

Blunt chest trauma—increased pulmonary capillary pressure—extravasation of blood cells, plasma and serum proteins into interstitium and alveoli

What is the physiologic result of this injury?

Intrapulmonary shunting (and hypoxia), reduced pulmonary compliance (and hypercarbia due to hypoventilation)

What is the classic finding on CXR?

Hazy infiltrate in region of blunt trauma

How long after injury before CXR findings become evident?

Variable. In 70% of cases, findings are seen within several minutes versus 30% have a lag time up to 6 hours; regardless, over the next 24 hours, the size and density often dramatically increase.

What may mimic pulmonary contusion on CXR in the trauma patient?

1. Atelectasis distal to aspiration of foreign body (e.g., tooth, dentures, food)
2. Hemothorax in supine patient (generalized haziness over entire lung field)

What is the treatment of pulmonary contusion?

Most cases require only supplemental oxygen, but patients should be closely monitored for respiratory failure. **Judicious** use of IV fluids (Note: Do **not** restrict fluid.) **No** steroids or prophylactic antibiotics (advocated by some in the past)

Pulmonary Laceration

Recent studies have demonstrated that pulmonary lacerations are more common than previously believed. What are mechanisms for lacerations in blunt trauma?

Penetration of fractured ribs, vertebra, for example; shearing effect due to differential inertia of lung segments; avulsions due to pleural adhesions

What are the associated CXR findings?

Elliptical radiodensity or cyst (due to the elastic recoil of surrounding lung) with thin pseudomembrane lining ± air-fluid level (due to blood in cavity) or round uniform density mass (pulmonary hematoma)

What are the complications?

PTX, bronchopleural fistula, hemothorax, and air emboli (see *Miscellaneous Thoracic Trauma Topics* section for discussion of air embolism)

ESOPHAGEAL TRAUMA

What is the usual presentation of esophageal perforation?

Chest pain, dyspnea; fever, subcutaneous emphysema, Hamman's sign (auscultated secondary to mediastinal emphysema)

What are the associated CXR findings?

Pneumomediastinum, widening of mediastinum (due to edema), pleural effusion, subcutaneous emphysema, and occasionally pneumothorax

Which diagnostic studies should be performed?

Contrast esophagogram if patient is awake and cooperative; esophagoscopy if altered mental status or sedated

Which contrast agent should be used for screening esophagogram, and why?

Water-soluble contrast (Gastrografin) is the first-line agent. Experimental evidence suggests that it causes less inflammatory reaction than barium if it leaks into the mediastinum.

When is this first-line contrast agent contraindicated, and why?

Suspected esophagorespiratory fistula. Has high osmolarity and causes pulmonary edema and pneumonitis if aspirated.

What should be done if water-soluble esophagogram is negative, and why?

Perform barium esophagogram. Gastrografin misses 25% to 50% of esophageal perforation!

What is the treatment of cervical esophageal perforation?

Surgical placement of drain in prevertebral–retroesophageal space usually sufficient; however, if easily visualized and tissue edges appear viable, primary repair of esophageal defect is indicated.

What incision should be used for thoracic esophageal perforation?

1. Left posterolateral thoracotomy if injury in the proximal or distal third of esophagus is suspected
2. Right posterolateral thoracotomy if injury in the middle third of esophagus is suspected

What are the surgical options for thoracic esophageal perforation?

1. **Two-layer** closure of defect with pleural or intercostal muscle flap secured over suture line
2. Esophagectomy (if irreparable)
3. Rarely, exclusion–diversion technique (proximal and distal ends of esophagus divided/stapled, feeding gastrostomy placed)

See the *Esophageal Perforation* section for management of chronic esophageal perforation.

CARDIAC TRAUMA

See the *Cardiac Trauma* section in the Cardiac Surgery chapter.

AORTIC TRAUMA

See the *Vascular Trauma* section in the Vascular Surgery chapter.

MISCELLANEOUS THORACIC TRAUMA TOPICS

Traumatic Asphyxia

What is the mechanism of injury?

Crush injury to the thorax

What is the classic triad of physical findings?

Facial and upper torso edema with cyanotic appearance, subconjunctival hemorrhage, and petechiae (due to retrograde flow through the valveless veins of upper body associated with the sudden increase in intrathoracic pressure)

What is the treatment?

Observation, head elevation, and supplemental oxygen. Most treatment is directed toward the common associated thoracic or head injuries.

Gas Embolism

What is the most common cause?

Penetrating wound to chest resulting in injury to abutting pulmonary vessel and tracheobronchial lumen

What dramatically increases the risk of air embolus?

Positive pressure ventilation

Presentation?

1. Cerebral ischemia (e.g., seizures) and cardiac ischemia (infarction, arrhythmias) due to the resultant air emboli and platelet–fibrin aggregates
2. Coagulopathy and bronchospasm due to activation of inflammatory cascades

What is the treatment?

Left lateral decubitus position, feet elevated 30° to 60° (unfortunately often difficult in the trauma patient); aspirate air from CVP line; ideally, initiate cardiopulmonary bypass or hyperbaric oxygen

Diaphragm Trauma

Which hemidiaphragm is more frequently injured in penetrating trauma, and why?

Left (60%–80%), because liver protects right side and most assailants are right-handed

What surgical approach should be used for repair, and why?

1. If diagnosed at time of injury— Exploratory laparotomy should be performed first to exclude the frequent intraabdominal injuries (seen in 85% of left-sided penetrating injuries)
2. If diagnosed late (≥ 1 week after injury)—Posterolateral thoracotomy should be performed to facilitate lysis of adhesions between herniated abdominal viscera and thoracic structures.

What additional procedure is often recommended if the diaphragmatic injury includes the esophageal hiatus?

Antireflux procedure (i.e., Nissen fundoplication)

Diagnosis is not infrequently missed, especially in blunt trauma. How do missed patients commonly present later?

Bowel obstruction due to herniation through defect into chest

High-Velocity Missiles

What are high-velocity missiles?

Bullets with muzzle velocity ≥ 500 meters per second

Why do these bullets cause so much more injury than larger, low-velocity bullets?

Energy transmitted by a bullet is quantitated by the following formula: Kinetic energy = (Mass x Velocity^2) ÷ 2

LUNG TRANSPLANTATION

What are the indications?

Select patients with:
1. Emphysema
2. Cystic fibrosis
3. Pulmonary fibrosis
4. Primary pulmonary hypertension
5. Eisenmenger syndrome (secondary pulmonary hypertension)

What is an absolute criterion for patient to be a candidate for lung transplant?

No significant heart disease (or at least surgically correctable); in particular, right ventricular function must be carefully assessed (by MUGA).

What preoperative studies are performed to match donor with recipient?

Only ABO blood compatibility

What is the most common mechanical complication in the early postoperative period?

Dehiscence of tracheal or bronchial anastomosis (due to the ischemia associated with disruption of the bronchial arterial supply)

What may reduce incidence of this complication?

1. Omentopexy around anastomosis at time of transplant (possible collateral arterial supply)
2. Avoidance of steriod use during the first week postoperatively

What is the usual immunosuppression for lung transplantation?

Cyclosporin and azathioprine from time of transplant, antilymphocyte immuno-globulin for the first week, replaced with prednisone (Note: Regimen varies between institutions.)

What is the most common postoperative infection?

CMV (Cytomegalovirus)

What is administered as prophylaxis against this infection?

Acyclovir (PO) started as soon as oral intake tolerated

What is the treatment of CMV infection?

Ganciclovir (IV)

What is the best way to diagnose rejection in lung allograft?

Pulse dose of IV methylprednisolone. Improvement in pulmonary status (e.g., oxygenation, exercise tolerance) occurs within hours of steriod administration in the setting of rejection.

What study is used for standard rejection surveillance?

Bronchoscopy with transbronchial biopsy

What is the most common mechanical complication in the late postoperative period?

Stricture formation at tracheal anastomosis

During what period after lung transplantation is mortality rate highest?

First 2 months postoperatively (20%–25%)

What is the 1-year survival rate?

Between 60% and 75%

52

Transplant Immunology and Solid Organ Transplantation

Anne C. Fischer, MD

TRANSPLANT IMMUNOLOGY

Define the following terms:

Autografting

Transplantation within an individual (donor and recipient are the same)

Isografting

Transplantation between genetically identical individuals

Allografting

Transplantation between individuals of the same species

Xenografting

Transplantation between a donor and a recipient of different species

What is an antigen?

Molecule that is recognized as foreign, or nonself. An antigen can evoke an immune response when introduced into an individual.

What is a hapten?

Low–molecular-weight substance that is antigenic (immunogenic) only when it is bound to a larger carrier molecule

What are the characteristics of an antigen?

1. Multivalency with multiple epitopes
2. Immunogenicity

What are alloantigens?

Substances that are recognized as foreign on tissues from members of the same species

What are xenoantigens?	Substances that are recognized as foreign on tissues from members of a different species
What factors determine antigen immunogenicity relative to transplantation?	1. Foreignness: Xenogeneic > Allogeneic > Syngeneic 2. Complexity: Proteins > Carbohydrates > Nucleic acids > Lipids 3. Size > 5 Kd
What steps are involved in antigen processing?	1. Antigens are endocytosed by antigen-presenting cells (APCs) 2. Antigens are degraded by proteolytic enzymes in the phagolysosome 3. Antigenic peptides are associated with class II major histocompatibility complex (MHC) molecules because they are expressed on the cell surface
What are the phases of the immune response?	1. Cognitive phase: Recognition 2. Activation phase: Lymphocyte proliferation 3. Effector phase: Immunologic memory induction
How does a secondary response differ from a primary response?	Secondary response is: 1. More rapid, but still specific 2. More intense because of immunologic memory
What are the two effector arms of an immune response?	1. Humoral immunity: B cells (antibody-producing cells) 2. Cell-mediated immunity: T cells (recognition cells)
Where do these cell types mature and develop?	B cells: Bone marrow and fetal liver T cells: Thymus
In secondary lymphoid organs, which areas of a lymph node are dependent on the following: **Thymus?**	Paracortical and medullary area
Bursal equivalent?	Germinal centers

What cell type produces all components of the immune response?	Pluripotent bone marrow stem cells

B CELLS

What is the basic structure of an antibody?	1. Serum proteins with four polypeptide chains: Two heavy chains and two light chains stabilized by disulfide bonds 2. Two regions: Variable and constant
What is the role of the: **Variable region?**	Binds specifically to an antigen
Constant region?	Mediates complement fixation and monocyte binding
What process generates diversity of the variable region?	Genetic recombination: Heavy chain (V and D segments) and light chain (V and J segments)
What other mechanisms generate diversity in the B cell response?	1. Random V-region readout 2. Variable recombination 3. Somatic mutation
What is the order of events that produce antibody specificity?	1. Rearrangements of the V, D, and J segments of the heavy chain cause expression of a μ heavy chain in pre-B cells. 2. Light chain rearrangement (V and J segments) occurs first with the Vκ genes and then with the Vλ genes for one productive rearrangement. 3. The surface immunoglobulin M (IgM) can act as a functional antigen receptor on the immature B cell.
B cells are the precursors of what cells?	Plasma cells
Describe the process of differentiation.	B cells differentiate from lymphoid stem cells to virgin B cells which, on antigen stimulation, undergo proliferation, activation, and blast transformation to become plasma cells or memory cells.

What lymphokines initiate the process of B cell differentiation?

1. Interleukin-7 (IL-7)
2. IL-3
3. Low–molecular-weight BCGF (B cell growth factor)

What types of surface immunoglobulin (sIg) are expressed on:

Immature B cells?   Surface IgM⁺

Mature B cells?   Surface IgM⁺ and IgD⁺

Activated B cells?   Surface IgM⁺ and IgD⁻

Memory B cells?   Surface IgG⁺ and IgA⁺

Plasma cells?   Only cytoplasmic immunoglobulins are produced; surface Ig are lost by the plasma cell!

What class (or classes) of antibody:

Corresponds to the most prevalent serum immunoglobulin?   IgG

Is most prevalent in secretions?   IgA

Fixes complement?   IgG and IgM

Is the predominant class produced during a primary response?   IgM

Is the predominant class produced during a secondary response?   IgG

Mediates type I hypersensitivity reactions?   IgE

Has the greatest number of subclasses?   IgG (4) > IgA (2)

May play a role in antigen-triggered lymphocyte differentiation?	IgD
Is the only trace immunoglobulin in serum?	IgD (<1%)
Confers passive immunity in the newborn?	IgG

T CELLS

What are typical T cell responses?	1. Cellular immunity 2. Delayed-type hypersensitivity reactions 3. Antiviral activity 4. Allograft rejection 5. T cell help for antibody responses 6. Cytokine production
What are the types of T cells?	1. Cytotoxic (CD8⁺ cells) 2. Helper/inducer (CD4⁺ cells) 3. Suppressor

What are their corresponding roles?	Cytotoxic T cells (CTLs): Recognize antigens in context with class I MHC molecules and destroy the target cell
	Helper T cells (T_h):
	  1. Stimulate B cells to produce antibody
	  2. Induce the maturation of precytotoxic T cells
	  3. Stimulate macrophages to produce a nonspecific inflammatory response
	  4. Induce cytokine production
	Suppressor T cells: Suppress the activity of T and B cells

Which alloantigens primarily stimulate: CD4⁺ T cells?	Class II MHC antigens
CD8⁺ T cells?	Class I MHC antigens

What are the steps in T-cell activation?

1. Processing of antigen by macrophages (antigen-presenting cells; APCs)
2. Presentation of antigen to T and B cells by APCs in context with self-MHC
3. Highly specific antigen recognition by T cell clones
4. Release of IL-1 by macrophages
5. Stimulation of IL-2 receptors on T cells
6. Increased expression of IL-2 receptors on T cells (T cell activation and proliferation)
7. Interaction of T_h cells with B cells, followed by blastogenesis, plasma cell production, and antibody production

What is needed for T-cell recognition of an antigen?

1. MHC compatibility between the T cell and the APC
2. Presence of a T-cell receptor specific to the antigen

What constitutes the T-cell receptor complex?

1. T-cell receptor with an antigen-binding site
2. Associated transmembrane proteins (i.e., CD3)

Where do foreign antigens bind?

Groove of the T-cell receptor

How is the immune response activated?

CD3 signal transduction

What region of the T-cell receptor confers antigenic specificity?

Polymorphic variable region

What is the structure of the T-cell receptor?

Heterodimer of two polypeptide chains (α, β). Each chain has both a variable and a constant region, with V, D, and J regions in continuity.

What are δ/δ T cells?

Thymically mature T cells that localize to the skin or mucosal tissue

What classic cell–cell interactions occur during antigenic stimulation?	1. T_h cells secrete cytokines after antigenic stimulation (i.e., exposure to antigens presented on APC). 2. T_h cytokines are needed for antigen-stimulated B cell proliferation and antibody production. 3. T_h cytokines are needed for maturation of CTLs.

OTHER CELLS

What are natural killer (NK) cells?	Non-T, non-B lymphocytes with nonspecific immune reactivity
What is the role of NK cells?	Surveillance against foreign and tumor cells; nonspecific immune reactivity
How does the cytotoxicity of an NK cell or a macrophage differ from that of a T cell?	1. Not restricted by MHC 2. No previous antigenic exposure necessary
What are the two types of phagocytic cells?	1. Monocytes, which mature to macrophages in tissue 2. Neutrophils
Which type is the major phagocytic cell in tissue?	Neutrophils
What are the functions of a macrophage?	1. Phagocytosis 2. Production of immunomodulators
Which cytokines are produced by macrophages?	1. Tumor necrosis factor (TNF) 2. α-Interferon (α-IFN) 3. IL-1
What is the function of dendritic cells?	Presentation of antigen to T and B lymphocytes

CELLULAR COMMUNICATION

What soluble glycoproteins function as immune cell regulators?	Cytokines
How do they function?	1. Autocrine: Affect identical cell types 2. Paracrine: Stimulate other cell types

What are the characteristics of cytokines?	1. Small glycoproteins (< 80 Kd) 2. Potent (picomolar concentrations) 3. Nonconstitutively expressed
What cell types produce lymphokines, and in response to what stimulus?	Lymphocytes, in response to antigen
What cell types produce monokines, and in response to what stimulus?	Monocytes, in response to other cytokines or viruses
Which cytokines affect lineage maturation?	1. Stem cell factor (SCF) 2. IL-3 3. Granulocyte macrophage colony-stimulating factor (GM-CSF) 4. IL-1 5. Erythropoietin
Which cytokine is given to: **Neutropenic patients?**	GM-CSF or G-CSF
Anemic patients with end-stage renal disease (ESRD)?	Erythropoietin

Interleukin-1

What are the two forms of IL-1?	1. IL-1α 2. IL-β
What cells produce IL-1?	Cells of monocyte and macrophage lineage
What are the functions of IL-1?	1. Induces T and B cell proliferation and IL-2 production 2. Stimulates the thermoregulatory center in the hypothalamus 3. Induces endothelial cells to produce prostaglandins, platelet-activating factor, and plasminogen activator 4. Induces normal inflammatory response 5. Stimulates acute-phase protein production

Interleukin-2

What cells primarily produce IL-2?

Activated T cells in response to IL-1 **or** antigen

What are the functions of IL-2?

1. Promotes proliferation of activated T lymphocytes
2. Stimulates B lymphocyte proliferation and differentiation
3. Augments NK cell cytotoxicity
4. Activates macrophages: Increased TNF and colony-stimulating factor

What cytotoxic cells are stimulated with the coculture of IL-2 and:
1. **NK cells?**
2. **Lymphocytes in a tumor?**

1. Lymphocyte-activated killer (LAK) cells
2. Tumor-infiltrating lymphocytes (TILs)

Which cytotoxic cells have a greater antitumor effect, and why?

TILs > LAK cells because of the increased specificity of TILs

Interferons

What are the major types of interferons, and which cell type produces them?

1. α-IFN: Leukocytes (macrophages)
2. β-IFN: Fibroblasts and epithelial cells
3. δ-IFN: T lymphocytes

What are the two functions of interferons?

1. Direct antiproliferative effect
2. Direct antitumorigenic effect

MAJOR HISTOCOMPATIBILITY COMPLEX

What is the MHC?

Cluster of genes on the short arm of chromosome 6

What is this cluster called in humans?

Human leukocyte antigen (HLA)

What are the important characteristics of MHC (HLA) antigens?

1. Extreme polymorphism
2. Produced by closely linked subloci that form inheritable HLA haplotypes
3. Codominant expression of HLA (HLA antigens on the cell surface)

Where are the polymorphisms clustered?

Polymorphic amino acids are clustered in the peptide-binding site in the antigen-binding groove.

What are the three basic products of the MHC and the corresponding regions involved?

1. Class I antigen: HLA-A, -B, and -C
2. Class II antigen: HLA-D region, with DR, DQ, and DP
3. Class III antigens: Complement cascade

On what cell types are these MHC products expressed?

1. Class I antigens: All nucleated cells and platelets
2. Class II antigens: B lymphocytes, activated T cells, macrophages, and monocytes

What lymphocytes do not express class II antigens?

Resting T lymphocytes

What causes allograft rejection?

Foreign histocompatibility antigens on the graft and tissue

What antigens are histocompatibility antigens?

Any antigen that causes tissue incompatibility between donor and recipient

What histocompatibility antigens and antigens produce a transplant response?

1. MHC gene products
2. ABO blood group
3. Lewis blood group

What blood type is the universal recipient?

AB

What blood type is the universal donor?

O

What are the strongest transplantation antigens?

Antigens that express the MHC (HLA in humans)

What two tests detect HLA antigens?

1. Serologic testing with antigen-specific antisera
2. Mixed lymphocyte culture (MLC)

What does MLC detect?

Proliferative capacity of the host lymphocytes to antigens on the graft (MHC class II antigens, or D antigens)

Which classes of MHC genes significantly affect transplantation?	Classes I and II
What is the structure of class I and class II molecules?	Two polypeptide chains with variable and constant regions, similar to the immunoglobulin structure
What do class I genes encode for?	Transplantation antigens that are primary targets for CTLs in rejection; cell surface molecules that present certain antigens to CD8 T cells (i.e., viral antigens)
What do class II genes represent?	Immune response genes
Class I gene products are the primary target of which cells?	CTLs
Class II gene products are the primary target of which cells?	T_h cells
What are the minor transplantation antigens?	Antigens that express genes on other chromosomes that are capable of weaker, slower rejection. They are presented by class I and class II MHC determinants.
Which antigens cause rejection of grafts between HLA-identical siblings?	Minor transplantation antigens

GRAFT REJECTION

What factors cause rejection despite histocompatibility matching?	1. Preformed antibodies against the donor (positive crossmatch) 2. Minor transplantation antigens in HLA-matched siblings 3. ABO isohemagglutinins
What are the steps of the afferent arc of the immune response to a graft?	1. Direct recognition of the graft 2. Release of immunogenic histocompatibility antigens from the graft 3. APC processing and recognition of the immunogens (indirect recognition)

4. Stimulation of the responsive lymphoid cell populations

What three components mediate graft destruction?
1. Specifically sensitized CTLs
2. Alloantibodies
3. Complement activation, which mediates lytic destruction

What are the types and timing of graft rejection?
1. Hyperacute: In the OR
2. Accelerated: < 1 week
3. Acute: Within 1 week
4. Chronic: Months or years

Which type is the most common?
Acute

What test eliminates hyperacute rejection?
Pretransplant donor–recipient crossmatching

What mediates graft destruction in:
 Hyperacute rejection?
Preformed antibody: Activates a complement cascade and vasoactive mediators, leading to thrombosis

 Accelerated rejection?
T cells that are sensitized to donor-type antigens: Produces a secondary immune response

 Acute rejection?
T cell–dependent event: Activates CTLs and T_h cells

 Chronic rejection?
Combined antibody-mediated and cell-mediated components: Cause graft fibrosis and vascular damage

What is the treatment of hyperacute rejection?
Immediate retransplantation. A second allograft is rarely available.

What is the treatment of acute rejection?
Increased immunosuppression (i.e., pulse steroids, rescue OKT3)

What is the treatment of chronic rejection?
Uncertain

What three main enzymatic cascade pathways play a role in allograft rejection?	1. Complement cascade 2. Clotting cascade 3. Kinin-release pathway

Complement

What triggers the complement system?	1. Immune complexes (IgG, IgM) activate the Fc end and bind to C1. 2. Microbial surfaces trigger the alternate pathway.
What complement components function as: **Opsonins?**	C3b and C4b (immune adherence)
Kinins?	C4a and C2b
Chemoattractants?	C3a and C5a
Anaphylatoxins?	C3a and C5a
What is the role of activated C5b?	Formation of the membrane attack complex (C5b6789) to lyse cell membranes
What is the role of complement in rejection?	1. Releases kinins 2. Opsonizes damaged cells, initiating phagocytosis 3. Elicits the release of liposomal enzymes from macrophages 4. Causes polymorphonuclear leukocyte (PMN) chemotaxis, releasing vasoactive substances

Clotting

Which pathway of the clotting system is initiated with antigen–antibody interactions?	Intrinsic pathway
What is triggered by this interaction?	Antibody–antigen complexes activate Factor XII directly.
What triggers the extrinsic pathway?	Release of tissue thromboplastin after cells are damaged by complements or a lytic attack

What are the consequences of initiating the complement, clotting, and kinin pathways to the:	
Vascular system?	Spasm, increased permeability, and occlusion with fibrin
Cellular system?	Chemotaxis of macrophages or PMNs; increased release of vasoactive mediators
Target organs?	Damage to the basement membrane; cellular lysis

HYPERSENSITIVITY REACTIONS

What are the four types of hypersensitivity reactions?	Type I: Immediate hypersensitivity reactions Type II: Cytotoxic reactions Type III: Immune complex–mediated reactions Type IV: Delayed hypersensitivity reactions
What triggers the reaction of each type?	Type I: Antigens that react with IgE Type II: Reaction of IgG or IgM antibody with cell-bound antigen Type III: Deposition of an antibody–antigen complex from the circulation Type IV: Previously sensitized T cells and antigens

HISTORY OF TRANSPLANTATION

What three discoveries are critical to transplantation?	1. Vascular anastomosis described by Alexis Carrel 2. Initial work with autografts and xenografts in 1700 by John Hunter 3. Documentation of tolerance by Peter Brian Medawar
Who received a Nobel Prize in medicine for transplantation, and why?	J. E. Murray and E. D. Thomas in 1990. They performed the first renal transplant in a human in 1954.

IMMUNOSUPPRESSION

COMPLICATIONS

What is the most common complication of immunosuppression?	Infection

What is the most common cause of death in transplant recipients?	Infection
What are the other complications of immunosuppression?	1. Hypertension (HTN) 2. Cushing disease (steroid-induced diabetes, cataracts, myopathy, hyperlipemia, osteoporosis, and hypercholesterolemia) 3. Thrombophlebitis 4. Malignancy 5. Pancreatitis 6. Avascular necrosis (femoral head)

Infection

What are the most common types of fungal infection in immunosuppressed patients?	1. *Candida albicans* 2. *Aspergillus*
What is the most common protozoan infection in immunosuppressed patients?	*Pneumocystis carinii*
What drug is given prophylactically for this protozoal infection?	Trimethoprim and sulfamethoxazole (Bactrim)
What is the typical chest x-ray finding in a patient with:	
Aspergillus **infection?**	Upper-lobe cavities
Pneumocystis **infection?**	Alveolar infiltrates
What are the most common viral infections in transplant recipients?	Herpes group of DNA viruses: Cytomegalovirus (CMV) > Herpes simplex > Herpes zoster
What is the most common viral agent thought to elicit rejection?	CMV

What is the usual clinical presentation of CMV?	Fever, neutropenia, malaise, pneumonitis myocarditis, pancreatitis, and acute cecal ulceration
What is the treatment of the viral infections mentioned earlier?	CMV: Ganciclovir Herpes: Acyclovir
Which immunosuppressant increases the risk of CMV infection?	Antilymphocyte antibody
Which immunosuppressant decreases the risk of CMV infection, and why?	Cyclosporine, because of the sparing of sensitized T cells

Malignancy

Which malignancies often occur in immunosuppressed patients?	1. Immunoproliferative malignancies (i.e., B cell lymphomas) 2. Epithelial cancers 3. Malignancies with viral etiologies (i.e., cervical cancer)
What is the relative increased risk of these cancers in transplant patients?	1. Lymphoma: 350 x 2. Skin cancer: 40 x 3. Cervical cancer: 4 x
What is the viral etiology of polyclonal B cell lymphoproliferative disorder?	Epstein-Barr virus
What are three explanations for the increased risk of cancer associated with immunosuppression?	1. Decreased tumor immunosurveillance 2. Use of mutagenic immunosuppressive agents (i.e., azathioprine [AZA; Imuran]) 3. Increased susceptibility to herpes and increased exposure to viral promoters

IMMUNOSUPPRESSIVE AGENTS

What is the rationale for multimodality therapy?	Synergy allows maximum immunosuppression with minimum side effects and permits the use of lower doses of each drug.

What is the typical "three-drug regimen?"	1. AZA 2. Prednisone 3. Cyclosporine or FK-506

Antimetabolites

What are antimetabolites?	Purine, pyrimidine, and folic acid analogs that inhibit lymphocyte mitosis
What Nobel laureate pioneered work with these agents?	George Hit
What are the target cells of antimetabolites?	Proliferating and differentiating cells
What is the most commonly used purine analog?	AZA
What active compound is found in AZA?	6-Mercaptopurine
Where is the drug converted to its active form?	Liver
What is the mechanism of action of AZA?	Inhibits DNA and RNA production by inhibiting the conversion of inosine monophosphate (IMP) to essential purines (adenosine, guanine)
What are the primary side effects of AZA?	1. Severe bone marrow suppression 2. Hepatic toxicity
When is the dose of AZA decreased?	1. White blood cell count < 4000 2. Concurrent allopurinol usage
In addition to AZA, what two antimetabolites are available?	1. Purine analog: RS-61443 (mycophenolate mofetil) 2. Pyrimidine analog: Brequinar
Name, and give examples of, three other classes of antiproliferative therapies.	1. Alkylating agents: Nitrogen mustard, cyclophosphamide 2. Folic acid antagonists: Methotrexate 3. Irradiation: Therapeutic radiation

Why are these antiproliferative agents not routinely used for organ transplantation?	Too toxic and mutagenic for long-term immunosuppression for organ transplantation

Steroids

What is the general mechanism of action of steroids?	Bind intracellular receptors and inhibit the synthesis of DNA and RNA
What is the mechanism of immunosuppression?	1. Decrease in total T lymphocyte count 2. Antimacrophage properties (i.e., blocks IL-1 production)
What adverse side effects are associated with corticosteroid administration?	1. HTN 2. Peptic ulcer disease 3. Obesity 4. Hyperglycemia 5. Avascular necrosis of femoral head
What are the relative potencies of the available steroids?	Cortisol: 1 Prednisone: 4 Methylprednisolone: 5 Dexamethasone: 25

Cyclosporine (CsA)

What is the structure of CsA?	Cyclic peptide
What is the source of CsA?	Fungus (*Tolypocladium gams*)
What is the typical dosing regimen for CsA?	1 to 5 mg/kg/day IV 4 to 15 mg/kg/day PO
What is the therapeutic drug level?	> 200 g/ml, although it varies with the organ transplanted, the time after transplantation, and the transplant center
Are higher or lower levels of CsA maintained in the early postoperative period?	Higher (up to twice the maintenance levels)

What is the mechanism of immunosuppression?

Suppresses T cell activation and maturation by inhibiting messenger RNA encoding for the production of IL-2 and other cytokines

What is the intracellular receptor for CsA?

Cyclophilin

What adverse side effects are associated with CsA administration?

1. Hirsutism
2. Neurotoxicity
3. HTN
4. Hyperglycemia
5. Hepatotoxicity
6. Nephrotoxicity
7. Hyperkalemia

What is the most significant dose-limiting toxicity?

Nephrotoxicity

How is CsA metabolized?

Cytochrome P-450 system in the liver

What drugs increase CsA levels?

1. Erythromycin
2. Ketoconazole
3. Diltiazem
4. Cimetidine

What drugs decrease CsA levels?

1. Activators of the P-450 system
2. Phenobarbital
3. Phenytoin
4. Octreotide
5. Rifampin
6. Trimethoprim
7. Carbamazepine

Fk-506 (Tacrolimus)

What is the basic structure of FK-506?

Macrolide antibiotic

What is the source of FK-506?

Soil fungus (*Streptomyces tsukubaensis*)

What is the potency of FK-506 compared with that of CsA?

FK-506 is 500 times more potent than CsA.

What is the typical dosing regimen for FK-506?	0.05 mg/kg PO every 12 hours
What is the therapeutic drug level?	10 to 15 ng/ml
What is the mechanism of immunosuppressive action?	Inhibits T cell activation and maturation
What are the intracellular receptors for FK-506?	FK-binding proteins
What adverse side effects are associated with FK-506 administration?	1. Nephrotoxicity 2. Anorexia and weight loss 3. Neurotoxicity
What drugs increase FK-506 levels?	1. Verapamil 2. Ketoconazole 3. Erythromycin 4. Diltiazem 5. Fluconazole 6. Cimetidine
What drugs decrease FK-506 levels?	1. Phenytoin 2. Phenobarbital 3. Carbamazepine 4. Rifampin

Rapamycin (RAPA)

What is the structure of RAPA?	Macrolide antibiotic
What is the mechanism of immunosuppressive action?	1. Inhibits B cell and T cell activation and proliferation 2. Inhibits **activated** T cells 3. Blocks the ability of the IL-2 receptor to induce signal transduction
What intracellular receptor does RAPA bind?	FK-binding proteins
What action is inhibited by RAPA, but not by CsA and FK-506?	Activated cell proliferation induced by IL-2 and IL-4

Antilymphocyte Globulin (ALG)

What is ALG?   Polyclonal serum

How is ALG obtained?   By injecting human lymphocytes into
                                  different species and collecting antisera
                                  (e.g., rats: RATS; horses: ATGAM)

What is the mechanism of   Sera directed against mature T
immunosuppressive   lymphocytes
action?

What are the indications   1. Acute rejection
for ALG in some centers?   2. Induction therapy

What immunologic   T cell–mediated reactions (e.g., allograft
reactions are blocked by   rejection, graft-versus-host reaction,
ALG?   tuberculin sensitivity)

What adverse effects are   1. Anemia
associated with ALG   2. Thrombocytopenia
administration?

OKT3

What is OKT3?   Anti-CD3 monoclonal antibody that
                                  binds to the T cell receptor complex
                                  (CD3)

What is the mechanism of   Inhibits the signaling portion of the T
immunosuppressive   cell receptor complex, blocking the
action?   function of mature T lymphocytes and
                                  the opsonization of circulating T
                                  lymphocytes

What are the indications   1. Induction therapy
for OKT3?   2. Acute rejection

What are the clinical signs   Fever, chills, nausea, diarrhea,
of OKT3 toxicity?   bronchospasm, pulmonary edema,
                                  hypotension (peripheral vasodilatation),
                                  rash, and headache

What are the advantages   1. Specific immunosuppression (removes
of OKT3 over ALG?   only CD3⁺ T cells)
                                  2. More uniform potency of the
                                     monoclonal preparation

| What is the disadvantage of OKT3? | Induces rapid sensitization to xenogeneic antibodies, leading to neutralization of the monoclonal antibody preparation. Thus, its effectiveness decreases with each use. |

SOLID ORGAN TRANSPLANTATION

What is orthotopic transplantation?	Donor organ is placed in the correct anatomic position in the recipient
Provide some examples.	Liver, heart, lung, and heart–lung
What is heterotopic transplantation?	Donor organ is placed in a site distant from the correct anatomic position in the recipient
Provide some examples.	Kidney, pancreas and, rarely, heart

DONOR–RECIPIENT MATCHING

What general criteria are used for donor–recipient matching?	1. ABO typing 2. HLA typing 3. Lymphocytotoxic crossmatching 4. Donor–recipient size matching Depending on the type of organ transplant, one to four criteria are used.
What is the purpose of lymphocytotoxic crossmatching?	To directly detect recipient sensitization to donor HLA
How is lymphocytotoxic crossmatching performed?	In vitro mixing of recipient serum with donor lymphocytes (plus rabbit complement)
What is a "positive crossmatch"?	Presence of preformed circulating antibodies that bind to donor lymphocytes and lyse them in the presence of complement
What risk factors are associated with a positive crossmatch?	1. Previous transfusion that produced antidonor HLA antibodies 2. Pregnancy 3. Previous transplant 4. Cross-reactive antibodies

CONTRAINDICATIONS TO TRANSPLANTATION

What are the absolute contraindications to transplantation?

1. Human immunodeficiency virus (HIV) positivity
2. Irreversible infection
3. Malignancy
4. Irreversible brain damage
5. Irreversible multiple organ failure
6. Irreversible significant cardiopulmonary disease
7. Recurrent noncompliance with medical therapy

RENAL TRANSPLANTATION

RECIPIENT

What is the indication for kidney transplant?

Irreversible renal failure (ESRD)

What are the most common etiologies of ESRD?

1. Diabetes
2. Chronic glomerulonephritis

What are the other causes of ESRD?

1. Chronic pyelonephritis
2. Hypertensive nephrosclerosis
3. Goodpasture disease
4. Hereditary nephropathies (Alport syndrome, polycystic kidney disease)
5. Renal vascular disease
6. Tumors necessitating nephrectomy (Wilms tumor, renal cell carcinoma)
7. Congenital disorders
8. Cortical necrosis
9. Acute tubular necrosis (ATN)

What is renal failure?

Glomerular filtration rate < 10% of normal value

When is therapy for renal failure instituted?

1. Before uremic complications (e.g., HTN, neuropathy, pericarditis) occur
2. Creatinine > 15 mg/dl
3. Creatinine clearance < 3 ml/min

What clinical signs indicate the need for early dialysis or transplantation?

1. Uncontrolled HTN
2. Peripheral neuropathy

What are the relative contraindications to renal transplantation?

1. Liver disease
2. Recurring renal diseases
3. Psychosocial issues

Provide examples of recurring renal diseases.

1. Focal glomerulosclerosis
2. Hemolytic uremic syndrome
3. Membrane proliferative glomerulonephritis

What two standard operative procedures are used to prepare a patient for dialysis?

1. Arteriovenous fistula
2. Peritoneal dialysis catheter

What is the leading cause of sepsis in patients who are undergoing peritoneal dialysis?

Peritonitis secondary to *Staphylococcus epidermidis* or *Staphylococcus aureus* infection

What is the annual mortality rate for:
    Patients undergoing dialysis?

6% to 20%

    Diabetic patients undergoing dialysis?

11% to 25%

    Patients undergoing renal transplantation?

< 2%

What is the survival rate for recipients of:
    Living related kidney graft?

85% to 90% at 3 years

    Cadaver kidney graft?

75% to 80% at 3 years

    Diabetic recipients (living related or cadaver graft)?

70% at 5 years

PREOPERATIVE EVALUATION

What should be done within 24 hours before transplantation?

Dialysis (to optimize the recipient's body chemistry)

When is nephrectomy indicated before transplantation?

1. Chronic renal infection
2. Uncontrollable HTN
3. Symptomatic cystic disease
4. Renal cancer

What preoperative test is used to evaluate the:

    Urinary tract, and why?

Voiding cystogram to evaluate outflow and detect ureterovesical reflux

    GI tract, and why?

GI endoscopy to identify peptic ulcer disease and malignancies, both of which may be exacerbated by immunosuppression

What tests are used to assess immunologic compatibility for renal transplantation?

1. Negative T cell crossmatch
2. ABO compatibility
3. HLA typing

What types of donor grafts are preferred, in decreasing order?

1. Living related donor: HLA-identical graft (>95%)
2. Living related donor: HLA-nonidentical graft
3. Cadaver donor: Six-antigen matched graft
4. Cadaver donor: Randomly matched graft

Why are siblings preferred matches for living related kidney donors?

Mendelian inheritance of histocompatibility antigens ensures the chance for a haploidentical match

What is the probability of any two siblings:

    Having HLA identity?

25%

    Sharing one HLA chromosome?

50%

    Having HLA disparity?

25%

What factors enhance allograft survival?

1. HLA matching
2. Donor-specific blood transfusions

What is the effect of multiple blood transfusions?

Pretransplant transfusions to a recipient treated with AZA and prednisone improves survival.

What is the immunologic mechanism of this effect?

Removes immunologic hyperresponders from the recipient and provides complex idiotypic regulation

What serologic results are absolute requirements for cadaver transplant?

1. ABO compatibility
2. Current negative T cell crossmatch

What characteristics are desirable in a donor?

1. Youth (> 2 years)
2. Normotensive
3. No infection or malignancy
4. Minimal warm ischemia time (≤ 1 hour)
5. Left donor kidney

Why are left kidneys more desirable than right kidneys?

Anatomically longer renal vein in the left kidney

TECHNICAL ASPECTS

What position is used for implantation?

Heterotopic, retroperitoneal position, near the iliac vessels

Why is the heterotopic position preferred over the orthotopic position in renal transplantation?

1. Easier access to the recipient vessels (iliac versus aorta and inferior vena cava [IVC])
2. Closer to the bladder to facilitate ureterocystostomy
3. Easy access for biopsy
4. Reduced risk of hemorrhage because retroperitoneal dissection in the region of the native kidney is avoided

What type of incision is used?

Oblique incision, just above the inguinal ligament

What anastomoses are used for kidney transplantation?

1. Renal artery to the common or internal iliac artery (hypogastric artery)
2. Renal vein to the common or external iliac vein
3. Urinary continuity

What are the surgical options for urinary continuity, and which is the most common?

1. Ureteroneocystostomy (most common)
2. Pyeloureterostomy
3. Ureteroureterostomy

How and why is ureteroneocystostomy performed?

With a submucosal tunnel to reduce the incidence of reflux

What are the indications for recipient nephrectomy?

1. Uncontrollable HTN
2. Ongoing renal sepsis

What paralytic agent is avoided during renal transplantation in patients undergoing dialysis, and why?

Succinylcholine. Hemodialysis breaks down serum cholinesterases (i.e., prolonged action of the agent).

POSTOPERATIVE COURSE

How long after surgery before kidney function returns to normal?

1. Living related graft: 3 to 5 days
2. Cadaver graft: 7 to 15 days

What is the standard immunosuppression regimen for renal transplantation?

1. FK-506 or CsA with prednisone
2. ALG or AZA until normal renal function returns

What is the standard therapy for rejection?

Steroids (i.e., prednisone, methylprednisone)

What is the therapy for steroid-resistant rejection?

OKT3

What are the causes of post-transplant HTN?

1. Rejection
2. Direct effects of CsA on the vasculature
3. Renal artery stenosis (in the transplant)
4. Recurrent disease in the allograft

What factors cause a large postoperative diuresis?

1. Osmotic stimuli (urea, glucose)
2. Tubular dysfunction secondary to allograft ischemia

Which is preferable: diuresis or oliguria?

Diuresis, because rejection or obstruction can be detected

What are the causes of post-transplant oliguria?

1. ATN (because of allograft ischemia)
2. Hyperacute rejection
3. Nephrotoxicity
4. Technical complications: Compression of the kidney or obstruction of flow

What is the most common cause of early post-transplant oliguria?

ATN

What is the best method to evaluate early post-transplant oliguria?

Doppler ultrasound

What are the clinical signs of deteriorating renal function?

1. Decreased urinary output
2. Elevation in diastolic blood pressure
3. Slow weight gain
4. Peripheral edema
5. Increase in creatinine value

What are the potential causes of early allograft dysfunction?

1. Rejection
2. Renal artery stenosis
3. Technical (e.g., vascular, urinary)
4. CsA toxicity
5. Infection

What studies are used to evaluate allograft dysfunction, and what information is obtained from each?

1. Doppler ultrasound: Flow through the vessels; the presence of hydronephrosis or perinephric fluid collections
2. Radionuclide scan: Renal function; flow through the vessels
3. Renal biopsy: Rejection versus CsA toxicity

What is the treatment of early renal dysfunction?

Empiric reduction of nephrotoxic therapies, ± increased immunosuppression

What is the treatment of renal artery stenosis?

Percutaneous angioplasty

What is the treatment of hydronephrosis?

1. Endourologic technique for antegrade shunt placement or balloon dilation
2. Surgical ureteroneocystostomy repair of ureteral stenosis

What is the usual cause of urinary extravasation?	Distal ureteral necrosis secondary to a short ureter, tension, or a hematoma
What are the options for surgical repair?	1. Reimplantation of the ureter 2. Pyeloureterostomy to the host ureter Both options require a temporary nephrostomy.
What test distinguishes between ATN and rejection?	Renal biopsy
What is the most significant pathologic characteristic of ATN?	Hydropic changes
What are the clinical signs of rejection?	1. Fever 2. Oliguria 3. Enlarged, tender graft 4. HTN 5. Leukocytosis
What is the most important laboratory parameter corresponding to rejection?	Creatinine clearance
What does new onset of proteinuria often suggest?	Venous thrombosis
What is the most common cause of urinary obstruction from extrinsic compression of the ureter?	Lymphocele caused by disruption of the lymphatics during implantation of the allograft

LIVER TRANSPLANTATION

RECIPIENT

What are the signs of chronic liver failure on physical examination?	Jaundice, palmar erythema, vascular spiders, testicular atrophy, gynecomastia, Dupuytren contracture, parotid enlargement, and ascites

What is the Child classification of liver failure?

Child Class	A	B	C
Bilirubin (mg/dl)	< 2	2–3	> 3
Ascites	Absent	Slight	Moderate
Albumin (g/dl)	> 3.5	2.8–3.5	< 2.8
Prothrombin time prolongation (seconds)	1–4	4–6	> 6
Hepatic encephalopathy	None	Mild (confusion, drowsiness)	Severe (significant confusion to coma)

What are the general classes of indications for liver transplantation?

1. Chronic liver disease (hepatocellular, cholestatic)
2. Fulminant or subfulminant hepatic failure
3. Budd-Chiari syndrome
4. Inborn errors in metabolism (i.e., α_1-antitrypsin deficiency)
5. Certain unresectable hepatic malignancies, but not cholangiocarcinoma or gallbladder carcinoma

What are the most common causes of liver failure in adults, in descending order?

1. Chronic active hepatitis (27%)
2. Cholestatic liver disease, including primary biliary cirrhosis and sclerosing cholangitis (21%)
3. Biliary atresia (16%)
4. Alcoholic cirrhosis (8.5%)

What are the relative contraindications to orthotopic liver transplant (OLTx)?

1. Recurrent alcoholism
2. HB_sAG or HB_eAG antigenemia
3. Active ulcerative colitis
4. Portal vein thrombosis

What is a surgical variation in OLTx that may be used in cases of portal vein thrombosis?

Vein grafts from a patent segment of mesenteric vein (superior mesenteric vein, inferior mesenteric vein, and large portal collateral) to the donor portal vein

What is the preoperative management of ascites?

1. Low-sodium diet (2 g/day) ± fluid restriction (< 1 L/day) if sodium level is < 130 mEq/L

2. Diuretic therapy (spironolactone ± furosemide)
3. Large-volume paracentesis in cases of tense ascites, respiratory insufficiency, and renal insufficiency
4. ± Prophylaxis for spontaneous bacterial peritonitis (i.e., norfloxacin)

What is the preoperative management of hepatic encephalopathy?

1. Treatment of the precipitating event (e.g., sepsis, GI bleed, renal failure, electrolyte disturbance)
2. Protein-restricted diet (< 1 g/kg/day)
3. Lactulose (orally or rectally)

PREOPERATIVE EVALUATION

What are the components of preoperative evaluation?

1. Assessment of hepatocellular function
2. Assessment of extrahepatic organ dysfunction
3. Investigation for tumor
4. Vascular (portal vein) patency
5. **Medical compliance**

What aspects of hepatocellular function are evaluated, and what tests are used?

1. Hepatitis screening
2. Occult tumors: α-Fetoprotein, computed tomography (CT), hepatic ultrasound
3. Biliary calculi: Radionucleotide excretion scan
4. Varices: Endoscopy (sclerotherapy may be performed)
5. Portal vein patency: CT or duplex ultrasound, magnetic resonance imaging (MRI), angiogram
6. Functional capacity: Coagulation profile

What laboratory value is a poor prognostic sign for OLTx?

Uncorrectable prothrombin time

Why are pulmonary function tests important?

To determine respiratory reserve for postoperative respirator dependence

What test is used to assess immunologic compatibility?

ABO compatibility

Liver transplantation can cross which immunologic barriers?

1. ABO. In an emergency, bloodlines may be crossed!
2. HLA

In addition to immunocompatibility testing, what factor is involved in donor–recipient matching?

Weight. Donor and recipient weights should match by ± 20%.

TECHNICAL ASPECTS

What is the standard recipient incision?

Transverse abdominal incision

This incision compromises which organ system postoperatively?

Respiratory

What factor significantly decreases the morbidity and mortality rates of the anhepatic phase of the OLTx procedure (i.e., after hepatectomy and before the completion of implantation)?

Heparin-free venoveno bypass. The cannula drains the IVC, and the centrifugal pump returns blood to the axillary vein.

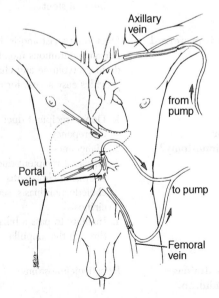

**What standard
anastomoses are used for
OLTx?**

1. Suprahepatic IVC and infrahepatic IVC anastomoses
2. Portal vein anastomosis
3. Hepatic (splenic) artery anastomosis
4. Anastomosis for biliary drainage

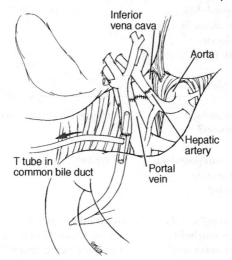

**What are the surgical
options for biliary
drainage in adults?**

1. Donor–recipient bile duct anastomosis over a T-tube stent
2. Choledochojejunostomy over a small internal stent

**Which option is preferred,
and why?**

Duct–duct anastomosis, because it permits continuous monitoring of bile drainage (volume and character) and provides easy access for cholangiogram

**What are the
indications for
choledochojejunostomy?**

1. Donor–recipient duct size discrepancy
2. Malignancy
3. Diseased recipient duct (i.e., primary sclerosing cholangitis, choledocholithiasis, secondary biliary cirrhosis)
4. Inability to pass a biliary probe through the ampulla

**How is biliary drainage
achieved in children?**

Hepaticojejunostomy

Why is splenectomy avoided?	Disrupts the portosystemic collateral pathway
What are the important intraoperative precautions for OLTx?	1. Avoidance of splenectomy 2. Dissection is minimized retroperitoneally and around the distal common duct 3. As much length as possible is preserved on the superior vena cava, portal vein, hepatic artery, and IVC to facilitate anastomoses
What are the standard locations of drains placed during OLTx?	1. Left subhepatic space 2. Right subdiaphragmatic region 3. Right subhepatic region, near the biliary anastomosis
What is the most common arterial anomaly?	Double (or multiple) hepatic artery
What two other commonly encountered variations in hepatic artery anatomy are important during procurement and implantation of the allograft?	1. Left hepatic artery originating from the left gastric artery (palpable in the gastrohepatic omentum): 15% of individuals 2. Right hepatic artery originating from the superior mesenteric artery (palpable posterior and to the right of the portal vein in the porta hepatis): 12% of individuals
What percentage of hepatic blood flow is supplied by the portal vein?	75%
What anatomic region depends on the hepatic artery for its blood supply?	Biliary tract

POSTOPERATIVE COURSE

What is the standard immunosuppression regimen?	CsA or FK-506 and prednisone
What regimen is used in patients with poor renal function?	AZA, ALG, steroid, and OKT3

What findings suggest good liver function in the immediate postoperative period?

1. Improving coagulation profile and glucose tolerance
2. Hemodynamic stability
3. Adequate bile output; golden brown color
4. Good renal function
5. Awakening from anesthesia

What laboratory values are monitored postoperatively?

Coagulation parameters and serum bilirubin, transaminase, alkaline phosphatase, ammonia, pH, and HCO_3- values

Ischemic preservation leads to unavoidable liver allograft injury as manifested by increased transaminase levels. When do these levels normally peak?

48 to 72 hours postoperatively

What peak transaminase level indicates severe injury?

> 2000 U/L

What is included in the differential diagnosis of abnormal coagulation parameters in a patient with OLTx?

1. Rejection
2. Ischemia
3. Infection
4. Obstruction
5. Cholangitis

What tests are used to evaluate the biliary system?

1. Radionucleotide excretory cholangiogram
2. T-tube cholangiogram
3. Transhepatic cholangiogram
4. Endoscopic retrograde cholangiopancreatography (ERCP)

What are the most serious complications?

1. Primary hepatic nonfunction
2. Infection

What are the early signs of nonfunction?

1. Failure of Factor V level to return to normal
2. Abnormal coagulation profile
3. Decreased bile output

What percentage of recipients have an episode of rejection in the early postoperative period?

40% to 50%

What complications necessitate retransplantation?

1. Primary hepatic nonfunction
2. Recurrent disease
3. Untreatable or chronic rejection

What are the clinical signs of hepatic artery, portal vein, or vena cava thrombosis?

1. Rapid deterioration of hepatic function ± fulminant hepatic failure and hemodynamic instability
2. No liver extraction during a liver scan
3. Elevated liver function test results, elevated bilirubin level, coagulopathy, hypoglycemia, and hyperkalemia
4. Decreased bile output

Thrombosis is most common in what vessel?

Hepatic artery. Portal vein thrombosis is rare.

What biliary complications are associated with acute versus chronic hepatic artery thrombosis?

Acute: Bile duct leak
Chronic: Bile duct strictures

What are the clinical signs of caval stenosis?

1. Lower extremity edema
2. Ascites
3. Renal insufficiency

What are the treatment options for vascular thrombotic occlusion?

1. Angioplasty
2. Stent placement
3. Retransplantation

Hepatic abscesses are a common presentation of what complication?

Hepatic artery thrombosis

What other complications occur after OLTx?

1. Respiratory insufficiency as a result of effusions, ascites, atelectasis, and diaphragmatic dysfunction
2. Renal dysfunction
3. Infection (CMV, gram-negative sepsis, fungus)
4. Neurologic dysfunction

What procedure differentiates among rejection, ischemia, viral infection, and cholangitis?	Liver biopsy
What histologic findings suggest rejection?	Mixed inflammatory cell infiltrate of the portal triads, bile duct injury, and endothelialitis
What histolgic finding suggests cholangitis?	PMN infiltration of the portal triads
What are the treatment options for:	
Rejection?	IV steroids, OKT3, ALG, and/or substitution of FK-506 for CsA
CMV hepatitis?	Ganciclovir, IV immunoglobulin
Cholangitis?	IV antibiotics, treatment of the biliary stricture or occlusion, and biliary drainage
What complications are related to duct–duct reconstruction over a T-tube?	1. Ampullary dysfunction 2. Bile duct stricture
Hepatic arterial thrombosis causes ischemia to what region?	Biliary tree
What are the consequences of biliary tree ischemia?	1. Bile duct necrosis 2. Cholestasis 3. Hepatic abscess
What is the most common cause of renal failure after OLTx?	Preoperative hepatorenal syndrome. Other causes include hypotension, sepsis, and CsA toxicity.
What are the survival rates at 1 year and 5 years?	1 year: 80% 5 year: 65%
What percentage of patients undergo retransplantation?	20%

PEDIATRIC LIVER FAILURE

What is the most common indication for OLTx in children?	Extrahepatic biliary atresia (> inborn errors in metabolism)
How does extrahepatic biliary atresia present clinically?	Persistence of conjugated hyperbilirubinemia > 2 weeks after birth
What are the surgical options for congenital biliary atresia?	1. Kasai procedure (portoenterostomy) 2. Size-reduction liver transplant 3. Living related liver transplant Size-reduction liver transplant and living related liver transplant employing segments from adult donors are necessary because of the difficulty in finding child donors.

PANCREAS TRANSPLANTATION

What is the usual indication for pancreas transplantation?	Diabetes, usually type I, with early secondary (end-stage) complications: Neuropathy, retinopathy, and nephropathy
What is the indication for combined kidney–pancreas transplantation?	ESRD secondary to diabetic nephropathy
Does pancreatic transplantation decrease diabetic end-organ disease?	Yes. It improves the neuropathy and decreases retinopathy and nephropathy.
Despite experimental success with pancreatic islet grafts, what feature of these cells prevents their clinical application?	Increased antigenicity of islet cells
What other factor contributes to the failure of islet cell transplantation?	Difficulty in obtaining sufficient quantities of islet cells (< 2% of the mass of the pancreas is composed of islet cells)

TECHNICAL ASPECTS

What position is used for implantation?

Heterotopic, retroperitoneal position, near the iliac vessels. An oblique cutaneous incision is made above the inguinal ligament (same as for the kidney).

What primary technical problems are associated with pancreatic transplantation?

1. Drainage of the pancreatic duct
2. Portal vein thrombosis

What are the surgical options for exocrine drainage?

1. Bladder drainage
2. Ductal injection with polymer
3. Enteric drainage

What is the favored surgical approach for exocrine drainage, and why?

Bladder drainage, because it permits continuous gross monitoring of pancreatic function through measurement of the level of amylase in the urine

What standard anastomoses are used for pancreas transplant?

1. Arteries: Splenic artery and superior mesenteric artery to iliac artery (often through the donor iliac artery "Y")
2. Veins: Portal vein to iliac vein
3. Duct drainage: Duodenocystostomy (or duodenoileostomy)

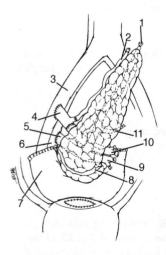

1. Splenic vein
2. Splenic artery
3. Common iliac artery
4. Donor iliac artery "Y" (with external iliac artery anastomosed to SMA and internal iliac artery to splenic artery)
5. Portal vein
6. Common iliac vein
7. Duodenum (with duodenocystostomy)
8. Gastroduodenal artery
9. SMV
10. SMA
11. IMV

POSTOPERATIVE COURSE

What methods are used to detect rejection?

1. Decrease in the urinary amylase level (if bladder drainage is employed)
2. Increase in the serum creatinine in a combined kidney–pancreas transplant
3. Percutaneous needle biopsy
4. Increase in the serum glucose level (late)

Why are the following parameters not useful indicators of rejection: Glucose levels?

Changes occur when rejection is too advanced for intervention.

Serum amylase levels?

Levels are usually unchanged.

Decrease in the urine amylase level precedes hyperglycemia by how long?

24 hours!

What other common complication may present with increasing serum glucose levels and decreasing urinary amylase levels?

Graft thrombosis (either arterial and venous) is responsible for as many as 20% of allograft losses.

What is the suspected etiology of this complication?

Low outflow phenomenon. Large vessels with the distal ends ligated (celiac and splenic artery) are left to drain small pancreatic vessels. Many centers use anticoagulation in the early postoperative period to reduce the risk of thrombosis.

What is the most common complication associated with bladder-drained pancreatic grafts?

Metabolic acidosis

What is the etiology of this complication?

Loss of bicarbonate in the urine. A benefit of enteric drainage is the conservation of bicarbonate.

What complications are associated with enteric drainage?	1. Bowel obstruction 2. Leak at the pancreaticojejunostomy
What is the 3-year success rate for: Pancreas transplants?	> 60%
Combined kidney–pancreas transplants?	> 89%

GASTROINTESTINAL TRACT TRANSPLANTATION

What are cluster transplants?	Transplants of multiple abdominal viscera
Provide examples of cluster transplants.	1. Liver–intestine en bloc 2. Liver, duodenum, and pancreas
What are the indications for small bowel transplantation?	Short gut because of necrotizing enterocolitis or malrotation with midgut volvulus (i.e., pediatric patients requiring chronic hyperalimentation)
What are the complications of chronic hyperalimentation?	1. Cirrhosis 2. Liver failure 3. Vascular access complications
What factor complicates rejection in small bowel transplantation?	In addition to classic allograft rejection, recipients may also experience graft-versus-host disease (GVHD) from donor lymphocytes.
How is the bowel pretreated to reduce the risk of GVHD?	Radiation
What is the complication of this therapy?	Radiation enteritis

REVIEW OF SELECTED TOPICS

What are the pretransplant requirements for each solid organ graft?	Kidney: ABO compatibility, negative crossmatch, HLA match preferred Liver: ABO compatibility Pancreas: ABO compatibility, negative crossmatch, HLA match preferred

What are the 1-year survival rates for kidney, liver, and pancreas transplants?	Organ	Survival Rate
	Kidney	
	HLA-identical graft	95%
	One-haplotype graft	90%
	Cadaver graft	80%
	Liver	80%
	Pancreas	65%

ORGAN PRESERVATION

What is the maximum acceptable ischemia time for:

Kidney?

48 hours with cold preservation; longer with continuous perfusion systems

Pancreas or liver?

18 to 24 hours

What is the main obstacle to optimal organ preservation?

Hypoxia and the reperfusion injury that occurs with restoration of blood flow

What are the basic principles of organ preservation?

1. Maintain optimal organ function in vivo beyond brain death. Preservation actually begins **before** organs are harvested!
2. Minimize warm ischemia time.
3. Perform surgical dissection rapidly to avoid vasospasm.
4. Use an "ideal" preservation solution (± perfusion systems). Despite two decades of intensive research, much debate remains regarding the components of the ideal solution.

What are the basic components of the ideal preservation solution?

1. Hypothermia (4°C)
2. Metabolites
3. Cellular impermeants: Lactobionate, gluconic acid, and saccharides

Why are these considerations important?

1. Hypothermia decreases metabolic activity and catabolism.
2. Metabolites are used as nutrients to regenerate compounds that are critical for survival (ATP, glutathione).
3. Impermeants minimize cellular swelling.

What is the most commonly used preservation solution?	University of Wisconsin (UW) solution
What are the constituents of UW solution?	Potassium phosphate, adenosine, insulin, lactobionate, raffinose, starch, buffers, and electrolytes

BRAIN DEATH

What are the clinical signs of brain death?	1. Fixed, dilated pupils 2. No brain stem function 3. Apnea lasting 3 minutes without ventilator support, with increased PCO_2 values 4. No reversible causes of cerebral dysfunction
What are the reversible causes of cerebral dysfunction?	1. Hypothermia 2. Drug overdose 3. Barbiturate therapy

53

Gynecologic Oncology

Gauri Bedi, MD

GYNECOLOGIC ANATOMY

PELVIS

What are the greater and lesser sciatic foramina?

The sacrotuberous and sacrospinous ligaments convert the greater and lesser sciatic notches (situated above and below the ischial spine, respectively) into the greater and lesser sciatic foramina.

What is the obturator canal?

A fibrous obturator membrane covers the entire obturator foramen, except for a gap above it. This membrane converts the obturator notch into a canal, through which the obturator nerves and vessels pass.

What are the origin and insertion of the obturator internus muscle?

The muscle arises from the obturator membrane, the bony margins of the obturator foramen, and the flat surface of the ischium. It is fan-shaped, and the fibers converge toward the lesser sciatic notch, through which the tendon passes, makes a right-angled turn, and inserts into the greater trochanter of the femur.

Which muscle passes through the greater sciatic notch?

The piriformis muscle arises from the middle three pieces of the sacrum and inserts into the greater trochanter.

What is the pelvic floor?

A sheet of muscle (the levator ani and coccygeus) and its covering fascia form the pelvic floor. The muscle fibers from the two sides slope downward and backward to the midline, forming a gutter that slopes downward and forward.

| What is the fascia of Waldeyer? | It is the part of the pelvic fascia that extends from the hollow of the sacrum to the ampulla of the rectum. Spinal nerves lie external to it; vessels lie internal. |

LEVATOR ANI

| What is the white line or arcus tendineus? | This line is a thickening across the obturator fascia, from the ischial spine to the body of the pubis. It is also the origin of the fibres of the levator ani muscle. |

List the muscular parts of the levator ani and the general location of each:

1. Ileococcygeus	Posterior fibers, inserted into the side of coccyx and anococcygeal raphe
2. Pubococcygeus	Intermediate fibers, inserted into the tip of coccyx and anococcygeal raphe
3. Puborectalis	Anterior fibers, form a U-shaped sling around the anorectal junction
4. Pubovaginalis or sphincter vaginae	Form a U-shaped sling behind vagina, forming part of the perineal body

| What is the nerve supply? | Perineal branch of S4, inferior rectal nerve, and perineal branch of pudendal nerve |

| Name the functions of the levator ani? | 1. Muscular sling that supports the pelvic viscera
2. Resistance to increase in intrapelvic pressure during straining by abdominal muscles, thereby maintaining continence
3. Important anorectal junction sphincter
4. Sphincter of the vagina |

UTERUS

| What is its embryologic origin? | Paramesonephric (Müllerian) ducts |

What is its normal shape and position?

Anteflexion (concave forward) and anteversion (forward at a right angle to the vagina)

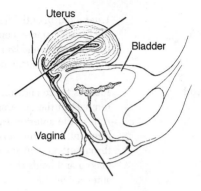

Which artery has the uterine artery as a branch?

Internal iliac artery

What is the relationship of the uterine artery to the ureter?

The uterine artery lies in the base of the broad ligament, **above** the ureter.

What are the labeled structures?

1. Round ligament of uterus
2. Internal iliac artery
3. Ovarian artery
4. Uterine artery
5. Ureter
6. Vaginal artery
7. Internal pudenal artery
8. Perineal branch of internal pudenal artery

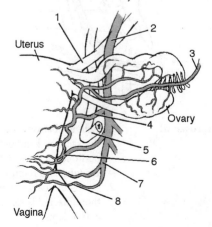

What is the broad ligament?	A double fold of peritoneum, lateral to the uterus, extending to the sidewall of the pelvis
What is the infundibulopelvic ligament?	Lateral fourth of the free superior edge of the broad ligament, containing the ovarian vessels and lymphatics; also called the suspensory ligament of the ovary
What is the round ligament?	Fibrous tissue and smooth muscle remnant of the gubernaculum, which runs in the anterior leaf of the broad ligament, from the cornua of the uterus through the inguinal canal to the labium majora and holds the uterus in anteversion
What are the labeled structures?	1. Oviduct 2. Mesosalpinx 3. Mesovarium 4. Round ligament 5. Broad ligament 6. Uterine artery 7. Ureter

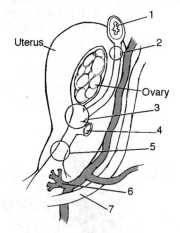

What is the uterosacral ligament?	1. Extends backward from the cervix to the sacrum, lying below the pelvic peritoneum, next to the pouch of Douglas and rectum 2. Keeps the cervix braced back, and therefore holds the uterus in anteversion

What are the lateral ligaments of Mackenrodt?	Condensed connective tissue around uterine vessels in the base of the broad ligament that extend laterally from the cervix to the side wall of the pelvis, helping to stabilize the cervix

OVARY

What is the embryologic origin of the ovary?	The paramesonephric ridge of the intermediate cell mass
Is the ovary covered by serosa?	The ovary is not invested with a peritoneal covering, although the surface is covered by low columnar epithelium.
Why is ovarian pain often referred down the inner side of the thigh?	The ovary lies on the sidewall of the pelvis, on the obturator nerve. The parietal peritoneum here is supplied by the obturator nerve, and its cutaneous distribution is the inner side of the thigh down to the knee.
What is the relationship of the ovarian artery to the ureter?	Arising from the aorta, just below the renal artery, the ovarian artery crosses the ureter on the psoas muscle above the pelvic brim.

PERINEUM

What are the boundaries of the perineum?	The perineum is the part of the pelvic outlet below the pelvic diaphragm. This diamond-shaped region is bounded by the symphysis pubis anteriorly, the tip of the coccyx posteriorly, and the ischial tuberosities laterally.
What is the urogenital triangle?	This triangle is the anterior part of the perineum, bounded posteriorly by a line through the ischial tuberosities.
What is the urogenital diaphragm?	This deep perineal space is bounded superiorly by a layer of fascia below the levator ani, and inferiorly by another layer of fascia, called the perineal membrane.

What are the contents of the deep perineal pouch?

This pouch contains parts of the urethra and vagina, the sphincter urethrae muscle, the deep transverse perineal muscles, internal pudendal vessels and their branches, and the dorsal nerves of the clitoris.

What is the perineal body?

This structure is a mass of fibrous tissue along with interdigitating fibers of the pubovaginalis, and additional fibers from the transverse perinei muscles and the superficial part of the external anal sphincter. It extends from the pelvic floor to the skin of the perineum.

What is the function of the perineal body?

The perineal body is integral to the stability of the pelvic organs and helps support the levator ani.

What is Alcock's canal?

This fibrous canal lies between the fascia of the obturator internus above and the falciform part of the sacrotuberous ligament below. It extends from the lesser sciatic foramen to the posterior edge of the perineal membrane anteriorly and lies along the lateral wall of the ischiorectal fossa. Also called the pudendal canal.

What are the contents of the pudendal canal?

The pudendal nerve and internal pudendal vessels

Internal pudendal artery

Where does it arise?

From the anterior branch of the internal iliac artery.

What does it supply?

This artery of the perineum supplies the anal triangle and the external genitalia.

What is the course of the pudendal artery?

This artery pierces the parietal pelvic fascia, passing out of the pelvis through the greater sciatic foramen, then passes anteriorly into the lesser sciatic foramen. Here it supplies the inferior rectal artery (which supplies not the rectum, but the contents of the anal triangle). The artery then enters the pudendal canal and runs forward to supply the external genitalia.

Pudendal nerve

From which nerve roots does it originate?

S2, 3, 4

What does the pudendal nerve supply?

The pelvic floor and perineum

What are its three branches, and what does each supply?

1. Inferior rectal nerve: This branch runs along with the inferior rectal vessels, supplying the levator ani and the external anal sphincter.
2. Perineal nerve: This terminal branch, supplies the urogenital triangle and the anterior part of the levator ani.
3. Dorsal nerve of the clitoris: This terminal branch supplies the urogenital triangle.

Label:

1. Common iliac artery
2. Iliolumbar artery
3. Internal iliac artery
4. Lateral sacral artery
5. Superior gluteal artery
6. Inferior gluteal artery
7. Pudendal nerve
8. Middle rectal artery
9. Perineal artery
10. Internal pudendal artery
11. Superior vesical artery
12. Uterine artery
13. Obturator artery and nerve
14. Inferior epigastric artery
15. External iliac artery

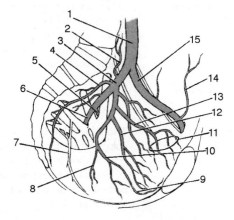

CARCINOMA OF THE CERVIX

What is the peak age of incidence?

Between 48 and 55 years for invasive cervical carcinoma
Between 25 and 40 years for carcinoma-in-situ

What are the risk factors?

1. Low socioeconomic status
2. First intercourse at an early age
3. Promiscuity, prostitution
4. Early parity
5. Increasing parity
6. HPV infection

Is an infectious etiology present?

Yes, human papillomavirus (HPV) types 16 and 18 are implicated. Herpesvirus type 2 (HSV-2) and other sexually transmitted disease such as chlamydia are not.

What are the pathologic types?

1. Squamous cell carcinomas (arising from the squamocolumnar junction of the cervix)—80%
2. Adenocarcinomas—15%

What are the precursor lesions?

Cervical intraepithelial neoplasia (CIN), which are divided into high- and low-grade squamous intraepithelial lesions

Over what period of time do these lesions progress to invasive carcinoma?

From 10 to 20 years, although it can progress more quickly

Are metastases more commonly hematogenous or lymphatic?

Lymphatic. The rich lymphatic network of the cervix interconnects with that of the uterus and upper vagina, then drains into large collecting trunks that drain into lymph nodes along the major arteries and veins.

Which are the sentinel nodes?

The obturator nodes

What is the basis for the staging system?

The Fédération Internationale de Gynécologie et d'Obstétrique (FIGO) classification is based on clinical evaluation of extent of spread. Lymph node involvement is **not** part of this evaluation.

What is stage 0?

Carcinoma in situ

What is stage I?

Disease is confined to the cervix. Stage IA is microinvasive carcinoma.
Stage IB is all other tumors confined to the cervix.

What are the main criteria distinguishing stages II, III, and IV?

Stage II: Parametrial spread, and confined to upper two-thirds of vagina
Stage III: Spread to lowest third of vagina or pelvic sidewall, ureteral obstruction or nonfunctioning kidney
Stage IV: Invasion of mucosa of bladder or rectum or distant metastases

What are the prognostic factors?

1. Stage
2. Lymphatic spread in the early stages, which is related to tumor size, depth of invasion, lymphovascular invasion, and histologic grade
3. Histology
Other possible variables under investigation are increased S-phase, c-myc overexpression, overexpression of HER2/neu.

Which histology has the worst prognosis?

Adenocarcinoma

What is the incidence of positive lymph nodes with each stage?

Stage I—15%
Stage II—35%
Stage III—50%

What are the most commonly involved distant sites?

1. Lung
2. Para-aortic, mediastinal and supraclavicular lymph nodes
3. Liver
4. Bone

What is the 5-year survival rate by stage?

Stage I—90%
Stage II—70%
Stage III—30%
Stage IV— < 10%

PRESENTATION AND DIAGNOSIS OF CERVICAL CANCER

What are the common presenting symptoms?

1. Vaginal discharge or bleeding, commonly postcoital spotting with early lesions

2. Dull pelvic pain, leg swelling, urinary or rectal symptoms with late disease

What are the guidelines for performing Pap smears?

Begin annual tests when a woman becomes sexually active or reaches 18 years of age. (Once three consecutive tests are normal, some say that the tests may be performed less frequently.)

What is the correct technique for obtaining a Pap smear?

The transformation zone should be gently scraped with a brush, and the fluid in the posterior fornix aspirated, then smeared onto a glass slide and immediately fixed to prevent drying.

How sensitive is the Pap smear?

The false-negative rate is 15% to 25%, but an optimally obtained smear can diminish this rate. However, a frankly invasive tumor can also yield a false-negative result due to associated inflammation.

Can a patient be treated based on a positive Pap smear?

No, a biopsy is mandatory for proper histologic diagnosis.

What is the further workup if a Pap smear is positive?

Colposcopy (vascular patterns visualized under a green light with magnification) and an appropriate biopsy are performed. When no lesion is grossly visible and colposcopy is inadequate, cervical conization is performed.

What is the standard clinical evaluation for staging?

Pelvic examination (preferably under anaesthesia) with cystoscopy and proctosigmoidoscopy, biochemical liver and renal function tests, CXR, and CT scan with contrast

Is an IVP required?

Although imaging of the kidneys and ureters is essential, an IVP is not required if a CT scan with contrast is obtained.

TREATMENT OF CERVICAL CANCER

How is carcinoma in situ (CIN-3) treated?

Conization or loop electrosurgical excision procedure (LEEP) of the cervix is the definitive therapy.

What is LEEP?

In this technique, a thin wire loop electrode is used to excise the cervical lesion. The procedure is used in the diagnosis and management of preinvasive cervical lesions, as an alternative to cold-knife conization.

What are the advantages of LEEP?

Well-tolerated, easy, quick, and low-cost office procedure

What are the disadvantages of LEEP?

Possible coagulation artifacts and specimen fragmentation

What is the treatment of cervical cancer?

1. Radiation therapy can be used to treat all stages.
2. Early lesions can be treated by radical surgery.

What is the treatment of microinvasive carcinoma (Stage IA)?

Confirm the depth of invasion with a cone biopsy.
   1. If invasion is less than 3 mm, total abdominal or vaginal hysterectomy is performed when preservation of fertility is not a consideration.
   2. If the patient wants to have children, close follow-up may be adequate in selected patients if the margins of resection are negative.

What is the Wertheim operation?

Radical abdominal hysterectomy with bilateral pelvic lymphadenectomy. The parametrial, paracervical, and upper paravaginal tissues are completely removed along with the upper third of the vagina.

What are the indications for this procedure?

Stages IB and IIA of cervical carcinoma

Most common complications of this procedure?

1. Neurogenic bladder dysfunction
2. Urinary tract fistulae

Does surgery have a role in advanced disease?

Yes, in stage IVA, when the bladder or rectum is involved, but **no** pelvic sidewall invasion is present, pelvic exenteration may be performed. However, with improved radiation therapy, this procedure is used less frequently today.

What are the indications for radiation therapy (XRT)?	1. Any stage of cervical cancer 2. Stage IIB–IV cancer (treatment of choice) 3. An alternative to radical hysterectomy for stages IB/IIA (both modalities have the same cure rate)
What form of radiation therapy is used?	Combination of brachytherapy (intracavitary and interstitial radiation) and external beam irradiation is necessary for successful therapy.

What is the most commonly used isotope for:

Intracavitary therapy?	^{137}Cs (Cesium)
Interstitial therapy?	^{192}Ir (Iridium)
What are the complications of XRT, and when are they seen after therapy?	1. Intestinal (e.g., proctitis and small bowel obstruction) complications are generally evident 2 years after therapy. 2. Urinary tract complications (e.g., chronic cystitis, ulceration of the bladder) may not be seen for 3 to 4.
Is there a role for combined XRT and surgery?	1. Generally not, because results are the same as with XRT alone 2. The role of postoperative XRT after a radical hysterectomy with positive nodes is controversial.
What is the role of chemotherapy in cervical cancer?	Very little, because responses are usually partial and of short duration. It is used as salvage therapy.
Which agents are most effective?	1. Cisplatinum 2. Ifosfamide

ENDOMETRIAL CANCER

What is its claim to fame?	1. Most common malignancy of the female genital tract 2. Fourth most common malignancy in women

Is it more common before or after menopause?

Mainly occurs after menopause, with peak incidence in the sixth decade. It is very uncommon before 40 years of age.

The incidence of endometrial cancer is more than that of ovarian cancer. Is the death rate proportional, and why?

The death rate is lower for endometrial cancer because of more frequent diagnosis at a very early stage.

What are the risk factors?

Multiple! Obesity, late first pregnancy, nulliparity, late menopause, polycystic ovary disease, estrogen-secreting ovarian tumors, exogenous estrogen use, diabetes, hypertension, hypothyroidism, and chronic anovulatory states

Do combination estrogen and progesterone contraceptive pills increase risk?

No, the concomitant use of progestins negates the effect of the estrogens, and the risk of endometrial cancer is actually lowered.

Do tumors arising in the setting of unopposed estrogen have a better or worse prognosis than those arising in the setting of endometrial atrophy?

Tumors arising in the setting of endometrial hyperplasia are better differentiated, and have a better prognosis than tumors arising in the setting of endometrial atrophy.

Which histologic types have the worst prognosis?

1. Serous papillary carcinoma
2. Clear cell carcinoma

Does endometrial hyperplasia always progress to malignancy?

No, it can also be physiological in certain settings.

Of the types of endometrial hyperplasia, which has the greatest malignant potential?

Atypical complex hyperplasia

What is the basis for the staging system?

The FIGO classification is now a surgical staging system. It is based on the operative findings, histologic grade, depth of myometrial invasion, peritoneal cytology, pelvic and para-aortic lymph node status, and evaluation of extrauterine and distant spread.

What are the prognostic factors?	1. Increasing age and stage at diagnosis are poor prognostic factors.
	2. Most significant are the histologic grade, the depth of myometrial invasion, and the lymph nodal status.

PRESENTATION AND DIAGNOSIS OF ENDOMETRIAL CANCER

What is the typical presentation?	Vaginal bleeding in a postmenopausal woman
What are the diagnostic procedures?	1. Fractional dilatation and curettage
	2. Endometrial biopsy
What is a good screening procedure?	None. The Pap smear is **not** reliable.
Is there a specific tumor marker?	No. CA 125 is not specific for endometrial carcinoma, but it may be elevated, and thus useful for follow-up **after** therapy.

TREATMENT OF ENDOMETRIAL CANCER

What is the usual treatment modality?	Surgery: Total abdominal hysterectomy and bilateral salpingo-oophorectomy with appropriate evaluations for surgical staging which usually involves sampling of the pelvic and para-aortic nodes

Radiation Therapy (XRT)

What is its role in the adjuvant setting?	1. Stage I tumors confined to the uterine corpus
	2. High-grade tumors
	3. Deep myometrial invasion
What are other indications for XRT?	1. Postoperative pelvic radiation for serosal or adnexal spread, extension to the cervix, or pelvic nodal metastasis
	2. Primary treatment for vaginal metastasis

Hormonal therapy

What is the agent of choice?	Progestogen, when receptor status is high

Does it improve survival in the adjuvant setting?	No
What is the indication for hormonal therapy?	Recurrent disease
What is the response rate?	About one-third respond. Well-differentiated tumors with a positive progesterone receptor status respond more frequently.
Although of little role in therapy, which chemotherapy agents have some response?	1. Cisplatin 2. Doxorubicin

OVARIAN CANCER

How common is ovarian cancer?	1. Second most common gynecologic malignancy, accounting for 25% 2. Accounts for only 4% of all visceral malignancies in women
What is its claim to fame?	Leading cause of gynecologic cancer death (responsible for 50%); almost 14,000 women in 1994
What is the lifetime risk for a woman to develop ovarian cancer:	
If no family members have ovarian cancer?	Between 1% and 2%
If one first-degree relative has ovarian cancer?	Approximately 5 %
If two or more first-degree relatives have ovarian cancer?	Approximately 7 %
If a member of a family has a hereditary ovarian cancer syndrome?	Approximately 40%

What factors are associated with increased risk?	1. Family history of ovarian cancer (most important) 2. Others—nulliparity, fewer pregnancies, history of infertility, advancing age, North American or Northern European descent, a personal history of breast, endometrial or colon cancer, talc use (dusting powder on tampons)
Is therapeutic pelvic irradiation associated with increased risk of ovarian cancer?	No
Are oral contraceptives risk factors?	Combination pills are **protective** (50% reduction in risk). They are thought to act by providing respite to the ovarian surface epithelium from the constant stimulation that occurs during ovulation.

What ovarian tumors are associated with:

Long-term anticonvulsant therapy?	Ovarian thecomas
Peutz-Jeghers syndrome?	Granulosa cell tumors
Inherited basal cell nevus syndrome?	Benign fibromas
Gonadal dysgenesis (46XY)?	Gonadoblastomas
Turner syndrome (45XO)?	None
What are the three hereditary ovarian cancer syndromes, and what is their mode of inheritance?	All three have an autosomal dominant inheritance with incomplete penetrance. They are: 1. Site-specific ovarian cancer 2. Breast–ovarian cancer syndrome 3. Lynch syndrome II

What is the increase in relative risk with these syndromes?

1. Site-specific ovarian cancer: 20-fold
2. Breast–ovarian cancer syndrome: 13-fold
3. Lynch syndrome II: 10-fold

What is Lynch syndrome II?

Also known as hereditary nonpolyposis colorectal cancer (HNPCC), this syndrome includes early onset colorectal cancer, endometrial cancer, cancer of the upper GI tract, urothelial carcinomas of the renal pelvis and ureters, and ovarian cancer.

What is the underlying genetic defect in:
    HNPCC?

Mutations in the mismatch–repair genes: MSH2, MLH1, PMS 1 and 2

    Breast-ovarian cancer syndrome?

BRCA-1 most commonly, BRCA-2 in a smaller proportion

What is the current recommendation for a woman from a hereditary ovarian cancer syndrome family?

1. Annual screening with rectovaginal pelvic examination, CA-125 levels, and transvaginal sonogram
2. When childbearing is complete, or by age 35, prophylactic bilateral oophorectomy is recommended. This surgery reduces the risk, but does not exclude the small risk of developing peritoneal carcinomatosis, which arises from the coelomic epithelium and is clinically similar to advanced ovarian cancer.

Of the molecular genetic lesions in ovarian cancer, which:
    Is most common?

Mutations of the p53 tumor suppressor gene

    Proto-oncogenes are implicated?

MYC, EGFR and ERBB2

    Are associated with RAS mutations?

Mucinous carcinomas

Are most ovarian tumors malignant transformations in the ovum?

No, the most common ovarian tumors are **epithelial** and represent malignant transformation of the surface epithelium covering the ovary.

What are the most frequent sites of spread?

Peritoneum, omentum, bowel surfaces, and retroperitoneal lymph nodes

What are the most common methods of dissemination?

The most common is transperitoneal dissemination, next is lymphatic spread, and last is hematogenous.

Can transperitoneal dissemination occur with the ovarian capsule intact?

Yes, by exfoliation of surface cells

What is the pathway for clearance of the cells shed into the peritoneum?

Paracolic gutters to lymphatic channels of the diaphragm (more commonly on the right side) to lymphatic channels on the pleural surface of the diaphragm to anterior mediastinal lymph nodes.

What are the pathways of lymphatic drainage from the ovary?

From the subovarian plexus at the ovarian hilus, there are three drainage pathways:
1. Along the ovarian blood vessels, into para-aortic nodes
2. Along the broad ligaments into the upper external iliac and hypogastric nodes
3. Along the round ligaments into the external iliac and inguinal nodes
   Pelvic nodes are the most frequently involved, the para-aortic less often, and the inguinal infrequently.

What are Krukenberg tumors?

They are ovarian metastases from gastric, colorectal, and breast cancers. Ovaries are usually involved bilaterally.

Which type of breast cancer most frequently involves the ovaries?

Invasive lobular carcinoma

What are the main classifications of ovarian tumors?

There are three major types:
1. Epithelial tumors: serous, mucinous, endometrioid, clear cell, and brenner tumors
2. Sex cord–stromal tumors: granulosa cell and Sertoli-Leydig cell tumors
3. Germ cell tumors: dysgerminoma, teratoma, endodermal sinus tumor, and embryonal carcinoma

What is the most common ovarian tumor overall?

Epithelial tumors (70%)

What is the most common malignant ovarian tumor?

Serous cystadenocarcinomas (42%)

What is the most common type of tumor in patients under 20 years of age?

Germ cell tumors (Epithelial tumors account for less than one-fifth of tumors in this age-group.)

What percentage of epithelial tumors are malignant?

1. Serous—20%
2. Mucinous—10%
3. Endometrioid—99%

What is the most important prognostic factor of epithelial tumors?

Histologic grade

Which type is associated with pseudomyxoma peritonei?

Malignant mucinous cystadenocarcinoma

Which type has pathognomonic "hobnail" cells?

Clear cell carcinoma

Which type is associated with a poorer prognosis?

Clear cell carcinoma

Which tumor is associated with:
Call-Exner bodies?

Granulosa cell tumors may contain these folliculoid structures.

Schiller-Duval bodies?

Endodermal sinus tumors often contain these papillary formations.

Hyperthyroidism?	Struma ovarii: a dermoid cyst with thyroid tissue as a component
Coombs' positive hemolytic anemia?	Mature cystic teratoma (dermoid cyst)
Masculinization?	Sertoli-Leydig cell tumors
Precocious puberty?	Granulosa and theca cell tumors
Bilaterality?	Dysgerminomas (10%) and dermoid cysts (15%)
Exquisite radiosensitivity?	Dysgerminomas
Elevated hCG?	Choriocarcinoma
Elevated AFP?	Endodermal sinus tumor
Basis of the staging system?	The FIGO classification is a surgical staging system: Stage I: Growth limited to the ovaries Stage II: Pelvic extension of the tumor Stage III: Peritoneal implants outside the pelvis, positive retroperitoneal or inguinal nodes Stage IV: Distant metastasis
What characterizes subdivision C in stages I and II?	Tumor on the surface of the ovary, capsule rupture, ascites with malignant cells, or positive peritoneal washings
What is the stage of a patient with tumor in one ovary, extension to the uterus, and a single superficial liver metastasis?	Stage III

DIAGNOSIS OF OVARIAN TUMORS

What is the management of an adnexal mass in a: Premenarchal girl?	Ultrasound (U/S), usually followed by exploratory laparotomy and conservative surgery

Premenopausal woman?

These masses are usually benign. Ultrasonographic assessment should be followed by surgical exploration if any of the following features are present: > 8 cm, complex structure on U/S, irregular, solid, bilateral, or associated ascites. Close follow-up with repeat pelvic exam and U/S if none of these features are present. If no regression in three menstrual cycles on follow-up, perform exploratory laparotomy.

Postmenopausal woman?

Ovarian tumors have a very high suspicion for malignancy. Ultrasonography and CA-125 level for assessment. A simple cystic structure < 5 cm in size, and CA-125 level < 35 U/ml may be followed serially (risk of malignancy is 1%). All other masses, and CA-125 > 35 U/ml, require surgical exploration.

What ovary size on pelvic exam warrants further investigation in postmenopausal women?

A palpable ovary

What is the role of laparoscopy in diagnosis of ovarian cancers?

Controversial. The standard recommendation is that if ovarian cancer is suspected preoperatively, the procedure should be an exploratory laparotomy.

Is transvaginal sonography superior to the transabdominal procedure in evaluation of the ovaries?

Yes. There is better resolution of architectural detail because the tip of the probe is closer to the ovaries, there is less operator-dependent variability, and the patient does not require a full bladder. If color flow Doppler imaging is also used to detect increased flow with lower impedance in tumors, the sensitivity is further increased.

What tumor markers are useful?

1. CEA
2. CA-125

Which tumors show elevated CEA?

1. > 50% of stage III epithelial cancers
2. Mucinous tumors most frequently

Is CEA specific?

No. It is elevated in cirrhosis, COPD, heavy smoking history, etc., and therefore has a limited diagnostic role. It can be useful for monitoring after therapy.

Which tumors show elevated CA-125?

Eighty percent of epithelial ovarian cancers (more commonly elevated with serous than mucinous varieties)

Is CA-125 specific?

Though more specific than CEA, it is also elevated with benign disease, with other malignancies (endometrial, pancreatic, colon, breast, lung), and in 1% of healthy people.

Is CA-125 useful as a screening test?

No, because of two problems:
1. Large number of false positives mean low predictive value.
2. Only 50% of patients with stage I ovarian cancer have elevated CA-125.

Is CA-125 useful for follow-up after therapy?

It is of some benefit. If elevated, it definitely indicates residual disease or a recurrence. However, it may fall within the normal range in the presence of disease.

TREATMENT OF EPITHELIAL TUMORS

What does an adequate staging laparotomy involve?

The following procedures may be performed by an experienced gynecologic oncologist:
1. Total abdominal hysterectomy with bilateral salpingo-oophorectomy (If the patient desires further childbearing, and there is no evidence of disease outside one ovary, unilateral salpingo-oophorectomy may be performed.)
2. Careful inspection and biopsies of the paracolic gutter peritoneum, infundibulopelvic ligament and lateral pelvic peritoneum, rectal and bladder serosa, and cul de sac peritoneum
3. Inspection and palpation of the small and large bowel, mesentery,

surfaces of the liver, spleen and diaphragm, and biopsy of the diaphragm
4. Omentectomy
5. Ascitic fluid or cell washings for cytological evaluation
6. Appropriate surgical debulking of tumor
7. If no more than minimal residual disease remains after all the above, biopsies of pelvic and para-aortic nodes. Nodes removed only to stage, or debulk if enlarged

Is there any difference in survival between patients with low-volume disease pre-operatively and those debulked to minimal residual disease?

Yes. Although debulking tumor to less than 1 cm of residual disease improves survival, it is still not as good as survival for those presenting with low-volume disease.

Should every tumor be aggressively debulked?

No. In every patient, the surgeon has to weigh the pros and cons of each procedure. If it is possible to safely leave little or no tumor, this is the goal. Even in stage IV, an attempt at debulking will increase disease-free survival.

Chemotherapy for Epithelial Tumors

What are the most effective agents?

Platinum analogs and Taxol

What adjuvant therapies are currently in use?

The standard is a single platinum analog. Melphalan and intraperitoneal 32P are being tried on protocol.

Which patients should receive adjuvant therapy?

Of the stage I patients, those with well-differentiated tumors in stage I A/B do not require adjuvant treatment. The rest of stage I and all stage II patients should receive adjuvant therapy.

What postoperative therapy is used for patients with advanced disease (stage III or IV)?

Platinum-based combination chemotherapy (Taxol and cisplatin being the most commonly used combination)

What is the role of CA-125 after primary treatment?

CA-125 levels should be obtained monthly on follow-up after surgery. Failure to normalize within three cycles of chemotherapy indicates chemoresistant disease. Normalization of values does **not** assure freedom from disease. Similarly, if the value falls and then goes up again, it has a 96% predictive value for recurrence.

After initial treatment using surgery with or without follow-up chemotherapy, what is the role of second-look surgery?

Fifty percent of patients with no clinical evidence of residual disease have residual disease at second-look surgery. These patients have a poor prognosis. Of those who have a negative second look, 40% develop a recurrence. Therefore, routine second-look surgery is falling out of favor. It is, however, important in the objective evaluation of new agents as second-line therapies.

What is the prognosis of patients who relapse after primary chemotherapy?

Extremely poor. Most salvage therapy is not curative.

What is the role of platinum compounds in second-line chemotherapy?

Platinum compounds may still be effective, response is **inversely** proportional to the interval to relapse. It is very poor in early (< 6 months) relapses.

What is the second-line chemotherapy of choice?

Taxol (paclitaxel), which is derived from the western yew plant *Taxus brevifolia*. It is not cross-resistant to platinum because of its unique mechanism of action. It binds to microtubules during mitosis, resulting in their stabilization and preventing them from disassembly.

What is the overall response rate with Taxol?

Approximately 35%

What are toxicities associated with Taxol?

Myelosuppression, peripheral neuropathy, alopecia, myalgias, and arthralgias

What is the current status of intraperitoneal chemotherapy and which agent is the drug of choice?

Experimental. Cisplatin is the drug of choice for this "belly bath." There is a definite pharmacologic advantage in the slow peritoneal clearance of high molecular weight compounds with a low lipid solubility. However, no survival benefit has been shown.

Radiation Therapy (XRT) for Epithelial Tumors

What are the indications for XRT in epithelial ovarian tumors?

1. Adjuvant after surgical debulking
2. Treatment of inoperable tumors that are chemoresistant
3. Salvage therapy for persistent disease
4. Palliation in advanced disease

What agent and route are frequently used?

Intraperitoneal 32P

What are the limitations of this therapy?

1. Only minimal residual disease can be treated because the β particles can penetrate only 3 to 4 mm.
2. Adhesions can cause uneven distribution.

What is the primary advantage of this therapy?

Limited toxicity

What is the current recommendation for its use?

Microscopic disease, though falling out of favor

What is the most important prognostic variable?

Amount of residual disease after initial surgery

GERM CELL TUMORS: DYSGERMINOMAS

What is the male counterpart?

Seminoma

What is the usual age at onset?

Usually less than 20 years old.

What is the treatment if only one ovary is involved?

1. Unilateral salpingo-oophorectomy with staging
2. The contralateral ovary should be examined very closely, because 10% are bilateral. If there is any doubt, it should be bivalved, with wedge biopsies sent for frozen section.

Should surgery be followed by adjuvant therapy?

Adjuvant chemotherapy or radiotherapy is recommended because 20% of unilateral encapsulated tumors relapse. Occasionally, if very close follow-up is possible, adjuvant therapy may be omitted.

Should a hysterectomy be performed if bilateral ovarian disease is present?

No; the uterus should be removed only if it is involved with disease. Further spread should be completely debulked.

What is the role of chemotherapy?

Nearly every patient receives chemotherapy (as adjuvant therapy) for residual disease, bulky adenopathy, or metastatic disease.

What is the role of XRT?

It is as effective as chemotherapy in most situations, but has greater toxicity, and almost always results in sterility. Therefore, it is reserved mainly for the occasional chemoresistant tumor.

What is the most frequent pathology of a large residual retroperitoneal mass after completion of chemotherapy?

Fibrosis, with no tumor

What is the cure rate for Stage IV disease?

More than 90%!

GRANULOSA AND THECA CELL TUMORS

Are they aggressive tumors?

No; they have a fairly indolent course.

What is the presentation in young patients?

Usually present as precocious feminization

What is the treatment?	1. Unilateral salpingo-oophorectomy for localized disease
	2. Chemotherapy or radiotherapy is **not** very effective. Therefore, if the tumor has spread, it should be aggressively surgically excised.

GESTATIONAL TROPHOBLASTIC DISEASE

What is gestational trophoblastic disease?	It is a spectrum of tumors that arise in the fetal chorion of the placenta.
What are the four types?	1. Complete hydatidiform mole
	2. Partial hydatidiform mole
	3. Gestational choriocarcinoma
	4. Placental-site trophoblastic tumor
Which of the preceding four are true neoplasms?	Only the latter two are true neoplasms. Molar pregnancies are merely pathologic products of conception.
What is the incidence?	1 in 1200 pregnancies in the United States; higher in Asia and South America
Do increasing age at pregnancy and greater parity increase risk?	Older age at pregnancy, especially over age 40 does, but greater parity does not
Which trophoblastic tumor develops after an abortion?	Choriocarcinomas
Which trophoblastic tumors develop after a normal pregnancy?	Choriocarcinomas. Hydatidiform moles **cannot** develop after abortion or term pregnancies.
What tumor marker is elevated in all types of gestational trophoblastic disease?	hCG
What is essential for accurate level measurement of this marker?	Measure the β subunit by radioimmunoassay for accurate levels.

COMPLETE HYDATIDIFORM MOLE

What are the pathologic characteristics?	Clusters of hydropic villi, absent fetal vessels, and trophoblastic proliferation. No evidence of fetus or amniotic tissues.
What are the cytogenetics?	Diploid, 46 XX, with both X-chromosomes paternal in origin
What are the clinical features?	1. Vaginal bleeding 2. Large-for-date uterus 3. hCG titers high for the duration of gestation 4. Absence of fetal heart sounds and other evidence of fetus 5. Theca lutein ovarian cysts 6. Occasionally, early toxemia of pregnancy or expulsion of grape-like villi
What are the sonographic features?	Large-for-date uterus filled with grape-like structures
What follow-up is necessary after evacuation?	1. Weekly hCG levels, until they are normal 2. Regular physical examination 3. Evaluation of any clinical symptoms 4. CXR every 1 to 2 months until hCG levels normalize
What percentage of patients develop postmolar gestational trophoblastic tumors?	40% with high-risk moles, 4% with low-risk moles High-risk features are: large-for-date uterine size, high hCG levels, large ovarian thecalutein cysts, toxemia, coagulopathy, trophoblastic embolization, and hyperthyroidism.

PARTIAL HYDATIDIFORM MOLE

How is this mole different from the complete form?	1. Fetal and amniotic tissues are present; focal distribution of hydropic villi and trophoblastic proliferation 2. Cytogenetic analysis: triploid, generally 69 XXY or 69 XYY

3. Uterus generally not enlarged
4. Malignant sequelae rare, though possible
Partial hydatidiform moles are most frequently diagnosed as incomplete abortion with hydropic degeneration

What follow-up is necessary after evacuation?

Same follow-up as required for the complete molar pregnancy

CHORIOCARCINOMA

What pathologic features are present?

Malignant trophoblastic tissue with cytotrophoblastic and syncytiotrophoblastic cells, and no evidence of villi; vascular invasion very common; frequent hemorrhage and necrosis of tumor.

What is the mode of metastatic spread?

Hematogenous

What are the common metastatic sites?

Lungs (80%), vagina (30%), liver (10%), brain (10%), GI tract, and kidneys

What is the staging system for choriocarcinoma?

Stage 0: Molar pregnancy (low risk or high risk)
Stage I: Confined to uterine corpus
Stage II: Metastases to pelvis and vagina
Stage III: Metastases to lung
Stage IV: Other distant metastases

What hCG titers are associated with high risk?

Greater than 100,000 IU/ml

What are the indications for surgery in choriocarcinoma?

1. Hysterectomy in stage I patients who do not desire to retain fertility
2. Selective use after chemotherapy, when a single focus in the lung or uterus is only residual disease

What are the indications for chemotherapy?

1. All patients with choriocarcinoma
2. Patients with hydatidiform mole if hCG levels are persistently high (plateaued or rising)

What chemotherapeutic regimens are used?	1. For low-risk patients: Single agent; methotrexate with leucovorin rescue or dactinomycin 2. For high-risk patients: Combination chemotherapy; methotrexate, dactinomycin, and an alkylating agent being the standard regimen. Etoposide is a new effective agent.
What are the indications for radiotherapy?	Local irradiation for patients with brain or liver metastases
What are the cure rates?	1. Nearly 100% for low and medium-risk disease 2. For high-risk disease, 80%
What is the outcome of subsequent pregnancies?	Expectation of normal pregnancy **same** as unaffected women, with no increase in congenital malformations or secondary infertility. Pregnancy allowed 1 year after completion of treatment.
What is the risk of another molar pregnancy?	Less than 1% (1 in 120)

PLACENTAL SITE TROPHOBLASTIC TUMOR

What are the pathologic features?	Composed of only one cell type, the intermediate trophoblast
Which types of pregnancy does tumor follow?	Any type
What are the tumor markers?	1. hCG levels are variable, and may be absent, but are usually lower than expected 2. Human placental lactogen levels are elevated more reliably.
What is the treatment?	Early hysterectomy once the diagnosis is established

CARCINOMA OF THE VULVA

What are risk factors?	1. Low socioeconomic class 2. Various medical illnesses (hypertension, obesity, diabetes, and cardiovascular disease)

3. Sexually transmitted diseases
4. Occupational history in the laundry and cleaning industry

What are the two most histopathologic types?

1. Squamous cell carcinomas (90%)
2. Malignant melanoma (10%)
Others include basal cell carcinoma, sarcoma, verrucous carcinoma, and Paget's disease

What are the two types of intraepithelial neoplasia?

1. Carcinoma in situ
2. Paget disease

What is the histologic appearance of Paget disease?

Large, round, vacuolated cells in nests surrounded by small hyperchromatic basaloid cells

What percentage of Paget disease is associated with malignancy?

In 33% of cases, there is an underlying adenocarcinoma arising in an adnexal structure.

What is verrucous carcinoma?

A rare type of well-differentiated squamous cell carcinoma that resembles condylomata acuminata; locally invasive, rarely metastatic

What is the mode of spread of vulvar carcinoma?

Slow growing; spread to adjacent tissues in continuity; lymphatic spread to inguinal lymph nodes

What is the staging of vulvar carcinoma?

Stage I : Tumor confined to the vulva/ perineum, < 2cm in size
Stage II : Tumor confined to the vulva/ perineum, > 2cm in size
Stage III : Tumor spread to lower urethra, vagina, anus, or unilateral inguinal nodes
Stage IVA : Invasion of upper urethra, bladder or rectal mucosa, pelvic bone, inguinal nodes
Stage IVB : Distant metastases, including pelvic lymph nodes

TREATMENT

What is the treatment of: Carcinoma in situ?

Wide local excision followed by primary closure, skin flaps, or skin graft as required

Paget disease?   Wide excision, down to underlying fat to
                                    remove all adnexal structures

Stage I?   Modified radical hemivulvectomy/
                                    vulvectomy and ipsilateral inguinal–
                                    femoral lymphadenectomy (bilateral
                                    node dissection for midline lesions).
                                    Recently, some surgeons have
                                    performed radical local excision instead
                                    of vulvectomy with equivalent results.

Stage II and III?   Radical vulvectomy and bilateral
                                    inguinal–femoral lymphadenectomy. If
                                    inguinal lymph nodes are positive,
                                    adjuvant pelvic irradiation is the choice.

Stage IV?   Pelvic exenteration may be required.
                                    Preoperative chemoradiation is used to
                                    shrink tumor and avoid exenteration.

CARCINOMA OF THE VAGINA

**What is the most common   Squamous cell carcinomas (80%–90%)
histopathologic type?**

**What is the most common   Common in the postmenopausal ages
age at onset?**

What is the treatment?   1. Mainstay of therapy is XRT (a
                                       combination of brachytherapy and
                                       external-beam irradiation).
                                    2. In disease limited to the vaginal wall
                                       (stage I), surgery can be considered
                                       (radical hysterectomy, partial
                                       vaginectomy, and pelvic
                                       lymphadenectomy).

CLEAR CELL CARCINOMA

What is the cause?   In utero exposure to DES by maternal
                                    ingestion of the agent during pregnancy

**At what age does the   19 years
incidence peak?**

VAGINAL ADENOSIS

Describe its appearance. Red, velvety, grape-like clusters in the vagina

Represents remnants of what tissue? Mullerian glandular epithelium

What is the cause? DES. It is the most common DES-associated histologic abnormality.

54

Neurosurgery

Mark Watts, MD

NEUROANATOMY

What are the five layers of the scalp?

The five layers can be remembered with the SCALP pneumonic:
1. **S**kin
2. **C**onnective tissue
3. **G**alea **a**poneurotica
4. **L**oose connective tissue
5. **P**eriosteum

What is the greatest risk associated with most scalp wounds?

Bleeding. The rich blood supply of the scalp can result in copious bleeding after laceration. Children in particular can potentially exsanguinate from a significant scalp wound.

Why are scalp wounds readily resistant to infection?

The rich vascular supply of the scalp provides a significant barrier against an infection.

What method is used to close a laceration of the scalp?

Closure of a scalp wound after debridement and irrigation includes deep monofilament sutures that encompass the galea. This method helps to prevent subgaleal hematoma.

What is the pterion?

It is the H-shaped junction of the frontal, parietal, temporal, and greater wing of the sphenoid bones. Its location is roughly 2.5 cm above the zygomatic arch and 1.5 cm behind the zygomatic process of the frontal bone.

Why is the pterion important?

Its position represents the central focus of one of the more common craniotomies in neurosurgery.

What is the largest foramen of the skull? — Foramen magnum located at the base of the skull

What does each foramen in the skull contain?

Foramen magnum? — Spinal cord and medulla, the anterior and posterior spinal arteries, the spinal accessory nerve (cranial nerve 11), and the vertebral arteries

Foramen ovale? — Mandibular branch of cranial nerve 5 and the motor branches to the jaw musculature

Jugular foramen? — Internal jugular vein and cranial nerves 9, 10, and 11

Foramen lacerum? — Although the foramen lacerum appears large when viewing the base of the skull, usually **no** structures enter or exit from this foramen.

What constitutes the base of the skull?
1. Orbital roofs of frontal bones
2. Cribriform plate of ethmoid bones
3. Sphenoid bone
4. Squamous and petrous portions of temporal bones
5. Occipital bones

What are the major anatomic divisions of the brain?
1. Two cerebral hemispheres
2. Brain stem
3. Cerebellum

What are the lobes of the cerebral hemispheres?
1. Frontal lobes
2. Parietal lobes
3. Temporal lobes
4. Occipital lobes

What are the three divisions of the brain stem?
1. Midbrain
2. Pons
3. Medulla

What are the functions of the frontal lobes? — The frontal lobes govern the planning and sequencing of movement, voluntary eye movements, and emotional affect.

What are the functions of the parietal lobes?

The parietal lobes subserve motor control and cortical sensation. The dominant parietal lobe governs motor programs, whereas the nondominant lobe governs spatial orientation.

What are the functions of the occipital lobes?

The occipital lobes govern visual perception and involuntary eye movements.

What are the functions of the temporal lobes?

The temporal lobes subserve olfaction, memory, and certain components of auditory and visual perception.

What region of the brain governs the comprehension of speech and in which lobe is it located?

Wernicke's area governs speech comprehension and is located in the dominant temporal lobe of the brain.

What region of the brain governs the motor component of speech and in which lobe is it located?

Broca's area lies within the posterior portion of the dominant frontal lobe.

What are the major vessels supplying blood to the brain and their branches?

1. The anterior circulation of the brain consists of the **internal carotid arteries** which further divide into the anterior cerebral artery and the middle cerebral artery.
2. The posterior circulation consists of the **vertebral arteries**, which join to form the basilar artery, which divides into the two posterior cerebral arteries. The vertebral arteries also give off the anterior spinal artery of the spinal cord and the posterior inferior cerebellar artery (PICA), whereas the basilar artery gives off the anterior inferior cerebellar artery (AICA) and the superior cerebellar artery (SCA).

What is the "circle of Willis"?

An arterial anastomosis of vessels that enables the entire brain to be reliably vascularized from one main feeding vessel. The **anterior communicating artery** between the two anterior cerebral arteries, and the two **posterior communicating arteries** between the internal carotid artery and the posterior cerebral arteries serve as the main conduits between the anterior and posterior circulatory systems as well as the right- and left-sided circulatory systems.

What are the main draining vessels of the brain?

The venous drainage systems of the brain are divided into superficial and deep systems:

1. In the superficial system, the **superior sagittal sinus** joins the **straight sinus** at the confluence of the sinuses, known as the torcular. Blood then drains from the cranial vault via the **transverse and sigmoid sinuses** to exit the skull via the **internal jugular veins**.

2. The deep system starts with the **internal cerebral veins** and **inferior sagittal sinus** draining into the straight sinus.

What is the cavernous sinus?

The cavernous sinus is a plexus of veins located on both sides of the bony sella turcica. A number of veins, including orbital and cortical vessels, contribute to its flow.

Which nerves travel within the lateral walls of the cavernous sinus?

Cranial nerves III, IV, and the ophthalmic and maxillary divisions of cranial nerve V

Which nerve and artery travel within the sinus itself?

Cranial nerve VI and the carotid artery

What is a carotid cavernous fistula?

Carotid cavernous fistulas are the general arterialization of the cavernous sinus. The fistulae are of two types: traumatic and spontaneous.

What symptoms are associated with carotid cavernous fistulas?

Headache, orbital pain, and diplopia

What signs are associated with carotid cavernous fistulas?

Ophthalmoplegia, arterialization of the conjunctiva (chemosis), and ocular or cranial bruit

What is the treatment of carotid cavernous fistulas?

Although some low-flow lesions may spontaneously thrombose, high-flow lesions often require balloon embolization.

Where is cerebrospinal fluid produced?

The bulk of CSF is produced by the choroid plexus, which is located in the lateral and fourth ventricles. Small amounts are also produced in the interstitial spaces, the ependymal linings of the ventricles, and the dural root sleeves.

How much CSF is produced daily in the adult?

Typically, 500 to 750 ml of CSF are produced daily (0.35 ml/min).

What is the pathway for CSF egress from the lateral ventricles to the surface of the brain?

CSF produced in the choroid plexus of the lateral ventricles travels first through the **foramen of Monro** of the lateral ventricles into the midline third ventricle. From the third ventricle CSF travels through the narrow **aqueduct of Sylvius** to the fourth ventricle. CSF then exits the brain via the **midline foramen of Magendie** or the **lateral foramina of Luschka**. Once over the surface of the brain, CSF is primarily absorbed by the arachnoid granulations located in continuity with the superior sagittal sinus.

INTRACRANIAL PRESSURE

What are the principles of the Monro-Kellie doctrine?

The Monro-Kellie doctrine states that in order for intracranial pressure to remain constant, the sum of the volumes of the intracranial contents (brain, blood, CSF) must remain constant. The addition of another component (e.g., tumor or hematoma) requires that the volume of the other cranial components be reduced in order for pressure to remain constant. This theory assumes a fixed, inelastic space (the skull), and also requires that pressure be distributed evenly throughout the space. In reality it is not clear that pressure is the same throughout the skull, given the presence of leaves of dura separating the hemispheres (falx) and the hemispheres and cerebellum (tentorium cerebelli). In addition, the brain itself is compliant.

What are the indications for intracranial pressure monitoring?

Indications for ICP monitoring include a Glasgow Coma Scale (GCS) less than or equal to 7 (i.e., a patient who does not speak, open eyes, or move purposefully to pain), a patient with altered level of consciousness and multisystem trauma requiring extensive intervention. Relative contraindications include coagulopathy and any patient who can be followed with serial neurologic exams.

What systems are available for measurement of ICP?

1. Historically, the Richmond screw (subarachnoid bolt) was the mainstay of ICP monitoring.
2. Today a considerable array of electronic and fiberoptic devices can be used to measure ICP in the subdural and epidural spaces and within the parenchyma of the brain itself.
3. ICP can also be measured with a ventricular drain.

What is the added advantage of a ventricular drain?

Enables the drainage of CSF to lower ICP

What is the management of elevated ICP?

1. Raising the head of the patient's bed to 30 degrees, with the head in a neutral position
2. Hyperventilation (only effective for approximately 24 hours)
3. Intravenous diuretics including mannitol and furosemide
4. Barbiturate coma (Note: No role for steroids in intracranial edema)

What is the target endpoint for hyperventilation?

P_{CO_2} = 26 to 28

What is the target endpoint for diuretic therapy?	Serum osmolality of 310 or serum sodium of 150
What is the importance of ICP?	ICP is a reflection of the more important entity, **cerebral perfusion pressure** (CPP). CPP = Mean Arterial Pressure (MAP) - ICP. CPP is, in turn, a reflection of **cerebral blood flow** (CBF).
What is the normal CPP and how is it maintained?	The brain, through autoregulation, maintains the CPP at greater than or equal to 50 mm Hg.
What is normal CBF?	CBF in the normal resting brain is 50 ml/100 mg brain/min.
At what CBF does the electroencephalogram become flatline?	At 25 ml/100 mg brain/min
At what CBF does neuronal cell death ensue?	At 10 ml/100 mg brain/min.
What is the end result of uncontrolled increases in ICP?	Herniation: Shifting of brain tissue through relatively rigid structures of the cranium (e.g., foramina or dural leaves).
What classic triad can be observed in the late stages of herniation?	Cushing's triad: 1. Hypertension 2. Bradycardia 3. Respiratory irregularity
How frequently is the full triad observed?	Only one-third of the time

CRANIAL TRAUMA

What is the Glasgow Coma Scale?	The Glasgow Coma Scale is a general measure of consciousness that is easily repeatable in serial exams and between examiners with a wide variety of backgrounds.
For which age-group is the scale applicable?	Patients 4 years of age or older

What is the range of scores?	From 3 to 15 points
What are the components of the GCS and how is each component scored?	
Best Eye Opening	4 Spontaneous 3 To speech 2 To pain 1 None
Best Verbal	5 Oriented 4 Confused 3 Inappropriate speech 2 Incomprehensible speech 1 None
Best Motor	6 Obeys Commands 5 Localizes Pain 4 Withdraws to pain 3 Flexor (decorticate) posturing 2 Extensor (decerebrate) posturing 1 None
What are the two general purposes for intubating a head-injury patient?	1. Protection of airway to prevent airway obstruction and aspiration 2. Need for hyperventilation to reduce intracranial pressure (ICP)
What is the significance of a linear skull fracture on plain skull radiographs after trauma?	The presence of a linear skull fracture is an indication of the amount of energy transferred to the cranium during trauma. The presence of a skull fracture, however, does **not** correlate with the presence or absence of underlying brain injury. Thus, plain radiographs are of **no** use in the management of acute head trauma.
What is the mainstay of radiographic examination of the head-injured patient?	Computed tomography (CT) scanning without intravenous contrast
What is the general indication for surgery in depressed skull fractures?	Bone fragments depressed lower than the inner table of calvarium to a depth greater than skull thickness. Debridement and elevation of fragments usually performed in these cases.

What skull fracture is classically associated with CSF leak?

Basilar skull fracture is associated with CSF rhinorrhea and/or otorrhea in 5% to 10% of cases.

What is the treatment of these CSF fistulas?

Lumbar spinal drainage for 7 days. If leak persists, surgical intervention is usually indicated.

What is the significance of hemotympanum?

Hemotympanum may be the only sign of basilar skull fracture.

What is often necessary to diagnose these fractures?

CT often misses the fracture unless fine cuts through the temporal bones are specified.

What is the usual treatment for these fractures?

Generally, no specific treatment is necessary for basilar skull fractures.

What is an epidural hematoma?

Epidural hematomas are collections of blood between the skull and dura.

What is the usual source of bleeding in epidural hematoma?

Arterial bleed, usually the middle meningeal artery (Note: The hematoma can also be the result of dural sinus bleeds in up to 15% of series.)

What is the radiographic appearance of epidural hematoma?

A hyperdense, biconvex (lenticular shape) fluid collection displacing the brain on CT scan

What is the classic presentation of an epidural hematoma?

A brief loss of consciousness is followed by a several-hour **"lucid interval,"** followed by rapid decline in consciousness, ipsilateral pupillary dilation, contralateral hemiparesis, and Cushing's triad due to midbrain compression from temporal lobe herniation.

How frequently are the classic lucid intervals seen?

The phenomenon is seen in less than 25% of epidural hematomas.

What is Kernohan's phenomenon?

Contralateral cerebral peduncle compression against the tentorial notch, resulting in contralateral dilated pupil and ipsilateral hemiparesis, is seen in 10% to 20% of epidural hematomas.

What is the treatment of epidural hematoma?

Craniotomy to control bleeding and evacuate hematoma

What is a subdural hematoma?

A subdural hematoma is a collection of blood below the dura and above the subarachnoid membranes.

What is the usual source of bleeding in subdural hematoma?

Bleeding is usually the result of the tearing of small bridging veins that traverse the brain to the dural sinuses. In the elderly, trauma as insignificant as stepping off a curb can result in subdural hematoma.

What is the radiographic appearance of subdural hematoma?

A hyperdense, crescent-shaped fluid collection displacing the brain on CT scan. Over several weeks, the hematoma becomes more isodense, with the brain parenchyma making it more difficult to visualize.

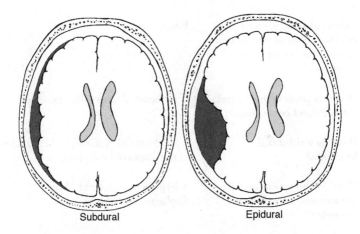

Subdural   Epidural

What distinguishes a simple from a complex subdural hematoma, and how does this affect mortality?

Simple subdural hematomas are not associated with any brain injury and have a mortality rate of about 20%.Complex subdural hematomas are often associated with frontotemporal contrecoup parenchymal lesions and have a mortality rate of 50% to 90%.

What is the treatment of an acute subdural hematoma?

Immediate surgical evaluation of hematoma by trephination (burr holes). (Note: Surgical intervention may not be indicated in some subacute or chronic subdural hematomas.)

What are the common cranial findings associated with child abuse?	1. Subdural hematomas of varying ages and often in layers 2. Retinal hemorrhages 3. Multiple skull fractures
What is the cause of axonal shear injury?	Axonal shear injury is the result of angular acceleration–deceleration injuries, typically seen in motor vehicle accidents. Shearing of deep white-matter tracts leaves the patient with a very low GCS and profound coma.
What are the usual findings of axonal shear injury on CT scan?	Minimal significant findings are seen on CT scan; instead, MRI is often helpful in delineating areas of shear injury.
What are the most common sites of cerebral contusions?	1. Temporal lobes 2. Undersurface of frontal lobes
Cerebral contusion of which region of the brain carries the worst prognosis?	Brain stem
When is surgery indicated for cerebral contusions?	If intracranial mass effect develops
What is a subdural hygroma?	A subdural fluid collection due to a tear in the arachnoid membrane
What is the radiographic appearance of subdural hygroma?	A **hypodense** crescent of fluid displacing brain tissue

SPINAL INJURIES AND INTERVERTEBRAL DISK DISEASE

Are neurologic deficits more common with cervical or thoracolumbar vertebral fractures, and why?	Thoracolumbar fractures. Spinal canal is smaller at more caudal levels.

How is motor strength graded on physical examination?

Table 54–1

Grade	Strength
0	No contraction
1	Muscle contracts
2	Movement without gravity
3	Movement against gravity
4	Movement against resistance
5	Normal strength

Which sensory levels correspond to the shoulders, nipples, umbilicus, knees, and perianal region?

Shoulders: C4
Nipples: T4
Umbilicus: T10
Knees: L3
Perianal region: S5

What are the general options available for stabilization of unstable spinal fractures?

1. Immobilization with halo device
2. Surgical fusion

What is the significance of a small chip of bone near the anteroinferior aspect of the vertebral body?

1. This chip may represent a benign avulsion injury in which the anterior longitudinal ligament is avulsed.
2. It also may be related to a fracture to the vertebral body secondary to a severe flexion injury. This type of injury is **unstable**.

What are the three types of incomplete spinal cord lesions?

1. Central cord syndrome
2. Anterior cord syndrome
3. Brown-Séquard syndrome (hemicord injury)

What pharmacologic intervention has reduced the severity of permanent neurologic deficits in spinal injury?

Intravenous methylprednisolone for 24 hours

Why may patients with spinal injury require large amounts of intravenous fluids?

Neurogenic shock resulting from a sympathectomized state with significant peripheral vasodilatation. (Note: This does **not** occur with isolated head trauma! Hypotension in these patients usually implies an intra-abdominal or intrathoracic injury.)

CERVICAL SPINE

What are the three functional columns of the cervical spine and the ligamentous complexes of each column:

Anterior column?

1. Anterior half of vertebral body and disk
2. Anterior longitudinal ligament and anulus fibrosus

Middle column?

1. Posterior half of vertebral body and disk
2. Posterior longitudinal ligament and anulus fibrosus

Posterior column?

1. Lamina, pedicles, spinous processes, and facet joints
2. Interspinous ligaments and facet capsules

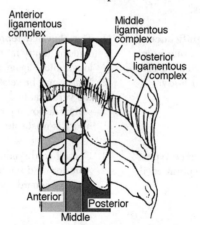

When is a cervical spine generally considered unstable?

When two or more of these functional columns are damaged

What are the names given to the first two cervical vertebrae (C1 and C2)?

C1 is the atlas.
C2 is the axis (has an anterior protuberance called the odontoid).

What is the usual mechanism of C1 versus C2 fracture?

C1: Axial loading
C2 (including odontoid): Hyperextension

What is a hangman's fracture?

Fracture through pedicles of C2 at the pars interarticularis

What is a Jefferson fracture?

A fracture of the ring of C1 at more than one site

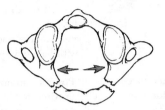

What is the radiographic criterion for a Jefferson fracture?

The "rule of Spence" provides that if the sum of the overhang of both lateral masses is greater than or equal to 7 mm (on AP view), an abnormality exists at the level of C1.

Are neurologic deficits common with this injury and why?

Given the large size of the spinal canal at this level, there is rarely any neurologic deficit if this lesion occurs in isolation.

What is the treatment of a Jefferson fracture?

External fixation in a Halo device.

What are the three types of odontoid fractures?

Type I: Fracture of the apical portion of the dens
Type II: Fracture of the dens at its base
Type III: Fracture of the dens extending into the body of C2

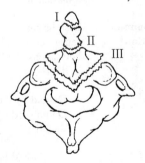

What is the treatment of odontoid fractures?

Type 1: Stable fracture; treatment rarely necessary

Type 2: **Unstable** fracture; surgical fusion

Type 3: Stable fracture; immobilization with halo device

What surgical procedures are used for fixation of odontoid fracture?

1. Posterior approach: C1 can be plated or wired to C2.
2. Anterior approach: A screw can be placed into the body of C2 through the axis of the dens.

Which of these approaches preserves rotation of the head?

The anterior approach preserves rotation, which at C1 to C2 represents 50% of all rotation of the head at the neck. This technique is generally reserved for younger individuals.

How many cervical nerve roots are there?

There are eight cervical nerve roots numbered C1 to C8, but only seven cervical vertebrae.

What nerve root exits between vertebra C3 and C4?

Nerve root C4

What are the clinical components of a radiculopathy?

Weakness, reflex changes, and dermatomal sensory changes ascribed to a particular nerve root

What is the most common cervical disk herniation and its associated radiculopathy?

Disk herniations at the C6 to C7 interval represent roughly two-thirds of all disk herniations. A C7 radiculopathy develops in these cases.

What are the clinical correlates of a C5 radiculopathy?

1. Deltoid weakness
2. Diminished sensation over the shoulder

What are the clinical correlates of a C5 radiculopathy?

1. Diminished biceps reflex
2. Biceps weakness
3. Decreased sensation over the upper arm, radial forearm, and thumb

What are the clinical correlates of a C7 radiculopathy?

1. Diminished triceps reflex
2. Triceps muscle weakness

What is the usual treatment of cervical disk herniation?

Over 95% of cervical disk herniation radiculopathies heal spontaneously.

What are the surgical approaches for those that fail to heal?

1. Anterior cervical diskectomy (ACDF) with or without fusion
2. Posterior foraminotomy and disk excision

What is cervical spondylosis?

A degenerative disease of the spine associated with osteophytic spurs, hardening of the intervertebral disks, and hypertrophy of the vertebral ligaments, particularly the posterior longitudinal ligament

How does cervical spondylosis present?

Neck pain and the physical findings associated with cervical spondylitic myelopathy (CSM)

What is CSM?

CSM is a syndrome commonly associated with a constellation of clinical findings including hyperreflexia, spasticity, weakness of the hands, proximal lower extremity weakness, and a paucity of sensory changes.

What is the physiologic basis for CSM?

Repetitive trauma to the spinal cord by a narrowed canal and associated with normal movement, ischemia of the cord associated with vascular compression with a narrow canal, or direct cord compression.

What is the treatment of CSM?

Treatment is aimed at the physiologic decompression of the cord, which may be achieved by cervical laminectomy. Despite the sound theory, some patients have progression of disease and confinement to a wheelchair.

LUMBAR SPINE

How many lumbar nerve roots are there?

There are five lumbar nerve roots (and five lumbar vertebrae).

What is the relationship of a nerve root to a vertebra of the same number?

The root exits between the vertebral bodies of its own number and the one below. Thus, the L4 root exits between L4 and L5.

A herniated disk between L4 and L5 generally affects which nerve root?

A herniated disk between vertebra L4 and L5 impinges the **L5** nerve root. Anatomically, the L4 nerve root has exited the spinal canal before the disk herniation. The shoulder of the L5 root, however, is readily impinged.

Can an L4 disk ever impinge on an L4 nerve root?

Yes. This is known as a far lateral disk herniation.

What is pain traveling down the lower extremity associated with nerve root impingement called?

Sciatica

What are the main components of an L4 radiculopathy?

1. Diminished knee jerk
2. Weakness of knee extension
3. Decreased sensation over the medial malleolus

What are the main components of an L5 radiculopathy?

1. Weakness in dorsiflexion of the great toe and foot
2. Decreased sensation at the web space of the great and second toes

What are the main components of an S1 radiculopathy?

1. Diminished ankle jerk
2. Plantar flexion weakness at the foot
3. Decreased sensation over the lateral foot

What is the treatment for acute disk herniation?

85% of patients with acute lumbar disk herniation improve **without** surgical intervention. Conservative care includes:
1. **Not more than** 1 or 2 weeks of bed rest (only a few days if axial back pain is the predominant pain)
2. A short course of analgesics (nonsteroidals and/or narcotics)
3. Education to protect the patient's back
4. After recovery is underway, physical therapy or a supervised exercise regimen may be beneficial for some patients.

What are the indications for emergent surgery in the setting of acute disk herniation?	1. Acute or progressive development of motor weakness 2. Cauda equina syndrome

NEURO-ONCOLOGY

What are the most common presentations of brain tumors?	1. Progressive neurologic deficit 2. Headache 3. Seizure
What is the difference between an intra-axial and an extra-axial mass?	An intra-axial mass is within the substance of the brain itself, whereas an extra-axial mass impinges on the brain.
What is the most common location of brain tumors in adults versus children?	Adults: Supratentorial (anterior or middle fossa) Children: Infratentorial (posterior fossa)
Which group has the higher incidence of seizures?	Supratentorial tumors (adults)
What is the most common intra-axial primary brain tumor in adults?	1. Astrocytoma 2. Meningioma
What is the most common intra-axial primary tumor in children?	1. Astrocytoma (#1) 2. Medulloblastoma

ASTROCYTOMA

How are astrocytomas graded?	There are a number of astrocytoma grading systems, but the most commonly used is a three-tiered system with:
	  Grade 1: Low-grade astrocytoma
	  Grade 2: Anaplastic astrocytoma
	  Grade 3: Glioblastoma multiforme (GBM)

Which grade is most common in adults versus children?	Grade 3 (GBM) is by far the most common primary brain tumor in adults. Grade 1 is most common in children.

What MRI findings are typical in low-grade glioma?

Low-grade gliomas typically do not enhance with contrast. High signal on the T2 or proton density images is always present. High-grade gliomas typically enhance on T1-weighted images. GBM's often have cysts or obvious areas of necrosis.

How do primary gliomas spread?

Spread is primarily through the white matter tracts of the brain and through the CSF pathways.

What is the cure rate for GBM?

There is no cure.

What is the treatment of GBM?

Chemotherapy and external beam radiation

What is the 1- and 2-year survival rate?

The 1-year survival rate is approximately 33%, whereas the 2-year survival rate is approximately 10%.

MENINGIOMA

What are the most common locations for a meningioma?

Parasagittal region and sphenoid bone

Is this tumor usually benign or malignant?

Benign

How does it cause focal neurologic deficits?

Compression (rather than invasion) of adjacent neural structures (an extra-axial tumor). Examples include unilateral exophthalmos and optic nerve compression.

What is the peak age of incidence for meningioma?

Age 45

What is the treatment of meningioma?

Surgical removal

What is the 5-year survival rate?

More than 90%. However, recurrences are common and often necessitate additional surgical interventions.

ACOUSTIC NEUROMA

What histologic type are the cells of an acoustic neuroma?

The term acoustic neuroma is actually a misnomer. The tumor cells are actually Schwann cells that typically arise from the vestibular portion, **not** the cochlear portion of cranial nerve 8.

What are the most common symptoms associated with acoustic neuroma?

1. Hearing loss (virtually all patients)
2. Tinnitus
3. Dysequilibrium

Other than hearing loss, what is the most common physical finding?

Roughly one-third of patients has loss of the corneal reflex.

Treatment of acoustic neuroma?

Surgical removal (via craniotomy and/or translabyrinthine approach)

PITUITARY TUMORS

What are the two general presentations of pituitary tumors?

1. Endocrine disturbance (excess ACTH, growth hormone, or prolactin)
2. Neurologic deficits due to mass effect

Do pituitary tumors most commonly arise in the anterior or posterior pituitary?

Anterior pituitary

Pituitary tumors are associated with what endocrine syndrome?

Multiple endocrine neoplasia I (MEN I).

What are the components of this syndrome?

1. Pancreatic islet-cell tumors
2. Nonsecretory pituitary adenomas
3. Parathyroid tumors

What is the common visual field defect associated with pituitary adenomas?

Bitemporal hemianopsia (due to compression of the medial retinal fibers at the chiasm)

What is the difference between Cushing syndrome and Cushing disease?	1. **Cushing syndrome** is the result of hypercortisolism. The findings include centripetal obesity (moon facies and buffalo hump), hirsutism and amenorrhea in women, thin fragile skin, hypertension, and glucose intolerance. 2. **Cushing disease** is caused by overproduction of ACTH by a pituitary adenoma.
What are the treatments for pituitary tumors?	1. For tumors that secrete prolactin, medical treatment with bromocriptine (dopamine agonist) is often helpful. 2. Otherwise, transsphenoidal surgery or open craniotomy, with or without adjuvant external beam irradiation, is the choice.

NEUROCUTANEOUS DISORDERS

What are the principal neurocutaneous disorders?	1. Neurofibromatosis (NF) 2. Tuberous sclerosis 3. von Hippel-Lindau disease 4. Sturge-Weber syndrome
Which of these disorders usually initially present with seizures?	Tuberous sclerosis, von Hippel-Lindau disease, and Sturge-Weber syndrome
Which is the most common NF?	NF-1, also called von Recklinghausen disease, represents 90% of cases of NF.
What is the inheritance pattern of this syndrome?	NF-1 has an autosomal dominant inheritance with nearly 100% penetrance.
What are the clinical features of this syndrome?	Café au lait spots, optic gliomas, cutaneous neurofibromas, and Schwann-cell tumors on any nerve.
What is the hallmark of NF-2?	Bilateral acoustic neuromas, which are virtually never seen in NF-1 patients
What is the most common cutaneous lesion in tuberous sclerosis?	Adenoma sebaceum (reddened nodules on face)

Where are the vascular malformations located in von Hippel-Lindau disease?

1. Retina (results in progressive vision loss)
2. Cerebellum (results in progressive ataxia)

What are the clinical features of Sturge-Weber syndrome?

1. Unilateral, cutaneous capillary angioma (a nevus flammeus or port-wine stain of upper face)
2. Leptomeningeal venous hemangiomas with intracranial calcification (classic "railroad track" appearance on x-ray)

ASSORTED NEURO-ONCOLOGY TOPICS

Where do chordomas commonly arise?

Chordomas are tumors of the notochord remnant. They typically arise at either end of the notochord (i.e., at the clivus and at the sacrum/coccyx)

What is a PNET and what is the most common type?

PNET stands for primitive neuroectodermal tumor. The most common type is the medulloblastoma, which accounts for about 20% of all intracranial tumors in children.

What are the most common metastases to the brain?

In descending order of frequency, they are:
1. Lung
2. Breast
3. Renal
4. Gastointestinal
5. Melanoma

Which primary brain tumors have potential to spread systemically?

Although brain tumors **rarely** spread systemically, medulloblastoma, meningioma, pineoblastomas, and choroid plexus tumors have the potential for systemic spread.

Which tumor generally arises from the roof of the fourth ventricle?

Medulloblastoma

Which tumor arises from the remnants of Rathke's pouch above the sella?

Craniopharyngioma (results in bitemporal field defects)

What are false lateralizing signs?

Clinical findings that are due to tumors but are not due to direct infiltration or compression of tumor. This situation may result in false localization of the primary tumor.

What are examples of false lateralizing signs?

1. CN III or CN VI palsy secondary to herniation syndromes
2. Ipsilateral hemiparesis secondary to compression of the contralateral cerebral peduncle against the tentorial ridge

CEREBROVASCULAR DISEASE

SUBARACHNOID HEMORRHAGE

What is its claim to fame?

Subarachnoid hemorrhage (SAH) is the most common type of intracranial hemorrhage (second most common being subdural hematoma). Fortunately, these hemorrhages are often of relatively little clinical significance.

What is the most common cause of SAH?

Trauma

What is the most common cause of spontaneous SAH?

Ruptured aneurysms represent nearly 80% of spontaneous SAH.

What are other causes of spontaneous SAH?

Arteriovenous malformation, tumor, vasculitides, and carotid artery dissection

Of patients with aneurysmal rupture, what is the 30-day mortality rate?

Approximately 50%!

Of survivors how many return to their premorbid level of function?

Only about 33%

What are the clinical features of SAH?

1. Sudden onset of "worst headache in life"
2. Nausea and vomiting
3. Syncope
4. Meningismus
5. Photophobia
6. Focal cranial nerve deficits
7. Bizarre behavior

What kinds of ocular hemorrhages accompany SAH?

Retinal hemorrhage, preretinal hemorrhage, and vitreal hemorrhage (Terson syndrome)

What other abnormalities accompany SAH?

Cardiac arrhythmias, ST- and T-wave changes on electrocardiogram, hyponatremia, and hydrocephalus

What is the workup for patients with a history suggestive of SAH?

CT scan (detects 95% of SAHs). If CT is negative, lumbar puncture (LP) is the most sensitive test for SAH.

How can a traumatic LP be distinguished from SAH?

1. Bloody CSF associated with a traumatic tap will clear in successive tubes.
2. Xanthochromia (yellow discoloration of CSF) will appear in most cases of SAH after 1 to 2 days.
3. The opening pressure in SAH is often high, whereas in a traumatic tap it is usually normal.

How useful is MRI in detecting SAH?

Not useful at all in the first 24 to 48 hours

What is the gold standard for imaging intracranial aneurysms?

Angiography

What is the most common location for an intracranial aneurysm?

Anterior communicating artery

What are the basic components of the initial therapy in SAH?

1. Telemetry and blood pressure monitoring with judicious blood pressure control
2. Seizure prophylaxis
3. Intravenous steroids (dexamethasone)
4. Analgesia
5. Calcium channel blockers
6. H$_2$-blockers

What is the usual cause of the delayed ischemic neurologic deficit that may be seen following SAH?	Vasospasm
When is the peak incidence of vasospasm after aneurysmal SAH?	The peak frequency of vasospasm is 6 to 8 days after SAH, but it can occur as early as day 1 and as late as day 17.
How common is vasospasm?	Symptomatic vasospasm can be seen in roughly 33% of aneurysmal SAH patients. (Up to 70% of angiograms show some degree of vasospasm after SAH.)
What are the clinical hallmarks of vasospasm?	Agitation, confusion, neurologic deficit (motor or speech), and/or decrease in level of consciousness
What is the treatment for vasospasm?	1. Hypervolemic therapy can lower the viscosity of the blood and hypertensive therapy can raise the blood pressure, with the goal of maximizing cerebral perfusion through spastic cerebral vessels. 2. In extreme cases, balloon angioplasty can be helpful.
What is a late complication of SAH?	Communicating hydrocephalus

NEUROVASCULAR MALFORMATIONS

What are the basic types of vascular malformations?	1. Venous angioma 2. Capillary telangiectasias 3. Cavernous angioma 4. Arteriovenous malformations (AVM)
What is the histological appearance of AVMs?	A tangle of abnormal vessels that do not have normal brain tissue between the vessels
What is the common presentation of AVMs?	Hemorrhage (peak age 15–20) and seizure are the most common features. Headache is rare.

| What are the treatment options for AVMs? | 1. Surgical excision
2. Intra-arterial embolization for AVMs that are not surgically accessible |

HYDROCEPHALUS

| What is hydrocephalus? | Hydrocephalus is the enlargement of cerebrospinal fluid (CSF) compartments of the brain and generally results from the obstruction of the reabsorption of CSF. |

| What are examples of congenital and acquired etiologies of hydrocephalus? | Congenital: Aqueductal stenosis, myelomeningocele, and Dandy-Walker syndrome
Acquired: Meningitis, intraventricular hemorrhage, and obstruction of CSF passage by tumor |

| How often is hydrocephalus due to overproduction of CSF? | Very rarely (e.g., choroid plexus papilloma) |

| What are the signs and symptoms of hydrocephalus? | Presentation of increasing ICP with headache, nausea, vomiting, and papilledema. Late signs of impending herniation include lethargy and diplopia. |

| What is the level of obstruction in communicating versus noncommunicating hydrocephalus? | Communicating: At the level of the arachnoid granulations
Noncommunicating: Proximal to the level of the arachnoid granulations |

| Why is it important to distinguish communicating from noncommunicating hydrocephalus? | The importance of this distinction is that pressure engendered by an obstruction can be relieved by lumbar puncture in the case of communicating hydrocephalus, whereas noncommunicating hydrocephalus generally requires ventricular drainage. |

| How is persistent hydrocephalus treated? | Ventriculoperitoneal shunting, or alternatively ventriculopleural, ventriculoatrial, or ventriculoureteral shunting |

CONGENITAL NEUROMALFORMATIONS

What is the most common congenital neuromalformation?

Spina bifida occulta

What is the most common form of neural tube defect?

Myelomeningocele (due to failure of closure of **posterior** neuropore)

What is spina bifida?

Congenital absence of posterior elements of spinal vertebra (e.g., spinous processes and lamina)

What differentiates spina bifida occulta from spina bifida aperta?

Occulta form has skin overlying the spinous defect.

What is an encephalocele?

Protrusion of neural tissue through a cranial defect (due to failure of closure of **anterior** neuropore)

What is the most common site of encephalocele?

Occipital region

What is a meningocele?

A membrane or skin-covered, cystic, posterior midline mass containing CSF and meninges (no neural elements)

What is the most common site of meningocele?

Lumbosacral region

INFECTIONS

BRAIN ABSCESS

What are the predisposing factors for brain abscess?

1. Systemic infection
2. Immunosuppression (AIDS, etc.)
3. Localized sinus infection
4. Cranial trauma
5. Pulmonary arteriovenous fistulae (Osler-Weber-Rendu syndrome).

What is the most common systemic source?

Pulmonary infections are the most common source, but in 25% of cases no source is identified.

What is the most common bacterial organism?	1. In adults, *Streptococcus* species predominate, but in 80% of cases, multiple organisms (often anaerobes like *Bacteroides*) are cultured. 2. In trauma, *Staphylococcus* is the most common pathogen. 3. In infants, gram-negative organisms predominate.
What is the most common organism in patients with AIDS?	*Toxoplasmosis*
What is the usual treatment of brain abscess?	Medical management of a **6- to 8-week** course of intravenous antibiotics is effective in many cases.
When is surgical intervention for abscess indicated?	1. If abscess exhibits significant mass effect (evidence of increased ICP or neurologic deficit) 2. If abscess approaches the ventricles (ventricular rupture carries high mortality)

SUBDURAL EMPYEMA

What are the most common sources?	1. Paranasal sinus infection 2. Otitis infection
With what dangerous vascular complication is subdural empyema associated?	Thrombophlebitis of the cerebral veins
What is the treatment?	Intravenous antibiotics and **emergent** surgical evacuation

PAIN SYNDROMES

What are the symptoms associated with trigeminal neuralgia (TN)?	The symptoms of trigeminal neuralgia (tic douloureux) are episodes of severe lancinating pain lasting only a few minutes. It is often triggered by facial or oral sensory stimuli.

Which divisions of the trigeminal nerve (CN V) are most commonly involved in TN?

V2 and V3 combined are most commonly involved, followed by V2 alone and V3 alone.

What are the major treatment modalities of TN?

1. Lesioning of the trigeminal nerves with radio frequency, glycerol, or balloon inflation has proved reliable.
2. Posterior microvascular decompression of the nerve from associated arteries and veins has also proved reliable.

What is a cordotomy?

Cordotomy is the interruption of the lateral spinothalamic tracts. It may be performed as an open procedure anywhere along the spinal cord or percutaneously at the level of C1–C2.

When is cordotomy useful?

It is most useful for unilateral pain below the nipple.

What nerve is trapped in carpal tunnel syndrome?

The median nerve

Under what structure is the nerve trapped?

The transverse carpal ligament

Which fingers typically experience decreased pinprick sensation in carpal tunnel syndrome?

The thumb and first and second fingers

What is Tinel's sign?

Tinel's sign is the production of pain or paresthesia in the aforementioned digits by gentle tapping over the transverse carpal ligament.

What is meralgia paresthetica?

MP is pain over the anterior lateral aspect of the thigh associated with entrapment of the lateral femoral cutaneous sensory nerve.

Which patients are at risk of meralgia paresthetica?

1. Obese patients
2. Patients undergoing iliac bone graft harvesting or abdominal surgery near the iliac crest

55

Urology

Sean P. Hedican, MD

SCROTUM AND SPERMATIC CORD

ANATOMY

What are the six major layers of the scrotal sac and the corresponding layers of the abdominal wall?

1. Skin
2. Dartos muscle
3. External spermatic fascia—Derived from external oblique
4. Cremaster muscle—Derived from internal oblique and transversus abdominis
5. Internal spermatic fascia—Derived from transversalis fascia
6. Tunica vaginalis—Derived from peritoneum

Which nerves receive sensory information from the scrotum?

1. Anterior scrotum
   Ilioinguinal nerve
   Genitofemoral nerve
2. Posterior scrotum
   Perineal division of the pudendal nerve
   Posterior femoral cutaneous nerve

What common surgical procedure can result in anesthesia of the scrotum, and why?

Inguinal hernia repair complicated by injury to the ilioinguinal nerve

INFECTIOUS DISORDERS

Fournier's Gangrene

What is Fournier's gangrene

Rapidly progressive gangrenous infection that usually involves scrotum, penis, and perineum (may extend up the abdominal wall)

What is the bacteriology?	Usually mixed infection of gram negatives and anaerobes
What is the most common origin of the infection?	Urinary tract (usually the urethra)
What are other origins?	Perianal, external genitalia, intra-abdominal process, and retroperitoneum
What is the clinical presentation?	Abrupt onset of severe pain and erythema of the scrotum, penis, and perineum. The patient often declines rapidly into florid sepsis.
What are the classic physical findings?	Erythema, induration, necrosis and crepitance of involved regions. Foul odor with a grayish discharge.
What is the mortality rate?	Fifty percent

What are the predisposing conditions?

1. Diabetes mellitus
2. Corticosteroid usage
3. Immune compromise
4. Alcohol abuse
5. Obesity
6. Trauma or surgery

What is the treatment?

1. Immediate surgical debridement— Possible diverting colostomy and/or suprapubic tube depending on the extent of debridement
2. Immediate initiation of triple IV antibiotic coverage (e.g., ampicillin, gentamicin, and flagyl)

CONGENITAL AND ACQUIRED DISORDERS

Hydrocele

Where does fluid accumulate in a hydrocele in relation to the layers of the scrotum?	Within the tunica vaginalis surrounding the testis; occasionally within the spermatic cord only
What is the clinical presentation?	Cystic scrotal mass that transilluminates; painless unless associated inflammation is present

What distinguishes a communicating from a noncommunicating hydrocele?

A communicating hydrocele is caused by a patent processus vaginalis that communicates with the peritoneal cavity

What are the unique features in the clinical presentation of a communicating hydrocele?

A congenital lesion that presents in infancy. The scrotal mass often enlarges at night because of the peritoneal connection

After what age does spontaneous closure of an infant hydrocele become unlikely?

After 1 year

What are the causes of a noncommunicating hydrocele?

1. Idiopathic
2. Epididymitis
3. Orchitis
4. Trauma
5. Neoplasm
6. Radiation

In a patient whose testicle is difficult to palpate, which additional study should be considered when evaluating a hydrocele, and why?

Scrotal ultrasound (U/S)—to rule out the possibility of an underlying testicular malignancy

What are the indications for treatment?

1. Tense hydrocele with vascular compromise of the testis
2. Scrotal discomfort
3. Cosmesis

What are the treatment options?

1. Definitive surgical repair to drain and evaginate the tunica vaginalis
2. Sclerotherapy (using a mixture of tetracycline dissolved in 5% bupivacaine)

What is a varicocele?

Abnormal dilatation of pampiniform plexus and internal spermatic veins of the spermatic cord

What are the physical findings?

A palpable "bag of worms" scrotal swelling; more prominent with standing or Valsalva maneuver

On which side does a varicocele occur, and why?

Left. Due to the more direct course of drainage into the renal vein and the increased incidence of incompetent venous valves

What is the clinical significance of a varicocele?

An association with infertility. Sperm counts and motility are decreased in 70% of subjects.

What are the indications for treatment?

1. Tender symptomatic varicocele
2. Ipsilateral testicular growth retardation
3. Decreased sperm motility
4. Oligospermia

What are the treatment options?

1. Open ligation (through either an inguinal or scrotal approach)
2. Percutaneous sclerosis, embolization, or balloon occlusion
3. Laparoscopic high ligation of the internal spermatic vein

What is the difference between neonatal torsion and torsion seen later in life?

Neonatal torsion involves the entire tunica vaginalis and enclosed spermatic cord structures (**extra**vaginal); later in life, the spermatic cord torses within the tunica vaginalis (**intra**vaginal).

Which classic abnormality seen in the scrotal layers makes a patient prone to torsion?

"Bell clapper deformity"—Horizontal position of the testis and high attachment of the tunica vaginalis to the spermatic cord resulting in a voluminous chamber in which the testicle can rotate. (Note: This deformity occurs bilaterally; thus, the contralateral testicle has an increased risk of torsion.)

What is the classic presentation?

1. Acute scrotal pain
2. Shortening and edema of the spermatic cord
3. Elevation of the testicle
4. Absent cremasteric reflex

What is the differential diagnosis?

1. Acute epididymitis—Usually associated with pyuria; rare prepubertally
2. Acute orchitis
3. Torsion of appendices testis or epididymis
4. Incarcerated hernia

In which direction does a testicle torse? Why is this important?

Toward the penis; the left testicle should be rotated clockwise and the right testicle rotated counterclockwise if a person is standing at the patient's feet attempting manual detorsion.

How is the torsion diagnosed?

1. Emergent surgical exploration—If suspicion is high, the best chance of preserving testicular viability is detorsion within the first 6 hours
2. Duplex Doppler U/S—Documents decreased intratesticular flow versus increased flow seen with epididymitis/orchitis
3. ^{99m}Tc-petechnetate scintillation scan—A 95% accuracy in documenting decreased uptake in a torsed testicle

What is the treatment?

Manual detorsion—This treatment may be attempted but rarely succeeds Delayed fixation of both testicles (orchiopexy) should still be performed to prevent subsequent torsion events
Surgical exploration:
1. If viable-appearing testicle on detorsion—Perform bilateral orchiopexy.
2. If nonviable appearing testicle—Perform ipsilateral simple orchiectomy and contralateral orchiopexy

TUMORS OF THE SPERMATIC CORD

What is the most common benign tumor of the spermatic cord?

Lipoma

What is the most common malignant tumor of the spermatic cord?

Rhabdomyosarcoma

What is the usual pathologic cell type of paratesticular rhabdomyosarcoma?

Embryonal

What is a common site of early metastasis?	Retroperitoneal LN
What is the treatment for paratesticular rhabdomyosarcoma?	Inguinal orchiectomy and radiologic evaluation of retroperitoneal lymph node (LN) status 1. If LN negative—Chemotherapy only (using vincristine and dactinomycin). No radiation. 2. If LN positive—Unilateral retroperitoneal lymph node dissection (RPLND). Chemotherapy using vincristine, dactinomycin and cyclophosphamide. Radiation therapy dependent upon the amount of residual local or nodal disease

PENIS AND MALE URETHRA

ANATOMY

What are the three erectile bodies of the penis and where does each originate?	1. Paired (2) corpora cavernosa—Just anterior to the ischial tuberosities 2. Corpora spongiosum—At the urogenital diaphragm and expands distally to form the glans penis
Within which corporal body does the urethra run?	Corpora spongiosum
What are the covering layers of the penis?	1. Tunica albuginea—Surrounds each corpora 2. Buck's fascia—Envelops all three corpora 3. Colles' fascia—Lies beneath the skin of the penis from the base of the glans to the urogenital diaphragm; continuous with Scarpa's fascia of the abdominal wall 4. Skin

What are the labeled structures or layers in the cross section of the penis?

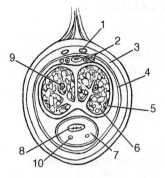

1. Cutaneous dorsal vein
2. Deep dorsal vein, artery, and nerve
3. Colles' fascia
4. Buck's fascia
5. Tunica albuginea
6. Corpora cavernosa
7. Corpus spongiosum
8. Urethra
9. Cavernosal artery and vein
10. Bulbourethral artery and vein

What are the three regional segments of the male urethra?

1. Prostatic urethra—Begins at the bladder neck, traverses the prostate and ends at the urogenital (UG) diaphragm; approximately 3 cm in length
2. Membranous urethra—Portion that traverses the UG diaphragm; these encircling muscles function as the external (voluntary) urethral sphincter; approximately 2 to 2.5 cm in length.
3. Penile urethra—Begins after the UG diaphragm and extends to the external meatus; often subdivided into bulbous and pendulous portions; approximately 15 cm in length.

Which branch of the hypogastric artery supplies the majority of blood to the penis?

Internal pudendal artery

What are the four main branches of the previously mentioned artery that supply the penis?

1. Deep cavernosal artery of the penis
2. Deep dorsal artery of the penis
3. Bulbar artery
4. Urethral artery

INFECTIOUS DISORDERS

Urethritis

What is the classic presentation of gonococcal urethritis?

Thick, yellow urethral discharge with dysuria

How long is the incubation period?

Usually 1 to 5 days

What is the causative organism?

Neisseria gonorrhoeae

How is gonorrhea diagnosed?

1. Positive Gram stain (urethral swab showing gram-negative diplococci within PMNs), **and/or**
2. Positive culture growth on a modified Thayer-Martin culture plate

What are the treatment options for gonococcal urethritis?

1. Procaine penicillin G IM with probenecid PO, or ceftriaxone IM, **plus**
2. Tetracycline PO for 7 days

What is the classic presentation of nongonococcal urethritis?

Thin, white, mucoid discharge with or without dysuria

How long is the incubation period?

From 1 to 3 weeks

What is the causative organism?

1. *Chlamydia trachomatis* (most common)
2. *Ureaplasma urealyticum*
3. *Mycoplasma hominis*
4. *Trichomona vaginalis*

How is nongonococcal urethritis diagnosed?

1. More than 4 PMNs per hpf in a urethral swab, **and**
2. Exclusion of gonococcal urethritis by Gram stain and culture

How can the presence of chlamydia be confirmed?

Conjugated monoclonal antibody test (sensitivity 93%; specificity 96%)

What are the treatment options for nongonococcal urethritis?

Seven-day course of tetracycline, minocycline, doxycycline, or erythromycin

What percentage of patients has treatment failure?

Between 20% and 40%

What are the complications of urethritis?	1. Urethral stricture 2. Epididymitis 3. Prostatitis 4. Impaired fertility

Genital Herpes

What is the classic presentation?	1. Primary infection—Grouped vesicles followed by painful shallow erosion lasting 4 days to 2 weeks; often associated fever, myalgias, and/or lymphadenopathy. Urinary retention can occur because of local pain. 2. Secondary infection—Usually constitutional and local symptoms less severe; reappearance of classic painful vesicles and ulcerations
What is the causative organism?	Herpes simplex virus (HSV) Type I or II
What is the regional predilection of each type?	In general, Type II infects the genital region and Type I infects the oral mucosal surface, but either organism can infect the external genitalia.
Where does the virus establish its latent infection?	Dorsal root ganglion
When does viral shedding occur?	When vesicles rupture; it can also occur when the patient is asymptomatic
Which diagnostic test is used?	1. Tzanck prep of a skin lesion often reveals the virus. 2. If Tzanck is negative, a viral culture should be obtained.
What is the treatment?	Seven-day course of acyclovir can be used to decrease severity and duration of primary and secondary infections.

Syphilis

What is the causative organism?	The spirochete *Treponema pallidum*

What is the incubation period?	Usually 2 to 4 weeks
What is the classic presentation?	1. Primary syphilis—Shallow painless ulcer with rolled borders (chancre) lasting 1 to 5 weeks; nontender uni- or bilateral inguinal adenopathy 2. Secondary syphilis—Copper-colored maculopapular lesions on the palms, soles, oral and anogenital region; generalized lymphadenopathy 3. Tertiary (latent) syphilis—No outward signs of disease; all organs of the body are now infected. Late manifestations in the CNS, peripheral nerves (tabes dorsalis), and/or aortic arch (aortitis)
How is syphilis diagnosed?	1. Demonstration of spirochetes on dark-field exam of chancre scrapings 2. Rapid plasma reagin (RPR) serology test for syphilis may be negative for up to 3 weeks after appearance of the chancre. 3. Fluorescent treponema antibody–absorption (FTA–ABS) test
What is the most sensitive test available?	FTA-ABS
What is the treatment of the following diseases: **Primary syphilis?**	Benzathine penicillin G 2.4 x 10^6 U IM (one dose)
Secondary syphilis?	Same as previously described
Neurosyphilis?	Administer one dose a week for 3 weeks

Chancroid

What is the clinical presentation?	Deep, ragged, painful ulcer or ulcers; foul smelling with unilateral or bilateral adenopathy
What is the causative organism?	*Haemophilus ducreyi*

How long is the incubation period?	From 1 to 5 days following exposure (usually intercourse)
How is chancroid diagnosed?	Usually clinical. Occasionally the organism grows from cultures of the ulcer.
What is the treatment?	Erythromycin PO for 7 days or ceftriaxone IM x 1 dose

Lymphogranuloma Venereum

What is the classic presentation?	Painless primary papule or vesicles that ulcerate, then heal; fixed matted unilateral adenopathy develops and can form multiple draining fistulae.
What is the causative agent?	*Chlamydia trachomatis* (an obligate intracellular organism)
How long is the incubation period?	From 1 week to 3 months following exposure (usually intercourse)
What are the associated complications from deep extension of the disease?	Extension to deep pelvic nodes can cause proctitis, rectal strictures, proctocutaneous or proctovaginal fistulae.
How is lymphogranuloma venereum diagnosed?	Immunofluorescent serologic testing
What is the treatment?	Tetracycline (or erythromycin) PO 3 weeks

CONGENITAL AND ACQUIRED DISORDERS

Hypospadias

What is hypospadias and why does it occur?	Meatal opening on ventral surface of the penis proximal to the tip of the glans; occurs due to abnormal fusion of urethral folds
What are the different types?	Defined by location of the meatal opening: glanular (proximal glans), coronal (coronal sulcus), penile (shaft of the penis), penoscrotal, and perineal

What is the incidence?	About 1 in 300 male births
With what other condition is hypospadias usually associated?	Chordee—Curvature of the penis due to asymmetric corporal length
What other tests should be performed in children with penoscrotal or perineal hypospadias?	1. Karyotyping to determine genetic sex 2. Electrolyte and cortisol testing to exclude adrenogenital syndrome
What structures can be used to reconstruct the urethra?	1. Foreskin and local penile skin (most common) 2. Free dermal skin graft 3. Bladder mucosa 4. Buccal mucosa
Which two substances released from a normal fetal testis are required for virilization of the internal ductal system, what cells produce them, and what is the function of each?	1. Müllerian inhibiting substance—Produced by the Sertoli cells; causes regression of the female ductal (müllerian) system 2. Testosterone—Produced by the Leydig cells; causes ipsilateral wolffian duct to develop into the epididymis, vas deferens, and seminal vesicle
At what week of gestation does phenotypic differentiation of the external genitalia occur?	Eighth week (i.e., the external genitalia are identical up until that point)
In the absence of gonads or appropriate hormonal stimulus, into which phenotype do the external genitalia differentiate?	Female
Which three elements are required for virilization of the external genitalia?	1. Production of testosterone 2. Conversion to 5-dihydrotestosterone 3. Normal androgen receptor activity
What are the four major classifications of ambiguous genitalia in order of frequency, and what are their corresponding karyotypes?	1. Female pseudohermaphroditism—46XX female exposed to exogenous or endogenous androgen in utero 2. Mixed gonadal dysgenesis—Most have the mosaic karyotype 45XO/46XY and a streak gonad on one side with a testis on the other

3. Male pseudohermaphroditism—46XY male with deficient testosterone production, decreased 5-α reductase, or abnormal androgen receptor activity

4. True hermaphrodite—Most are 46XX but 46XY mosaic patterns are also seen. Gonadal tissue of both sexes must be present.

Which type of female pseudohermaphroditism is most common?

Congenital adrenal hyperplasia

Which enzyme defect in cortisol synthesis is most commonly associated with this condition?

21-OH (hydroxylase) deficiency

Which life-threatening condition can be seen in association with this disorder?

Addisonian crisis—80% may have severe mineralocorticoid deficiency with resultant hyponatremia, hyperkalemia, hypoglycemia, and eventually life-threatening acidosis, dehydration, and hypovolemic shock.

What is the acute treatment of this disorder?

1. Normal saline fluid replacement
2. Appropriate electrolyte and glucose replacement after volume stabilization
3. Hydrocortisone sodium hemisuccinate (HSH) bolus with an additional HSH added to saline infusion
4. Desoxycorticosterone acetate IM if hyponatremia and hyperkalemia present

What is the chronic treatment of this disorder?

1. Maintenance glucocorticoids—Hydrocortisone PO
2. Mineralocorticoids (fludrocortisone) and increased dietary salt for salt losers
3. Surgical repair of ambiguous genitalia prior to 1 year of age

What is included in the evaluation of a child with ambiguous genitalia?

1. History—Information about prior pregnancies, family history of abnormal sexual development, medications during pregnancy, etc.

2. Physical exam—Checking for palpable gonads, uterus on rectal exam, and evidence of congenital adrenal hyperplasia such as dehydration, hypertension, and hyperpigmentation
3. Plasma measurements:
   17-OH-progesterone
   11-deoxycortisol
   Testosterone (before and after HCG stimulation should be evaluated in male pseudohermaphrodites)
4. Urinary measurements:
   17-OH ketosteroids
   Tetrahydro-11-deoxycortisol
5. Radiographic evaluation:
   Ultrasound—Evaluation of internal ductal system and the presence of a uterus.
   Genitogram—Injection of contrast into the urogenital sinus to further define the anatomy as well as the internal ductal system
6. Chromosomal analysis—Either karyotyping of peripheral leukocytes or Barr body analysis of the buccal smear

Which enzyme deficiency is usually associated with presentation of dehydration versus hypertension?

Dehydration—21-OH deficiency
Hypertension—11-b-OH deficiency

Which measurements are elevated in 11-b-OH deficiency?

11-deoxycortisol in plasma and tetrahydro-11-deoxycortisol in urine

Which measurements are elevated in 21-OH deficiency?

17-OH progesterone in plasma and 17-OH ketosteroids

Urethral Stricture

What are the common causes of stricture disease in the male urethra?

1. Prior episodes of urethritis
2. Infection and mucosal ischemia from indwelling urethral catheters
3. Mucosal trauma from prior urologic instrumentation or surgery
4. External trauma—Pelvic fracture, straddle injury, gunshot wound, etc.

Which region of the urethra is most commonly strictured as a result of cystoscopy?

Fossa navicularis from traumatic introduction of the cystoscope

What are the common presenting complaints?

1. Decreased urinary stream
2. Post-void dribbling, spraying, or splayed stream
3. Chronic urethral discharge
4. Symptoms of infection
5. Dysuria

What are the complications of stricture disease?

1. Varying degrees of obstruction to urine flow, which can progress to obstructive nephropathy
2. Recurrent bouts of cystitis and prostatitis due to urinary stasis
3. Periurethral abscesses and urethral fistula
4. Bladder calculi

How are strictures evaluated?

1. Physical exam—Assessment of the degree of induration of the urethra and extent of fibrosis extending into the corpora
2. Retrograde urethrogram or voiding cystourethrogram
3. Ultrasound evaluation of the upper tracts (if evidence of renal compromise)
4. Cystoscopic evaluation—Determining the extent and location of the narrowing

What are the treatment options?

1. Dilation (A narrow hollow cannula with a screw attachment at the end (filiform) can be passed blindly or under direct cystoscopic vision through the stricture, and followers of increasing size are sequentially attached and passed through the stricture.
2. Direct vision internal urethrotomy (DVIU)—A cold knife is used to incise the stricture at 12 o'clock if it is short, and a catheter is then placed. The patient is taught intermittent catheterization to maintain patency.

3. Surgical reconstruction—Depending on the site and the length this procedure may involve primary anastomosis, a patch graft urethroplasty, or a free urethral graft.

Paraphimosis

What is paraphimosis?

A foreskin with a narrowed opening that forms a tight band behind the coronal ridge when retracted, leading to inflammation and inability to pull the foreskin back over the glans

What is the primary sequela?

Further painful swelling of the glans and foreskin, which can lead to decreased arterial flow and necrosis of the glans

What is the treatment?

1. Manual compression of the glans for 5 to 10 minutes after a penile block with 1% lidocaine may reduce its size enough to allow the foreskin to be pulled back into place.
2. If this fails, a dorsal slit is made in the constricting foreskin followed by a formal circumcision when inflammation has resolved. Antibiotics should also be administered.

Priapism

What is priapism

Prolonged, often painful, erection not associated with sexual desire and lasting 4 or more hours

What are the etiologic classifications?

1. Primary (idiopathic)
2. Secondary
   Intracavernous injections for impotence (PGE, phentolamine, papaverine)
   Hematologic (sickle-cell disease, leukemia, hypercoagulable states)
   Oral agents (alcohol, psychotropics, antihypertensives)
   Neurogenic (anesthesia and spinal cord injury)
   Traumatic injury of cavernosal artery within corporal tissue causing traumatic arteriovenous (A-V) fistula

(pelvic fracture or laceration from injection therapy)
Malignant metastasis to the corpora

What are the two most common causes?

1. Primary (> 50%)
2. Intracavernous injections for impotence

What are the differences between classic low-flow priapism and the high-flow priapism associated with pelvic trauma?

Low-flow priapism
1. Usually painful
2. Dark, poorly oxygenated, blood obtained on corporal aspiration
3. Associated with sludging, thrombosis, and fibrosis if not treated within 24 hours

High-flow priapism:
1. Usually painless
2. Red, well oxygenated blood obtained on corporal aspiration
3. An A-V fistula exists between the injured cavernosal artery and the corpora resulting in a persistent erection without associated sludging and thrombosis

What are the classic treatment approaches to priapism associated with sickle cell disease?

1. Oxygenation
2. Hydration
3. Alkalinization
4. Needle corporal aspiration followed by intracavernous injection of a dilute α-adrenergic compound (e.g., phenylephrine or epinephrine)
5. Blood transfusion to increase Hgb to > 10 mg/dl and decrease Hgb S to < 30%

What is the general treatment approach to other types of low-flow priapism?

1. Aspiration of 10 to 20 ml of corporal blood followed by injection of dilute α-adrenergic compound every 5 minutes up to 10 doses (Note: Blood pressure and heart rate should be monitored; use caution in patients with cardiac or cerebrovascular disease.)
2. Surgical shunting (Multiple procedures have been described to shunt blood from the corpora cavernosa to the spongiosum or directly to the venous system.)

What is a simple, effective shunting procedure?

Winter's shunt—Shunt generated by passing a 16-gauge IV or Tru-Cut needle several times through the glans into the cavernosal bodies

Peyronie Disease

What is Peyronie disease?

Fibrosis and plaque formation in the tunica albuginea of the corpora cavernosa, often associated with pain and a bending deformity with erection

What are the common etiologic theories?

1. Vasculitic immune-mediated process
2. Repeated microtrauma to the tunica during intercourse

What percentage of these conditions will resolve spontaneously?

Approximately 50%

What is the medical treatment if no resolution?

1. Vitamin E
2. Potassium para-aminobenzoate (Potaba)
3. Dimethyl sulfoxide (DMSO)
4. Intralesional steroids (triamcinolone 40 mg)

What is the surgical treatment?

Excision of plaque and placement of a dermal patch graft with or without a penile prosthesis
(Note: This treatment is usually reserved for patients with angulation too severe for successful intercourse.)

URETHRAL TRAUMA

Which part of the urethra is usually injured in association with a pelvic fracture?

Membranous urethra; separation from the apex of the prostate due to shear forces at the prostatomembranous junction

Which physical findings are usually present in this situation?

1. Abdominal tenderness
2. Blood at the urethral meatus
3. A pelvic hematoma on rectal exam, with an associated "high-riding" prostate due to the displacing force of the expanding hematoma

Which procedure should be performed if blood is present at the urethral meatus?

Retrograde urethrogram with water-soluble contrast (Note: Catheterization should **not** be attempted in this situation because it can convert a partial disruption into a complete one, increase pelvic bleeding, or introduce infectious organisms into the hematoma.)

What is the treatment?

1. Open placement of a suprapubic catheter and inspection of the bladder for areas of rupture; perioperative antibiotic coverage
2. Delayed primary urethral reconstruction via a perineal approach after 3 months of suprapubic diversion

(Note: Immediate open reconstruction is advocated by some authors; however, persistent bleeding and tissue edema from the acute injury make this approach more difficult.)

What complications are seen from membranous urethral injury, and how does the acuity of repair (delayed vs. immediate) affect the observed incidence of each complication?

1. Stricture: Delayed repair 5% Immediate repair: 50%
2. Incontinence: Delayed repair: < 5% Immediate repair: 33%
3. Impotence: Delayed repair: 10% Immediate repair: 50%

What portion of the urethra is usually injured with straddle injuries?

Bulbous urethra

To what level can extravasation of urine and blood extend, and what limits it?

Into the perineum in a butterfly distribution and along the abdominal wall. Spread is limited only by Colles' fascia.

What is the treatment of minor urethral lacerations?

Open or percutaneous suprapubic cystotomy with voiding study performed 7 days after injury

What is the treatment of major urethral lacerations?

1. Drainage of scrotum, perineum, or lower abdomen if massive urinary extravasation
2. IV antibiotic coverage

3. Suprapubic cystotomy; should be left in place for 2 to 3 weeks prior to a voiding study

TUMORS

Urethral Cancer

What is the most common histologic type?

Squamous cell carcinoma

What are the risk factors?

1. Stricture disease
2. Chronic irritation and infection

What is included in the evaluation?

1. Urethroscopy with transurethral biopsy or brushings
2. Pelvic CT to evaluate lymph node status
3. Chest x-ray

What is the difference in pattern of nodal drainage between anterior and posterior tumors?

Anterior (distal) tumors—Drain to the inguinal chain.
Posterior tumors—Drain to the pelvic nodes (e.g., external iliac, obturator, and hypogastric).

What are the treatment options?

1. Transurethral resection—For superficial, low-grade lesions of the proximal penile or prostatic urethra
2. Segmental urethrectomy and reanastomosis—For superficial, low-grade cancers of the penile urethra
3. Partial penectomy—For invasive lesions of the distal urethra
4. Extended en bloc cystectomy including proximal urethrectomy with excision of the pubic symphysis and subsymphyseal soft tissue—For proximal invasive bulbous or membranous urethral lesions

Is therapeutic lymph node dissection effective?

Occasional long-term survivors with inguinal or pelvic lymph node metastases have been reported following lymphadenectomy.

Penile Cancer

What is the incidence of penile cancer in:

    United States males?   < 1% of all malignancies

    African males?   10% to 20%

What is the theoretic cause for this difference?   Difference in circumcision rates and hygiene. Exposure to smegma buildup is thought to be carcinogenic.

What is another name for squamous cell carcinoma in situ?   Bowen disease

What is its appearance?   Red plaque with encrustations

What is the incidence of visceral malignancy in association with this condition?   Approximately 25%

What is the most common location of invasive penile squamous cell carcinoma?   Glans

What is the primary route of dissemination?   Lymphatic

How does location of the primary tumor affect its pattern of spread?
1. Prepuce and shaft—Superficial inguinal nodes
2. Glans and corporal bodies—Superficial and deep inguinal nodes

(Note: Due to extensive cross-communications, penile lymphatic drainage is bilateral.)

What percentage of patients present with palpable nodes?   > 50%

What percentage of this enlargement is secondary to inflammation?   Approximately 50%

What is the classic Jackson staging system for penile cancer?

Stage I: Tumor involving glans or prepuce only
Stage II: Tumor involving the penile shaft
Stage III: Operable nodal involvement
Stage IV: Inoperable local, nodal, or distant metastasis

What does the metastatic workup include?

1. CXR
2. Bone scan
3. Abdominal pelvic CT scan

What is the treatment of:
  CIS?

Conservative treatment with fluorouracil cream or neodymium/Yag laser

  Carcinoma of prepuce?

Circumcision only—provided the margin is adequate

  Carcinoma of glans or distal penile shaft?

Distal penectomy with a 2-cm margin

  Proximal lesions?

If unable to maintain enough length for direction of urinary stream or sexual function, then total penectomy with perineal urethrostomy

What is the management of regional lymphadenopathy?

Antibiotics for 4 weeks; if still palpable, bilateral ilioinguinal node dissection

What is the management of nonpalpable lymph nodes in the setting of penile carcinoma?

Low-stage tumor—Nodal observation
High-stage tumor—Limited sentinel node biopsy

TESTIS AND EPIDIDYMIS

ANATOMY

From the epithelial lining of what structures within the testis do spermatozoa develop?

Seminiferous tubules

What is the arterial blood supply to the testis?

1. Internal spermatic artery
2. Cremasteric artery
3. Artery of the vas

What is the clinical significance of this collateral blood supply?	Blood flow via the collaterals is often sufficient to allow ligation and division of the internal spermatic artery to gain extra length during orchiopexy (Fowler-Stephens orchiopexy)
What are the primary lymphatic drainage sites of the:	
Right testicle?	Interaortocaval LNs followed by precaval, pre-aortic, and paracaval LN's
Left testicle?	Left para-aortic LNs followed by the preaortic LNs
Where is the epididymis located in relation to the normal testicle?	Along the posterolateral surface of the testis

INFECTIOUS DISORDERS

Acute Epididymitis

What are the two main etiologies of epididymitis and the respective organisms associated with each?	1. Retrograde spread of the sexually transmitted diseases *Chlamydia trachomatis* and/or *Neisseria gonorrhoeae* 2. Reflux of infected urine through the ejaculatory ducts and vas deferens during voiding. Infected urine results from an initial bout of cystitis or prostatitis caused primarily by *Enterobacteriaceae* or *Pseudomonas*.
What is the classic presentation?	1. Acute onset of severe pain and swelling of the epididymis 2. Fever 3. Cloudy, infected urine 4. Delayed swelling and tenderness of the entire testicle
What are the laboratory findings?	1. Elevated WBC count with a left shift 2. Pyuria 3. Gram-negative diplococci seen within the WBC's in patients with gonorrhea

In contrast to torsion, does elevation of the testicle toward the pubic symphysis worsen or lessen the pain of epididymitis?

Pain is lessened with epididymitis and worsened with torsion (Prehn's sign).

What are the complications of epididymitis?

1. Epididymal and possible testicular abscess formation
2. Chronic epididymitis

What is the treatment of acute epididymitis in young, sexually active, men?

Ceftriaxone IM, followed by doxycycline, tetracycline, or ciprofloxacin PO for 3 weeks (Note: For nongonococcal causes, erythromycin is another alternative.)

What is the treatment of nonsexually transmitted infections?

Trimethoprim-sulfamethoxazole PO for 4 weeks or ciprofloxacin PO for 3 weeks

Acute Orchitis (not associated with acute epididymitis)

What viral infection occurs most commonly in association with acute orchitis?

Mumps (seen in 20%–35% of patients with parotitis)

What percentage of these cases are bilateral?

Only 10%

Does orchitis occur in prepubertal patients with mumps?

No

What are the classic presenting symptoms?

1. Swollen, tender testicle and scrotum; the epididymis is not involved initially
2. Fever
3. Symptoms of orchitis begin 3 to 4 days after the onset of parotitis.

[Note: In contrast to epididymo-orchitis, the urinalysis (UA) is typically normal.]

What medical advance has made this disease much less common?

Development and routine administration of mumps vaccine

What are the complications?

1. Impaired spermatogenesis (in 30% of patients)
2. Testicular atrophy

What is the treatment?

1. Symptomatic treatment such as scrotal support, heat, and anti-inflammatory agents
2. Administration of corticosteroids is believed to have an advantageous effect on decreasing the inflammatory destruction of the seminiferous tubules.

ACQUIRED AND CONGENITAL DISORDERS

Ectopic Testis

What is the difference between an ectopic testis and a cryptorchid testis?

An **ectopic** testis has descended along an abnormal path, whereas a **cryptorchid** testis has descended along the normal course but has not made it out of the inguinal canal.

What are some observed ectopic positions and which is most common?

1. Superficial inguinal (most common)—Migrates cephalad and lateral to the external ring
2. Femoral—Lies in the superficial femoral triangle
3. Perineal—Lies in the perineum anterior and lateral to the anus
4. Penile—Lies subcutaneously at the base of the penis
5. Crossed descent—Both testicles descending through the same inguinal canal

Cryptorchid Testis

What are the etiologic theories?

1. Deficient maternal gonadotropin stimulation
2. Intrinsic gonadal defect, making the testicle nonresponsive to gonadotropin stimulation
3. Abnormal gubernaculum formation

Why is it important for the testicles to descend?

The scrotal location is 1 to 2 degrees cooler than the rest of the body, a condition that is necessary for normal spermatogenesis to occur.

What is the incidence of cryptorchidism in:
    Preterm infant?

30%

Full-term infant?	3.5%
1 year?	0.8%
Adulthood?	0.8%

What is the single most common factor that causes a misdiagnosis of a cryptorchid testis?	A retractile testis from cremasteric contraction
If a testis is not retractile or ectopic and it cannot be palpated, what are the possible locations?	1. Canalicular—Located between the internal and external rings 2. Intraabdominal—Located proximal to the internal ring 3. Absent
How is bilateral cryptorchidism distinguished from bilateral anorchia?	Baseline testosterone levels are obtained. Then human chorionic gonadotropin (hCG) is given for 3 days; if testicular tissue is present, an elevation in serum testosterone will be seen
By what age should intervention for a cryptorchid testis be initiated, and why?	By 1 year of age; after this: 1. Spontaneous descent is extremely unlikely 2. Significant histologic changes (fibrosis) occur, greatly increasing the risk of diminished fertility of the involved testis
What is the incidence of neoplasm formation in a cryptorchid testis versus a normally descended testis?	35 to 50 times greater in a cryptorchid testis
Does the timing of orchiopexy affect the risk of neoplasm formation in a cryptorchid testis?	No (Note: However, it improves the ability to examine the testis.)
Due to its abnormal position and lie, what other complication can be seen in association with an undescended testis?	Torsion (especially in the enlarged postpubertal testis)

What is the medical treatment of cryptorchid testes?

1. hCG stimulation—Increasing testicular testosterone production, which may stimulate testicular descent Note: Varying success rates range from 15% to 50%.
2. Gonadotropin-releasing hormone (Gn-RH), specifically luteinizing hormone-releasing hormone (LH-RH), which is theorized to overcome the low basal LH levels seen in association with cryptorchidism (for 4 weeks delivered as a nasal spray) Note: Varying success rates range from 6% to 70%.

What is the surgical treatment of cryptorchid testes?

1. Standard orchiopexy—Incision is made in the groin, the external oblique muscle is split, the peritoneum of the hernia sac is dissected off the vessels and ligated, and the testicle is delivered to the base of the scrotum through a separate skin incision. (Note: A Prentiss maneuver may be performed by opening the floor of the inguinal canal and dividing the inferior epigastric vessels to gain additional length.)
2. Fowler-Stephens orchiopexy—In cases with insufficient length to bring the testicle into the scrotum, the internal spermatic artery is clamped and, if adequate testicular collateral blood supply is demonstrated, the artery is divided and the testis is brought into the scrotum.
3. Laparoscopic orchiopexy
4. Testicular autotransplantation—The testicular artery is anastomosed to the inferior epigastric artery and the testicle is transplanted into the scrotum. (Note: This technically difficult procedure has relatively poor success rates.)

TUMORS

Epididymal Adenomatoid Tumors

At what age do these tumors usually present?	Third and fourth decades
What is the classic presentation?	Round discrete, usually painless, mass that can be found in any region of the epididymis
In what other regions are these lesions found?	1. Tunica albuginea of the testicle 2. Spermatic cord
What is the histologic appearance?	Acidophilic epithelial-like cells in a collagenized stroma
What are the theories of etiology?	1. Reaction to injury 2. Some ultrastructural similarities to mesotheliomas
What is the lifetime probability of a white United States male developing a testicular tumor?	Approximately 0.2%
What percentage of these are germ-cell tumors?	From 90% to 95%
On which side is testicular cancer more common?	Right
What percentage of men with testicular cancer have a history of unilateral or bilateral cryptorchidism?	Approximately 10%
In which age-group is testicular cancer most common?	Between 20 and 40 years old
What is the classic presentation?	**Painless** testicular swelling or nodularity noted incidentally in a young man
What percentage have metastatic disease at presentation?	Approximately 50%

What are the two main divisions of germ-cell tumors?

1. Seminomatous
2. Nonseminomatous

What are the different histologic germ-cell tumors as they relate to patterns of normal germ-cell development?

1. **Unfertilized Gamete**—Seminoma: Malignant spermatogonia
2. **Fertilized Gamete (Intraembryonic differentiation)** Embryonal: Malignant germ cell at the embryo stage Teratoma: Malignant germ cell at the more differentiated fetal stage
3. **Fertilized gamete (Extraembryonic differentiation)** Choriocarcinoma: Malignant germ cell developing along a placental pathway Yolk Sac Tumor: Malignant germ cell developing along a yolk sac pathway

What percentage of tumors are of a single histologic type?

Approximately 60%

What are the stages in the modified Boden-Gibb staging system?

Stage A (I): Tumor involving testis and cord only
Stage B (II): Tumor metastasis to regional nodes only
Stage C (III): Distant lymphatic or soft tissue metastases

What are the three subtypes of seminomas and the relative incidences of each?

1. Classic seminoma (85%)—Sheets of large clear cells
2. Anaplastic seminoma (5 to 10%)— Increased nuclear pleomorphism with three or more mitoses per high-power field
3. Spermatocytic seminoma (5%–10%)—Condensed chromatin and round nuclei

What are the normal cells of origin, values, half-life, and cancer types in which the following tumor markers are elevated: Human chorionic gonadotropin (hCG)?

1. Normally produced by syncytiotrophoblast cells of the placenta

2. Normal values < 5 mIU/ml
3. Half-life of 24 hours
4. Elevated in all patients with choriocarcinoma, 40 to 60% with embryonal, and 5 to 10% of seminomas

Alpha-fetoprotein?

1. Normally produced by the fetal yolk sac
2. Normal values < 40 ng/ml
3. Half-life 5 to 7 days
4. Produced by embryonal carcinoma and yolk sac tumors (Note: It is not made by pure choriocarcinoma or seminoma.)

What is the most frequent mixed cell type?

Teratocarcinoma (a mixture of teratoma and embryonal carcinoma)

What is the most frequent cell type seen in children?

Yolk sac tumor

What is the typical pattern of regional LN metastases for:

Right testicular cancer?

Interaortocaval LNs followed by precaval and preaortic LNs at the level of the renal hilum

Left testicular cancer?

Para-aortic and preaortic LNs at the level of the renal hilum
(Note: Right to left crossover metastases are unusual; retrograde spread to the iliacs can be seen with advanced right- or left-sided disease.)

Why is the incision for radical orchiectomy made in the groin rather than transcrotally?

Incision of the scrotal skin and tumor spillage could, theoretically, result in early inguinal metastases. This incision also allows high ligation of the spermatic cord as it enters the internal ring.

What is included in the evaluation of a patient with testicular cancer?

1. CXR
2. Abdominal CT
3. hCG (pre-orchiectomy and 1 week post-op)
4. AFP (pre-orchiectomy and 4 weeks post-op)
5. Radical orchiectomy for local control and tissue diagnosis

What is the percentage of false-negative metastatic evaluations?	From 20% to 30%
What is the treatment based on stage in seminoma?	Stage I: Radical orchiectomy, external beam radiation to the periaortic and ipsilateral pelvic nodes Stage II: Radical orchiectomy, external beam radiation. If nodal disease > 10 cm is present, the patient is treated with primary BEP chemotherapy (bleomycin, etoposide, and *cis*-platinum). Stage III: Radical orchiectomy and primary BEP chemotherapy (Note: Residual retroperitoneal masses > 3 cm after chemotherapy will contain cancer in approximately 40% of cases and RPLND should be performed.)
What is the treatment based on stage in nonseminomatous germ cell tumors?	Stage I: Radical orchiectomy followed by modified RPLND or surveillance. If microscopic nodal metastases are discovered in the specimen, the patient should receive two cycles of BEP chemotherapy Stage II: Radical orchiectomy, followed by BEP (3 to 4 cycles); if a residual mass > 3 cm and normalization of tumor markers occurs then RPLND is performed [Note: If tumor markers do not normalize salvage chemotherapy (*cis*-platinum, VP-16, bleomycin, and ifosfamide) should be administered followed by RPLND] Stage III: Radical orchiectomy, followed by BEP (3 to 4 cycles); a RPLND is performed for residual bulky disease. Salvage chemotherapy is performed as described previously.
When is surveillance considered in stage I nonseminomatous germ cell tumors?	1. The patient is reliable. 2. Tumor is confined within the tunica albuginea. 3. No vascular invasion is present. 4. Tumor markers normalize following orchiectomy. 5. No radiographic evidence of metastatic disease is present.

KIDNEYS

ANATOMY

What are the dimensions of a normal adult kidney?	Vertical: 10 to 12 cm Transverse: 5 to 7 cm Anteroposterior: 3 to 4 cm

Which intra-abdominal organs are in contact with the labeled regions of anterior surface of the kidneys?

1. Adrenal gland
2. Liver
3. Colon
4. Ileum
5. Adrenal gland
6. Stomach
7. Pancreas
8. Ileum
9. Spleen
10. Colon

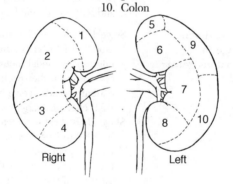

Right   Left

What is the normal location of the upper pole of each kidney relative to the:
1. **Vertebral bodies?**
2. **Ribs?**

1. Left: T12; Right: Top of L1
2. Left: To 11th rib; Right: To 11th interspace

What is the clinical significance of the location of the upper pole with regard to:

Penetrating chest trauma?

Stab wounds to the lower chest require renal evaluation

Surgical incision?

Inadvertent entry into the pleural space can occur during a standard flank incision (Obtain a post-operative CXR)

Access to large renal tumors can be facilitated by a thoracoabdominal incision which enters the chest and splits the diaphragm to expose the upper pole.

Which structures are contained within Gerota's fascia?
1. Perirenal fat
2. Kidney
3. Adrenal gland
4. Ureter
5. Gonadal vessels

What is the order of structures in the renal hilum (anterior to posterior)?
Renal vein > Renal artery > Renal pelvis

The main renal artery:
Arises at which vertebral level?
L2. Just below the takeoff of the superior mesenteric artery

Divides into what five segmental branches?
Anterior division: Apical, upper, middle, and lower;
Posterior division: Posterior
Segmental divisions are named after the region of parenchyma they supply)

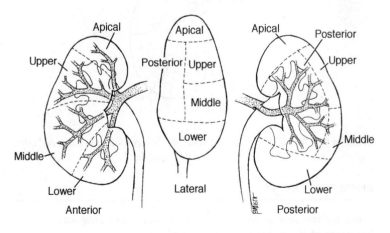

Which segmental branch is the first and most constant branch?
Posterior

What collateral drainage exists to the left renal vein?	1. Left inferior phrenic vein 2. Left adrenal vein 3. Left ascending lumbar vein 4. Left gonadal vein
What is the clinical significance of collaterals?	Surgical ligation or occlusion of the left renal vein by tumor thrombus may be tolerated in some cases.
What are the components of the intrarenal collecting system?	1. Minor (tertiary) calyx—seven to nine cup-shaped structures surrounding the papilla of each renal pyramid 2. Infundibula—The narrowing of each minor calyx, which coalesces to form a major calyx 3. Major calyx—The coalescence of several infundibula to form these two or three larger drainage channels 4. Renal pelvis—Main collection chamber, which can be completely contained within the substance of the kidney or can be a large saccular extrarenal structure

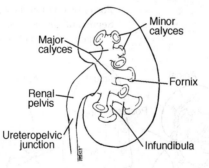

What is the fornix?	The delicate rim of each calyx or "edge of the wineglass"

RENAL PHYSIOLOGY

What are the four major functions of the kidney?	1. Excretion of metabolic waste products 2. Reabsorption of necessary solutes 3. Secretion of unnecessary solutes 4. Endocrine function (e.g., erythropoietin, renin, and vitamin D)

What percentage of normal cardiac output do the kidneys receive?	From 20% to 25%
What is renal clearance?	Rate at which the kidney excretes a substance in relation to its plasma concentration (ml/min)
What does clearance indirectly measure?	Glomerular filtration
How is clearance calculated?	C = (U x V)/P C = clearance (ml/min) U = urine concentration of index substance (e.g., inulin or Cr) P = plasma concentration of index substance V = volume of urine flow in 1 minute [Note: To compare values for persons of different size, GFR is standardized per unit of body surface (1.73 m^2)]
Which formula allows a quick calculation of creatinine (Cr) clearance based on serum Cr?	[(140 - age) x (weight)]/(72 x SCr) SCr = serum creatinine (mg/dl)
How is the calculation altered for women?	Multiply by 0.85
What is the normal adult value for Cr clearance?	75 to 120 ml/min
Where is most filtered sodium reabsorbed in the nephron?	Proximal tubule (70%–80% of the filtered load)
Is this an active or passive process?	Active. The energy for the function of the Na$^+$ K$^+$-pump comes from aerobic metabolism.
Where is renin produced, and what stimulates its release?	The myoepithelial (juxtaglomerular) cells of the afferent arteriole. Release is stimulated by: 1. Decreased renal perfusion 2. β-adrenergic stimulation 3. Decreased salt delivery to the distal tubule

What is the major effect of renin?

Renin converts angiotensinogen to angiotensin I which is then converted to angiotensin II in the lung. Angiotensin II is a potent vasoconstrictor and also stimulates the release of aldosterone.

Where is aldosterone produced, and what are its major effects?

Zona glomerulosa of the adrenal cortex; it acts upon the collecting tubule causing:
1. Increased Na^+ reabsorption
2. Increased H^+ secretion
3. Increased K^+ secretion

How much acid must the kidney excrete per day to maintain acid–base balance?

0.3 to 1.0 mEq/kg/day

How does the kidney accomplish this task, and in what part of the nephron do these mechanisms occur?

1. Reclamation of filtered HCO_3^-—Primarily in the proximal tubule
2. Generation of new HCO_3^-—Via net acid excretion (The collecting tubule secretes H^+ ions, which are then bound to titratable buffers, e.g., PO_4 and NH_4^+.)

INFECTIOUS DISEASES

Acute Pyelonephritis

What is the classic clinical presentation?

Chills, fever, unilateral or bilateral costovertebral angle tenderness, tachycardia, and irritative voiding symptoms are often present (urgency, frequency, and dysuria).

What is seen on urinalysis (UA)?

Increased levels of WBC's, RBC's, and WBC casts. Bacterial rods or cocci are often seen.

What causative agents are isolated from the urine?

E. coli (most common), *Klebsiella, Proteus, Enterobacter, Pseudomonas, Serratia, Citrobacter, Streptococcus faecalis,* and *Staphylococcus aureus*

What is found on the surface of many bacteria that infect the urinary tract?

Pili or fimbriae that facilitate binding to the urothelium

Is an intravenous pyelogram (IVP) indicated in patients with presumed pyelonephritis?

Only if there is a possibility of obstruction

What percentage of IVPs are abnormal?

Approximately 25%

Which IVP abnormalities may be seen?

1. General or localized parenchymal enlargement
2. Delayed contrast excretion
3. Nonobstructive collecting system dilation (may be due to endotoxin paralysis of ureteral motility)
4. Cortical striations (possibly due to intratubular occlusion by purulent debris)

What is the treatment of uncomplicated infection in a healthy patient?

1. Hydration
2. Fluoroquinolone or trimethoprim-sulfamethoxazole if outpatient therapy can be attempted (2-week course)
3. Adjustment of antibiotics if necessary based on organism sensitivities from urine culture and clinical response
4. Follow-up urine culture before discontinuing antibiotics

What is the treatment of uncomplicated infection in a debilitated patient or hospital/catheter-associated infection?

1. Hydration as tolerated
2. Rapid treatment of complicating conditions (e.g., stone or obstruction)
3. IV ampicillin and aminoglycoside versus third-generation cephalosporin (2-week course)
4. Adjustment of antibiotics if necessary based on sensitivities or response
5. Follow-up urine culture before discontinuing antibiotics

Chronic Pyelonephritis

In contrast to acute pyelonephritis, how is this chronic process defined and diagnosed?

Small, contracted, scarred kidney associated with tubulointerstitial disease due to repeated bacterial infections. This diagnosis is radiologic rather than clinical.

With what condition is chronic pyelonephritis most often associated?

Childhood vesicoureteral reflux (VUR)

What is the clinical presentation?	May be asymptomatic, present with recurrent acute infectious episodes, or display signs of renal insufficiency (e.g., hypertension)
What are the IVP findings?	Atrophic kidney with cortical scarring and calyceal clubbing

Pyonephrosis

What is pyonephrosis?	An obstructed, infected, hydronephrotic kidney filled with purulent debris
What is the clinical presentation?	Flank pain, fever, and chills. Patients are often floridly septic.
What is the treatment?	1. Emergent drainage via percutaneous nephrostomy 2. Triple IV antibiotic coverage (e.g., ampicillin, aminoglycoside, and flagyl)

Xanthogranulomatous Pyelonephritis

What is xanthogranulomatous pyelonephritis?	A chronic bacterial infection of the kidney associated with calculi and often partial obstruction/dilation of the collecting system
What is the classic histology?	Localized yellow nodules composed of inflammatory infiltrate and foamy macrophages
What is the target population?	Middle-aged or older women
What is the usual presentation?	Fever, flank tenderness, anorexia, or malaise
What are the common laboratory findings?	1. Anemia—65% 2. Leukocytosis—50% 3. Pyuria 4. Microhematuria 5. Positive urine culture (*P. mirabilis* and *E. coli* are the most often isolated organisms)

What other disease process of the kidney is this mistaken for, both clinically and radiographically?	Renal cell carcinoma
What is the treatment?	Simple nephrectomy (Note: Partial nephrectomy may be attempted in cases of isolated polar involvement.)

CONGENITAL AND ACQUIRED DISORDERS

Renal Tubular Acidosis (RTA)

From what defect does type I renal tubular acidosis (RTA) result?	Distal tubule is unable to secrete H^+ ions across a large gradient (Note: Proximal tubule's ability to absorb HCO_3^- is not affected.)
What are the clinical features?	1. Systemic acidosis 2. Inappropriately alkaline urine 3. Hypokalemia/hyperchloremia 4. Calcium phosphate stone formation (70%) due to hypercalciuria in the setting of low urinary citrate levels
What is the treatment?	1. Increased fluid intake 2. Sodium bicarbonate or potassium citrate to alkalinize the urine (Note: Effect can be monitored by measuring urinary citrate.)
From what defect does type II RTA result?	Proximal tubule decreased HCO_3^- reabsorptive ability, which causes ECF contraction, Cl⁻ reabsorption, and acidosis
What are the clinical features?	1. Acidosis 2. Initially, due to increased HCO_3^- loss, the urine is alkaline; but as metabolic acidosis (i.e., whole body HCO_3^- loss) worsens, the urine will acidify. 3. Hypokalemia/hyperchloremia 4. No nephrocalcinosis since citrate excretion is relatively normal
What is the treatment?	Sodium bicarbonate or potassium citrate to correct HCO_3^- loss

Pelvic Kidney

What is the incidence of pelvic kidney?

1:500 to 1:1000 (the most common location of ectopic kidney)

In which sex and on which side is this condition found most commonly?

Boys. Left side

Are these kidneys normal?

Approximately 50% are pathologic with poor function. Reflux is common.

What is the treatment?

Correction of the reflux, if possible. Most remain asymptomatic or require nephrectomy.

Adult Polycystic Kidney Disease

What is the pattern of inheritance?

Autosomal dominant—100% penetrance

What are the classic clinical findings?

1. Bilateral flank masses—Large cystic enlargement of both kidneys
2. Hypertension (65%)
3. Renal failure
4. Lumbar pain
5. Recurrent pyelonephritis—Infection of cysts is also common.

What are two associated nonrenal lesions and what is the incidence of each?

1. Hepatic cysts (33%)
2. Aneurysm of the circle of Willis (10% to 40%)

What is the treatment?

1. General conservative measures (e.g., low protein diet—0.5 to 0.75 g/kg/day)
2. Cyst decompression or drainage—Indicated for infection, obstruction, or severe distension and compression of the diaphragm
3. Nephrectomy—Indicated in a few patients with severe hemorrhage, complicated infections, or obstruction
4. Dialysis versus renal transplant (progression to renal failure common)

Infantile Polycystic Kidney Disease

What is the genetic mode of transmission and the sex predilection?

Autosomal recessive; no sex predilection

What is the incidence?

1 in 40,000 live births

What are the appearance and onset of cystic disease?

Bilateral small subcapsular and cortical cysts, which enlarge and become spherical as the child ages.

When does it present?

Always becomes evident during childhood

How does the age at onset of symptoms correlate with the severity of disease?

Patients who present early tend to have worse disease with early-onset renal failure.

What other organ is also always involved, and what are the associated lesions?

Liver—Biliary ectasia or periportal fibrosis

What is the treatment?

Management of renal and hepatic failure, which may include renal transplant and portal systemic shunting if the child survives

Multicystic Dysplastic Kidney Disease (MCKD)

What is the typical renal appearance in this order?

Grape-like cystic structures replace the kidney, which has little true stroma and no calyceal system.

What are the etiologic theories?

1. Severe hydronephrosis secondary to atresia of the ureter or pelvis
2. Failure of union between the ureteric bud and metanephric blastema

On which side is this disorder more typically seen?

Left

What is the presentation of MCKD?

Diagnosis may be via prenatal ultrasound or later in life on evaluation of abdominal pain, hematuria, or hypertension

What abnormalities of the contralateral kidney are associated with MCKD?	1. Ureteropelvic junction obstruction 2. Obstructive megaureter
What name is given to the syndrome of bilateral MCKD?	Potter syndrome
What are the clinical features of this syndrome?	1. Classic facial appearance (blunted nose, prominent skinfold beneath each eye, depression between lower lip and chin, and broad ear lobes) 2. Bilateral multicystic dysplastic kidneys 3. Oligohydraminos
What is the prognosis of this syndrome?	Incompatible with life
What test is most useful in differentiating MCKD from severe hydronephrosis?	Dimercaptosuccinic acid (DMSA) renal scan—Function (i.e., radioisotope clearance) is usually present with hydronephrosis and not with MCKD.
What is the treatment?	Controversial. Most advocate conservative management unless severe flank pain is present. Then the best management is with simple nephrectomy. (Note: Current literature does not show convincing evidence of increased risk of Wilms' tumor or hypertension [HTN] in these patients.)

Renal Artery Stenosis

What is renovascular HTN?	Renin-dependent HTN that is reversible with surgical correction of the renal arterial lesion
What degree of stenosis is usually required?	Critical stenosis > 70%
What are the two major pathologic lesions that produce renal artery stenosis?	1. Atherosclerosis (60%) 2. Fibromuscular disease (40%)

Which region is most commonly diseased with atherosclerosis?

Orifice and proximal 2 cm of the renal artery

What are the three types of FMD?

1. Medial fibroplasia
2. Perimedial fibroplasia
3. Intimal fibroplasia

Which types of FMD are commonly progressive?

Perimedial and intimal fibroplasia

Which type of FMD is most common and what is the target population?

Medial fibroplasia. Women 20 to 50 years old

What is the classic appearance on angiography?

"String of beads" appearance

Which type of FMD may be seen in children?

Intimal fibroplasia (involves the midportion of the renal artery)

What are some clues that hypertension may be due to renovascular disease?

1. Age of onset < age 25 or > age 45
2. No family history of HTN
3. Accelerated, treatment refractory, HTN
4. Systemic evidence of atherosclerosis
5. Evidence of renal insufficiency in association with angiotensin-converting enzyme (ACE) inhibitors
6. Hypokalemia due to elevated aldosterone production

Identify and describe the diagnostic studies used to evaluate for renal HTN.

1. Plasma renin activity profile—Plasma renin plotted against 24-hour urine sodium excretion while on a normal diet. (Antihypertensives must be discontinued 2 weeks prior to study.)
2. Captopril challenge test—Plasma renin measured before and after captopril PO administered
3. Captopril renogram—After captopril administration, a decrease in ^{99m}Tc-DTPA uptake in the affected kidney is noted, with preservation of ^{131}I-hippuran and ^{99m}Tc-DTPA in the normal kidney.
4. Renal vein renin sampling—Each renal vein and the IVC are sampled;

in the diseased kidney, renin increase is documented by (RV-IVC) / IVC > 0.50 whereas in the contralateral normal kidney (RV-IVC) / IVC = 0.
5. Arteriogram or digital subtraction imaging—Performed for surgical planning or during angioplasty

What percentage of patients with renovascular HTN will have elevations in plasma renin?

Approximately 80%

What are the criteria for a positive captopril stimulation test?

Renovascular HTN can be diagnosed with a specificity of 100% and sensitivity of 95% if:
1. Stimulated plasma renin activity >12 ng/ml/hr,
2. Increase in plasma renin activity of > 10 ng/mL/hr, *and*
3. 150% increase of plasma renin activity or 400% increase if initial value < 3 ng/ml/hr

What is the medical treatment of renovascular HTN?

1. ACE inhibitors are the most effective agents, but can lead to renal insufficiency if bilateral disease exists
2. Calcium channel blockers
(Note: Medical therapy is usually limited to patients not amenable to surgery.)

What are the surgical treatment options for renovascular HTN?

1. Angioplasty
2. Surgical vascular reconstruction
3. Nephrectomy

Which lesions are best treated with angioplasty?

1. FMD
2. Nonosteal atherosclerotic lesions

Which lesions are best treated with surgical vascular reconstruction?

Osteal or complex lesions not amenable to or failing angioplasty

Which lesions are best treated with nephrectomy?

1. Patients with absent function and failed revascularization in the diseased kidney and normal function on the opposite side
2. Patients who are not candidates for revascularization and are at high risk from their uncontrolled HTN

RENAL TRAUMA

Which physical exam findings suggest the presence of a renal injury?

1. Flank tenderness
2. Fractures of the lower ribs or transverse processes of the lumbar spine
3. Flank ecchymosis or crepitance
4. Gunshot or stab wound over lower rib cage

Which studies are used for the evaluation of renal trauma?

1. Intravenous pyelogram (IVP)—A scout KUB film should be taken, followed by injection of 1 to 2 ml/kg of contrast. A film is taken at 5 minutes, with delayed images if the patient's condition allows.
2. Abdominal CT—Should be obtained if the patient's condition is stable and other injuries are suspect

How accurately does the IVP stage renal injuries?

From 60% to 80%

What are the three classes of renal trauma and what is the relative percentage of each?

Class I (minor parenchymal injury)— Contusion, subcapsular hematoma. (65%–70% of injuries)

Class II (major parenchymal injury)— Complex parenchymal laceration often with a resultant perirenal hematoma *or* extension into the collecting system (10% to 15%)

Class III (shattered kidney *or* a major pedicle injury)—This condition can be a vascular thrombosis or disruption (10%).

What are the absolute indications for renal exploration?

1. Persistent hypotension with an expanding flank mass
2. Pulsatile or expanding retroperitoneal hematoma found at laparotomy
3. Major renal vasculature injury in a solitary kidney or in both kidneys

Which structures should be isolated first during renal exploration, and how is this achieved?

The renal vessels in the retroperitoneum by making an incision over the aorta just superior to the inferior mesenteric vein

TUMORS

Wilms' Tumor

What percentage of pediatric GU malignancies are Wilms' tumors?	Approximately 95%
What is the median age at diagnosis?	Age 3
What structures in the kidney proliferate abnormally and are thought to give rise to Wilms' tumor?	Metanephric blastemas
Do "favorable" or "unfavorable" cell types dominate?	Favorable (90% of cases)
What are the favorable cell types?	1. Multilocular cysts (MLC) 2. Congenital mesoblastic nephroma 3. Rhabdomyosarcoma
What are the unfavorable cell types?	1. Anaplastic 2. Rhabdoid 3. Clear cell sarcoma ("bone-metastasizing" Wilms' tumor)
What are the main predictors of poor prognosis?	1. Unfavorable histology 2. Stage
What are the classic presenting signs?	1. Large abdominal or flank mass 2. Hypertension (60%) 3. Hematuria (25%)
What is the classic staging system?	Stage I—Kidney only with complete excision Stage II—Beyond kidney with complete excision Stage III—Residual nonhematogenously spread tumor in the abdomen (positive LN or massive tumor spillage) Stage IV—Distant hematogenous metastases Stage V—Bilateral renal involvement

What does treatment of tumor depend on?	Stage and histology

What is the treatment of:

Stage I and favorable histology?	Simple nephrectomy then double agent chemotherapy (actinomycin D and vincristine)
Stage I unfavorable and stages II to V favorable histology?	Simple nephrectomy, 1080 cGy plus a boost dependent upon residual disease, and triple drug chemotherapy (addition of adriamycin)
Stage II to IV unfavorable histology?	Simple nephrectomy, radiation dose on a sliding scale dependent upon age, and triple drug chemotherapy (Addition of cyclophosphamide if diffuse anaplastic histology)
Stage IV?	Renal sparing surgery together with combination chemotherapy and radiation therapy (Note: In the presence of lung metastasis, patients also receive whole lung irradiation, 1200 cGy]

Oncocytoma

What is the distinguishing histologic feature?	Uniform cells with eosinophilic granular cytoplasm due to increased number of mitochondria
Are the cells benign or malignant?	Benign
Which characteristic angiographic feature is often noted?	"Spoke wheel" configuration of arterioles (Note: This appearance can also be seen in renal cell cancers.)
What is the treatment?	Due to the similar radiographic and clinical appearance with renal cell cancer, these lesions are usually treated with nephrectomy.

Renal Cell Carcinoma (RCCa)

What percentage of solid renal tumors are RCCa?	Ninety percent!

What are the cells of origin in the kidney?	Proximal convoluted tubule
What are the classic presenting signs?	1. Hematuria (60%) 2. Pain (40%) 3. Weight loss (35%) 4. Anemia (30%) 5. Flank mass (25%) 6. HTN (20%)
What is the staging system of RCCa?	Stage I: Tumor confined to kidney Stage II: Tumor extending into the perinephric fat but contained within Gerota's fascia Stage IIIA: Tumor thrombus within the renal vein or inferior vena cava (IVC) Stage IIIB: Tumor involving regional LN Stage IIIC: Tumor thrombus within renal vein or IVC and regional LN involvement Stage IVA: Tumor extending into adjacent organs other than the adrenal Stage IVB: Distant metastases
What is the single best diagnostic study?	Abdominal CT with contrast
Which feature is this study helpful in detecting?	Perirenal spread, LN spread (80% sensitivity), renal vein involvement (90%), and IVC extension (95%)
Which methods are best for determining the extent of tumor thrombus extension?	1. Magnetic resonance imaging (MRI) is excellent in most cases. 2. Cavogram remains the gold standard for those cases that are equivocal on MRI.
What is the treatment of: **Stage I and II cancers?**	Radical nephrectomy (Note: Partial nephrectomy can be attempted in cases of single renal units or small polar lesions)
Stage III cancers?	Radical nephrectomy (Note: Cardiac bypass techniques and hypothermic arrest can be used to remove tumors with caval extension)

Stage IV?	Palliative nephrectomy or embolization can be performed for severe pain, bleeding, or paraneoplastic syndromes (Note: Spontaneous regression of metastases has been reported in < 1% of patients undergoing nephrectomy.)
What is removed in a radical nephrectomy?	All structures contained within Gerota's fascia, including regional LNs.
What is the 5-year survival rate in the presence of positive lymph nodes?	Fifteen percent
What is the 5-year survival rate in the presence of caval extension?	Fifty-five percent
When is chemotherapy effective against RCCa?	It is never effective as RCCa is extremely chemoresistant.
Which clinical trials for advanced RCCa are currently being investigated?	Tumor debulking via radical nephrectomy in addition to: 1. Interleukin-2, 2. γ-interferon, or 3. Gene therapy: granulocyte macrophage colony-stimulating factor (GM-CSF) producing tumor vaccine

ADRENALS

ANATOMY

Which arteries supply the adrenals and where does each originate?	1. Superior adrenal artery—Arises from the inferior phrenic artery 2. Middle adrenal artery—From the aorta 3. Inferior adrenal artery—From the renal artery
Which feature of the right adrenal vein makes surgical removal of the right adrenal gland more difficult than the left?	It is short and empties directly into the IVC, whereas the left adrenal vein empties into the left renal vein.

What is the zonal anatomy of the adrenal, including the major steroid product of each zone?

1. Zona glomerulosa (outer cortical zone)—Produces aldosterone in response to angiotensin II or hyperkalemia
2. Zona fasciculata (middle cortical zone)—Produces cortisol in response to ACTH
3. Zona reticularis (inner cortical zone)—Produces dehydroepiandrosterone (DHEA) in response to ACTH
4. Adrenal medulla—Functions like a presynaptic sympathetic nerve ending secreting norepinephrine (20%) and epinephrine (80%)

CONGENITAL AND ACQUIRED DISORDERS

Cushing Syndrome

What steroid product is overproduced in this syndrome?

Cortisol

What are the characteristic features?

1. Truncal obesity
2. Moon facies
3. Cutaneous striae
4. Easy bruisability
5. HTN
6. Osteoporosis
7. Hypokalemia

What are the major etiologies of Cushing syndrome and the relative frequencies of each?

1. Cushing disease (50%–60% of cases)
2. Cortisol-producing adrenal adenoma or adenocarcinoma (30%–40%)
3. Ectopic ACTH (< 5%)

Why are cortisol levels increased in each etiology?

1. Cushing disease: Overproduction of ACTH by a pituitary adenoma resistant to cortisol feedback leads to bilateral adrenal hyperplasia. High-dose dexamethasone suppression test will result in a reduction of cortisol production.
2. Adenoma or adenocarcinoma: Cortisol production is not regulated by ACTH levels.

3. Ectopic ACTH: Extra-adrenal tumors of the lung, breast, thymus, and pancreas produce ACTH, which is not responsive to even high-dose dexamethasone suppression.

What is the treatment of each etiology?

1. Cushing disease: Transsphenoidal hypophysectomy
2. Adenoma or adenocarcinoma: Adrenalectomy
3. Ectopic ACTH: Surgical excision of the tumor

TUMORS

Adrenocortical Carcinoma

What percentage of adrenocortical carcinomas are functioning?

Eighty percent

What are the clinical manifestations?

1. Cushing syndrome
2. Virilization in women

Where do these lesions usually metastasize?

Lungs, liver, and LN

What is the only effective form of therapy?

Complete surgical excision

Pheochromocytoma

What is the cell of origin?

Neural crest cells

What percentage arise in extra-adrenal sites, and what are examples of these sites?

Fifteen percent. Near the renal pedicle, the organ of Zuckerkandl, or the bladder wall

What percentage of these are malignant?

Five percent

What situation determines malignancy?

Metastases in the bone, lungs, or liver

What is the classic presentation?	1. Hypertension—Either sustained (66%) or paroxysmal (33%) 2. Anxiety episodes (sudden anxiety, diaphoresis, and palpitations) 3. Headaches (in association with blood pressure elevations)
Which diagnostic studies and results are seen with pheochromocytoma?	1. 24-hour urinary catecholamine metabolites—Elevated levels of vanillylmandelic acid (VMA), normetanephrine, and metanephrine 2. Plasma catecholamines—Elevations of epinephrine, norepinephrine, or both may be seen. 3. Abdominal CT—Most lesions are > 2 cm. 4. Metaiodobenzylguanidine (MIBG) scan—A guanethidine derivative which concentrates in neuroendocrine tissue also helps isolate extra-adrenal disease.
What does an isolated elevation of plasma epinephrine suggest, and why?	The methylating enzyme necessary for converting norepinephrine to epinephrine is present only in medullary tissue. Isolated elevations of epinephrine imply that the tumor arises in the adrenal medulla, ectopic medullary tissue, or the organ of Zuckerkandl.
What is the treatment of pheochromocytoma?	1. Preoperative α-blockade (prazosin or phentolamine) and volume expansion 2. Surgical excision

Neuroblastoma

What is its claim to fame?	Most common solid tumor in children
What percentage are diagnosed in the first year of life?	Fifty percent
From what cells of origin do they arise?	Neural crest cells of the adrenal medulla or sympathetic ganglia
What percentage of patients present with metastatic disease?	Sixty percent

Sites of metastases?	Bone marrow (most common), liver, LN, lung, and orbit
What is the classic presentation?	Pain (40%), abdominal distention, weight loss, malaise, proptosis from metastasis to the orbit, and anemia
Which substances are usually elevated in a neuroblastoma patient's urine?	1. Dopamine 2. VMA 3. Homovanillic acid (HVA)
What is the treatment of patients with distant metastasis?	Surgical excision, local radiation, and combination chemotherapy (cisplatin, etoposide, doxorubicin, and cyclophosphamide)

PROSTATE

ANATOMY

What percentage of the prostate gland is: **Fibromuscular stroma?**	Forty percent
Glandular epithelial tissue?	Sixty percent
From what embryonic structures does the prostate originate?	Urogenital sinus (with the exception of the central zone and ejaculatory ducts, which are of wolffian origin)
What are the major zones of the prostate?	1. Peripheral zone—Together with the central zone, it makes up 95% of the gland. 2. Central zone—Surrounds the ejaculatory ducts and is found in the posterior portion of the gland 3. Transition zone—Surrounds the urethra and verumontanum 4. Anterior fibromuscular area—Forms a cap over the anterior surface of the prostate and has some sphincteric action
In which zone does benign hyperplasia arise?	Transition zone

In which zones do adenocarcinomas arise?	Peripheral (60%–70%), transition (10%–20%), and central (5%–10%) zones
Which vessel supplies the majority of blood to the prostate?	Inferior vesical artery. Branches supply the seminal vesicle, then the artery divides into the urethral group (supplying bladder neck and periurethral gland) and the capsular group (supplying the outer prostate).
Which nerve roots contribute autonomic innervation to the prostate and seminal vesicles?	Parasympathetic visceral efferents from S2 to S4 and sympathetics from T11 through L2
Which structures mark the macroscopic location of the nerves supplying innervation to the cavernosal bodies?	The lateral pedicle of the inferior vesical artery marks the location of the "neurovascular bundle," which runs dorsolaterally (outside Denonvillier's fascia) in the lateral pelvic fascia

INFECTIOUS DISORDERS

Acute Bacterial Prostatitis

What are the causative organisms?	1. *E. coli* 2. *Pseudomonas* species 3. *Streptococcus faecalis*
What are the routes of infectious spread?	1. Retrograde ascent up the urethra 2. Reflux of infected urine into the prostatic ducts 3. Direct lymphatic spread from the rectum 4. Blood-borne infection
What are the usual presenting symptoms?	Perineal or low sacral pain, fever, chills, irritative voiding symptoms, and varying degrees of obstruction
What is found on digital rectal exam?	Swollen, firm, indurated, and extremely tender prostate
Should a prostatic massage be performed to express the infecting pathogen, and why?	No. Vigorous prostatic manipulation can result in significant bacteremia, and urine cultures alone are often positive.

If the patient cannot empty his bladder completely, should a Foley catheter be inserted?	No, for the reason mentioned previously. If significant residual urine exists, a percutaneous *suprapubic* tube should be placed.
What are the complications of prostatitis?	1. Septic shock 2. Pyelonephritis 3. Epididymitis 4. Prostatic abscess
What is the treatment of prostatitis in an uncompromised patient?	Trimethoprim-sulfamethoxazole PO for 30 days (Note: Antibiotics are altered if cultures show lack of sensitivity or if a poor clinical response is noted.)
What is the treatment of prostatitis in a septic or otherwise compromised patient?	1. Gentamicin IV or IM and ampicillin IV for 1 week 2. Thereafter, oral agents for 30 days

Prostatic Abscess

What is the difference between causative organisms seen today and those seen prior to widespread antibiotic use?	The primary causative agent is now *E. coli* whereas *N. gonococcus* predominated in the pre-antibiotic era.
What is the etiology?	Usually a complication of acute bacterial prostatitis
What are the clinical symptoms?	Identical to those of acute prostatitis
What are the findings on digital rectal exam?	Tender, fluctuant prostate with asymmetric enlargement
What is the best imaging modality for confirming the diagnosis?	Transrectal ultrasound
Which patient group has a much higher incidence of abscess formation?	AIDS patients
What is the treatment of prostatic abscess?	1. Surgical drainage via transurethral unroofing or transperineal drainage 2. Antibiotic coverage—Similar to that for acute prostatitis

CONGENITAL AND ACQUIRED DISORDERS

Benign Prostatic Hyperplasia (BPH)

What is BPH?	Hyperplastic growth of prostatic adenoma in the transition zone of the prostate, causing varying degrees of obstructive and irritative voiding symptoms.
In which age-group does the disease usually first become manifest?	Age 60 to 69
What are the histologic findings?	Fibrostromal, acinar, and fibroadenomal nodule formation in the periurethral (transition) zone
What are the etiologic theories?	1. Renewed ability of the urogenital sinus mesenchyme to proliferate 2. Altered relationship between the levels of estrogen and testosterone, which can lead to stromal proliferation and subsequent epithelial proliferation
Which two mechanisms are responsible for the symptoms associated with BPH?	1. Static enlargement of the gland 2. Increased smooth muscle tone within the prostate mediated by α-receptors
What is the presentation of BPH?	1. Diminished caliber and force of the urinary stream 2. Intermittency of urination 3. Hesitancy of urination 4. Incomplete voiding 5. Post-void dribbling 6. Urinary retention 7. Recurrent infections
Which substances or events can trigger urinary retention in someone with an enlarged prostate?	1. Alcohol consumption 2. Hypothermia 3. Anticholinergic agents 4. Psychotropic drugs 5. α-adrenergic agonists

What is the most dangerous late complication of severe prostatic obstruction?

Obstructive nephropathy—Renal insufficiency secondary to prolonged obstruction

What are the classic findings on digital rectal exam?

Large, flat, elevated smooth prostate

Does size correlate with the degree of obstruction?

No. Patients with normal size glands can have significant symptoms.

What should laboratory evaluation of patients with significant BPH include?

1. Serum electrolytes (BUN/Cr)
2. UA and culture
3. Prostate-specific antigen (PSA)—Early evaluations reveal a 10-fold greater contribution to PSA by prostate cancer versus BPH, although significant elevations can be seen with BPH alone.

What is the indication for biopsy of prostate?

PSA > 4.0 ng/ml (to rule out prostate cancer)

What is the most useful noninvasive study for proving significant obstruction?

Flow rate study—In the absence of neuropathic changes, a maximum flow of < 10 ml/s when voided volumes are > 100 ml implies that significant intravesical obstruction exists.

What are the goals of radiologic evaluation in patients with evidence of obstruction?

1. Calculate the volume of BPH.
2. Evaluate the upper tracts for obstruction or tumors.
3. Calculate residual urine volume.

Which radiologic study is used most commonly?

Ultrasonography

Why should cystourethroscopy be performed in men who choose surgical treatment?

1. To rule out stricture disease
2. To assess prostate size and configuration

What are the medical management options and the rationale for their use?

1. Alpha blockade—To decrease smooth muscle tone (e.g., prazosin and terazosin)
2. Hormonal manipulation—Based on the initial observation that reduction in prostate size secondary to

castration improved the symptoms of BPH

5-α–reductase blockade (e.g., proscar)—Inhibits conversion of testosterone to dihydrotestosterone

Antiandrogen (e.g., flutamide)— Blocks nuclear androgen receptor

LHRH agonists (e.g., Lupron)— Suppresses pituitary release of LH

What are the absolute indications for definitive surgical therapy for BPH?

1. Urinary retention
2. Hydronephrosis
3. Recurrent urinary tract infections
4. Bladder calculi

What are the surgical options?

1. Open prostatectomy—Enucleation of hyperplastic tissue
2. Transurethral resection of the prostate with electrical current (TURP)
3. Transurethral vaporization of the prostate with electrical current or laser
4. Transurethral incision of the prostate (TUIP)—For small obstructing glands two deep cuts can be made at 5 and 7 o'clock instead of a formal resection
5. High-intensity focused ultrasound (HIFU)—A rectal source is used to focus a high-intensity ultrasonic beam to ablate the prostate. (Under experimental investigation)

Which surgical treatment remains the gold standard?

TURP

What conditions are best managed by simple open prostatectomy?

1. Glands that are > 100 g or prostatic urethra > 6 cm
2. Significant bladder calculi and a large gland
3. Need for diverticulectomy

What are the acute complications following TURP?

1. TURP syndrome (2%)—Due to opening of venous sinuses and excess absorption of irrigant causing hyponatremia, hypervolemia, cerebral edema, and seizures (if serum sodium < 120 mEq/L)

2. Postoperative hemorrhage (4%)
3. Clot retention (3%)
4. Urinary tract infection (2%)

What are the delayed complications following TURP?

1. Retrograde ejaculation
2. Impotence (4% to 30%)

TUMORS

Prostate Cancer

What is its claim to fame?

Most common malignancy in American men

How does it rank in cancer-related deaths?

Second most common cause of cancer mortality in American men

What are the major risk factors?

1. Age
2. Race—African-Americans have a twofold increased risk
3. Family history

Based on autopsy findings, what percentage of men age 70 to 79 have undetected prostate cancer?

Thirty percent

What percentage of men age 80 to 89?

Sixty-five percent

What is the Gleason scoring system?

Evaluation of glandular architecture under low-power magnification and grading of 1 to 5 based on the degree of differentiation. The most representative and second most representative areas of cancer are assigned grades, and these are added together to give a Gleason score between 2 and 10, which is predictive of the extent of disease.

Which stages are based on the modified AUA Jewett system?

Stage A (T1): Microscopic disease found at simple prostatectomy for benign disease
Stage B (T2): Palpable disease confined to the prostate
Stage C (T3): Extracapsular extension into periprostatic tissue or seminal vesicle
Stage D (T4): Metastatic disease

In the TMN classification system, what is the designation given nonpalpable, sonographically negative cancers diagnosed on biopsy for elevated PSA?

T1c lesion

Where is the most common site of:

Lymphatic spread?

Obturator LNs

Hematogenous spread?

Bone (Lumbar spine > pelvis > proximal femur > thoracic spine > ribs > sternum > skull)

Are prostate-cancer bone metastases osteoblastic or osteolytic?

More than 90% are osteoblastic.

How is prostate cancer diagnosed?

TRUS-guided prostate biopsy

What are the indications for prostate biopsy?

Abnormal DRE or PSA elevation

What is PSA?

A protease produced by the prostatic epithelium; a serum elevation > 4 ng/ml is associated with an increased risk of prostate cancer.

What is the standard workup for a patient with presumed organ-confined disease?

1. DRE—Most accurate method for determining local extent of disease
2. TRUS—Hypoechoic lesions are more likely to represent cancer. Distortion of normal anatomy suggests locally advanced disease.
3. Pelvic CT—Performed to access LN status in patients at high risk for metastasis (accuracy of 60%–80%)
4. PSA—Correlates directly with the extent of disease
5. Bone scan—^{99m}Technetium-labeled methylene diphosphonate is taken up selectively by metastatic bone lesions. (Note: False positives (2%) are a result of metabolic or traumatic bone disease.)

What PSA level suggests that the cancer is confined to the gland?

PSA < 10 ng/ml

By how many months do positive bone scan findings usually precede plain-film changes?

From 2 to 6 months

What are the treatment options for a patient with localized prostate cancer?

1. Radical retropubic or perineal prostatectomy
2. External beam radiotherapy—6600 cGy to the prostate and an additional 4500 cGy to the pelvic LNs over 6 to 7 weeks
3. Watchful waiting—estimated 10-year mortality is as high as 20% depending on the series.

(Note: Most appropriate for men with < 10-year life expectancy)

What is the mean 10-year disease-free survival for a stage B cancer treated with options 1 and 2?

1. Seventy percent
2. Fifty percent

What are the complications of radical retropubic prostatectomy?

1. Hemorrhage
2. Rectal injury
3. Deep venous thrombosis
4. Pulmonary embolus
5. Bladder neck contracture
6. Incontinence
7. Impotence
8. Mortality (< 1%)

What are the complications of external beam therapy?

1. Radiation proctitis (includes diarrhea, radiation ulcers, and strictures)
2. Irritative voiding symptoms
3. Urethral strictures
4. Incontinence
5. Impotence

What is the management of stage D disease?

Androgen deprivation therapy (ADT). Results in temporary regression of prostate cancer

What are the options for ADT?

1. Inhibition of androgen production:
   Bilateral orchiectomy—simplest and most cost-effective
   LHRH agonist (lupron) with or without the antiandrogen flutamide, or low-dose estrogen–diethylstilbestrol (DES) 1 mg orally each day
2. Inhibition of androgen action with antiandrogens (e.g., flutamide)—Sometimes added to block adrenal androgens

What are some indications for immediate ADT in patients with metastatic prostate cancer?

1. Spinal cord compression
2. Impending pathologic fracture
3. Bladder or ureteral obstruction
4. Significant lower extremity edema from nodal involvement

Which emergent options are available for patients presenting with spinal cord compression from untreated metastatic prostate cancer?

Steroids (Decadron PO) **and** either:
1. Bilateral orchiectomy
2. Eulexin (flutamide)
3. External beam radiotherapy to metastatic site
4. Emergent decompression laminectomy

BLADDER

ANATOMY

What is the capacity of the normal adult bladder?

From 350 to 450 ml

What is the urachus?

The fibrous remnant of the allantois, which joins the dome of the bladder with the umbilicus

What is the clinical significance?

1. Varying degrees of patency can result in urachal cysts, diverticula, or sinuses.
2. Often the site of origin of bladder adenocarcinoma

What is the main muscle of the bladder and how are its fibers arranged?

Detrusor muscle
1. Inner—Longitudinal
2. Middle—Circular
3. Outer—Longitudinal

In the male bladder, from what vessels does the major arterial blood supply come?	The superior, middle, and inferior vesical arteries, which arise from the anterior division of the hypogastric artery (Minor branches arise from the obturator and inferior gluteal artery.)
Where is the major lymphatic drainage of the bladder?	External iliac, common iliac, and hypogastric LNs
Which nerve fibers supply the contractile innervation of the detrusor muscle?	Parasympathetic fibers via S2 to S4
What supplies the motor innervation of the trigone and bladder neck sphincter?	Sympathetic fibers from T11 to T12 and L1 to L2

INFECTIOUS DISORDERS

Acute Cystitis

What are the most common causative organisms?	1. Coliform bacteria (*E. coli*—most common) 2. Gram-positive organisms are also occasionally found (e.g., Enterococci and *Staphylococcus saprophyticus*).
How do these organisms gain access to the bladder?	Ascending infections from the urethra
What viral infection is reported to cause hemorrhagic cystitis in children?	Adenoviral infection
Are men or women more commonly affected?	Women
What is the clinical presentation?	1. Irritative voiding symptoms (e.g., frequency, urgency, and dysuria) 2. Suprapubic discomfort 3. Hematuria or foul-smelling urine
What are the laboratory findings?	1. CBC may show mild WBC elevation with a left shift. 2. UA shows WBCs, RBCs, and bacteria.

What are the complications?	1. Ascending pyelonephritis 2. Epididymitis 3. Prostatitis
What is the treatment?	1. Hydration 2. In uncomplicated patients, oral antibiotic therapy for 1 to 3 days is usually adequate (e.g., ampicillin, nitrofurantoin, or trimethroprim-sulfamethoxazole). 3. In complicated patients (e.g., associated calculi, diabetes, or immunocompromise), intravenous therapy may be necessary.

CONGENITAL AND ACQUIRED DISORDERS

Interstitial Cystitis

What is interstitial cystitis?	Chronic irritative process of the bladder wall leads to fibrosis, pelvic pain, and irritative voiding symptoms.
Which group of patients does it tend to affect?	Middle-aged women
What are the etiologic theories?	1. Autoimmune collagen disease 2. Hypersensitivity response to food allergens 3. Obstruction of the pelvic lymphatics secondary to surgery causing fibrosis 4. Fibrosis secondary to thrombophlebitis from recurrent bladder infections 5. Arteriolar spasm secondary to vasculitic or psychogenic impulses
What is the clinical presentation?	1. Worsening irritative voiding symptoms (e.g., frequency, urgency, and nocturia) 2. Suprapubic pain made worse by bladder distention and relieved with voiding 3. Microscopic hematuria, which may progress to gross hematuria with bladder overdistention

What are the classic cystoscopic findings?

Areas of punctate hemorrhage (i.e., glomerulations), stellate splitting of the dome, and occasional areas of ulceration (i.e., Hunner's ulcer)

What is the treatment?

No definitive treatment; the goal is symptomatic pain relief. The following methods have been tried with varying degrees of success:
1. Hydraulic distention under anesthesia
2. Instillations of dimethyl sulfoxide (DMSO) every 2 weeks
3. Irrigations with 0.4% oxychlorosene sodium (Clorpactin)
4. Corticosteroids (unpredictable results)
5. Surgical therapies such as augmentation and loop diversion (unpredictable results)

Hemorrhagic Cystitis

What chemotherapeutic agent is most often associated with this condition?

Cyclophosphamide (the urotoxic metabolite acrolein is the etiologic agent.)

What percentage of patients being treated with this agent may have this complication?

2% to 40%

What severity of bleeding is typically seen?

The sterile hemorrhage seen with this condition ranges from minimal gross hematuria to life-threatening hemorrhage.

What is one of the most effective preventive measures?

Either saline diuresis or irrigation during the period of cyclophosphamide therapy reduces the contact time of metabolites with the urothelium and greatly reduces the risk of occurrence.

Which treatment measures (from least to most aggressive) are used if hemorrhagic cystitis occurs?

1. Clot evacuation and continuous saline bladder irrigation
2. Continuous bladder irrigation with 1% alum solution
3. After confirming that no ureteral reflux exists, 1% silver nitrate or instillation of 4% formalin may be attempted.

4. Surgical intervention—Selective embolization of the internal iliacs, transuretheral cauterization, open laser coagulation, open packing, and even simple cystectomy

What are the four main categories of incontinence, and how is each defined?

1. Total incontinence—Continuous involuntary loss of urine as seen with ectopic ureters below the sphincteric mechanism, major sphincteric abnormalities, or vesicovaginal fistula
2. Stress incontinence—Involuntary loss of urine associated with increases in abdominal pressure (e.g., coughing, sneezing, Valsalva)
3. Urge incontinence—Involuntary loss of urine associated with an intense desire to void corresponding to an uncontrolled detrusor contraction
4. Overflow incontinence—Detrusor weakness, or outlet obstruction, can lead to significant bladder overfilling and involuntary loss of urine as pressure within the bladder overcomes sphincteric control.

What is the evaluation for incontinence?

1. History—Characterization of the incontinence, obstetric-gynecologic history, medications, for example
2. Physical—In addition to DRE of the prostate, a full pelvic exam including stress maneuvers, and a thorough neurologic evaluation
3. UA and culture—To rule out possible infection
4. Blood tests—Electrolyte panel and fasting glucose
5. Postvoid residual—To differentiate between a failure to empty and a failure to store
6. Special studies (obtained based upon the individual patient)—Including uroflow, urethral pressure profile, cystometrogram, voiding cystourethrogram (VCUG), and cystoscopy

What is the treatment of total incontinence?

Requires repair of the underlying primary disorder whether it is an ectopic ureter, vesicovaginal fistula, or damaged sphincter

What is the treatment of stress urinary incontinence?

1. Pharmacologic increase of outlet resistance (e.g., ephedrine, phentolamine)
2. Bladder neck suspension (e.g., Burch, Marshall-Marchetti Krantz, Stamey)
3. Sling procedures when intrinsic urethral damage is present

What is the treatment of urge incontinence?

1. Pharmacologic treatment of detrusor instability (e.g., oxybutinin, imipramine)
2. A small, poorly compliant bladder may benefit from an augmentation cystoplasty.

What is the treatment of overflow incontinence?

1. Surgical relief of obstructing prostatic tissue, bladder neck contracture, or stricture disease
2. Clean intermittent catheterization can be used in patients with detrusor weakness.

What are some examples of the following neuropathic conditions?

    Sensory neurogenic bladder?

Diabetes mellitus, tabes dorsalis, and pernicious anemia

    Motor paralytic bladder?

Pelvic surgery or trauma and herpes zoster

    Uninhibited neurogenic bladder?

Cerebrovascular accident, tumors of the spinal cord or brain, and demyelinating spinal cord diseases

    Reflex neurogenic bladder?

Spinal cord injury after resolution of spinal shock and transverse myelitis

    Autonomous neurogenic bladder?

Acute spinal shock

What are the classic detrusor and sphincter findings of each of these neuropathic conditions?

1. Sensory neurogenic bladder— Impaired sensation with resultant detrusor decompensation; synergistic sphincter function
2. Motor paralytic bladder—Destruction of the parasympathetic innervation of the bladder with poor detrusor function
3. Uninhibited neurogenic bladder— Normal sensation with hyperreflexic detrusor and variable sphincter synergy
4. Reflex neurogenic bladder— Complete interruption of the motor and sensory pathway resulting in a hyperreflexic detrusor, sphincter dyssynergia, and loss of sensation.
5. Autonomous neurogenic bladder— Complete motor and sensory separation of the bladder from the sacral spinal cord; detrusor areflexia, loss of sensation, and poor sphincter function

BLADDER TRAUMA

What are the three major categories of bladder rupture?

1. Intraperitoneal bladder rupture— Urine extravasates into the peritoneal cavity.
2. Extraperitoneal bladder rupture— Urine extravasates into the perivesical space.
3. Concomitant intra- and extraperitoneal bladder rupture

What are the typical blunt trauma scenarios that cause bladder rupture?

1. Intraperitoneal bladder rupture usually results from a compressive force on a full bladder causing the dome to rupture into the peritoneal cavity.
2. Extraperitoneal bladder rupture usually occurs in association with a pelvic fracture due to shear forces on the wall of the bladder or direct puncture by the fractured bone.

What percentage of patients with a bladder rupture present with gross hematuria?	Ninety-five percent
What study is used to confirm the existence and location of a bladder perforation?	Cystogram
What film is often most helpful in distinguishing subtle extraperitoneal extravasation versus intraperitoneal rupture?	Postvoid film

What is the treatment of:

1. **Small extraperitoneal rupture?**
2. **Large extraperitoneal rupture?**
3. **Intraperitoneal rupture?**

1. Catheter drainage for 1 to 2 weeks
2. Exploration, debridement, repair, and placement of a suprapubic tube
3. Exploration, debridement, repair, and placement of a suprapubic tube

TUMORS

Adenocarcinoma of the Bladder

What percentage of bladder cancer does adenocarcinoma represent?	< 2%

What are the three possible sites of origin?

1. Primary bladder adenocarcinoma arising from the base of the bladder
2. Urachal remnant
3. Metastatic adenocarcinoma from the gastrointestinal or the female gynecologic tract

What developmental abnormality is associated with increased risk of this condition?	Classic bladder extrophy
What is the treatment?	Preoperative radiotherapy with 3000 cGy followed by radical cystectomy

Squamous Cell Carcinoma (SCCa) Of The Bladder

What percentage of bladder lesions does SCCa represent?

< 8%

What are the risk factors?

1. Chronic indwelling catheter or other foreign body irritation
2. Vesical calculi
3. Stricture disease
4. Infection with *Schistosoma haematobium*

What is the treatment?

1. Superficial well-differentiated tumors can be treated with transurethral resection or partial cystectomy.
2. Locally invasive lesions should receive preoperative radiotherapy with 3000 cGy and radical cystectomy.
3. There is no effective chemotherapy for metastatic squamous cancers.

Transitional Cell Carcinoma (TCCa) Of The Bladder

What are the classic demographics in terms of age, sex, and race?

1. Mean age 65 years
2. Male-to-female ratio of 2.7:1
3. White to African-American ratio of 4:1

What are the known occupational risk factors?

Exposure to the aromatic amines:
1. Benzidine
2. β-naphthylamine
3. 4-aminobiphenyl
(Note: These substances are most commonly encountered in the manufacturing of dyes, rubber, textiles, and plastics.)

What are the known nonoccupational risk factors?

1. Cigarette smoking—This risk factor is present in 50% of men and 30% of women.
2. Dietary nitrosamines
3. Cytoxan exposure
(Note: Other controversial risk factors include caffeine and artificial sweeteners.)

What are the TMN stage groupings of TCCa of the bladder?

T0—Papillary lesion confined to the mucosa

TIS—Carcinoma in situ (CIS)

T1—Tumor invading submucosa or lamina propria

T2—Tumor invading superficial muscle

T3—Tumor invading deep muscle or perivesical fat; LN negative

T4—Tumor extending into adjacent organs, LN involvement, or distant metastasis

Which histologic features determine the grade of a lesion, and how does this correlate with tumor invasiveness?

Grade is determined by:
1. Cellular atypia
2. Nuclear abnormalities
3. Number of mitotic figures
   Grade 1: well differentiated (10% are invasive)
   Grade 2: moderately differentiated (50% are invasive)
   Grade 3: poorly differentiated (> 80% are invasive)

What is the most common presenting sign of bladder cancer?

Hematuria, either gross or microscopic (present in 85%–90%)

What is another common presenting complaint more often seen in association with diffuse CIS?

Irritative voiding symptoms such as dysuria, frequency, and urgency

What is the evaluation?

1. UA, culture, and bladder washings for cytology
2. Bimanual exam (usually performed under anesthesia at the time of cystoscopy and deep bladder biopsy)
3. Intravenous pyelogram to rule out concomitant upper tract disease
4. Cystoscopy with directed deep biopsy of any suspicious lesions and random cold-cup biopsies of the four walls, trigone, and prostatic urethra
5. CT scan to determine presence of intra-abdominal metastases and nodal involvement > 1.5 cm

What is the treatment of CIS?

1. Due to the high risk of progression to invasive disease (50%–75%), these

lesions are treated with intravesical bacillus Calmette-Guérin, BCG (an attenuated strain of *Mycobacterium bovis*)

2. Recurrences can be treated by a repeat course of BCG or radical cystectomy.

What is the treatment of stage T0 and T1?

1. Transurethral resection of the bladder tumor (TURBt)
2. Recurrences can be treated with repeat TURBt with or without intravesical chemotherapy.

What are the indications for intravesical chemotherapy in superficial bladder TCCa?

1. CIS
2. Multicentricity
3. Rapid recurrence
4. Progression to higher grade

What are the most common intravesical agents?

1. Thiotepa
2. Mitomycin C
3. Doxorubicin
4. BCG

How often should superficial lesions be followed with repeat cystoscopy and cytology?

Every 3 months

What is the treatment of stage T2 and T3 (muscle-invasive) TCCa?

1. Radical cystectomy with bilateral pelvic LN dissection and urinary diversion.
2. Preoperative radiotherapy (3000 cGy) is controversial; some studies have shown a decrease in the incidence of recurrence in patients with full-thickness muscle invasion.
3. Partial cystectomy may be performed for isolated lesions of the posterior wall, lateral wall, dome, or within a diverticulum in the absence of CIS.

What is the treatment of stage T4?

1. Combination methotrexate, vinblastine, adriamycin, and cisplatin (MVAC)
2. A cystectomy may be performed for uncontrolled bleeding but does not improve overall survival rate.

COLLECTING SYSTEM AND URETERS

ANATOMY

From what major vessels does the ureter receive its arterial blood supply?	1. Upper and middle ureter—Renal, gonadal, aorta, and common iliac arteries 2. Distal ureter—Internal iliac, superior vesical, uterine and vaginal (in females), middle rectal, and inferior vesical arteries
What are the three anatomic narrowings of the ureter and their usual calibers?	1. Ureteropelvic junction—2 mm 2. Iliac vessel crossing—4 mm 3. Ureterovesical junction—3 to 4 mm
What is the significance of these narrowings?	They are the most common sites of stone obstruction.

CONGENITAL AND ACQUIRED DISORDERS

Ureteropelvic Junction Obstruction

What are the etiologies?	1. Intrinsic circular smooth muscle disorder 2. Compression due to a crossing vessel from the lower pole of the kidney 3. High insertion of the ureter on the renal pelvis 4. Valvular fold of mucosa (rare)
What is the male to female ratio?	2.5:1
What are the usual presenting symptoms?	1. Infants usually present with an asymptomatic flank mass, evaluation of hydronephrosis detected on prenatal U/S, or urosepsis. 2. Children and adults usually present with episodic flank pain with or without associated vomiting.
What percentage present during the first year of life?	Twenty-five percent

Which studies are included in the evaluation?

1. Intravenous pyelogram (IVP) can usually establish the diagnosis.
2. Diuretic DTPA renogram is useful in equivocal cases.
3. Retrograde pyelogram is often attempted to further define the region of obstruction.

What are the treatment options?

1. Open pyeloplasty (gold standard therapy)
2. Laparoscopic pyeloplasty
3. Antegrade or retrograde pyelotomy

Vesicoureteral Reflux (VUR)

What is VUR?

Abnormal backward flow of urine from the bladder up the ureter (and possibly into the intrarenal collecting system)

What are the complications?

1. Recurrent infections
2. Renal parenchymal scarring
3. Renal damage (reflux nephropathy)

Which factors contribute to the occurrence of reflux?

1. Shortened intramural segment of ureter (less than a 4:1 ratio of intramural segment to ureteral diameter)
2. Abnormal ureteral orifice due to varying degrees of diminished supporting musculature (i.e., stadium orifice or golf hole)
3. Ectopic lateral displacement of the ureter
4. Edema secondary to infection or inflammation
5. Displacement from a diverticulum or from the ureterocele of a duplicated ureter

What is the gold standard diagnostic test for VUR?

Voiding cystourethrogram

What is the radiographic grading system for VUR?

Grade I: Ureter only
Grade II: Into the intrarenal collecting system without dilation
Grade III: Reflux into the calyceal system with loss of the fornices
Grade IV: Moderate dilation of the renal

pelvis, calyces, and ureter with or
without ureteral tortuosity

Grade V: Severe dilation of the ureter,
renal pelvis, and calyces with a
markedly tortuous ureter

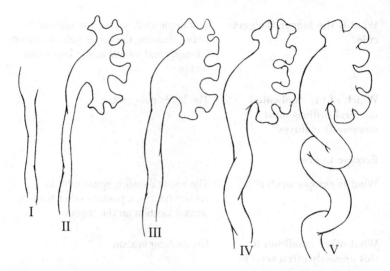

**What is the medical
treatment of VUR?**

Low-dose suppressive antibiotics,
frequent urine culture, yearly nuclear or
voiding cystourethrogram, and an IVP
every 2 years

**What are the indications
for medical treatment?**

Young patients without evidence of
progressive renal damage and a normal
appearing ureteral orifice

**What is the surgical
treatment of VUR?**

Ureteral reimplantation (Of the many
techniques, the primary principle of
each is to increase the length of the
intravesical ureter.)

**What are the indications
for surgical treatment?**

1. Progressive scarring or pyelonephritis
   despite medical therapy
2. Poor compliance with medical
   therapy
3. Reflux in association with a significant
   anatomic abnormality such as a
   diverticulum, duplication, ureterocele,
   or ectopic location

What is its claim to fame?	Most common anomaly of the urinary tract
What is the female-to-male ratio?	2:1
What is the Meyer-Weigert rule?	In a duplicated system, the ureteral orifice draining the upper pole is located inferiorly and medial to the lower pole ureter
Which of the duplicated ureteral orifices most commonly refluxes?	The lower pole ureter

Ectopic Ureter

What is ectopic ureter?	The ureteral orifice opens into the urinary tract in a position other than its normal location on the trigone.
What other condition is this anomaly often seen in association with?	Ureteral duplication
What are the most common extravesical ectopic sites in men?	1. Posterior urethra 2. Seminal vesicle
What are the most common extravesical ectopic sites in women?	1. Urethra 2. Vestibule 3. Vagina
What is the treatment?	1. Partial nephroureterectomy if the ectopic ureter drains a nonfunctioning renal segment 2. Pyelopyeloplasty and distal ureterectomy if the renal moiety is functioning 3. A primary reimplantation if a single ureter is ectopic

Idiopathic Retroperitoneal Fibrosis

What is idiopathic retroperitoneal fibrosis?	A chronic inflammatory process in the retroperitoneum, which can encompass the ureters

What is the primary complication?

Ureteral obstruction and hydroureteronephrosis

What are the etiologies?

1. Primary: idiopathic
2. Secondary:
   Cancer (e.g., breast, ovarian, prostate)
   Several drugs/medications (e.g., methysergide, hydralazine, β-blocker)
   Infections (e.g., tuberculosis, syphilis)
   Radiation exposure
   Inflammatory processes (e.g., leaking aortic aneurysm, inflammatory bowel disease)

What is the usual presentation?

Flank or abdominal pain

What is the most useful diagnostic modality for evaluating this condition?

Abdominal and pelvic CT scan with contrast to define the extent of involvement and to evaluate for the existence of underlying malignancy

What is the treatment?

Diagnostic biopsy of the retroperitoneal process followed by ureteral lysis and intraperitonealization of the ureters (Note: Some surgeons advocate wrapping the ureters with segments of omentum to keep them from becoming reincorporated in the process.)

Calculus Disease

What are the three major theories of stone formation?

1. Nucleation theory—Urine is supersaturated with crystal-forming salts, and stone formation is initiated by deposition of a crystal or foreign body.
2. Stone matrix theory—Crystallization occurs due to the presence of an organic protein matrix in the urine.
3. Lowered urinary crystallization inhibitors—Low levels of crystal inhibitors (e.g., magnesium, pyrophosphate, citrate, mucoproteins)

What is the classic region of pain and area of radiation experienced during passage of a renal stone?

An upper ureteral stone often presents as severe colicky flank or costovertebral angle pain as the ureter contracts against the obstructing stone. As the stone travels down the ureter, pain often radiates to the ipsilateral scrotum or labia.

What are the associated nonrenal symptoms?

Nausea, vomiting, abdominal distention, ileus, and urinary retention (infrequent)

What percentage of stones are radiopaque?

Ninety percent

What are the most common compositions of these stones?

1. Calcium phosphate
2. Calcium oxalate
3. Magnesium ammonium phosphate
4. Cystine (slightly opaque)

What stone compositions are nonradiopaque?

1. Uric acid
2. Xanthine

In what percentage of stones is calcium oxalate the sole or major component?

Eighty percent

What is included in the evaluation of patients with presumed renal colic?

1. UA and urine culture—To evaluate for signs of infection
2. Abdominal x-ray—90% of stones will be radiopaque; this study also helps to evaluate for other types of pathology (e.g., gallstones, visceral perforation)
3. IVP—To determine the degree of delay in visualization of the kidney (i.e., obstruction) and the region to which contrast columnates (i.e., location of the stone)
4. Ultrasound—To look for hydronephrosis and the presence of renal or UPJ stones if contrast cannot be given (e.g., renal insufficiency, pregnancy, etc.)
5. Retrograde pyelogram—To define the level of obstruction, often done in conjunction with ureteroscopic stone extraction

What type of stones is most often seen in association with infection?

Magnesium ammonium phosphate (i.e., struvite) stones

What is the typical urinary pH associated with these infections, and what is the source of its alteration?

> 7.0 because of the presence of urea-splitting organisms such as *Proteus, Klebsiella, Pseudomonas,* and *E. coli*

What are the four major categories of uric acid stone disease?

1. Idiopathic
2. Hyperuricemia (in association with such conditions as gout, myeloproliferative disorders, and Lesch-Nyan)
3. Chronic dehydration (from diarrhea or high ileostomy output)
4. Hyperuricosuria without hyperuricemia (can be caused by drugs such as thiazide diuretics or salicylates)

What are some examples of these categories?

1. Hyperuricemia—Gout, myeloproliferative disorders, Lesch-Nyan, etc.
2. Chronic dehydration—Diarrhea or high ileostomy output
3. Hyperuricosuria without hyperuricemia—Drugs such as thiazide diuretics or salicylates

What are common indications for surgical intervention for stone disease?

1. Infection
2. Complete obstruction
3. Intractable pain
4. Debilitating underlying conditions (diabetes, immune compromise)
5. Progressive renal damage (especially high-grade obstruction of a solitary renal unit)

What are the surgical treatment options for staghorn or large pelvic stone?

1. Primary percutaneous nephrolithotripsy (PCNL)
2. Combination PCNL and extracorporeal shock wave lithotripsy (ESWL)

What are the surgical treatment options for calyceal stones?

Most can be treated effectively with ESWL

What are the surgical treatment options for ureteropelvic junction stones?	1. ESWL 2. PCNL (if the stone is large) 3. Retrograde ureteroscopic extraction
What are the surgical treatment options for ureteral stones?	1. Expectant therapy—Most stones < 5mm in diameter will pass spontaneously. 2. ESWL—Effective in the treatment of almost all forms of ureteral stones although stones of dense crystallization (e.g., cystine) are often hard to fragment 3. Ureteroscopic stone extraction—Used most frequently for stones in the distal third of the ureter (although flexible ureteroscopes have made all regions of the ureter more accessible) 4. Ureterolithotomy—Usually reserved for stones that have failed both ESWL and ureteroscopic procedures

URETERAL TRAUMA

What is the incidence in association with a gunshot wound to the abdomen?	From 2% to 5%
In what percentage of hysterectomies does an injury of the ureter occur?	< 1%
What percentage of ureteral injuries have another associated intra-abdominal injury?	Ninety-two percent
What is the best way of evaluating a patient with a possible ureteral injury?	IVP—extravasation of contrast is seen in up to 90% of cases.
What is the treatment of proximal ureteral injury?	1. A ureteropelvic junction avulsion is best treated with a pyeloplasty or a ureteropyelostomy over a ureteral stent. 2. If enough ureter is present, a primary ureteroureterostomy over an indwelling stent is performed with renal mobilization if extra length is needed

3. If a large segment of ureter is missing, a transureteroureterostomy (TUU), ureterocalycostomy, or ileal ureter can be performed in a delayed fashion. The proximal ureter is ligated and nephrostomy drainage is secured at the initial exploration.

What is the treatment of mid-ureteral injury?

1. Ureteroureterostomy over a ureteral stent
2. TUU or ileal ureter may be necessary if a large segment of ureter is missing.

What is the treatment of distal ureteral injury ?

1. Ureteroneocystostomy
2. To gain extra length, a tubular flap of bladder (Boari flap) can be raised, or the bladder can be elevated and secured to the psoas muscle (psoas hitch) prior to reimplantation of the ureter.

What is essential to prevent urinoma formation and infection postoperatively?

Adequate retroperitoneal closed-suction drainage

TUMORS

Transition Cell Carcinoma (TCCa) of the Renal Pelvis or Ureter

What percentage of TCCa tumors are located in either the renal pelvis or ureter?

Approximately 4%

What percentage of patients with an upper tract tumor will develop a lesion in the lower tract?

33%

What are the most common presenting complaints?

1. Hematuria—Most common (70%–80%)
2. Flank pain—Due to obstruction from clot or tumor

**What studies and
procedures are included in
the evaluation?**

1. UA with cytology
2. IVP—Often the initial study; to also
   evaluate the contralateral collecting
   system
3. Cystoscopy with retrograde
   pyelogram and selective ureteral
   washings —To further define the
   lesion and to gain a pathologic
   diagnosis. Cystoscopy is necessary to
   rule out concomitant disease in the
   bladder.
4. Ureteropyeloscopy with brush
   biopsies (occasionally necessary)
5. Abdominal and pelvic CT scan—To
   evaluate for obvious metastases
6. Chest x-ray

**What is the staging
system?**

Stage 0: CIS or superficial papillary
    cancer
Stage I: Invasion of the lamina propria
Stage II: Invasion of the underlying
    smooth muscle
Stage III: Invasion of the peripelvic fat,
    periureteral fat or renal parenchyma
Stage IV: Invasion through the renal
    capsule, into adjacent organs or
    metastasis to LN or distant organs

**What is the treatment of:
  Low-stage, low-grade
  distal ureteral tumor?**

Distal ureterectomy, excision of a cuff of
bladder and ureteral reimplantation

** Stage I to III tumors?**

Nephroureterectomy (Note: In patients
with a solitary renal unit, more
conservative therapy such as segmental
ureteral resection or endoscopic pelvic
resections followed by chemotherapeutic
instillations have all been tried with
variable results.)

** Stage IV tumors?**

Combination chemotherapy using
methotrexate, vinblastine, adriamycin,
and cisplatin (MVAC)

56

Ophthalmology

Kirk J. Fleischer, MD

ANATOMY

What are the labeled ocular structures?

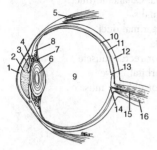

1. Cornea
2. Anterior chamber
3. Iris
4. Posterior chamber
5. Conjunctiva
6. Lens
7. Zonular fibers
8. Ciliary body
9. Vitreous humor
10. Retina
11. Choroid
12. Sclera
13. Macula
14. Optic disk
15. Retinal artery and vein
16. Optic nerve

**What are the labeled
structures in this anterior
view of the dissected
orbital cavity?**

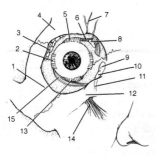

1. Zygomatic bone
2. Lateral rectus muscle
3. Lacrimal gland
4. Frontal bone
5. Superior rectus muscle
6. Superior oblique tendon
7. Supraorbital muscle
8. Trochea
9. Lacrimal canaliculi (duct)
10. Lacrimal sac
11. Nasolacrimal duct
12. Maxilla
13. Inferior rectus muscle
14. Infraorbital nerve
15. Inferior oblique muscle

OPHTHALMOLOGIC EXAMINATION

**What are the basic
components of the bedside
ophthalmologic
examination?**

Systematically evaluate structures from
anterior to posterior:
Orbital rim—palpate for crepitus, step-
off deformities; test for periorbital
hypesthesia.
Eyelid—inspect lid for lacerations/
foreign bodies (examination should
include careful lid eversion).
Visual acuity—test with counting of
fingers (or reading of card eye chart).
Globe—test extraocular muscles; inspect
for laceration or rupture.
Conjunctiva—inspect for subconjunctival
hemorrhage, laceration, emphysema,
or foreign body

Anterior chamber—inspect for hyphema
and chamber depth (tangential
lighting).
Iris—inspect for shape and reactiveness.
Lens—inspect for transparency and
position (dislocated?); red reflex?
Vitreous humor—inspect for
transparency.
Retina—inspect for hemorrhage and
detachment.

What may absence of red
reflex suggest?

Cataract, vitreous hemorrhage, or retinal
detachment

What may lid ptosis
suggest?

Injury to levator palpebrae or its
innervation (CN III)

NONTRAUMATIC OCULAR EMERGENCIES

ORBITAL CELLULITIS

What are the most
common microbial
etiologies?

Gram-positive cocci (*Streptococcus*,
Staphylococcus); *Haemophilus influenzae*
(in children < age 5)

What are the routes to
orbit?

Direct extension via paranasal sinuses,
vascular drainage from periorbital soft
tissue, and occasionally hematogenous
spread from distant site

What is the usual
presentation?

Acute onset of severe orbital pain,
reduced mobility of eye, conjunctival
chemosis (edema), reduced vision,
malaise, fever, and in some cases,
marked periorbital erythema and edema

What are the sequelae?

Cavernous sinus thrombosis due to
thrombophlebitis of the orbital veins,
blindness due to optic neuritis, spread of
infection to brain or meninges

What is the treatment?

Hospitalization, systemic antibiotics,
warm packs, bed rest; occasionally,
surgical drainage indicated (Note: Most
experts recommend CT scan of orbit to
exclude abscess.)

ACUTE ANGLE-CLOSURE GLAUCOMA

Presentation?

Severe ocular pain, headache, blurred vision, nausea ± vomiting (Note: Acute angle-closure glaucoma is actually a relatively rare diagnosis.)

What are the findings on examination?

Shallow anterior chamber as determined by tangential lighting of the anterior globe, corneal chemosis, pupil fixed in midposition

What can precipitate the development of glaucoma in patient with acute angle closure of iris?

Any drug that will dilate the pupil and thus reduce the normal circulation of the aqueous humor in the anterior chamber. Classically, this occurs with anticholinergic agents used by anesthesiologists preoperatively (e.g., atropine, scopolamine). It is safe, however, to premedicate patients with **chronic** history of glaucoma (**open-angle**) with these agents.

What is the goal of acute treatment of acute angle closure glaucoma?

Reduction of intraocular pressure

What is the acute treatment?

Timolol (to reduce aqueous humor formation), pilocarpine (to resolve pupillary block), acetazolamide and hyperosmotic agent (isosorbide or glycerol) [to further decrease intraocular pressure]

What are the surgical treatment options?

Laser iridotomy (Note: The contralateral eye is also prophylactically treated.)

TRAUMATIC OCULAR EMERGENCIES

MECHANICAL OCULAR TRAUMA

In addition to examination of the periorbital region and globe, what test should be performed on all patients early in their evaluation?

Visual acuity of both eyes (to document baseline)

What percentage of patients with facial fractures have associated ocular injuries?

Between 60% and 70% (Note: They are often difficult to diagnose initially because of associated injuries and/or decreased mental status of patient. A high index of suspicion is necessary for early ophthalmologic consultation to prevent potential vision loss.)

Most common fracture associated with ocular injury?

Frontal bone (> nasal and midfacial fractures)

What percentage have permanent physiologic or visual sequela?

Twenty percent. Less than 5% are blind. (Note: Most of these are associated with midfacial fractures.)

In fractures of the orbital floor ("blow-out" fractures), what are the classic ocular symptoms and etiology?

Diplopia with upward (or downward) gaze; due to herniation and entrapment of extraocular muscle (usually inferior rectus or inferior oblique muscle) through fracture site

What is the classic tactile sensory deficit and etiology?

Hypesthesia over the ipsilateral upper lip and cheek. The infraorbital nerve is frequently damaged as it traverses the floor of the orbit.

What is the classic sign on physical exam?

Enophthalmos—Posterior displacement of the globe (Note: Very specific but often difficult to detect acutely to significant periorbital edema.)

What is the best view to demonstrate fracture on x-ray?

Waters' view

Which patients require emergent surgery?

Those with suspected entrapment of extraocular muscle (to avoid resultant ischemia)

Corneal Abrasions

How is the diagnosis of corneal abrasions made?

Corneal epithelial defect visualized with fluorescein stain under ultraviolet light

What is the treatment?

Topical antibiotic (e.g., tobramycin, gentamycin, sulfacetamide), update of tetanus prophylaxis, ± patch eye (Note: All patients should be reexamined in 24–36 hours to rule out infection.)

Hyphema

What is hyphema?

Hemorrhage into anterior chamber of the eye; seen as meniscus or layering of blood anterior to iris

What percentage of patients rebleed?

Between 10% and 30% rebleed in the first week post-trauma.

Medical management of hyphema?

Controversial; the most conservative treatment involves elevation of head for 5 to 7 days (± admission to hospital), bed rest, daily examination and tonometry (to ensure absorption of blood without development of glaucoma).

What are the indications for surgical washout of hyphema?

Blood staining of cornea, secondary glaucoma

Conjunctival Emphysema

What is the usual etiology of conjunctival emphysema?

Fracture of sinus (often the lamina papyracea of the ethmoid bone) permitting air to dissect under the conjunctiva

What special instructions should be given to the patient?

Patient should not blow nose, because acute increases in sinus pressure result in further dissection.

Lens Dislocation

What is the mechanism of lens dislocation?

Disruption of > 25% of zonular fibers (anchored to ciliary body) which hold lens to posterior surface of iris

What is the usual presentation?

Blurred vision (often subtle)

Which general type of lens dislocation is a surgical emergency, and why?	Anterior. Can cause acute glaucoma. (Note: Posterior dislocation into vitreous humor is treated electively after resolution of inflammation.)
What is the classic LATE complication of blunt trauma?	Retinal detachment (due to retinal tear)
What is the usual presentation?	Decreased visual acuity (due to slowly progressive and painless dissection of retina from choroid)
What is the treatment?	Cryosurgery and/or scleral buckling (performed **emergently** if the macula is threatened because it can prevent permanent loss of central vision)

Penetrating Ocular Trauma

In penetrating ocular trauma, what is the key point regarding physical examination?	Do not manipulate the periorbital tissue. Any manipulation may result in additional prolapse of intraocular contents.
What is the key point regarding diagnostic studies?	Do not perform MRI if metallic intraocular foreign body may be present.
What are the key points regarding acute management of globe lacerations or rupture?	1. Place rigid *nonpressure* protective eye shield (not eye pads) to avoid increasing global pressures with resultant extrusion of intraocular contents. 2. Do not apply topical antibiotics.
What are the other aspects of management?	Broad-spectrum IV antibiotics, update of tetanus prophylaxis, and emergency ophthalmologic referral

OCULAR BURNS

Which chemical burns (acid vs. alkali) frequently do NOT initially present with obvious ocular injury despite their more destructive nature?	Alkali (often result in significant liquefaction necrosis and scarring with no acute signs)

What is the treatment of acid versus alkali burns?	1. Topical anesthetic, then copious irrigation (2–3 liters) with **neutral pH solution** (normal saline or lactated Ringer's) 2. Topical antibiotics 3. Update tetanus prophylaxis 4. ± Corticosteroid ointment (Note: **All alkali** ocular exposures should be referred to an ophthalmologist immediately after irrigation even if examination is unremarkable.)
What is the best way to neutralize acid versus alkali ocular burns?	Do **not** try to neutralize the acid or alkali with its chemical counterpart because the resultant heat causes further injury.

SYMPATHETIC OPHTHALMIA

What is sympathetic ophthalmia	Rare autoimmune process occurring in the setting of penetrating injury to the globe whereby a destructive uveitis initially occurs in the injured eye and then progresses to involve the uninjured globe.
How can this condition be prevented?	Enucleate **irreversibly** injured globes within 2 weeks of trauma.

ASSORTED OPHTHALMOLOGIC TOPICS

What are the terms used to describe the constriction and dilatation of the iris?	Miosis—parasympathetic-mediated constriction Mydriasis—sympathetic-mediated dilatation
What type of ophthalmologic medication should not be given to the patient for outpatient use, and why?	Local anesthetics. Patient may further injure eye without realizing it, and these agents often delay healing.
What drugs are used to reduce the spasm of the ciliary muscle frequently seen with ocular injuries?	Cycloplegic–anticholinergic agents (e.g., atropine drops)

What are the untoward sequelae of topical corticosteroids?	Herpes simplex keratitis, cataract formation, fungal infection, and acute-angle glaucoma
Which injuries to the eye classically first present with symptoms 4 to 12 hours after injury?	Ultraviolet burns of cornea (e.g., welding arc, "snow blindness")
What is the associated finding on examination?	Diffuse punctate fluorescein staining of corneas
What is the treatment?	Topical corticosteroids, oral analgesia (Note: Resolution of symptoms in 1–2 days without sequela)
Which lacerations to the eyelid should be repaired by an ophthalmologist or plastic surgeon?	Lacerations involving: 1. Medial canthal region 2. Deep or through-and-through laceration involving the tarsal plate) 3. Edge of lid (risk of obvious lid notching)
What is a cataract?	Opacification of the lens
What are the etiologies?	Age, blunt trauma, and congenital
What is anisocoria?	Unequal pupil size
What are the etiologies?	Normal variant, trauma, iritis, temporal herniation, and syphilis
What is dacrocystitis?	Infection of the lacrimal sac
What is the usual etiology?	Obstruction of nasolacrimal duct with resultant *Streptococcus pneumoniae* infection (In infants, *Haemophilus influenzae* is the responsible organism.)

References

Abbas AK, Lichtman AH, Pober JS: *Cellular and Molecular Immunology.* Philadelphia, WB Saunders, 1991. **(Transplant Surgery)**

Abbott ME: Coarctation of the aorta of the adult type II: A statistical study and historical retrospect of 200 recorded cases, with autopsy, or stenosis or obliteration of the descending arch in subjects above the age of two years. *Am Heart J* 3:574, 1928.

Abcarian H, Alexander-Williams J, Christiansen J, et al: Benign anorectal disease: Definition, characterization, and analysis of treatment. *Am J Gastroenterol* 89:S182–S193, 1994.

American College of Surgeons: *Advanced Trauma Life Support Course.* Chicago, American College of Surgeons, 1989. **(Thoracic, Vascular, and Cardiac Surgery)**

Anderson JE: *Grant's Atlas of Anatomy,* 9th ed. Baltimore, Williams & Wilkins, 1991. **(Plastic Surgery)**

Appuzzo, M: *Brain Surgery Complication Avoidance and Management.* New York, Churchill Livingstone, 1993. **(Neurosurgery)**

Armstrong P, Wastie M: *Xray Diagnosis,* 1st ed. Oxford, Blackwell Scientific Publications, 1981.

Ahlman H: Midgut carcinoid tumors. *Surg Annual* 18:65–93, 1986.

Armitage, JO: Treatment of non-Hodgkin's lymphoma. *N Engl J Med* 328:1023–1029, 1993.

Arsenio, et al: Management of penetrating neck injuries: Contemporary problems in trauma surgery. *Surg Clin North Am* 71:267–296, 1991.

Auda SP, Brennan MF, Gill JG: Evolution of the surgical management to primary hyperaldosteronism. *Ann Surg* 191:1, 1980.

Austin KF: Diseases of immediate type hypersensitivity. In *Harrison's Principles of Internal Medicine,* 12th ed. Edited by Wilson JD. New York, McGraw-Hill, 1991, pp 1422–1427.

Bailey BJ, et al: *Head and Neck Surgery—Otolaryngology.* Philadelphia, JB Lippincott, 1993. **(Otolaryngology, Head and Neck Surgery)**

Baker JP, Detsky AS, Stewart S, et al: A randomized trial of total parenteral nutrition in critically ill patients: Metabolic effects of varying glucose-lipid ratios as the energy source. *Gastroenterology* 87:53–59, 1984.

Bates B: *A Guide to Physical Examination and History Taking.* Philadelphia, JB Lippincott, 1991.

Balch CM, Singletary SE, Bland KI: Clinical decision-making in early breast cancer. *Ann Surg* 217:207–225, 1994.

Balthazar EJ, Robinson DL, Megibow AJ, et al: Acute pancreatitis: Value of CT in establishing prognosis. *Radiology* 174:331–336, 1990.

Baltimore Regional Burn Center: *Manual for house officers*. Baltimore, Bayview Medical Center and the Department of Surgery, Johns Hopkins University School of Medicine, 1990. **(Plastic Surgery)**

Basson MD, et al: Biology and management of the midgut carcinoid. *Am J Surg* 165:288–297, 1993.

Baumgartner WA, Owens SG, Cameron DE, et al (eds): *The Johns Hopkins Manual of Cardiac Surgical Care*. St. Louis, Mosby-Year Book, 1994. **(Cardiac Surgery)**

Baumgartner WA, Reitz BA: *Heart and Heart-Lung Transplantation*. Philadelphia, WB Saunders, 1990. **(Cardiac Surgery)**

Beahrs OH (ed): *American Joint Committee on Cancer Manual for Staging Cancer*, 4th ed. Philadelphia, JB Lippincott, 1992.

Becker JM: Pancreatic pseudocyst. In *Current Surgical Therapy*. Edited by Cameron JL. St. Louis, Mosby-Year Book, 1992, pp 423–426.

Becker JM, Moody FG: The colon and rectum: VII. Ulcerative colitis. In *Textbook of Surgery: The Biological Basis of Modern Surgical Practice*, 14th ed. Edited by Sabiston DC. Philadelphia, WB Saunders, 1993, pp 927–940.

Beebe DS, McNevin MP, Crain JM, et al: Thermal injury of the posterior duodenum during laparoscopic cholecystectomy. *Surgical Endoscopy* 8(3):197–200, 1994.

Beger HG, Buchler M: Acute pancreatitis. In *Current Surgical Therapy*. Edited by Cameron JL. St. Louis, Mosby-Year Book, 1992, pp 405–410.

Berl T: Treating hyponatremia: Damned if we do and damned if we don't. *Kidney Int* 37:1006–1018, 1990.

Bernstein JM, Erk SD: Choice of antibiotics, pharmacokinetics, and dose adjustments in acute and chronic renal failure. *Med Clin North Am* 74(4):1059–1076,1990.

Berger RE: Sexually transmitted diseases. In *Campbell's Urology*. Edited by Walsh PC, Retik AB, Stamey TA, et al. Philadelphia, WB Saunders, 1992, p 823. **(Urologic Surgery)**

Beutler B, Grau GE: Tumor necrosis factor in the pathogenesis of infectious diseases. *Crit Care Med* 21:S423–S435,1993.

Billiar TR, Hoffman RA, Curan RD, et al: A role for inducible nitric oxide biosynthesis in the liver in inflammation and in the allogeneic immune response. *J Lab Clin Med* 120:192–197, 1992.

Blackbourne LH, Earnhardt R, et al: The sensitivity and role of ultrasound in the evaluation of biliary obstruction. *Am Surg* 60(9):683–690, 1994.

Bland KI, Copeland EM (eds): *The Breast*. Philadelphia, WB Saunders, 1991.

Bone RC: Sepsis and its complications: The clinical problem. *Crit Care Med* 22:S8–S11,1994.

Bojar RM: *Manual of Perioperative Care in Cardiac and Thoracic Surgery*, 2nd ed. Cambridge, MA, Blackwell Scientific Publications, 1994. **(Thoracic, Cardiac Surgery)**

Boswell WC, Odom JW, Rudolph R, et al: A method for controlling bleeding from the abdominal wall puncture site after laparoscopic surgery. *Surgical Laparoscopy and Endoscopy* 3(1):47–48, 1993.

Bradley EL: A fifteen year experience with open drainage for infected pancreatic necrosis. *Surg Gynecol Obstet* 177:215–222, 1993.

Bradley EL: Pancreatic abscess. In *Current Surgical Therapy*. Edited by Cameron JL. St. Louis, Mosby-Year Book, 1992, pp 419–422.

Bradley EL, Allen KA: A prospective longitudinal study of observation versus surgical intervention in the management of necrotizing pancreatitis. *Am J Surg* 161:19–24, 1991.

Braunwald E, et al: *Harrison's Principles of Internal Medicine*, 11th ed. New York, McGraw-Hill, 1987.

Bravo EL, Gifford RW Jr: Pheochromocytoma: Diagnosis, localization and management. *N Engl J Med* 311(20):1298–1303, 1984.

Bravo EL, Tarazi RC, Duson HP, et al: The changing clinical spectrum of primary aldosteronism. *Am J Med* 74:641, 1983.

Brennan MF: Adrenocortical carcinoma. *Cancer* 37:348, 1987.

Burke DJ, Alverdy JC, Aoys E, et al: Glutamine-supplemented total parenteral nutrition improves gut immune function. *Arch Surg* 124:1396–1399, 1989.

Cameron J: *Atlas of Biliary Tract Surgery*. New York, Churchill Livingstone, 1993.

Cameron JL (ed): *Current Surgical Therapy*, 3rd ed. St. Louis, BC Decker, 1989. **(Thoracic, Vascular Surgery)**

Cameron JL (ed): *Current Surgical Therapy*, 4th ed. St. Louis, Mosby-Year Book, 1992. **(Thoracic, Vascular Surgery)**

Cameron J (ed): *Current Surgical Therapy*, 5th ed. St Louis, Mosby, 1995.

Campbell DB, Waldhausen JA, Peirce WS, et al: Should elective repair of coarctation of the aorta be done in infancy? *J Thorac Cardiovasc Surg* 89:128, 1985.

Cancer Facts and Figures 1994. American Cancer Society, Inc, 1994.

Cance WG, Wells SA Jr: Multiple endocrine neoplasia type IIa. *Current Problems in Surgery* 22:1, 1985.

Cannistra SA: Cancer of the ovary. *N Engl J Med* 329:1550–1558, 1993. **Gynecologic Oncology)**

Capo L: Cushing's syndrome: A review of diagnostic tests. *Metabolism* 28:955, 1979.

Carducci, et al: *Ann Emerg Med* 15:208–221,1986.

Carpenter M: *Neuroanatomy*, 4th ed. Baltimore, Williams & Wilkins, 1991. **(Neurosurgery)**

Carrico CJ, Maier RV: Developments in the resuscitation of critically ill surgical patients. *Advances in Surgery* 19:271–378, 1986.

Carrol PR: Urothelial carcinoma: Cancers of the bladder, ureter, and renal pelvis. In *Smith's General Urology*. Edited by Tanagho EA, McAninch JW. Norwalk, CT, Appleton & Lange, 1992, p 341. **(Urologic Surgery)**

Casson AG, et al: Five year survival after pulmonary metastasectomy for adult soft tissue sarcoma. *Cancer* 69:662–668, 1992.

Cattey RP: Nobel prize winners in surgery: Completing the list. *Surgery* 109(6):804–805, 1991.

Champion V: Relationship of age to mammography compliance. *Cancer* 74:329–335, 1994.

Chandler J. The history of the surgical treatment of portal hypertension. *Arch Surg* 128(8):925–940, 1992.

Cheek W: *Pediatric Neurosurgery: Surgery of the Developing Nervous System*, 3rd ed. Philadelphia, WB Saunders, 1994. **(Neurosurgery)**

Chen TS, Chen PS: The Whipples and their legacies in medicine. *Surg Gynecol Obstet* 176(5):501–506,1993.

Chisholm GD: Renal function: Physiology and investigation. In *Scientific Foundations of Surgery*. Edited by Kyle J, Carey LC. Chicago, Year Book, 1989, pp 484–493.

Cirocco WC, Schwartzman A, Golub RW: Abdominal wall recurrence after laparoscopic colectomy for colon cancer. *Surgery* 116(5):842–846, 1994.

Clemente CD: *Anatomy: A Regional Atlas of the Human Body*, 3rd ed. Baltimore, Urban and Schwartzenberg, 1987. **(Orthopedic, Vascular, Thoracic, and Cardiac Surgery)**

Cline RW, Poulos E, Clifford EJ: An assessment of potential complications caused by intraperitoneal gallstones. *Am Surg* 60(5):303–305, 1994.

Cohen JR: *Vascular Surgery for the House Officer*, 2nd ed. Baltimore, Williams & Wilkins, 1992.

Cohn K, Gottesman L, Brennan MF: Adrenocortical carcinoma. *Surgery* 100:1170, 1986.

Cooper DS, Ridgeway EC: Clinical management of patients with hyperthyroidism. *Med Clin North Am* 69(5), 1985.

Cope LH: Radiological, ultrasound and isotope studies. In *Practical Renal Medicine*. Edited by Gabriel R. Oxford, Blackwell Scientific Publications, 1993, pp 67–89.

Cotran RS, Kumar V, Robbins SL: *Robbins Pathologic Basis of Disease*, 4th ed. Philadelphia, WB Saunders, 1989. **(Plastic Surgery)**

Cowgill LD (ed.): *Cardiac Surgery State of the Art Reviews: Cyanotic Congenital Heart Disease*, Vol. 3, No. 1. Philadelphia, Hanley and Belfus, 1989. **(Cardiac Surgery)**

Crenshaw AH: *Campbell's Operative Orthopaedics*, 7th ed. St. Louis, CV Mosby, 1987. **(Orthopedic Surgery)**

Creutzfeldt W, Stockmann F: Carcinoids and carcinoid syndrome. *Am J Med* 82(5B):4–16,1987.

Crist D, Gadacz T: Complications in laparoscopic surgery. *Surg Clin North Am* 73 (2)265–289, 1993.

Cummings CW, et al: *Otolaryngology—Head and Neck Surgery*, 2nd ed. St. Louis, Mosby-Year Book, 1993. **(Otolaryngology, Head and Neck Surgery)**

Daniel WW: *Applied Nonparametric Statistics*, 2nd ed. Boston, PWS-Kent, 1990.

Darnell JE: *Molecular Cell Biology*. New York, Scientific American Books, 1986.

Davidson NE, Martin D, Abeloff MD: Adjuvant therapy of breast cancer. *World J Surg* 19:112–116, 1994.

Davis JH: Some thoughts of a trauma surgeon. *Archiv Surg* 128(5):489–493, 1993.

Dawson-Saunders B, Trapp R: *Basic and Clinical Biostatistics*. Norwalk, CT, Appleton & Lang, 1990.

Dean RH: Indications for operative management of renovascular hypertension. *JSC Med Assoc* 73:523, 1977.

DeBakey ME: A surgical perspective. *Ann Surg* 213(6):499–531, 1991.

DeCosse JJ, Tsioulias GJ, Jacobson JS: Colorectal cancer: Detection, treatment, and rehabilitation. *CA Cancer J Clin* 44:27–42, 1994.

DeMarkles MP, Murphy JR: Acute lower gastrointestinal bleeding. *Med Clin North Am* 77:1085–1100, 1993.

Detsky AS, McLaughlin JR, Baker JP, et al: What is subjective global assessment of nutritional status? *J Parenter Enter Nutr* 11(1):8–13, 1987.

DeVita VT, Hellman S, Rosenberg SA (eds): *Cancer: Principles and Practice of Oncology*. Philadelphia, JB Lippincott, 1989.

DeVries EGE, et al: Recent developments in diagnosis and treatment of metastatic carcinoid tumors. *Scand J Gastroenterol* 28(200):87–93, 1993.

Dimaio VJM. *Gunshot Wounds*. Boca Raton, FL, CRC Press, 1993.

Domsky MF, Wilson RF: Hemodynamic resuscitation. *Critical Care Clinics* 10(4), 715–726, 1993.

Donohue JH, van Heerden JA, Monson JRT (eds.): *Atlas of Surgical Oncology*. Cambridge, MA, Blackwell Scientific Publications, 1995.

Donovan AJ: Explorers. Christopher Columbus and Leonardo daVinci. *Arch Surg* 128(7):725–729, 1993. **(Cardiac, Vascular, and Thoracic Surgery)**

Donovan AJ: *Trauma Surgery: Techniques in Thoracic, Abdominal and Vascular Surgery*. St. Louis, Mosby-Year Book, 1994.

Dougherty SH, Simmons RL: The biology and practice of surgical drains. *Current Problems in Surgery* 29(8):559–730, 1992.

Dreicer R, Williams RD: Renal parenchymal neoplasms. In *Smith's General Urology*, 13th ed. Edited by Tanagho EA, McAninch JW. Norwalk, CT, Appleton & Lange, 1992, p 359. **(Urologic Surgery)**

Dreznik Z, Soper NJ: Trocar site abscess due to spilled gallstones: An unusual late complication of laparoscopic cholecystectomy. *Surgical Laparoscopy and Endoscopy* 3(3):223–224, 1993.

Dubois F, Berthelot G, Levard H: Laparoscopic cholecystectomy: Historic perspective and personal experience. *Surgical Laparoscopy and Endoscopy* 1(1):52–57, 1991.

Dunham CM, Cowley RA: *Shock Trauma/Critical Care Manual*. Gaithersburg, MD, Aspen Publishers, pp 3-1:1–3-1:9, 1991.

Earnhardt RC, McQuone SJ, Minasi JS, et al: Intraoperative fine needle aspiration of pancreatic and extrahepatic biliary masses. *Surg Gynecol Obstet* 177:147–152, 1993.

Eddy DM: Screening for cervical cancer. *Ann Intern Med* 113:214–226, 1990. **(Gynecologic Oncology)**

Eiseman B: The puzzle people: Memoirs of a transplant surgeon. *Arch Surg* 127(9):1009–1011, 1992.

Eisenberg R: *Diagnostic Imaging in Surgery*. New York, McGraw-Hill, 1987.

Eisenberg R: *Clinical Imaging*, 2nd ed. Gaithersburg, MD, Aspen Publishers, 1992.

El-Ashry E, Lippman ME: Molecular biology of breast carcinoma. *World J Surg* 18:12–20, 1994.

Elder JB: Inhibition of acid and gastric carcinoids. *Gut* 26:1279–1283, 1985.

Elston RC, Johnson WD: Essentials of Biostatistics, 2nd ed. Philadelphia, FA Davis, 1994.

Emergency Cardiac Care Committee and Subcommittees, American Heart Association: Guidelines for cardiopulmonary resuscitation and emergency cardiac care I: Introduction. *JAMA* 268:2172–2183, 1992.

Enzinger FM, Weiss SW: *Soft Tissue Tumors*. St Louis, Mosby-Year Book, 1995.

Ernst CB, Stanley JC (eds): *Current Therapy in Vascular Surgery*, 3rd ed. St. Louis, CV Mosby, 1995. **(Vascular Surgery)**

Evarts CM, Pelligrini VD Jr: Complications. In Rockwood and Green's *Fractures in Adults*, ed 3. Edited by Rockwood CA, Green DP, and Bucholz RW. Philadelphia, JB Lippincott, 1991, pp 390–396.

Farrar WB, LaValle GJ, Kim JA: Breast Cancer. In *Cancer Surgery*. Edited by McKenna RJ, Murphy GP. Philadelphia, JB Lippincott, 1994.

Farrington K: Management of acute renal failure. In *Practical Renal Medicine*. Edited by Gabriel R. Oxford, Blackwell Scientific Publications, 1993, pp 224–251.

Fazio VW: Surgery of the colon and rectum. *Am J Gastroenterol* 89:S106–S115, 1994.

Feliciano David V: Management of traumatic retroperitoneal hematoma. *Ann Surg* 211(2):109–123, 1990.

Feldman JF: Carcinoid tumors and the carcinoid syndrome. *Current Problems in Surgery* Dec:831–885, 1989.

Fengler SA, Pearl RK: Technical considerations in the surgical treatment of colon and rectal cancer. *Seminars in Surgical Oncology* 10:200–207, 1994.

Ferrara JJ, Steinberg SM, Flint LM: Myocardial failure in sepsis. *Surgical Rounds* 16:863–868, 1993.

Finch WT, Sawyer JL: A prospective study to determine efficacy of antibiotics in acute pancreatitis. *Ann Surg* 183:667–670, 1976.

Finn WF: Diagnosis and management of acute tubular necrosis. *Med Clin North Am* 74(4):873–891, 1990.

Fogarty TJ: Acute arterial occlusion. In *Textbook of Surgery*, ed 14. Edited by Sabiston DC Jr. Philadelphia, WB Saunders, 1994, pp 1624–1626.

Foster DW, McGarry JP: The metabolic derangements and treatment of diabetic ketoacidosis. *New Engl J Med* 309 (3), 1983, pp 159–169.

Freedom RM, Benson LN, Smallhorn JF: *Neonatal Heart Disease*. London, Springer-Verlag, 1992. **(Cardiac Surgery)**

Frey CF: Gallstone pancreatitis. In *Current Surgical Therapy*. Edited by Cameron JL. St. Louis, Mosby-Year Book, 1992, pp 410–414.

Frymoyer J: *The Adult Spine, Principles and Practice*. New York, Raven Press, 1991. **(Neurosurgery)**

Gabriel R: Clinical presentation of renal disease. *Med Clin North Am* 74(4):1–11, 1990.

Gay S, Sistrom C: Computed tomographic evaluation of blunt abdominal trauma. *Radiol Clin North Am* 30(2):367–388, 1992.

Georgiade GS, Georgiade NG, Riefkohl R, et al *(eds): Textbook of Plastic, Maxillofacial and Reconstructive Surgery,* vols I and II, 2nd ed. Baltimore: Williams & Wilkins, 1992. **(Plastic Surgery)**

Gerzoff SG, Banks PA, Robbins AH, et al: Early diagnosis of pancreatic infection by computed tomography-guided aspiration. *Gastroenterology* 93:1315–1320,1987.

Glassman JA: *Biliary Tract Surgery: Tactics and Techniques.* New York, MacMillan.

Godwin JD: Carcinoid tumors. *Cancer* 36:560–569, 1975.

Goldman L: Evaluation of the cardiac patient for noncardiac surgery. *ACC Current Journal Review* (Feb):60–63, 1994.

Goldman, et al: Multifactorial index of cardiac risk in noncardiac surgical procedures. *N Engl J Med* 297:845–850, 1977.

Goodale RL: Evidence of venous stasis after abdominal insufflation for laparoscopic cholecystectomy. Surg Gynecol Obstet 176(5):443–447, 1993.

Garfinkel L, Boring CC, Heath CW Jr: Changing trends: An overview of breast cancer incidence and mortality. *Cancer* 74:222–227, 1994.

Goodman AG, Rall TW, Nies AS, et al (eds): *Goodman and Gilman's The Pharmacologic Basis of Therapeutics,* 8th ed. New York, Pergamon, 1990.

Gordon LA, Shapiro SJ, Daykhousky L: Problem solving in laparoscopic surgery. *Surgical Endoscopy* 7:348–355, 1993.

Gordon RL, Shapiro HA: Nonoperative management of bile duct stones. *Surg Clin North Am* 70(6):1313–1328.

Gouma DJ, et al: Bile duct injury during laparoscopic and conventional cholecystectomy. *J Am Coll Surg* 178(3):229–233, 1994.

Govett GS, Amedee RG: Ocular trauma in otolaryngology. *LSMSJ* 144:187–191, 1992. **(Ophthalmology)**

Grahm TW, Zadrozny DB, Harrington T: The benefits of early jejunal hyperalimentation in the head-injured patient. *Neurosurgery* 25:729–735, 1989.

Gray RJ, Matloff JM (eds): *Medical Management of the Cardiac Surgical Patient.* Baltimore, Williams & Wilkins, 1990. **(Cardiac Surgery)**

Green RM, Ouriel K: Peripheral arterial disease. In *Principles of Surgery,* 6th ed. Edited by Schwartz SI. New York, McGraw-Hill, 945–949, 1994.

Greenberg M: *Handbook of Neurosurgery,* 3rd ed. Greenberg Graphics, 1994.

Greenfield L, et al: *Surgery: Scientific Principles and Practice,* 1st ed. Philadelphia, JB Lippincott, 1993.

Greenfield L (ed): Carcinoid tumors. In *Surgery: Scientific Principles and Practice,* 1st ed. Philadelphia, JB Lippincott, 1993, pp 760–763.

Gronbech JE, Soreide O, Bergan A: The role of resective surgery in the treatment of the carcinoid syndrome. *Scand J Gastroenterol* 27:433–437, 1992.

Guidelines for the use of parenteral and enteral nutrition in adult and pediatric patients. American Society of Parenteral and Enteral Nutrition (A.S.P.E.N.) Board of Directors. *J Parenter Enter Nutr* 17(Suppl), 1993.

Hall WD, Wollam GL, Tuttle EP Jr: Diagnostic evaluations of patient with hypertension. In *The Heart*. Edited by Hurst JW. New York, McGraw Hill, 1986, p 1057.

Hallet JW Jr, Brewster DC, Darling RC: *Patient Care in Vascular Surgery*, 2nd ed. Boston, Little, Brown, 1987. **(Vascular Surgery)**

Hansen KJ, Trible RW, Reavis SW, et al: Renal duplex sonography: Evaluation of clinical utility. *J Vasc Surg* 12:227, 1990.

Hansen KJ, Starr SM, Sands E, et al: Contemporary surgical management of renovascular disease. *J Vasc Surg* 16:319, 1992.

Harris JR, Lippman ME, Veronesi U, et al: Breast Cancer. *N Engl J Med* 327:319–328, 1992.

Harrison MR, Langer JC, et al: Correction of diaphragmatic hernia in utero: Initial clinical experience. *J Pediatr Surg* 25:47–55, 1990. **(Pediatric Surgery)**

Hart RO, Tamadon A, Fitzgibbons RJ Jr, et al: Open laparoscopic cholecystectomy in pregnancy. *Surgical Laparoscopy and Endoscopy* 3(1):13–16, 1993.

Hasel R, Arora SK, Hickey DR: Intraoperative complications of laparoscopic cholecystectomy. *Can J Anaesth* 40(5 Pt 1):459–464, 1993.

Hass BE, Daoud IM, Carlson JA: Management of the unexpected ovarian neoplasm at laparotomy for acute abdomen in patients younger than age 35. *Contemporary Surgery* 40:21–25, 1992. **(Gynecologic Oncology)**

Hedican SP, Berger RE: Sexually transmitted diseases. In *Campbell's Urology*, 6th ed. Edited by Walsh PC, Retik AB, Stamey TA, et al. Philadelphia, WB Saunders, 1992, p 823.

Heger K: *The Illustrated History of Surgery*. New York, Bell Publishing Co, 1988.

Hendren WH: Urinary tract refunctionalization after long-term diversion: A 20 year experience with 177 patients. *Ann Surg* 212:478–495, 1990. **(Pediatric Surgery)**

Henrich WL: The endothelium—A key regulator of vascular tone. *Am J Med Sci* 302:319–332, 1991.

Hills MW, Delprado AM, Deane SA, et al: Sternal fractures: Associated injuries and management. *J Trauma* 35(1):55–60, 1993.

Hiyama DT, Zimmer MJ: Fat embolism. In *Principles of Surgery*, 6th ed. Edited by Schwartz SI. New York, McGraw-Hill, 1995, pp 455–456.

Holzman M, Sharp K, Richards W: Hypercarbia during carbon dioxide gas insufflation for therapeutic laparoscopy: A note of caution. *Surgical Laparoscopy and Endoscopy* 2(1):11–14, 1992.

Howes R, Zuidema GD, Cameron JL: Evaluation of prophylactic antibiotics in acute pancreatitis. *J Surg Res* 18:197–200, 1975.

Howlett, et al: Cushing's syndrome. *Clin Endocrinol Metab* 14:911, 1985.

Huber PJ, Thal ER: Management of colon injuries. *Surg Clin North Am* 70 (3), 1990.

Idler RS, Manktelow RT, Lucas G, et al: *The Hand: Examination and Diagnosis*, 3rd ed. New York, Churchill Livingstone, 1990. (**Plastic Surgery**)

Idler RS, Manktelow RT, Lucas G, et al: *The Hand: Primary Care of Common Problems*, 2nd ed. New York, Churchill Livingstone, 1990. (**Plastic Surgery**)

Imbembo AL, Bailey RW: The colon and rectum: V. Diverticular disease of the colon. In *Textbook of Surgery: The Biological Basis of Modern Surgical Practice*, 14th ed. Edited by Sabiston DC. Philadelphia, WB Saunders, 1993, pp 910–920.

Imbembo AL, Fitzpatrick JL: The colon and rectum: VI. Benign neoplasms of the colon, including vascular malformations. In *Textbook of Surgery: The Biological Basis of Modern Surgical Practice*, 14th ed. Edited by Sabiston DC. Philadelphia, WB Saunders, 1993, pp 921–927.

Imbembo AL, Lefor AT: The colon and rectum: IX. Carcinoma of the colon, rectum, and anus. In *Textbook of Surgery: The Biological Basis of Modern Surgical Practice*, 14th ed. Edited by Sabiston DC. Philadelphia, WB Saunders, 1993, pp 944–958.

Imbembo AL, Zucker KA: The colon and rectum: VIII. Volvulus of the colon. In *Textbook of Surgery: The Biological Basis of Modern Surgical Practice*, 14th ed. Edited by Sabiston DC. Philadelphia, WB Saunders, 1993, pp 940–944.

Isselbacher KJ, Braunwald E, Wilson JD, et al (eds): *Harrison's Principles of Internal Medicine*, 13th ed. New York, McGraw-Hill, 1994. (**Vascular, Cardiac, Orthopedic, and Thoracic Surgery**)

Janda AM: Ocular trauma. *Postgrad Med* 90:51–60, 1991. (**Ophthalmology**)

Jarrell BE, Carabasi RA III: *NMS Surgery*, 2nd ed. Baltimore, Williams & Wilkins, 1991.

Jarrett F: Discoverer of penicillin was a surgeon. *Surgery* 109(6):805, 1991.

Jenkins JL, Loscalzo J: Trauma to eye and periorbital area. In *Manual of Emergency Medicine*. Edited by Jenkins JL, Loscalzo J: Boston, Little, Brown, 1990, pp 303–307. (**Ophthalmology**)

Johns ME, et al: *Atlas of Head and Neck Surgery*. Philadelphia, BC Decker, 1990. (**Otolaryngology, Head and Neck Surgery**)

Jones RS: *Atlas of Liver and Biliary Surgery*, 1st ed. Chicago, Year Book, 1990.

Jones RS: Carcinoma of the gallbladder. *Surg Clin North Am* 70(6):1419–1428, 1990.

Jones RS, Meyers WC: *Textbook of Liver and Biliary Surgery*, 1st ed. JB Lippincott, 1990.

Jones WG, Minei JP, Barber AE, et al: Elemental diet promotes spontaneous bacterial translocation and alters mortality after endotoxin challenge. *Surg Forum* 40:20–22,1989.

Jurkiewicz MJ, Krizek TJ, Mathes SJ, et al *(eds): Plastic Surgery: Principles and Practice*, vols I and II. Baltimore, CV Mosby, 1990. (**Plastic Surgery**)

Karakousis CP: Surgery for soft tissue sarcomas. In *Cancer Surgery*. Edited by McKenna and Murphy. Philadelphia, JB Lippincott, 1994, pp 577–599.

Kelly TR, Wagner DS: Gallstone pancreatitis: A prospective randomized trial of the timing of surgery. *Surgery* 104:600–605, 1988.

Keith RG: Pancreas divisum in Cameron JL (ed): *Current Surgical Therapy.* St. Louis, Mosby-Year Book, 1992, pp 414–418.

Kemshead JT, Pizer BL, Patel K: Neuroblastoma: Perspectives for future research. In *Neuroblastoma: Tumor Biology and Therapy.* Edited by Pochedly C. Boca Raton, FL: CRC Press, 1990, pp 381–395. **(Pediatric Surgery)**

King TC, Smith CR: Chest wall, pleura, and mediastinum. In *Principles of Surgery,* 6th ed. Edited by Schwartz S. New York, McGraw-Hill, 1994, pp 677, 704–707.

Kirby DF, DeLegge MH: Refeeding syndrome: Background, diagnosis, and management. Presented at the American Society of Parenteral and Enteral Nutrition 19th Clinical Congress, 1995.

Kirklin JW, Barrat-Boyes BG: *Cardiac Surgery,* 2nd ed. New York, Churchill Livingstone, 1993. **(Cardiac Surgery)**

Kissin MW: The patron saints of breast disease. *Aust N Z J Surg* 61(6):452–458, 1991.

Knutzen AM, Gisvold JJ: Likelihood of malignant diseases for various categories of mammographically detected nonpalpable breast lesions. *Mayo Clin Proc* 68:454–460, 1993.

Kvols LK, Reubi JC: Metastatic carcinoid tumors and the malignant carcinoid syndrome. *Acta Oncol* 32(2):197–201, 1993.

Krause WJ, Cutts JH: *Concise Text of Histology.* Baltimore, Williams & Wilkins, 1986.

Kronborg O: Optimal follow-up in colorectal cancer patients: What tests and how often? *Seminars in Surgical Oncology* 10:217–224, 1994.

Kryzywda EA, et al: Glucose response to abrupt initiation and discontinuation of total parenteral nutrition. *J Parenter Enter Nutr* 117:64–67, 1994.

Kudsk KA, Campbell SM, O'Brien T, et al: Postoperative jejunal feedings following complicated pancreatitis. *Nutrition in Clinical Practice* 5:14–17, 1990.

Landercasper J, Miller GJ, Strutt PJ, et al: Carbon dioxide embolization and laparoscopic cholecystectomy. *Surgical Laparoscopy and Endoscopy* 3(5):407–410, 1993.

Last RJ: *Anatomy Regional and Applied,* 7th ed. Edinburgh, Churchill Livingstone, 1984, p. 323. **(Gynecologic Oncology)**

Lavelle-Jones M, Mayer AD, Moossen AR: Surgical complications. In *Principles of Surgery,* 6th ed. Edited by Schwartz SI. New York, McGraw-Hill, 1994, pp 310–311, 315, 317–329.

Legorreta AP, Siber JH, Costantino GH, et al: Increased cholecystectomy rate after the introduction of laparoscopic cholecystectomy. *JAMA* 270(12):1429–1432, 1993.

Leibel, SA: Soft tissue sarcoma: Therapeutic results and rationale for conservative surgery and radiation therapy. *Radiation Oncology Annual* 1983. New York, Raven Press, 1984.

Leibenhaut, MH: The changing role of staging laparotomy in the management of Hodgkin's disease. *Cancer Treatment and Research* 66:1–19, 1993.

Leitch AM (ed): *Sarcomas and Lymphomas. Selected Readings in General Surgery* 20:1–64, 1993.

Levine BA, Copeland EM, Howard RJ, et al (eds): *Current Practice of Surgery.* New York, Churchill Livingstone, 1994. **(Thoracic, Vascular, and Cardiac Surgery)**

Levinsky NG: Fluids and electrolytes. In *Harrison's Principles of Internal Medicine,* 12th ed. Edited by Wilson JD. New York, McGraw-Hill, 1991, pp 242–253.

Lewis JL Jr: Diagnosis and management of gestational trophoblastic disease. *Cancer* 71S:1639–1647, 1993. **(Gynecologic Oncology)**

Lewis RP: Digitalis: A drug that refuses to die. *Crit Care Med* 18(1):5–13, 1990.

Lipsett PA, Pitt HA: Acute cholangitis. *Surg Clin North Am* 70(6):1297–1312, 1990.

Lopez-Viego MA (ed): *The Parkland Trauma Handbook.* St. Louis, CV Mosby, 1994. **(Ophthalmologic, Thoracic, Orthopedic, and Vascular Surgery)**

Lore, JM: *An Atlas of Head and Neck Surgery,* 3rd ed. Philadelphia, WB Saunders, 1988. **(Otolaryngology, Head and Neck Surgery)**

Lucas CE: Splenic trauma—Choice of management. *Ann Surg* 213(2):98–113, 1991.

Lyerly HK, Gaynor JW (eds): *Handbook of Surgical Intensive Care,* 3rd ed. St. Louis, Mosby-Year Book, 1992. **(Thoracic, Cardiac Surgery)**

Lynch K: Professor of Pharmacology. Lecture series in antibiotics. University of Virginia School of Medicine, Charlottesville, VA, 1993.

MacKinnon S, Dellon A: *Surgery of the Peripheral Nerve.* New York, Thieme, 1988. **(Neurosurgery)**

Mandell GL: Chairman: Infectious diseases department. Personal correspondence on infectious diseases consult service. University of Virginia Health Sciences Center, Charlottesville, VA, 1995.

Mandell GL, et al: *Principles and Practice of Infectious Diseases, Antimicrobial Therapy, 1993/1994.* New York, Churchill Livingstone, 1994.

Mandell GL, Gordon DR Jr, Bennett JE (eds): *Principles and Practice of Infectious Diseases,* 3rd ed. New York, Churchill Livingstone, 1990.

Manson PN: *Maxillofacial Injuries: Physical Signs, Radiographic Diagnosis, and Treatment.* Baltimore, Division of Plastic, Maxillofacial, and Reconstructive Surgery, Johns Hopkins School of Medicine, 1992. **(Plastic Surgery)**

Marino P, et al: *The ICU Book.* Philadelphia, Lea & Febiger, 1991.

Marshall JB, Bodnarchuk G: Carcinoid tumors of the gut. *J Clin Gastroenterol* 16(2):123–219, 1993.

Martin FM, Braasch JW: Primary sclerosing cholangitis. *Current Problems in Surgery* 29(3):133–193, 1992.

Martin M: Primary sclerosing cholangitis. *Annual Review of Medicine* 44:221–227, 1993.

Martindale RG: Gut issues in early enteral feeding. Presented at the American Society of Parenteral and Enteral Nutrition 19th Clinical Congress, 1995.

Martiny SS, Phelps SJ, Massey KL: Treatment of severe digitalis intoxication with digoxin specific antibody fragments: A clinical review. *Crit Care Med* 16(6):629–634, 1988.

Mashadi ZB, Amis AA: The effect of locking loops on the strength of tendon repair. *J Hand Surg* (Br) 16B:35–39, 1991. **(Plastic Surgery)**

Mazanet R, Antman K: Sarcomas of soft tissue and bone. *Cancer* 68:463–473, 1991.

McAninch JW: Disorders of the penis and male urethra. In *Smith's General Urology*, 13th ed. Edited by Tanagho EA, McAninch JW. Norwalk, CT, Appleton & Lange, 1992, p 594. **(Urologic Surgery)**

McAninch JW: Injuries to the genitourinary tract. In *Smith's General Urology*, 13th ed. Edited by Tanagho EA, McAninch JW. Norwalk, CT, Appleton & Lange, 1992, p 308. **(Urologic Surgery)**

McClelland RN, et al: *Selected Readings in General Surgery* Jan/Feb/Mar 1993.

McClelland RN, et al: *Selected Readings in General Surgery* 20(8) August 1993.

McClelland RN, et al: *Selected Readings in General Surgery* 21(5–6) May 1994.

McClelland RN, Weigelt JA, et al: *Selected Readings in General Surgery*. June–September, 1994.

McClelland RN, et al: *Selected Readings in General Surgery* 21(10–12), 1994.

McClelland RN: Selected readings in general surgery. *Stomach* 22:4–7, 1995.

McKenna RJ: The abnormal mammogram: Radiographic findings, diagnostic options, pathology, and stage of cancer diagnosis. *Cancer* 74:244–255, 1994.

Meier GH, Sumpio B, Black HR, et al: Captopril renal scintigraphy: An advance in the detection and treatment of renovascular hypertension. *J Vasc Surg* 11:770, 1990.

Merrell RC, Evans DB: Pancreatic islet cell tumors. In *Current Surgical Therapy*. Edited by Cameron JL. St. Louis, Mosby-Year Book, 1992, pp 451–457.

Merono-Cabajosa EA, Celdran-Uriarte A, Moreno-Caparros A, et al: Caroli's Disease: Study of six cases, including one with epithelial dysplasia. *Int Surg* 78(1):46–49, 1993.

Miles JM: Intravenous fat emulsions in nutrition support. *Curr Opin Gastroenterol* 7:306–311, 1991.

Mileski WJ: Sepsis: What is it and how to recognize it. *Surg Clin North Am* 71:749–764, 1991.

Miller MD (ed): *Review of Orthopaedics*. Philadelphia, WB Saunders, 1992. **(Orthopedic Surgery)**

Milsom SR, Espiner EA, Nicholls MG, et al: The blood pressure response to unilateral adrenalectomy in primary aldosteronism. *Q J Med* 61:1141, 1986.

Minard G: Enteral access. *Nutrition in Clinical Practice* 5:268–278, 1994.

Minard G, Kudsk KA: Is early feeding beneficial? How early is early? *New Horizon* 2(2):156–163, 1994.

Mistry P, Seymour CA: Primary biliary cirrhosis–from Thomas Addison to the 1990s. *Q J Med* 82(299):185–196, 1992.

Moertel CG: Chemotherapy for colorectal cancer. *N Engl J Med* 330:1136–1142, 1994.

Moertel CG, et al: Carcinoid tumor of the appendix: Treatment and prognosis. *N Engl J Med* 317:1699–1701, 1987.

Moldawer LL: Biology of proinflammatory cytokines and their antagonists. *Crit Care Med* 22:S3–S7, 1994.

Montecalvo MA, Steger KA, et al: Critical care research team. Nutritional outcome and pneumonia in critical care patients randomized to gastric versus jejunal tube feedings. *Crit Care Med* 29:1377–1387, 1992.

Moore DS, McCabe GP: *Introduction to the Practice of Statistics.* New York, W.H. Freeman and Company, 1989.

Moore EE, et al: Organ injury scaling, II: Pancreas, duodenum, small bowel, colon, and rectum. *J Trauma* 30:1427–1429, 1990.

Moore KL: *Clinically Oriented Anatomy,* 2nd ed. Baltimore, Williams & Wilkins, 1985.

Moossa AR, Easter DW: Unusual pancreatic tumors. In *Current Surgical Therapy.* Edited by Cameron JL. St. Louis, Mosby-Year Book, 1992, pp 448–451.

Moran BJ, Jackson AA: Function of the human colon. *Br J Surg* 79:1132–1137, 1992.

Morris JB, Schirmer WJ: The right stuff: 5 Nobel Prize-winning surgeons. *Surgery* 108:71–80, 1990.

Morris PJ (ed.): *Kidney Transplantation: Principles and Practice.* New York, Grune and Stratton, 1984. **(Transplant Surgery)**

Moskop RJ Jr, Lubarsky DA: Carbon dioxide embolism during laparoscopic cholecystectomy. *South Med J* 87(3):414–415, 1994.

Moss AJ, Parson VL: Current estimates from the national health interview survey, United States, 1985. Hyattsville, MD, National Center for Health Statistics, 1986, p 667. **(Otolaryngology, Head and Neck Surgery)**

Moylan JA: Fat embolism. In *Textbook of Surgery,* 14th ed. Edited by Sabiston DC Jr. Philadelphia, WB Saunders 1994, pp 1520–1522.

Mullan H, Roubenoff RA, et al: Risk of pulmonary aspiration among patients receiving enteral nutrition support. *J Parenter Enter Nutr* 16:160–164, 1992.

Nagy AG, Poulin EC, Girotti MJ, et al: History of laparoscopic surgery. *Canadian J Surg* 35(3):271–274, 1992.

Napolitano G, et al: An overview on the management of carcinoid tumors. *J Nucl Biol Med* 35:337–340, 1991.

Natanson C, Shelhamer JH, Parillo JE: Intubation of the trachea in the critical care setting. *JAMA* 253(8):1160–1165, 1985.

National Institutes of Health. *Ovarian cancer: Screening, Treatment, and Followup.* NIH Consensus Statement 12:1994. **(Gynecologic Oncology)**

References

Nelson DH, Meakin JW, Thorn GW: ACTH-producing pituitary tumors following adrenalectomy for Cushing's syndrome. *Ann Intern Med* 52:560, 1960.

Netter FH: *Atlas of Human Anatomy.* West Caldwell, Ciba-Geigy 334:1989. **(Gynecologic Oncology)**

Neuberger J, Lombard M, Galbraith R: Primary biliary cirrhosis. *Gut* Suppl:S73–S78, 1991.

NIH Consensus Conference: Gallstone and laparoscopic cholecystectomy. *JAMA* 269(8), 1993.

Nichols DG, Cameron DE, Greeley WJ, et al: *Critical Heart Disease in Infants and Children.* St. Louis, Mosby-Year Book, 1995. **(Cardiac Surgery)**

Nordback IH, Cameron JL: Periampullary cancer. In *Current Surgical Therapy.* Edited by Cameron JL. St. Louis, Mosby-Year Book, 1992, pp 441–448.

Norton RA, Foster EA: Bile duct cancer. *CA: Cancer J Clin* 40(4):225–233, 1990.

Nyhus LM, Baker RJ (eds): *Mastery of Surgery,* 2nd ed. Boston, Little, Brown, 1992. **(Thoracic Surgery)**

Oberg K, Eriksson B: Medical treatment of neuroendocrine gut and pancreatic tumors. *Acta Oncol* 28:425–431,1988.

O'Leary JP (ed): *The Physiologic Basis of Surgery,* 1st ed. Baltimore, Williams & Wilkins, 1993.

O'Neil JA: Choledochal cyst. *Current Problems in Surgery* 29(6):363–410, 1992.

Paksoy N, Lilleng R, et al: Diagnostic accuracy of FNA cytology in pancreatic lesions. A review of 77 cases. *Acta Cytol* 37:889–893, 1993.

Papel, ID, Nachlas, NE: *Facial Plastic and Reconstructive Surgery.* St. Louis, Mosby-Year Book, 1992. **(Otolaryngology, Head and Neck Surgery)**

Parker SH: Percutaneous large core breast biopsy. *Cancer* 74:256–262, 1994.

Paul WB: *Fundamental Immunology,* 2nd ed. New York, Raven Press, 1989. **(Transplant Surgery)**

Pederzoli P, Bassi C, Vesenti S, et al: A randomized multicenter clinical trial of antibiotic prophylaxis of septic complications in acute necrotizing pancreatitis with imipenem. *Surg Gynecol Obstet* 176:480–488,1993.

Pels RJ, Bor DH, Woolhandler S, et al: Dipstick urinalysis screening of asymptomatic adults for urinary tract disorders. II. Bacteriuria. *JAMA* 262(9):1221–1224, 1989.

Perry MO: Acute limb ischemia. In *Vascular Surgery,* 4th ed. Edited by Rutherford RB. Philadelphia, WB Saunders, 1995, pp 641–666.

Pisters PWT, Ranson JHC: Nutritional support for acute pancreatitis. *Surg Gynecol Obstet* 175:275–284, 1992.

Plaus WJ: Laparoscopic trocar site hernias. *Journal of Laparoendoscopic Surgery* 3(6):567–570, 1993.

Prieto J, Rodes J, Schafritz DA (eds): *Hepatobiliary Diseases.* New York, Springer-Verlag, 1992.

Pritchett ELC: Management of atrial fibrillation. *N Engl J Med* 326(19):1264–1271, 1992.

Qazi F, McGuire WP: The treatment of epithelial ovarian cancer. *CA Cancer J Clin* 45:88–101, 1995. **(Gynecologic Oncology)**

Quigley EMM, Sorrell MF: *The Gastrointestinal Surgical Patient.* Baltimore, Williams & Wilkins 1994.

Rajfer J: Congenital abnormalities of the testis. In *Campbell's Urology*, 6th ed. Edited by Walsh PC, Retik AB, Stamey TA, et al. Philadelphia, WB Saunders, 1992, p 1543. **(Urologic Surgery)**

Ranson JHC: Necrosis and abscess. In *Complications of Pancreatitis: Medical and Surgical Management.* Edited by Bradley EL. Philadelphia, WB Saunders, 1982, pp 72–95.

Ranson JHC: The current management of acute pancreatitis. *Advances in Surgery* 28:93–112, 1995.

Ranson JHC, Berman RS: Long peritoneal lavage decreases pancreatic sepsis in acute pancreatitis. *Ann Surg* 211:708–716, 1990.

Ranson JHC, Rifkind KM, Roses DF, et al: Prognostic signs and the role of operative management in acute pancreatitis. *Surg Gynecol Obstet* 139:69–81, 1974.

Reddick EJ, Olsen DO: Outpatient laparoscopic laser cholecystectomy. *Am J Surg* 160:485–489, 1990.

Regechary S, Wilkins R: *Principles of Neurosurgery.* Prescott, AZ, Wolfe, 1994. **(Neurosurgery)**

Ress AM, Sarr MG, Nagorney DM, et al: Spectrum and management of major complications of laparoscopic cholecystectomy. *Am J Surg* 165(6):655–662, 1993.

Reynolds WR, Brinkman JD, Haney BD, et al: Oriental cholangiohepatitis. *Mil Med* 159(2):158–160, 1994.

Richie JP: Neoplasms of the testis. In *Campbell's Urology*, 6th ed. Edited by Walsh PC, Retik AB, Stamey TA, et al. Philadelphia, WB Saunders, 1992, p 1222. **(Urologic Surgery)**

Rockwood CA, Green DP, Bucholz RW: *Fractures*, 3rd ed. Philadelphia, JB Lippincott, 1991. **(Orthopedic Surgery)**

Rodriguez J, Kasberg C, et al: CT-guided needle biopsy of the pancreas: A retrospective analysis of diagnostic accuracy. *Am J Gastroenterol* 87:1610–1613, 1992.

Roggo A, Wood WC, Ottinger LW: Carcinoid tumors of the appendix. *Ann Surg* 217(4):385–390, 1992.

Roitt IM, Brostoff J, Male DK: *Immunology.* St. Louis, CV Mosby, 1985. **(Transplant Surgery)**

Rombeau JL, Jacobs DO: Nasoenteric tube feedings. In *Enteral and Tube Feedings.* Edited by Rombeau JL, Caldwell MD. Philadelphia, WB Saunders, 1984, pp 261–274.

Roslyn JJ, Zinner MJ: *The colon and rectum: I. Surgical anatomy and operative procedures.* In *Textbook of Surgery: The Biological Basis of Modern Surgical Practice*, 14th ed. Edited by Sabiston DC. Philadelphia, WB Saunders, 1993, pp 899–903.

Roslyn JJ, Zinner MJ: The colon and rectum: II. Physiology. In *Textbook of Surgery: The Biological Basis of Modern Surgical Practice*, 14th ed. Edited by Sabiston DC. Philadelphia, WB Saunders, 1993, pp 903–904.

Rossi RL, Schirmer WJ: Chronic pancreatitis. In *Current Surgical Therapy*. Edited by Cameron JL. St. Louis, Mosby-Year Book, 1992, pp 431–441.

Roulet M, Detsky AS, Marliss EB, et al: A controlled trial of the effect of parenteral nutritional support on patients with respiratory failure and sepsis. *Clin Nutr* 2:97–105, 1983.

Rubino FA: Neurologic complications of alcoholism. *Psychiatric Clinics of North America* 15(2):359–371, 1992.

Rudolph AM, Hoffman JIE, Rudolph CD (eds): *Rudolph's Pediatrics*, 19th ed. Norwalk, CT, Appleton & Lange, 1991.

Rustgi AK: Hereditary gastrointestinal polyposis and nonpolyposis syndromes. *N Engl J Med* 331:1694–1702, 1994.

Rutherford RB (ed): *Vascular Surgery*, 4th ed. Philadelphia, WB Saunders, 1995.

Rutkow IM: How American surgeons introduced radiology into U.S. medicine. *Am J Surg* 165(2):252–257, 1993.

Saadia R, Schein M, MacFarlane C, et al: Gut barrier function and the surgeon. *Br J Surg* 77:487–492, 1990.

Sabiston DC Jr (ed): *Atlas of General Surgery*. Philadelphia, WB Saunders, 1994.

Sabiston DC Jr (ed): *Textbook of Surgery*, 14th ed. Philadelphia, WB Saunders, 1991. **(Transplant, Thoracic, Orthopedic, Vascular, and Cardiac Surgery)**

Sabiston DC Jr: Pulmonary embolism. In *Textbook of Surgery,*14th ed. Edited by Sabiston, DC Jr. Philadelphia, WB Saunders, 1994, pp 1502–1512.

Sabiston DC, Spencer FC: *Gibbon's Surgery of the Chest*, 5th ed. Philadelphia, WB Saunders, 1992. **(Thoracic Surgery)**

Safran DB, Orlando R: Physiologic effects of pneumoperitoneum. *Am J Surg* 167:281–286, 1994.

Saini A, Waxman J: Management of carcinoid syndrome. *Postgrad Med J* 67:506–508, 1991.

Sankaran, et al: *Surg Clin North Am* 57:139–150, 1977.

Saunders CE, Ho MT (eds): *Current Emergency Diagnosis and Treatment*, 4th ed. Norwalk, CT, Appleton & Lange, 1992. **(Orthopedic Surgery)**

Saunders KD, Cates JA, Roslyn JJ: Pathogenesis of gallstones. *Surg Clin North Am* 70(6):1197–1216, 1990.

Schaeffer, AJ: Infections of the Urinary Tract. In *Campbell's Urology*, 6th ed. Edited by Walsh PC, Retik AB, Stamey TA, et al. Philadelphia, WB Saunders, 1992, p 731. **(Urologic Surgery)**

Schirmer B: Current status of proximal gastric vagotomy. *Ann Surg* 209 (2):131–148, 1989.

Schneider RE: Genitourinary trauma. *Emergency Medicine Clinics of North America* 11(1):37–145, 1993.

Schroeder T, Sainio V, Kivisaari L, et al: Pancreatic resection versus peritoneal lavage in acute necrotizing pancreatitis. *Ann Surg* 214:663–666, 1991.

Schuster DP: A physiologic approach to initiating, maintaining, and withdrawing mechanical ventilatory support during acute respiratory failure. *Am J Med* 88:268–278, 1990.

Schwartz SI, Shires GT, Spencer FC (eds): *Principles of Surgery*, 6th ed. New York, McGraw-Hill, 1994. **(Plastic, Vascular, Thoracic, and Cardiac Surgery)**

Scott HW Jr, Oates JA, Niles AS, et al: Pheochromocytoma: Presentation, diagnosis and management. *Ann Surg* 183:587, 1976.

Sherlock S: Primary biliary cirrhosis: Clarifying the issues. *Am J Med* 96(1A):27S–33S, 1994.

Sherlock S, Dooley J (eds): *Diseases of the Liver and Biliary System*, 9th ed. London, Blackwell Scientific Publications, 1993.

Shields TW (ed): *General Thoracic Surgery*, 4th ed. Baltimore, Williams & Wilkins, 1994. **(Thoracic Surgery)**

Shiu MH, Brennan MF: *Surgical Management of Soft Tissue Sarcoma*. Philadelphia, Lea & Febiger, 1989.

Shutze WP, Halpern NP: Gastric lymphoma. *Surg Gynecol Obstet* 172:33–38, 1991.

Silverman H, Nunez L: Treatment of common eye emergencies. *Am Fam Physician* 45:2279–2287, 1992. **(Ophthalmology)**

Simmons RL, Finch NL (eds.): *Manual of Vascular Access, Organ Donation, and Transplantation*. New York, Springer-Verlag, 1984. **(Transplant Surgery)**

Sinanan MN: Acute cholangitis. *Infect Dis Clin North Am* 6(3):571–599, 1992.

Singer S, et al: Long-term salvageability of patients with locally recurrent soft tissue sarcoma. *Arch Surg* 127:548–554, 1992.

Singletary S, Ames FC, Buzdar AU: Management of inflammatory breast cancer. *World J Surg* 18:87–92, 1994.

Sirmon MD, Kirkpatrick WG: Acute renal failure. What to do until the nephrologist comes. *Postgrad Med* 87(3):55–62, 1990.

Slaff J, Jacobson D, Tillman CR, et al: Protease-specific suppression of pancreatic exocrine secretion. *Gastroenterology* 87:44–52, 1984.

Smith SD, Rowe MI: Physiology of the patient. In *Pediatric Surgery*, 2nd ed. Edited by Ashcraft K, Holder T. Philadelphia, WB Saunders, 1993, pp 1–18. **(Pediatric Surgery)**

Smith SJ, Wengrovitz MA, DeLong BS: Prospective validation of criteria, including age, for safe, nonsurgical management of the ruptured spleen. *J Trauma* 33(3):363–369, 1992.

Soave F: A new surgical technique for treatment of Hirschsprung's disease. *Surgery* 56:1007, 1964. **(Pediatric Surgery)**

Solomon SM, Kirby DF: The refeeding syndrome: A review. *J Parenter Enter Nutr* 14:90–97, 1990.

Soper NJ, Dunnegan DL: Routine versus selective intra-operative cholangiography during laparoscopic cholecystectomy. *World J Surg* 16(6):1133–1140, 1992.

Sosa JL, Sleeman D: Biliary complications related to endoscopic cholecystectomies [letter; comment]. *Surgical Laparoscopy and Endoscopy* 3(3):276–277, 1993.

Spaulding WB: Should you operate on your own mother? *Pharos AOA Honor Med Soc* 55(3):23, 1992.

Starzl TE, Shapero R, Simmons RL: *Atlas of Organ Transplantation.* New York, Gower, 1992. **(Transplant Surgery)**

Steinberg, et al: Acute pancreatitis. *N Engl J Med* 330:1198–1210, 1994.

Stiles DP, Stobo JD, Fudenbergh HH, et al: *Basic and Clinical Immunology.* Los Altos, CA, Lange Medical Publications, 1984. **(Transplant Surgery)**

Storm FK, Mahvi DM: Diagnosis and management of soft tissue sarcoma. What's New in General Surgery from the Division of Surgical Oncology, Department of Surgery, University of Wisconsin.

Strodel WE, et al: Surgical therapy for small bowel carcinoid tumors. *Arch Surg* 118:391–397,1983.

Strong RM, Condon SC, et al: Equal aspiration rates from postpylorus and intragastric-placed small-bore naso-enteric feeding tubes: A randomized, prospective study. *J Parenter Enter Nutr* 16:59–63, 1992.

Sutton JM: Evaluation of hematuria in adults. *JAMA* 263(18):2475–2480, 1990.

Tabbara KF: Eye emergencies. In *Current Emergency Diagnosis and Treatment.* Edited by Saunders CE, Ho MT. Norwalk, CT, Appleton & Lange, 1992, pp 405–426. **(Ophthalmology)**

Teneriello MG: Early detection of ovarian cancer. *CA Cancer J Clin* 45:71–87, 1995. **(Gynecologic Oncology)**

Thompson JPS, Akwari OE: The colon and rectum: X. Disorders of the anal canal. In *Textbook of Surgery: The Biological Basis of Modern Surgical Practice*, 14th ed. Edited by Sabiston DC. Philadelphia, WB Saunders, 1993, pp 958–972.

Thompson WD: Genetic epidemiology of breast cancer. *Cancer* 74:279–287, 1994.

Tomkins RK: Surgical management of bile duct stones. *Surg Clin North Am* 70(6):1329–1339, 1990.

Toribara NW, Sleisinger MH: Screening for colorectal cancer. *N Engl J Med* 332:861–867, 1995.

Touloukian RJ: Intestinal atresia and stenosis. In *Pediatric Surgery*, 2nd ed. Edited by Ashcraft K, Holder T. Philadelphia, WB Saunders, 1993, pp 305–309. **(Pediatric Surgery)**

Toouli J, (ed): *Surgery of the Biliary Tract.* New York, Churchill Livingstone, 1993.

Tuchschmidt J, Fried J, Astiz M, et al: Elevation of cardiac output and oxygen delivery improves outcome in septic shock. *Chest* 102(1):216–220, 1992.

Tuchschmidt J, Oblitas D, Fried JC: Oxygen consumption in sepsis and septic shock. *Crit Care Med* 19:664–670, 1991.

Tuggle D, Huber PJ: Management of rectal trauma. *Am J Surg* 148:806–808, 1984.

Turney SZ, Rodriguez A, Cowley RA (eds): *Management of Cardiothoracic Trauma*. Baltimore, Williams & Wilkins, 1990. **(Cardiac, Vascular, and Thoracic Surgery)**

Valimaki M, Pelkonen R, Porkka L, et al: Long-term results of adrenal surgery in patients with Cushing's syndrome due to adrenocortical adenoma. *Clin Endocrinol* 20:229, 1984.

Vander AJ: *Renal Physiology*, 5th ed. New York, McGraw Hill, 1995.

Von Allmen, Fischer JE: Metabolic complications. In *Total Parenteral Nutrition*. Boston, Little, Brown, 1991.

Van Heerdeen JA, Steps SG, Hamberger B, et al: Pheochromocytoma: Current status and changing trends. *Surgery* 91:367, 1982.

Vaughan DG: Ophthalmology. In *Current Surgical Diagnosis and Treatment*, 10th ed. Edited by Way LW. Norwalk, CT, Appleton & Lange, 1994, pp 814–824. **(Ophthalmology)**

Vinik Ai, et al: Clinical features, diagnosis, and localization of carcinoid tumors and their management. *Gastroent Clin North Am* 18(4):865–896, 1989.

Walsh PC: Benign prostatic hyperplasia. In *Campbell's Urology*, 6th ed. Edited by Walsh PC, Retik AB, Stamey TA, et al. Philadelphia, WB Saunders, 1992, p 1009. **(Urologic Surgery)**

Walsh PC: The differential diagnosis of ambiguous genitalia in the newborn. *Urol Clin North Am* 5:213–221, 1978. **(Urologic Surgery)**

Walt AJ: Pancreatic ascites and pancreatic pleural effusions. In *Current Surgical Therapy*. Edited by Cameron J. St. Louis, Mosby-Year Book, 1992, pp 427–430.

Wangensteen, OH: *The Rise of Surgery: From Empiric Craft to Scientific Discipline*. Minneapolis, University of Minnesota Press, 1978.

Walker LA: Using rapid sequence intubation to facilitate tracheal intubation. *Emergency Medicine Review* 14 (15):126–132, 1993.

Weigelt JA: Duodenal injuries. *Surg Clin North Am* 70(3):529–539, 1990.

Weigelt JA: Respiratory and cardiac management of surgical patients. *Selected Readings in General Surgery* 19(10), 1992.

Weingrad DW, Rosenberg SA: Early lymphatic spread of osteogenic and soft tissue sarcomas. *Surgery* 84:231–240,

Weinmann and Salzman. Deep vein thrombosis. *N Engl J Med* 331:1630–1641, 1994.

Weinshel EL, Peterson BA: Hodgkin's disease. *CA Cancer J Clin* 43:327–346, 1993.

Weiss AJ, Lackman RD: Therapy of desmoid tumors and related neoplasms. *Comprehensive Therapy* 17: 32–34, 1991.

Wheeler KH: Laparoscopic inguinal herniorrhaphy with mesh: An 18-month experience. *Journal of Laparoendoscopic Surgery* 3(2):265–289, 1993.

Whipple AO, Parsons WB, Mullins CR: Treatment of carcinoma of the ampulla of Vater. *Ann Surg* 102:763, 1935.

Williams RA, Wilson SE: Gastrointestinal disorders requiring surgical treatment in patients with AIDS. *Comprehensive Therapy* 18(8):9–12, 1992.

Wilmore DW, Brennan MF, Harken AH, et al (eds): *Care of the Surgical Patient.* New York, Scientific American, 1992. **(Thoracic Surgery)**

Wilmore DW, Smith RJ, O'Dwyer ST, et al: The gut: A central organ after surgical stress. *Surgery* 104:917–923, 1988.

Wilson RH, Moorehead RJ: The current management of trauma to the pancreas. *British Journal of Surgery* 78:1196–1202, 1991.

Wilson-Pauwels A, Akesson EJ, Stewart PA: *Cranial Nerves: Gross Anatomy and Clinical Comments.* Philadelphia, BC Decker, 1988. **(Plastic Surgery)**

Wong K, Henderson CH: Management of metastatic breast cancer. *World J Surg* 18:98–111, 1994.

Wood DE, Mathisen DJ: Late complications of tracheotomy. *Clinics in Chest Medicine* 12(3):597–609, 1991.

Woolhandler S, Pels RJ, Bor DH, et al: Dipstick urinalysis screening of asymptomatic adults for urinary tract disorders. I. Hematuria and proteinuria. *JAMA* 262(9):1214–1269, 1989.

Woolley M: Teratomas. In *Pediatric Surgery,* 2nd ed. Edited by Ashcraft, Holder T. Philadelphia, WB Saunders, 1993, pp 847–862. **(Pediatric Surgery)**

Wurman LH: Epistaxis. In *Current Treatment in Otolaryngology, Head and Neck Surgery,* 5th ed. Edited by Gates G. St. Louis, Mosby-Year Book, 1994, pp 354–358.

Yeo CJ, Pitt HA, Cameron JL: Cholangiocarcinoma. *Surg Clin North Am* 70(6):1427–1447, 1990.

Yeo CJ, Cameron JL: The pancreas. In *Textbook of Surgery: The Biological Basis of Modern Surgical Practice.* Edited by Sabiston DC Jr. Philadelphia, WB Saunders, 1991, pp 1076–1107.

Youmans J: *Neurological Surgery,* 4th ed. Philadelphia, WB Saunders, 1996. **(Neurosurgery)**

Young RC, Perez CA, Hoskins WJ: Cancer of the ovary. In DeVita VT Jr, Hellman S, Rosenberg SA (eds). *Cancer: Principles and Practice of Oncology,* 4th ed. Philadelphia, JB Lippincott, 1993. **(Gynecologic Oncology)**

Young RC, Perez CA, Hoskins WJ: Gynecologic tumors. In DeVita VT Jr, Hellman S, Rosenberg SA (eds.). Cancer: Principles and Practice of Oncology, 4th ed. Philadelphia, JB Lippincott, 1993. **(Gynecologic Oncology)**

Young WF, Klee GC: Primary aldosteronism. *Endocrinol Metab Clin North Am* 17:367, 1988.

Yu SC, Chen SC, Wang SM, et al: Is previous abdominal surgery a contraindication to laparoscopic cholecystectomy? *Journal of Laparoendoscopic Surgery* 4(1):31–35, 1994.

Zarilli L, et al: The surgical management of carcinoid tumors. *J Nucl Biol Med* 35:341–342, 1991.

Zeitels J, et al: Carcinoid tumors. *Arch Surg* 117:732–737,1982.

Zimberg YH: Pancreatitis: Principles of management. *Surg Clin North Am* 48:889–905, 1968.

Zimmaro DM, Rolandelli RH, Koruda MJ, et al: Isotonic tube feeding formula induces liquid stool in normal subjects: Reversal by pectin. *J Parenter Enter Nutr* 13:117–123, 1989.

Zollinger RM Jr, Zollinger RM: *Atlas of Surgical Operations,* 7th ed. New York, Macmillan, 1993. **(Vascular Surgery)**

Index

Italic page numbers indicate illustrations; page numbers with *t* indicate tables.

intra-aortic balloon pump, 752–753
left ventricular assist device, 754
open versus closed procedures in, 662
postoperative intensive care
management
cardiovascular drugs, 745
hemorrhage, 742–743
hyperdynamic myocardium
syndrome, 741–742
hypertension, 740–741
hypotension, 741
myocardial ischemia, 740
output, 737–739
Swan-Ganz catheter, 743–745
postpericardiotomy syndrome, 752
trauma to heart and great vessels
blunt, 748–750
penetrating, 745–748
traumatic aneurysms of thoracic
aorta, 750–752
tumors, 755–756
Cardiac tamponade, 327
Cardiac trauma, blunt, 748–750
Cardiac tumors, 755–756
benign, 755–756
Cardiac valves, three-dimensional relation
between, 719
Cardiogenic shock, 127, 700, 741
Cardiomyopathy, 256
Cardiopulmonary bypass (CPB), 78,
735–737
Cardiopulmonary compromise, degree of
curvature associated with, 922
Cardiovascular complications
arrhythmias, 116–118
bradycardia, 118
cardiac arrest, 118–119
Cardiovascular medications, 90–93, 745
Cardiovascular system in critical care
medicine, 652–653
Carmustine, 254
Caroli's disease, 485
Carotid arteries, 32, 33, 34
injury surgery/anatomy, 337–340
origins of, 781
surgical treatment of disease, 786
systemic heparinization during
traumatic repair, 338
Carotid bifurcation, 781
Carotid body tumor, 839
Carotid cavernous fistula, 1201–1202
Carotid disease, 783

Carotid endarterectomy, 22, 786
monitoring of postoperative levels, 249
tumors associated with, 249
Carpal tunnel syndrome, 1035–1036,
1226
Carpal-metacarpal (CM) dislocation,
treatment of, 1033
Carrel, Alexis, 19, 22, 23
Cat bites, pathogens in, 209
Cataract, 1317
Categoric variable, 268
Catharsis, 94
Cathepsin D, 534–535
Catheter contrast study, purpose of, 29
Cattel maneuver, 49, *49*
Caudal block, 242
Cava filter, indications for, 145
Caval stenosis, clinical signs of, 1157
Cavernous hemangioma, 456–457
Cavernous sinus, 1201
Cavitation, 331
C-cells, 246
Cecostomy
and comparison of end ileostomy, 420
indications for, 362
Cefazolin, 188
comparison of cefoxitin and, 93
Cefoperazone, 188
Cefotetan, 188, 198
Cefoxitin, 198
comparison of cefazolin and, 93
Ceftazidime, 188
Ceftriaxone, 188
association with cholestatic jaundice
and gallbladder sludge, 478
Celiac artery compression syndrome, 794
Celiac trunk, 600
Cell biology, 243–247
Cell cycle of tumors, duration of, 248
Cells
alpha, 246
amine precursor uptake decarboxylase,
290
B, 246, 1124–1126
beta, 246
C, 246
delta, 246
dendritic, 1128
endothelial, 84
eucaryotic, 243
follicular, 246
G, 245

Loop colostomy, 366
  versus end colostomy, 420
Loop electrosurgical excision procedure
  (LEEP), 1175
Loop ileostomy, 361
Low back pain, 927
Low cardiac output syndrome (LCOS),
  738–739
Lower extremity
  amputations in, 779–781
  chronic arterial occlusive disease of,
    768–774
  deep venous thrombosis in, 817–819
  varicosities in, 813–814
Lower gastrointestinal bleeding, 129
Ludwig's angina, 962
Lugol's solution, 539
Lumbar hernia, 307
Lumbar spine, 1213–1215
Lumbricals, function of, 1014
Lumpectomy, 528
Lunate dislocation, 1034
Lung
  abscess of, 1059–1060
  anatomy of, 1056–1057
  benign tumors, 1063–1064
  carcinoma of, 1065
    staging of, 1068–1069
  congenital lesions, 1057–1058
  infections of, 1059–1063
  lobes of, 180
  massive hemoptysis, 1063
  metastatic tumors, 1072–1073
  primary malignant tumors, 1064–1072
  segmental anatomy of, 1075
  solitary pulmonary nodules, 1073–1074
Lung sequestration, 1058
Lung transplantation, 23, 1120–1121
Lupus anticoagulant, 85
Lymphadenitis, cervical, 982
Lymphangiograms
  indications for, 617
  with oil-soluble contrast, 822
Lymphangioma, 944
Lymphangitis, 210
Lymphedema, 822–823
Lymphogranuloma venereum, 1237
Lymphoma, 249, 1081, 1084
  definition of, 616
  gastric, 381–382, 621–622
    therapeutic options for, 622
  Hodgkin disease, 616–620

Ann Arbor staging classification of,
  619
diagnosis of, 617
lymphangiograms in, 617
oophoropexy, 618
spread of, 617
staging laparotomy in, 617–618
treatment for, 620
incidence of, 616
non-Hodgkin, 620–621
pancreatic, 510
of small bowel, 395
Lymphoscintigraphy
  with 99mTc antimony sulfide, 822
  as guide to elective lymph node
    dissection, 644
Lynch syndrome, 1181
  types of, 250
Lynch tumors, 250
Lysosome, function of, 244

Mackenrodt's ligament, 42
Macrophages, 247, 1128
Mafenide acetate cream, side effects of,
  358
Major histocompatibility complex,
  1130–1132
Mal perforans ulcer, 838
Malabsorption syndromes, 397
Malignant fibrous histiocytoma (MFH),
  630
Malignant hyperthermia (MH), 234
Malignant potential, 248
Mallet toe, 927
Mallory-Weiss syndrome, 383–384
Malnutrition and surgical infection,
  182–183
Malpractice, avoiding, 7
Mammalian cell cycles, phases of, 243
Mammary artery, 34
Mammograms, 521–523
Mammography, screening, 520
Mandatory minute ventilation (MMV),
  description of, 650
Mandible, 33
  fracture of, 1008–1009
Mandibular nerve, 936
Mannitol, 70
Marcy treatment, 310
Marfan disease, 723
Marginal artery of Drummond, 420
Marginal ulcer, 378